# Sports Concussions

A Complete Guide to Recovery and Management

# Sports Concussions

## A Complete Guide to Recovery and Management

Edited by
Isabelle Gagnon
Alain Ptito

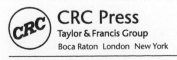

**CRC Press**
Taylor & Francis Group
Boca Raton London New York

CRC Press is an imprint of the
Taylor & Francis Group, an **informa** business

Cover art: Courtesy of Carolina Echeverria (www.carolinaecheverria.ca)

CRC Press
Taylor & Francis Group
6000 Broken Sound Parkway NW, Suite 300
Boca Raton, FL 33487-2742

First issued in paperback 2019

© 2018 by Taylor & Francis Group, LLC
CRC Press is an imprint of Taylor & Francis Group, an Informa business

No claim to original U.S. Government works

ISBN-13: 978-1-4987-0162-4 (hbk)
ISBN-13: 978-0-367-87145-1 (pbk)

**Visit the Taylor & Francis Web site at
http://www.taylorandfrancis.com**

**and the CRC Press Web site at
http://www.crcpress.com**

# Contents

# Editors

**Dr. Isabelle Gagnon** is a pediatric physical therapist and clinical scientist at the trauma center of The Montreal Children's Hospital, McGill University Health Center, and an associate professor in the School of Physical and Occupational Therapy of McGill University, Montreal, Quebec, Canada. In both these roles, she has participated in changing the landscape of concussion assessment and care, as well as in the inclusion of concussion awareness in the curriculum of future physical therapists.

She leads an innovative research program, which focuses on the consequences and the management of mild traumatic brain injuries or concussions in the pediatric and adolescent population. More specifically, she has investigated sensorimotor outcomes in children and adolescents, and how these can impact return to physical activities and self-confidence after traumatic injuries. Her work has also examined intervention programs and service organization for children and adolescents after a traumatic injury. As an author of several key publications in the field of pediatric concussions, she has participated in the creation of pediatric concussion management guidelines and in standardizing the assessment of children and teens who sustain concussions. As it has been since the beginning of her career, her goal remains to contribute to the well-being of children after they sustain injuries, placing evidence-based management at the heart of her approach.

**Dr. Alain Ptito** is professor of Neurology and Neurosurgery at McGill University. He has worked as a neuropsychologist at the Montreal Neurological Institute and Hospital since 1983 and he is now the director of the Psychology Department at the McGill University Health Centre (MUHC) and a medical scientist at the Research Institute of the MUHC. Dr. A. Ptito's research program involves the investigation of the mechanisms involved in cerebral reorganization and plasticity in patient populations (hemispherectomy, callosotomy, Parkinson's disease, stroke, and head injury) and his clinical work includes the neuropsychological assessment of these patients. One of his principal research focuses has been the investigation of the residual visual abilities (blindsight) of patients following a rare procedure called hemispherectomy, the surgical removal or disconnection of a cerebral hemisphere.

Dr. Ptito studied clinical psychology at the McGill University (1975) and obtained his postgraduate degrees in experimental psychology (1979) and neuropsychology (1986) from the Université de Montréal. His doctoral thesis examined residual vision in the blind field of patients who underwent a hemispherectomy. Dr. Ptito now delivers lectures throughout the world on residual vision and on traumatic brain injury (TBI). He is a member of the Order of Psychologists of the Province of Quebec and of the Société des Experts en Evaluation Médicolégale du Québec. Dr. Ptito has been a member of several consensus panels on guidelines for TBI.

In recent years, Dr. Ptito has explored new methods of using functional magnetic resonance imaging for examining brain trauma. In athletes, he has been using fMRI to investigate the neural mechanisms underlying the working memory. Thanks for the support from Canadian Institutes of Health Research (CIHR), he has been able to carry out baseline fMRI and neuropsychological testing with hockey and football varsity athletes and to repeat the tests immediately after concussion and subsequently until symptom resolution. His results show that fMRI is sensitive enough to detect abnormal activation patterns in symptomatic-concussed individuals and that it could provide an objective way to measure the severity of or recovery from a concussion. More recently, he has been investigating mild TBI (mTBI) in motor vehicle accident victims and in children with funding from CIHR, the Department of Defense, and the Ontario Neurotrauma Foundation. In addition, with the Natural Sciences and Engineering Research Council support, Dr. Ptito continues to investigate hemispherectomy and its effects on vision.

With the recent support from the Canadian Foundation for Innovation, his team will acquire an ultrahigh-performance MRI system (housed at the Montreal General Hospital) that will be able to carry out more applications than any existing MRI system and will help observe the brain's response to trauma with improved precision. This knowledge will allow the development of new diagnostic tools and treatments to help thousands of Canadians who suffer head injuries every year.

The editors wish to thank Dr. Michelle Keightley for proposing the idea and highlighting the need for this book.

# Contributors

**Ammar Al-Kashmiri**
Emergency Department
Khoula Hospital
and
Emergency Medicine Training
   Program
Oman Medical Specialty Board
and
College of Medicine & Health Sciences
Sultan Qaboos University
Muscat, Oman

**Vicki Anderson**
Psychology Department
RCH Mental Health
Royal Children's Hospital Melbourne
and
Clinical Sciences Research
Murdoch Childrens Research Institute
Parkville, Victoria, Australia
and
National Health and Medical Research
   Council
and
Psychological Sciences & Paediatrics
University of Melbourne
Melbourne, Victoria, Australia

**Amanda Black**
Sport Injury Prevention Research Centre
Faculty of Kinesiology
University of Calgary
and
Cumming School of Medicine
Hotchkiss Brain Institute
University of Calgary
and
Cumming School of Medicine
Alberta Children's Hospital Research
   Institute
University of Calgary
Calgary, Alberta, Canada

**Brian L. Brooks**
Neurosciences Program
Alberta Children's Hospital
and
Department of Paediatrics
Cumming School of Medicine
University of Calgary
and
Department of Clinical Neurosciences
Cumming School of Medicine
University of Calgary
and
Department of Psychology
Faculty of Arts
University of Calgary
and
Alberta Children's Hospital Research
   Institute
University of Calgary
Calgary, Alberta, Canada

**Jen-Kai Chen**
Cognitive Neuroscience Unit
Montreal Neurological Institute
McGill University
Montreal, Quebec, Canada

**J. Scott Delaney**
Department of Emergency Medicine
McGill University Health Centre
McGill Sport Medicine Clinic
Montreal, Quebec, Canada

**Carol DeMatteo**
School of Rehabilitation Science
McMaster University
and
CanChild Centre for Childhood Disability
    Research
McMaster University
Hamilton, Ontario, Canada

**Ruben J. Echemendia**
Concussion Care Clinic
University Orthopedics Center
State College, Pennsylvania

and

Department of Psychology
University of Missouri – Kansas City
Kansas City, Missouri

**Paul Eliason**
Sport Injury Prevention Research Centre
Faculty of Kinesiology
University of Calgary
and
Hotchkiss Brain Institute
University of Calgary
and
Alberta Children's Hospital Research
    Institute
Cumming School of Medicine
University of Calgary
Calgary, Alberta, Canada

**Carolyn Emery**
Sport Injury Prevention Research Centre
Faculty of Kinesiology
University of Calgary
and
Department of Pediatrics
Cumming School of Medicine
University of Calgary
and
Department of Community Health
    Sciences
Cumming School of Medicine
University of Calgary
and
Alberta Children's Hospital Research
    Institute
University of Calgary
and
Hotchkiss Brain Institute
University of Calgary
Calgary, Alberta, Canada

**Isabelle Gagnon**
School of Physical and Occupational
    Therapy/Pediatric Emergency Medicine
McGill University
Montreal, Quebec, Canada

**Gerard A. Gioia**
Division of Pediatric Neuropsychology
Safe Concussion Outcome Recovery &
    Education (SCORE) Program
Children's National Health System
and
Department of Psychiatry and Behavioral
    Sciences
George Washington University School of
    Medicine & Health Sciences
Washington, District of Columbia

**Robin Green**
Cognitive Neurorehabilitation Sciences
  Laboratory
Toronto Rehabilitation Institute
University Health Network
Toronto, Ontario, Canada

**Guido Guberman**
Cognitive Neuroscience Unit
Montreal Neurological Institute
McGill University
and
Concussion Research Laboratory
Trauma Center
McGill University
and
Integrated Program in Neuroscience
Faculty of Medicine
McGill University
Montreal, Quebec, Canada

**Scott A. Holmes**
Cognitive Neuroscience Unit
Montreal Neurological Institute
McGill University
and
Concussion Research Laboratory
Trauma Center
McGill University
Montreal, Quebec, Canada

**Blaine Hoshizaki**
Neurotrauma Impact Science Laboratory
University of Ottawa
Ottawa, Ontario, Canada

**Gillian Hotz**
KiDZ Neuroscience Center
UConcussion Program
Department of Neurosurgery
The Miami Project to Cure Paralysis
University of Miami Miller School of
  Medicine
Miami, Florida

**Grant L. Iverson**
Department of Physical Medicine and
  Rehabilitation
Harvard Medical School
and
Spaulding Rehabilitation Hospital
and
Sports Concussion Program
MassGeneral Hospital for Children
and
Home Base
A Red Sox Foundation and Massachusetts
  General Hospital Program
Boston, Massachusetts

**Clara Karton**
Neurotrauma Impact Science Laboratory
University of Ottawa
Ottawa, Ontario, Canada

**Marshall Kendall**
Neurotrauma Impact Science Laboratory
University of Ottawa
Ottawa, Ontario, Canada

**Michael W. Kirkwood**
Department of Physical Medicine and
  Rehabilitation
University of Colorado School of Medicine
  and Children's Hospital Colorado
Aurora, Colorado

**David Koncan**
Neurotrauma Impact Science Laboratory
University of Ottawa
Ottawa, Ontario, Canada

**Lisa Koski**
McGill University Health Centre
Brain Repair and Integrative Neuroscience
    Program
Research Institute of the MUHC
and
Departments of Neurology and
    Neurosurgery
McGill University
and
Department of Psychology
McGill University
Montreal, Quebec, Canada

**Maude Laguë-Beauvais**
Traumatic Brain Injury Program
McGill University Healthy Centre
Montreal General Hospital
Montreal, Quebec, Canada

**Geneviève Léveillé**
Traumatic Brain Injury Outpatient
    Rehabilitation Program
Lucie-Bruneau Rehabilitation
    Centre/CIUSSS
    Centre-Sud-de-l'Île-de-Montréal
Centre for Interdisciplinary Research in
    Rehabilitation of Greater Montreal
Montreal, Quebec, Canada

**Paul McCrory**
Florey Institute of Neuroscience and
    Mental Health
Parkville, Victoria, Australia

**Michelle McKerral**
Department of Psychology
Faculty of arts and Sciences
Université de Montréal
and
Lucie-Bruneau Rehabilitation
    Centre/CIUSSS
    Centre-Sud-de-l'Île-de-Montréal
Centre for Interdisciplinary Research in
    Rehabilitation of Greater Montreal
Montreal, Quebec, Canada

**Anna Oeur**
Neurotrauma Impact Science
    Laboratory
University of Ottawa
Ottawa, Ontario, Canada

**Linda Papa**
Academic Clinical Research
Orlando Regional Medical Center
and
University of Central Florida College
    of Medicine
Orlando, Florida

and

Florida State University College of
    Medicine
Tallahassee, Florida

and

University of Florida College of
    Medicine
Gainesville, Florida

and

Department of Neurology and
    Neurosurgery
McGill University
Montreal, Quebec, Canada

**Declan Patton**
Sports Injury Prevention Research Centre
    (SIPRC)
Faculty of Kinesiology
University of Calgary
Calgary, Alberta, Canada

and

Australian Collaboration for Research
    into Injury in Sport and its Prevention
    (ACRISP)
Federation University Australia
Ballarat, Victoria, Australia

and

Oslo Sports Trauma Research Centre (OSTRC)
Norwegian School of Sports Sciences
Oslo, Norway

**Vickie Plourde**
Faculty Saint-Jean
University of Alberta
Edmonton, Alberta, Canada

**Andrew Post**
St. Michael's Hospital
Division of Neurosurgery
and
Human Kinetics
University of Ottawa
Ottawa, Ontario, Canada

**Alain Ptito**
Department of Psychology
McGill University Health Center
and
Departments of Neurology and
    Neurosurgery
Montreal Neurological Institute and Hospital
McGill University
Montreal, Quebec, Canada

**Danielle Ransom**
Department of Neurology
Sports Medicine Institute Concussion
    Program
University of Miami
Miller School of Medicine
Miami, Florida

**Nick Reed**
Bloorview Research Institute
Holland Bloorview Kids Rehabilitation
    Hospital
and
Department of Occupational Science and
    Occupational Therapy
University of Toronto
and
Rehabilitation Sciences Institute
University of Toronto
Toronto, Ontario, Canada

**Philippe Rousseau**
Neurotrauma Impact Science Laboratory
School of Human Kinetics
Faculty of Health Sciences
University of Ottawa
Ottawa, Ontario, Canada

**Kathryn J. Schneider**
Sport Injury Prevention Research Centre
Faculty of Kinesiology
Alberta Children's Hospital Research
    Institute
University of Calgary
and
Hotchkiss Brain Institute
Calgary, Alberta, Canada

**Noah D. Silverberg**
Division of Physical Medicine and
    Rehabilitation
Department of Medicine
University of British Columbia
and
Rehabilitation Research Program
Vancouver Coastal Health Research
    Institute
Vancouver, British Columbia, Canada

and

Department of Physical Medicine and
    Rehabilitation
Harvard Medical School
and
Home Base
A Red Sox Foundation and Massachusetts
    General Hospital Program
Boston, Massachusetts

**Rajeet Singh Saluja**
McGill University Health Centre
Montreal General Hospital
and
Department of Neurology and
    Neurosurgery
McGill University
Montreal, Quebec, Canada

**Josh Stanley**
Faculty of Medicine
University of Ottawa
Ottawa, Ontario, Canada

**Kathy Stazyk**
McMaster University
Hamilton, Ontario, Canada

**Michael Takagi**
Child Neuropsychology
Emergency Research
Murdoch Children's Research Institute
and
Melbourne School of Psychological
    Sciences
University of Melbourne
Melbourne, Victoria, Australia

**Charles Tator**
Canadian Concussion Centre
Toronto Western Hospital
University Health Network
and
Division of Neurosurgery
Department of Surgery
University of Toronto
Toronto, Ontario, Canada

**Emma Thompson**
Child Neuropsychology
Emergency Research
Murdoch Children's Research Institute
University of Melbourne
Melbourne, Victoria, Australia

**Keith O. Yeates**
Department of Psychology
Faculty of Arts
University of Calgary
and
Departments of Paediatrics and Clinical
    Neurosciences
Cumming School of Medicine
University of Calgary
and
Department of Clinical Neurosciences
Cumming School of Medicine
University of Calgary
and
Alberta Children's Hospital Research
    Institute
University of Calgary
Calgary, Alberta, Canada

**Roger Zemek**
Department of Pediatrics and Emergency
    Medicine
Children's Hospital of Eastern Ontario
University of Ottawa
and
Children's Hospital of Eastern Ontario
    Research Institute
Ottawa, Ontario, Canada

*section one*

---

*What is a concussion?*

# chapter one

# Introduction

*Isabelle Gagnon, Scott A. Holmes, and Alain Ptito*

The adoption of *specialized* concussion care has been explored in the past 5 years in North America. With an increased awareness of the condition, brought by both media and athletes themselves, individuals have willingly come forward to report their injuries. More laws mandate organizations to develop concussion management plans and establish links with health-care providers for those members who need clearance before returning to sports. To meet this requirement, health-care providers have delivered a service of various scope and quality. What constitutes optimal care remains unclear in light of the fact that concussion care is complex.

The mission of *Sport Concussion: A Complete Guide to Recovery and Management* is to offer the clinician, who is interested in providing concussion care, up to date, evidence-based information to help in the task of setting up or upgrading individualized treatment programs. While concussion is often a sport-related injury, it is also an injury to the brain and this implies that the practitioner involved in the management of concussions needs knowledge and understanding of neuroanatomy, neurophysiology, as well as of rehabilitation of neurological conditions.

The pathophysiology underlying concussions has been a subject of continued research. It has been suggested that the impact of aberrant metabolic, hemodynamic, neurophysiologic, or structural properties may lead to post-concussive symptoms (Barkhoudarian et al. 2016; Choe et al. 2012). The following paragraphs provide a brief outline of microstructural damage resulting from a concussion, how structural damage leads to changes in neurophysiology, and how the immune system responds to a concussion.

A main focus of research on the pathophysiology of concussion has been centered on how the *microstructural environment* is affected. Post-concussion symptoms have been attributed to diffuse mechanical injury, which involves a shearing stress and deformation of brain tissue (Maruta et al. 2010), producing changes at the level of the cytoskeleton and neurofilaments (Barkhoudarian et al. 2016; Johnson et al. 2013), as well as impaired axonal transport and axonal swelling (Buki and Povlishock 2006). The term diffuse axonal injury can refer to a number of processes including the breaking of the axonal cytoskeleton, transport interruptions as well as swelling and proteolysis through secondary physiological changes (Johnson et al. 2013). With more severe forms of TBI, Wallerian degeneration, a process of neuronal deterioration, may follow wherein a damaged neuron decays at a distance from the spot of injury (Chen et al. 2009). In addition, not all regions are equally affected as axonal conduction deficits have been observed in unmyelinated fibers after a closed head injury, and not in their myelinated counterparts (Creed et al. 2011). This has important implications for pediatric populations who are undergoing myelination as a part of normal development (Ajao et al. 2012). In the chronic phase, amyloid beta deposition and tau protein aggregates released from damaged cells can accumulate in response to repeated concussive events, and this process has been linked to Chronic Traumatic

Encephalopathy (Jordan et al. 1995; McKee et al. 2009; see also the review by Seifert and Shipman (2015) on the pathophysiology of sport-related concussions).

Neurophysiologically, the stretching and deformation of axons caused by movement of the brain during a concussion may lead to the disruption of cellular membranes and an unregulated efflux of ions (Farkas et al. 2006). As a result of these ionic changes, a rapid depolarization occurs within cells, leading to an uncontrolled release of neurotransmitters, mainly glutamate (Faden et al. 1989). To restore the normal ionic balance, sodium-potassium pumps work excessively, causing a transient increase of glucose metabolism to generate ATP for these pumps (Giza and Hovda 2001; Peskind et al. 2011). This occurs in conjunction with reduced cerebral blood flow leading to a discrepancy between the demands and the supply of glucose stores (McKee et al. 2014). In parallel, an inefficient level of oxidative metabolism, believed to be the result of mitochondrial dysfunction (Verweij et al. 1997; Xiong et al. 1997), leads to a local increase in anaerobic glucose metabolism, which may lead to lactic acidosis and cerebral edema (Kawamata et al. 1995). Some researchers believe this mismatch in energy demand versus requirements may represent a phase of ongoing vulnerability to secondary injuries (Navarro et al. 2012). The precise pathophysiologic mechanism of decreased cerebral blood flow is unknown; however, possibilities may include the interruption of cerebral autoregulation, vasospasm, and/or disturbance of regional perfusion (Maugans et al. 2012; Prins et al. 2013; Seifert and Shipman 2015). Interestingly, there may be an effect of age as the observed cerebral blood flow alterations post-TBI may be limited to younger patients (Mandera et al. 2002). Further information regarding neurometabolic cascades occurring subsequent to an mTBI can be found in a review by Giza and Hovda (2014).

The neuroinflammatory response to concussion has been suggested to have a strong role in post-concussion symptoms (Rathbone et al. 2015). Following injury, there is an activation and infiltration of microglia (Kelley et al. 2007) and if sufficient forces are produced to damage the blood–brain barrier, circulating neutrophils, monocytes, and lymphocytes are able to leak through and release inflammatory factors that may become implicated in neuronal cell death (Ghirnikar et al. 1998). In both adult and immature rats, microarray studies report extensive up-regulation of cytokines—IL-6, IL-1ß, and TNF-α by mononuclear cells and IL-1ß by astrocytes (Holmin et al. 1997)—and inflammatory genes after TBI (Giza and Prins 2006; Li et al. 2004). However, the role of each inflammatory molecule, whether pro- or anti-inflammatory, may have positive or negative implications (see Patterson et al. 2012 for review). For example, Interleukin-1 may have a neuroprotective role in the brain being immediately upregulated in response to a brain injury (Dalgard et al. 2012; Shojo et al. 2010; Taupin et al. 1993); however, inhibition of IL-1B, a member of the IL-1 family, has been shown to reduce cerebral edema as well as the loss of tissue, improving overall cognitive outcome (Clausen et al. 2009, 2011). Indeed, the prolonged activation of neuroinflammatory mechanisms is associated with secondary damage from concussions, making this a viable target for developing treatments (Patterson and Holahan 2012). Further information regarding the role of inflammation in the brain subsequent to an mTBI can be found in Rathbone and colleagues' (2015) review of the literature.

Together, data suggest that the brain's response to a concussion is extensive and multifactorial. The structural injuries sustained diffuse and produce physiological challenges that the brain may be unable to meet. The immune system is directly implicated in this process as it attempts to repair neuronal damage, while itself producing further metabolic challenges for the brain. Though knowledge is increasing regarding the diversity of pathophysiology subsequent to concussion, further research is required in terms of how structural damage translates into the diversity of patient outcomes and whether neuroimaging can be used to visualize either microstructural damage or its physiological sequelae.

Fortunately, the majority of individuals with concussions will achieve rapid recovery, but it is only with a global understanding of the cerebral mechanisms involved that health professionals will be able to return athletes to function safely. Our book is divided into five parts; each chapter attempts to answer a question often raised by clinicians or by patients themselves.

Section I covers the essence of what a concussion is, starting with a historical perspective on the definition, and how approaches to its understanding have evolved. We then move on to a comprehensive portrait of the incidence and prevalence of the problem from a sport-specific perspective. This section ends with the process leading to making a diagnosis of concussion.

Section II presents management approaches from the perspective of various professionals and what they can bring to care. These chapters will contribute to the understanding of the global nature of what a concussion is and how it can be approached. Evaluations and treatments are presented, accompanied by case studies to illustrate concepts.

Section III deals with returning to life activities after having sustained one or more concussions. Specific chapters are devoted to returning to school, work, and sports, and we end with approaches to dealing with persistent difficulties when recovery does not happen as quickly as expected. Finally, we discuss long-term outcomes of one or multiple concussions.

Section IV presents special situations such as baseline evaluations and on-field assessment, as well as emerging diagnostic and treatment approaches.

The final section (Section V) proposes to put it all together to present a multilayered model of concussion care as well as additional cases illustrating simple and complex recovery courses post-injury.

## References

Ajao, D. O., V. Pop, J. E. Kamper, A. Adami, E. Rudobeck, L. Huang, R. Vlkolinsky et al. 2012. Traumatic brain injury in young rats leads to progressive behavioral deficits coincident with altered tissue properties in adulthood. *J Neurotrauma* 29 (11):2060–2074. doi: 10.1089/neu.2011.1883.

Barkhoudarian, G., D. A. Hovda, and C. C. Giza. 2016. The molecular pathophysiology of concussive brain injury—An update. *Phys Med Rehabil Clin N Am* 27 (2):373–393. doi: 10.1016/j.pmr.2016.01.003.

Buki, A. and J. T. Povlishock. 2006. All roads lead to disconnection?—Traumatic axonal injury revisited. *Acta Neurochir (Wien)* 148 (2):181–193; discussion 193–194. doi: 10.1007/s00701-005-0674-4.

Chen, X. H., V. E. Johnson, K. Uryu, J. Q. Trojanowski, and D. H. Smith. 2009. A lack of amyloid beta plaques despite persistent accumulation of amyloid beta in axons of long-term survivors of traumatic brain injury. *Brain Pathol* 19 (2):214–223. doi: 10.1111/j.1750-3639.2008.00176.x.

Choe, M. C., T. Babikian, J. DiFiori, D. A. Hovda, and C. C. Giza. 2012. A pediatric perspective on concussion pathophysiology. *Curr Opin Pediatr* 24 (6):689–695. doi: 10.1097/MOP.0b013e32835a1a44.

Clausen, F., A. Hanell, C. Israelsson, J. Hedin, T. Ebendal, A. K. Mir, H. Gram, and N. Marklund. 2011. Neutralization of interleukin-1beta reduces cerebral edema and tissue loss and improves late cognitive outcome following traumatic brain injury in mice. *Eur J Neurosci* 34 (1):110–123. doi: 10.1111/j.1460-9568.2011.07723.x.

Clausen, F., A. Hanell, M. Bjork, L. Hillered, A. K. Mir, H. Gram, and N. Marklund. 2009. Neutralization of interleukin-1beta modifies the inflammatory response and improves histological and cognitive outcome following traumatic brain injury in mice. *Eur J Neurosci* 30 (3):385–396. doi: 10.1111/j.1460-9568.2009.06820.x.

Creed, J. A., A. M. DiLeonardi, D. P. Fox, A. R. Tessler, and R. Raghupathi. 2011. Concussive brain trauma in the mouse results in acute cognitive deficits and sustained impairment of axonal function. *J Neurotrauma* 28 (4):547–563. doi: 10.1089/neu.2010.1729.

Dalgard, C. L., J. T. Cole, W. S. Kean, J. J. Lucky, G. Sukumar, D. C. McMullen, H. B. Pollard, and W. D. Watson. 2012. The cytokine temporal profile in rat cortex after controlled cortical impact. *Front Mol Neurosci* 5:6. doi: 10.3389/fnmol.2012.00006.

Faden, A. I., P. Demediuk, S. S. Panter, and R. Vink. 1989. The role of excitatory amino acids and NMDA receptors in traumatic brain injury. *Science* 244 (4906):798–800.

Farkas, O., J. Lifshitz, and J. T. Povlishock. 2006. Mechanoporation induced by diffuse traumatic brain injury: An irreversible or reversible response to injury? *J Neurosci* 26 (12):3130–3140. doi: 10.1523/JNEUROSCI.5119-05.2006.

Ghirnikar, R. S., Y. L. Lee, and L. F. Eng. 1998. Inflammation in traumatic brain injury: Role of cytokines and chemokines. *Neurochem Res* 23 (3):329–340.

Giza, C. C. and D. A. Hovda. 2001. The neurometabolic cascade of concussion. *J Athl Train* 36 (3):228–235.

Giza, C. C. and D. A. Hovda. 2014. The new neurometabolic cascade of concussion. *Neurosurgery* 75:S24–S33. doi: 10.1227/NEU.0000000000000505.

Giza, C. C. and M. L. Prins. 2006. Is being plastic fantastic? Mechanisms of altered plasticity after developmental traumatic brain injury. *Dev Neurosci* 28 (4–5):364–379. doi: 10.1159/000094163.

Holmin, S., M. Schalling, B. Hojeberg, A. S. Nordqvist, A. Skeftruna, and T. Mathiesen. 1997. Delayed cytokine expression in rat brain following experimental contusion. *J Neurosurg* 86:493–504.

Johnson, V. E., W. Stewart, and D. H. Smith. 2013. Axonal pathology in traumatic brain injury. *Exp Neurol* 246:35–43. doi: 10.1016/j.expneurol.2012.01.013.

Jordan, B. D., A. B. Kanik, M. S. Horwich, D. Sweeney, N. R. Relkin, C. K. Petito, and S. Gandy. 1995. Apolipoprotein E epsilon 4 and fatal cerebral amyloid angiopathy associated with dementia pugilistica. *Ann Neurol* 38 (4):698–699. doi: 10.1002/ana.410380429.

Kawamata, T., Y. Katayama, D. A. Hovda, A. Yoshino, and D. P. Becker. 1995. Lactate accumulation following concussive brain injury: The role of ionic fluxes induced by excitatory amino acids. *Brain Res* 674 (2):196–204.

Kelley, B. J., J. Lifshitz, and J. T. Povlishock. 2007. Neuroinflammatory responses after experimental diffuse traumatic brain injury. *J Neuropath Exp Neuro* 66 (11):989–1001.

Li, H. H., S. M. Lee, Y. Cai, R. L. Sutton, and D. A. Hovda. 2004. Differential gene expression in hippocampus following experimental brain trauma reveals distinct features of moderate and severe injuries. *J Neurotrauma* 21 (9):1141–1153.

Mandera, M., D. Larysz, and M. Wojtacha. 2002. Changes in cerebral hemodynamics assessed by transcranial doppler ultrasonography in children after head injury. *Childs Nerv Syst* 18 (3–4):124–128. doi: 10.1007/s00381-002-0572-5.

Maruta, J., S. W. Lee, E. F. Jacobs, and J. Ghajar. 2010. A unified science of concussion. *Ann N Y Acad Sci* 1208:58–66. doi: 10.1111/j.1749-6632.2010.05695.x.

Maugans, T. A., C. Farley, M. Altaye, J. Leach, and K. M. Cecil. 2012. Pediatric sports-related concussion produces cerebral blood flow alterations. *Pediatrics* 129 (1):28–37. doi: 10.1542/peds.2011-2083.

McKee, A. C., D. H. Daneshvar, V. E. Alvarez, and T. D. Stein. 2014. The neuropathology of sport. *Acta Neuropathol* 127 (1):29–51. doi: 10.1007/s00401-013-1230-6.

McKee, A. C., R. C. Cantu, C. J. Nowinski, E. T. Hedley-Whyte, B. E. Gavett, A. E. Budson, V. E. Santini, H. S. Lee, C. A. Kubilus, and R. A. Stern. 2009. Chronic traumatic encephalopathy in athletes: Progressive tauopathy after repetitive head injury. *J Neuropathol Exp Neurol* 68 (7):709–735. doi: 10.1097/NEN.0b013e3181a9d503.

Navarro, J. C., S. Pillai, L. Cherian, R. Garcia, R. J. Grill, and C. S. Robertson. 2012. Histopathological and behavioral effects of immediate and delayed hemorrhagic shock after mild traumatic brain injury in rats. *J Neurotrauma* 29 (2):322–334. doi: 10.1089/neu.2011.1979.

Patterson, Z. R. and M. R. Holahan. 2012. Understanding the neuroinflammatory response following concussion to develop treatment strategies. *Front Cell Neurosci* 6:58. doi: 10.3389/fncel.2012.00058.

Peskind, E. R., E. C. Petrie, D. J. Cross, K. Pagulayan, K. McCraw, D. Hoff, K. Hart, C. E. Yu, M. A. Raskind, D. G. Cook, and S. Minoshima. 2011. Cerebrocerebellar hypometabolism associated with repetitive blast exposure mild traumatic brain injury in 12 Iraq war Veterans with persistent post-concussive symptoms. *Neuroimage* 54 (1):S76–S82. doi: 10.1016/j.neuroimage.2010.04.008.

Prins, M., T. Greco, D. Alexander, and C. C. Giza. 2013. The pathophysiology of traumatic brain injury at a glance. *Dis Model Mech* 6 (6):1307–1315. doi: 10.1242/dmm.011585.

Rathbone, A. T., S. Tharmaradinam, S. Jiang, M. P. Rathbone, and D. A. Kumbhare. 2015. A review of the neuro- and systemic inflammatory responses in post concussion symptoms: Introduction of the "post-inflammatory brain syndrome" PIBS. *Brain Behav Immun* 46:1–16. doi: 10.1016/j. bbi.2015.02.009.

Seifert, T. and V. Shipman. 2015. The pathophysiology of sports concussion. *Curr Pain Headache Rep* 19 (8):36. doi: 10.1007/s11916-015-0513-0.

Shojo, H., Y. Kaneko, T. Mabuchi, K. Kibayashi, N. Adachi, and C. V. Borlongan. 2010. Genetic and histologic evidence implicates role of inflammation in traumatic brain injury-induced apoptosis in the rat cerebral cortex following moderate fluid percussion injury. *Neuroscience* 171 (4):1273–1282. doi: 10.1016/j.neuroscience.2010.10.018.

Taupin, V., S. Toulmond, A. Serrano, J. Benavides, and F. Zavala. 1993. Increase in IL-6, IL-1 and TNF levels in rat brain following traumatic lesion. *J Neuroimmunol* 42:177–186.

Verweij, B. H., J. P. Muizelaar, F. C. Vinas, P. L. Peterson, Y. Xiong, and C. P. Lee. 1997. Mitochondrial dysfunction after experimental and human brain injury and its possible reversal with a selective N-type calcium channel antagonist (SNX-111). *Neurol Res* 19 (3):334–339.

Xiong, Y., Q. Gu, P. L. Peterson, J. P. Muizelaar, and C. P. Lee. 1997. Mitochondrial dysfunction and calcium perturbation induced by traumatic brain injury. *J Neurotrauma* 14 (1):23–34. doi: 10.1089/neu.1997.14.23.

*chapter two*

# Concussion revisited: A historical perspective

## How has the focus on concussion evolved over the years?

*Paul McCrory*

### Contents

### Introduction

Concussion is a well-recognized clinical entity; however, the detailed understanding of its pathophysiologic basis is evolving. In the broadest clinical sense, concussion is often defined as representing the immediate and transient symptoms of traumatic brain injury; however, such operational definitions do not give an insight into the underlying processes through which the brain is impaired. This issue of understanding concussion and mTBI is clouded not only by the lack of critical data but also by confusion in definition and terminology. For over 100 years, various definitions of concussion and mild traumatic brain injury (mTBI) have been proposed by individual authors as well as international bodies; however, these definitions do not concur with one another, which makes understanding the epidemiology of these injuries difficult and management complicated (Ruff and Jurica 1999).

One key unresolved issue is whether concussion is part of a TBI injury spectrum and thus associated with lesser degrees of diffuse structural change that are seen in severe traumatic brain injury, or whether the concussive injury is the result of reversible functional changes.

Newer technological advances have opened the possibility that now we not only can separate different patterns of injury presentation but give important insights into the underlying pathophysiology and ultimately provide a platform to develop a clear definition, which is underpinned by evidence. It is likely that head injury and concussion will ultimately be defined by the severity of clinical signs, as well as genetic, epigenetic, metabolomic, proteomic, advanced imaging findings, and blood/cerebrospinal fluid (CSF) biomarkers in the same way that cancer and other medical disease is diagnosed. At this stage, however, we have only the nonspecific clinical signs and symptoms to try and provide the beginnings of that framework and we lack sufficient certainty in aspects of physiology, metabolomics, proteomics, genetics, and epigenetics to enable a complete understanding of the entity.

## Understanding the definition of concussion

Key elements of a *clinical or operational definition* of concussion must acknowledge that it is a subset of TBI and should include:

- Induced by direct or indirect trauma
- A defined physiological disruption of brain function
- An alteration in attention (mental state) at the time of the injury (e.g., confusion, disorientation, slowed thinking, alteration of consciousness, or mental state)
- A period of post-traumatic amnesia (PTA)
- A range of evolving clinical symptoms that may or may not involve loss of consciousness (LOC)

Despite many publications and definitional attempts (McCrory et al. 2017a), these considerations leave several issues unanswered, notably: Does being dazed, seeing stars, or feeling dizzy in the absence of unconsciousness constitute either concussion or mTBI? The millions of minor bumps to the head both in children and adults in which the victim is only momentarily dazed and is completely back to normal within a few seconds or minutes without later clinical sequelae, should remind us of the dangers of the overenthusiastic use of medical labels and their indiscriminate dissemination to the public.

## Historical context

The clinical manifestations of concussion as a transient neurological syndrome without structural brain injury have been known since the tenth century AD when the Arabian physician Rhazes first defined the condition (Rhazes 1497, McCrory and Berkovic 2001). Lanfrancus in 1306 taught that symptoms after a head injury could rapidly disappear and were the results of a transient paralysis of cerebral function caused by the brain being shaken (Lanfrancus 1565). Da Carpi in the sixteenth century developed Lanfrancus' concept of concussion, which he termed *cerebrum commotum* and was distinguished from more severe brain injuries, which he named *contusio* (bruising/hemorrhage) and *compressio* (brain swelling/oedema) (da Carpi 1535, Abbott 1961). In the sixteenth and seventeenth centuries, the term *commotio* (or commotion) of the brain was used interchangeably with *concussio* (or concussion), a term derived from the Latin verb *concutere*, which means to *shake violently* (McCrory and Berkovic 2001). In Europe, the term *brain commotion* (or *commotio cerebri*) is still used in place of concussion as well as in the current DSM5 criteria where concussion (S06.1) is still listed as commotio cerebri and there is no category for mTBI or any other descriptor of lesser severities of TBI. The historical evolutions of the concepts surrounding brain injury and concussion and the development of theoretical models have been extensively reviewed elsewhere (Courville 1944, 1967, McCrory and Berkovic 2001, Pearce 2007).

Since the 1970s, clinicians and scientists have begun to distinguish sport-related concussions (SRC) from other causes of concussion and mTBI, such as motor vehicle crashes, and so on. While this seems like an arbitrary separation from other forms of mTBI, which account for 80% of such injuries (Langlois and Sattin 2005, Langlois et al. 2006), it is largely driven by the need to have clear and practical guidelines to determine recovery and safe return to play for athletes suffering a SRC. In addition, SRC can be viewed as a research laboratory to study mTBI, given the detailed SRC phenotype data that is typically available in elite sports (Kelly and Rosenberg 1998). Having said that, it is critical to understand that the lessons derived from nonsporting mTBI research provides the understanding of SRC (and vice versa), and this arbitrary separation of sporting versus nonsporting TBI should not be viewed simply as a dichotomous or exclusive view of TBI.

This paper will focus on the evolution of SRC guidelines over the past 50 years. The author of this paper has been involved in the Concussion In Sport Group (CISG) consensus process.

## Concussion guidelines pre-1974

A key development in the history of SRC was in 1905 when President Theodore Roosevelt drew attention to the American football *death harvest*. In 1905 alone, at least 18 people died and more than 150 were injured playing football. People were especially shaken by the November 1905 death of Union College halfback Harold Moore, who died of a cerebral hemorrhage after being kicked in the head while trying to tackle a New York University player. President Theodore Roosevelt summoned coaches and athletic advisers from Harvard University, Yale University, and Princeton University to the White House to discuss how to improve the game of football. Soon after, rules started to change to reduce the amount and severity of head injuries in football (Miller 2011). Up until 1980, the primary focus regarding concussions was to exclude a potentially fatal intracranial hemorrhage. While more recent studies have become increasingly aware of long-term consequences of concussions in some individuals, the perception over many decades was that virtually all concussions would *clear* with time and rest (Dunn et al. 2006, Stone et al. 2014, Maroon et al. 2014).

A number of neurosurgically driven laboratories or surgically oriented neurologists began to examine mTBI more specifically, in part because of the military research programs and clinical exposure to brain trauma seen in various conflicts (Russell 1932, Denny-Brown and Russell 1941, Russell 1971). After World War II, other neurosurgeons took up the mantle, and a key figure during this period was Dr. Richard Schneider (1913–1986), a leading U.S. neurosurgeon, who published an influential book in 1973 examining head injuries in sport (Schneider 1973). This book did much to draw the focus of clinicians to the management of SRC.

At the same time, TBI researchers using primate models began to examine milder forms of brain injury to try and determine the pathophysiological basis of the clinical features (Ommaya et al. 1964, Ommaya and Gennarelli 1975, Gennarelli 1982).

## Concussion severity grading scales and guidelines 1974–2001

From the 1970s until the early 2000s, numerous authors proposed injury severity scales and return to sport recommendations for the management of concussions that occurred during sport. Neurosurgeons or orthopedic surgeons trying to use the same approach as was used in more severe TBI cases to SRC published most of these scales.

The published sport-related concussion severity scales can be broken down into a number of broad groupings. The details of these early scales have been reviewed elsewhere (Johnston et al. 2001). Table 2.1 gives illustrative examples of each category.

1. *Surrogate head injury scales*: Whereas the practical needs in the majority of concussions are for a scale, which is biased toward distinguishing the marginal clinical injury from the mild to moderate injury, most of the scales are biased toward the higher severity injuries. In some cases these include coma, persistent vegetative state, and death, far beyond the historical understanding of concussion (Ommaya and Gennarelli 1974, Ommaya 1990, Torg 1991, Gersoff 1991). The aim of these types of injury scales is to avoid missing the more severe brain injuries (e.g., cerebral hemorrhage) that may mimic concussion in their early stages. There is no evidence that these scales achieve this goal.

2. *Neurosurgical scales*: Traditional neurosurgical thinking is evident in the composition of each of these scales (Maroon et al. 1980, Hugenholtz and Richard 1982, Cantu 1986, Wilberger and Maroon 1989, Kelly et al. 1991, Roberts 1992, Polin et al. 1996). While the duration of LOC and PTA are important outcome predictors in severe brain injury, the extrapolation of such clinical features to milder grades of brain injury remains speculative. In each of these scales, an arbitrary separation is made between different grades of concussive injury.

3. *Sport-specific scales*: Sporting organizations throughout the world have responded to the needs of injury management within their given sport by the development of their own severity scales (Turner 1998). In most cases, these have been developed by designated medical officials within the sport and reflect the specific logistics and practicalities inherent within a particular sport. Most have not been published formally but exist as part of the medical regulations for the sport. As a result, these specific scales have much in common with category 2.

4. *Sporting injury scales*: In these cases the stated aim of the injury scales is to distinguish the mild injuries from more severe injuries (Kulund 1982, Nelson et al. 1984, Kolb 1989, Schneider 1973, Saal 1991, American Academy of Neurology 1997). In some cases, attempts have been made to amalgamate neurosurgical concepts within this framework but in general these types of scales are largely symptom-driven. Often terminology is used loosely (e.g., *extended* LOC or *prolonged* retrograde amnesia), which makes interpretation of the arbitrary subcategories difficult. Although this approach is more in keeping with the typical management

Table 2.1 Examples of early concussion grading scales

| Severity grade | Surrogate head injury scale (Torg 1991) | Neurosurgical scale (Cantu 1986) | Category | | |
| | | | Sport specific scale Jockey club (UK)(Turner 1998) | Sporting injury scale AAN(American Academy of Neurology 1997) | Unclassifiable scale (Parkinson 1977) |
|---|---|---|---|---|---|
| 1 | Confusion Momentary LOC Dazed appearance Unsteady gait | No LOC, PTA < 30 min | No LOC | Transient confusion No LOC Concussion symptoms or mental status abnormalities resolve > 15 min | Normal somatic mobility with impaired performance |
| 2 | Vertigo PTA | LOC < 5 min, PTA > 30 min | LOC < 60 s or any degree of PTA or if rider sent to hospital | Transient confusion No LOC Concussion symptoms or mental status abnormalities resolve > 15 min | Normal visceral mobility with impaired somatic mobility |
| 3 | Vertigo PTA RA | LOC > 5 min PTA > 24 h | LOC > 60 s | Any LOC | Return of irregular visceral mobility with continuing somatic immobility |
| 4 | PTA Immediate LOC | | | | Visceral (respiratory) immobility and somatic immobility |
| 5 | Paralytic coma CR arrest | | | | |
| 6 | Death | | | | |

LOC = loss of consciousness, PTA = post-traumatic amnesia, PVS = persistent vegetative state, RA = retrograde amnesia, CR = cardiorespiratory.

problems faced by sports medicine clinicians, no scientific validation has been attempted with any of these scales.

5. *Unclassifiable scales*: In this category, the scaling system proposed is more reflective of pathophysiological constructs than clinical management (Parkinson 1977).

At the First International Conference on Concussion in Sport, held in Vienna in 2001, one of the key outcomes was the recognition by the expert panel that none of the numerous concussion scales then published was scientifically valid. For this reason a seminal recommendation was made to assess individual *recovery* using a multimodality assessment upon which to determine safe return to play rather than rely on invalidated recommendations.

## Concussion consensus and agreement statements 2001–present

Since 2001, a variety of SRC guidelines have been published. These include:

1. Global initiatives with a formal consensus process and guidelines or recommendations (Aubry et al. 2002, McCrory et al. 2005, 2009, 2013, 2017b)
2. Sport-specific meetings with outcome papers (Smith et al. 2015, 2011)
3. Organization (Guskiewicz et al. 2004, Herring et al. 2006, Harmon et al. 2013, Giza et al. 2013, Broglio et al. 2014) or institutional (Collins et al. 2016) conferences that have led to systematic reviews, guidelines, and/or recommendations
4. Reports of various conferences or position statements

In many cases, the authors of various papers overlap; however, it is worth observing that the majority of sport-specific and institutional guidelines derive from North America and reflect the sports played on that continent.

The methodology for the various guidelines differs substantially, which in turn means that the published outcomes need to be considered in that context. In the case of the formal consensus meetings (Aubry et al. 2002, McCrory et al. 2005, 2009, 2013, 2017b) although the lead author is often cited, the opinions represent the agreed consensus view of the expert panel that are named in the paper. The consensus process attempts to define a more transparent method through which outcomes are developed. In the case of the CISG meetings, in addition to the summary paper, the group publishes formal systematic reviews on each of the questions under discussion (and meta-analyses where possible) upon which the summary recommendations are based and these should be read in conjunction with the summary papers.

### Formal consensus meetings

#### CISG guidelines

One of the most significant developments in SRC over the past two decades has been the establishment of the Concussion In Sport Group (CISG). This group has organized five consensus meetings to date and has published the guidelines and assessment tools that have become globally adopted. The outcome documents from the meetings are first and foremost, intended to guide clinical practice; however, they also help form the agenda for SRC research. All outcome papers and assessment tools have been made available copyright free to encourage dissemination. The first two meetings (2001 and 2004) were expert panel meetings but from 2008 onwards these meetings have adopted a U.S. National Institutes of Health Consensus meeting format with background systematic reviews of each of the topics under discussion published in conjunction with the summary paper of each meeting. The methodology of the meetings is described in detail in conjunction with each summary paper (Aubry et al. 2002, McCrory et al. 2005, 2009, 2013, 2017b, Meeuwisse et al. 2017).

*First CISG meeting Vienna, November 2001* (Aubry et al. 2002)    The Vienna conference was held in November 2001 and was supported and organized by the International Ice Hockey Federation (IIHF), Fédération Internationale de Football Association (FIFA), and the IOC Medical Commission, with a stated objective of providing recommendations for the improvement of the safety and health of athletes who suffer concussive injuries in ice hockey, soccer, and other sports. Part of the drive by sporting organizations to organize a specific meeting was the lack of a practical and valid management paradigm to diagnose and treat concussions seen in a sporting context. One particular catalyst for the meeting was the need for SRC guidelines leading into the 2002 Winter Olympic Games and, paradoxically, this occurred at a time when concussion in sport was not topical. Although consensus definitions for mTBI already existed, they were not related to the type of injuries seen in sport and did not provide practical guidance in regard to recovery and return to sport (ACRM 1993). For this reason, experts were invited to address issues involving epidemiology, basic and clinical science, grading systems, cognitive assessment, new research methods, protective equipment, management, prevention, and long-term outcome from SRC. At the conclusion of the conference, a small group of the experts was given the mandate to draft the summary document (Aubry et al. 2002) that was subsequently co-published in three sports medicine journals.

The key recommendations from the Vienna meeting were:

1. A new consensus definition of SRC (see the previous section)
2. The paradigm shift from the use of concussion grading scales to the multidimensional assessment of individualized SRC recovery
3. The critical role of neuropsychological or cognitive assessment in the management of SRC
4. The novel suggestion that return to sport should follow a stepwise graduated rehabilitation protocol
5. Highlighting the role of rule change and enforcement in the prevention of SRC
6. Acknowledging that the science of studying concussion was at an early stage and as a result, decisions regarding SRC management and return to play lie largely in the realm of clinical judgment and must be made on an individual basis

*Second CISG meeting Prague, November 2004* (McCrory et al. 2005)    This second international conference on concussion in sport was considerably more widely attended than the first and had a much greater representation from new groups, such as trauma surgeons and sports psychologists. There were some important recommendations made including:

1. That concussion severity should only be determined after clinical and cognitive recovery was complete and that that neuropsychological assessment following concussion should not be performed until all signs and symptoms have resolved.
2. Noting that LOC should not be relied on as a measure of concussion severity.
3. That pediatric SRC could be managed using guidelines similar to those used in caring for adult patients.

4. That cognitive rest may be an important management strategy where cognitive activities intensify or prolong post-concussion symptoms
5. That the number and duration of post-concussion symptoms were most important in determining concussion severity
6. The development of a new sideline concussion assessment tool (SCAT) for use by clinicians
7. The separation of SRC into simple concussion (symptoms < 10 days) and complex concussion (symptoms > 10 days or where the patient lost consciousness for longer than 1 min, had a convulsive concussion, or had repeated concussions involving diminishing force)
8. Described the motor phenomena of SRC (e.g., tonic posturing, convulsions) as benign but dramatic in presentation
9. Whenever a player shows any symptoms or signs of concussion, he or she should not be allowed to return to play in the current game or practice, should not be left alone, and should undergo serial reassessment for deterioration

At the conclusion of the conference, a small group of the experts was given the mandate to draft the summary document that was subsequently co-published in three sports medicine journals (McCrory et al. 2005).

*Third CISG meeting Zurich, November 2008* (McCrory et al. 2009)  The third International Conference on Concussion in Sport was held in Zurich, Switzerland, on October 29th and 30th, 2008 and was designed as a consensus meeting broadly following the organizational guidelines set forth by the U.S. National Institutes of Health (details of the consensus methodology can be obtained at: http://consensus.nih.gov/ABOUTCDP.htm). The principles governing the conduct of a consensus development conference include: a broad-based expert panel with full disclosure of conflicts of interest; development of specific questions to be addressed with a systematic review paper on each topic circulated to the panel in advance of the meeting; presentation of the data in an open public session followed by an executive session to prepare the summary statement, which serves as a scientific record of the meeting and is then disseminated.
    The key recommendations from this meeting included:

1. A minor change to the definition noting that SRC symptoms could be persistent or prolonged
2. Abandoning the simple versus complex SRC terminology
3. Reinforcing the need for a multidimensional SRC assessment
4. Reinforcing the *no same day return to play* approach
5. Highlighting the role of balance assessment in concussion management
6. Emphasizing the role of physical and cognitive rest in the acute stages after concussion followed by the graduated symptom limited rehabilitation protocol
7. Developing a list of modifying factors that may influence the investigation and management of SRC
8. Highlighting the issue of mental health sequelae following SRC
9. Highlighting the role of management of SRC in children and adolescents
10. Noting the developing literature on cognitive impairment in retired athletes but no consensus was reached of the significance of these observations
11. Updating the sideline concussion assessment tools—SCAT2 and pocket SCAT

At the conclusion of the conference, the summary document was co-published in seven sports medicine journals (McCrory et al. 2005, 2009).

*Fourth CISG meeting Zurich, November 2012* (McCrory et al. 2013)   The fourth International Conference On Concussion In Sport was held in Zurich, Switzerland, in November 2012. This meeting was designed to build on the principles outlined in the previous meetings and to develop further conceptual understanding of this problem using the formal consensus-based approach previously described.

The key recommendations from this meeting included:

1. The agreement that SRC was an evolving injury in the early stages with rapidly changing clinical signs and symptoms. This in turn makes the exclusion of the diagnosis on the sidelines problematic. For that reason it was recommended that all athletes who have transient neurological symptoms should be removed from play for a detailed assessment
2. No single sideline tool has sufficient sensitivity or specificity to make or exclude the diagnosis of SRC
3. A revision of the SCAT3 tools and publishing a new Child SCAT3 for assessment of young (<13 years) individuals
4. Emphasizing the role of trained neuropsychologists in the assessment of cognitive dysfunction in SRC
5. Acknowledging the developing literature on vestibular and cervical physiotherapy in the rehabilitation of symptomatic individuals
6. Highlighting the *difficult* concussion patient and the appropriate management
7. Reviewing the modifiers from the previous meeting in terms of strength of evidence
8. Discussing about the literature on chronic traumatic encephalopathy and noting the lack of prospective studies in this area
9. Highlighting the role of knowledge translation

At the conclusion of the conference, the summary document was co-published in seven sports medicine journals (McCrory et al. 2013).

*Fifth CISG meeting Berlin, October 2016* (McCrory et al. 2017b)   The fifth International Conference On Concussion In Sport was held in Berlin, Germany, on October 27–29, 2016. Once again, the meeting utilized a formal consensus approach to build on the principles outlined in the previous meetings and to develop further conceptual understanding of SRC. The details of the meeting and the consensus process have been published in a separate paper (Meeuwisse et al. 2017). It is worth noting that approximately 60,000 published articles were screened by the expert panels for the Berlin meeting as part of the review process. The meeting itself engaged more formally with experts from TBI research, dementia and neurodegenerative disease, genetics and biomarker research, as well as a range of peak sporting bodies.

The key outcomes from the meeting include:

1. A revision of the SRC definition highlighting that concussion should be seen as a subset of TBI and that the features of the injury cannot be explained by drug, alcohol, medication use, other injuries (such as cervical injuries, peripheral vestibular dysfunction etc.), or other comorbidities (e.g., psychological factors or coexisting medical conditions)

2. The limited clinical role of helmet-based or other sensor systems to clinically diagnose or assess SRC
3. A revision of the SCAT tools
4. Emphasizing the importance of a multidimensional assessment of SRC
5. Removal from play of an athlete with SRC and the importance of allowing adequate time for the medical assessment
6. Noting that advanced neuroimaging, fluid biomarkers, and genetic testing are important research tools, but require further validation to determine their clinical utility in evaluation of SRC
7. The role of symptom limited physical and cognitive rest (rather than complete rest) in the recovery phase
8. Recognizing the role of rehabilitation strategies in the recovery phase including: controlled subsymptom threshold, submaximal exercise programs, as well as psychological, cervical, and vestibular rehabilitation
9. Discussing about the definition and management strategies for persistent symptoms
10. Reviewing the evidence for concussion modifiers
11. Noting that modalities of measuring physiological change after SRC, while useful as research tools, are not ready for clinical management
12. Reviewing the graduated return to sport paradigm
13. Highlighting the importance of the correct management of children and adolescents with SRC
14. Reviewing the literature on neurobehavioral sequelae and long-term consequences of exposure to recurrent head trauma and noting that this is largely inconclusive at this stage
15. Reviewing injury prevention strategies

The outcome papers will be co-published in a number of journals (McCrory et al. 2017b).

## *Sport-specific meetings with outcome papers* (Smith et al. 2015, 2011)

While numerous sporting bodies have held conferences and symposia on SRC in their sport, few have published outcome or recommendation papers. In most cases, these meetings are didactic rather than consensus driven; however, one sport that has attempted to prioritize prevention strategies using a form of consensus is ice hockey.

Two conferences on SRC in ice hockey occurred in 2011 and 2013 and a third meeting is planned for September 2017. These meetings were an attempt to integrate the research on SRC in ice hockey and develop an action plan to reduce the risk, incidence, severity, and consequences of SRC in that sport. Topics for discussion were circulated in advance of the meetings and breakout groups formed to present the literature related to those topics. At the meeting, attendees voted using an *audience response system* to prioritize areas for future action planning. At the second meeting in 2013, progress in each of these action areas was reviewed and new developments identified. Brief summaries of each topic were presented to the audience for prioritization. While commendable in terms of knowledge translation, the outcome papers did not discuss how the literature was searched and the comprehensiveness of the process.

## Organization (Guskiewicz et al. 2004, Herring et al. 2006, Harmon et al. 2013, Giza et al. 2013, Broglio et al. 2014) and institutional (Collins et al. 2016) guidelines

### National athletic trainers' association position statement: Management of sport-related concussion 2004 & 2014 (Guskiewicz et al. 2004; Broglio et al. 2014)

This position statement, which was published in 2004 (Guskiewicz et al. 2004) and revised and updated in 2014 (Broglio et al. 2014) is a detailed and extensive narrative review of the published literature and intends to provide athletic trainers with best practice guidelines for SRC management based on an up-to-date research. The statement lists 36 specific recommendations and grades the strength of the recommendation using the strength of recommendation taxonomy (SORT) (Ebell et al. 2004). The recommendations cover areas such as recognizing concussion; making return-to-play decisions; and assessment tools, cognitive screening, postural assessment, and neuropsychological testing. It also contains sections on when to refer an athlete to a physician after a concussion and when to disqualify an athlete, as well as sections on special considerations for the young athlete, home care, and equipment issues.

### Concussion (Mild Traumatic Brain Injury) and the team physician: A consensus statement 2006 & 2011 (Herring et al. 2006, 2011)

In 2006, the American College of Sports Medicine published a consensus statement on SRC and specifically on the role of the team physician in this setting and focusing on the on-field and sideline management of SRC (Herring et al. 2006). This statement was updated in 2011 (Herring et al. 2011). The statement represented the collaborative effort of six major professional associations, including the American Academy of Family Physicians, the American Academy of Orthopedic Surgeons, the American College of Sports Medicine, the American Medical Society for Sports Medicine (AMSSM), the American Orthopedic Society for Sports Medicine, and the American Osteopathic Academy for Sports Medicine, and was endorsed by a number of additional organizations, including the American Osteopathic Association, the National Athletic Trainers' Association (NATA), the North American Spine Society, the National Collegiate Athletic Association, the National Youth Sports Safety Foundation, the American Academy of Podiatric Sports Medicine, and the American Kinesiotherapy Association.

The areas covered within the narrative review include: epidemiology, biomechanics, and pathophysiology, preseason planning and assessment, same day evaluation and treatment, post same day evaluation, diagnostic testing, return-to-play decisions, complications, prevention, as well as legislation and governance issues. Each section of the document includes the panel's consensus view on what is *essential* and what is *desirable* for the team physician to know and understand.

This statement was similar to the CISG statements in that it emphasized that concussion severity should be determined by the duration and number of post-concussion symptoms, not by whether there was brief LOC or even whether amnesia alone was one of the symptoms.

*American Medical Society for sports medicine position statement:*
*Concussion in sport 2013* (Harmon et al. 2013)

The purpose of this statement was to provide an evidence-based, best practice summary to assist physicians in the evaluation and management of SRC and to establish the level of evidence, knowledge gaps, and areas requiring additional research. The focus of the statement was for nonsurgical sports medicine physician with additional training in sports medicine. The recommendations derived from this narrative review were graded according to the strength of the recommendation using the SORT criteria (Ebell et al. 2004).

*American Academy of Neurology—evaluation and management of concussion in*
*sport—1997 & 2013* (American Academy of Neurology 1997, Giza et al. 2013)

This evidence-based guideline (Giza et al. 2013) replaced the 1997 American Academy of Neurology (AAN) practice parameter on the management of sports concussion (American Academy of Neurology 1997). This is one of the most comprehensive documents on SRC available. The multidisciplinary authors very clearly describe the systematic review process that was followed to search and extract data. The strength of the evidence was assessed according to the GRADE scale (Guyatt et al. 2011). The writing panel formulated recommendations on the basis of the evidence systematically reviewed and when evidence directly related to sports concussion was unavailable, from strong evidence derived from nonsport-related mTBI, similar to the CISG approach. The clinician level of obligation of recommendations was assigned using a modified Delphi process. The summary document is accompanied by extensive online data supplement (available at www. neurology.org).

This guideline addressed the following clinical questions: (1) For athletes, what factors increase or decrease SRC risk? (2) For athletes suspected of having sustained an SRC, what diagnostic tools are useful in identifying those with SRC? (3) For athletes suspected of having an SRC, what diagnostic tools are useful in identifying those at increased risk for severe or prolonged early impairments, neurologic catastrophe, or chronic neurobehavioral impairment? and (4) For athletes with SRC, what interventions enhance recovery, reduce the risk of recurrent concussion, or diminish long-term sequelae?

*Statements of agreement from the targeted evaluation and active*
*management approaches to treating concussion* (Collins et al. 2016)

A group of concussion experts was convened in Pittsburgh, Pennsylvania, on October 14–16, 2015, to determine areas of agreement regarding the current state of concussion treatment. The outcome document (Collins et al. 2016) presents the results of the meeting, which was designed to foster an understanding among clinicians, scientists, and laypeople that concussion symptoms and impairment are treatable with more active and targeted approaches than prescribed rest alone. In contrast to meetings such as the CISG meetings, which used formal consensus meeting guidelines, the targeted evaluation and active management (TEAM) meeting used a majority voting approach to determining agreement on each statement similar to that used by ice hockey summit described earlier (Smith et al. 2011, 2015).

Thirty-seven concussion experts from neuropsychology, neurology, neurosurgery, sports medicine, physical medicine and rehabilitation, physical therapy, athletic training, and research and 12 individuals representing sport, military, and public health organizations attended the meeting. A total of 16 statements of agreement were supported covering (1) summary of the current approach to treating concussion, (2) heterogeneity and evolving clinical profiles of concussion, (3) team approach to concussion treatment: specific strategies, and (4) future directions: a call to research.

## Reports of various conferences or position statements

Numerous organizations have published position statements or statements of practice with varying degrees of scientific rigor, stating how the data was derived upon which recommendations are based (Halstead et al. 2010, Echemendia et al. 2012, NCAA 2014, Moreau et al. 2015). While this list is not exhaustive, it highlights the need for organizations to develop methodologies that describe the process by which position/summary statements are developed and the strength of evidence of any recommendations provided.

## Conclusion

It is important to consider that all SRC need to be medically assessed given the potential for adverse outcomes. Embedded in that approach is the concept that diagnosing concussion is often not a *point in time* event but rather one that requires observation over time and exclusion of other conditions that may mimic a concussion. The role of evidence-based guidelines has evolved over the past 50 years driven by various sporting, cultural, political, and scientific agendas from a *neurosurgical era* of trying to rule out severe TBI to an *SRC era* of trying to diagnose the minimal injury and manage these using best practice strategies. The future challenge will be to unify the various groups and bodies who publish individual guideline statements in a global initiative.

## References

No author listed. 2005. SORT: The strength-of-recommendation taxonomy. *Am Fam Physician* 71 (1):19–20. http://www.aafp.org/dam/AAFP/documents/journals/afp/sortdef07.pdf (accessed September 5, 2017).

Abbott, K. H. 1961. Berengario on cerebral concussion. *Bull LA Neurol Sci* 26:97.

ACRM. 1993. American congress of rehabilitation medicine mild traumatic brain injury committee of the head injury interdisciplinary special interest group. Definition of mild traumatic brain injury. *J Head Trauma Rehabil* 8 (3):86–87.

American Academy of Neurology. 1997. Practice parameter: The management of concussion in sports (summary statement). *Neurology* 48:581–585.

Aubry, M., R. Cantu, J. Dvorak, T. Graf-Baumann, K. M. Johnston, J. Kelly, M. Lovell, P. McCrory, W. H. Meeuwisse, and P. Schamasch. 2002. Summary and agreement statement of the 1st international symposium on concussion in sport, Vienna 2001. *Clin J Sport Med* 12 (1):6–11.

Broglio, S. P., R. C. Cantu, G. A. Gioia, K. M. Guskiewicz, J. Kutcher, M. Palm, T. C. Valovich McLeod, and Association National Athletic Trainer's. 2014. National athletic trainers' association position statement: Management of sport concussion. *J Athl Train* 49 (2):245–265. doi: 10.4085/1062-6050-49.1.07.

Cantu, R. C. 1986. Guidelines for return to contact sports after cerebral concussion. *Phys Sportsmed* 14:75–83.

Collins, M. W., A. P. Kontos, D. O. Okonkwo, J. Almquist, J. Bailes, M. Barisa, J. Bazarian et al. 2016. Statements of agreement from the targeted evaluation and active management (TEAM) approaches to treating concussion meeting held in Pittsburgh, PA October 15–16, 2015. *Neurosurgery* 79 (6):912–929. doi: 10.1227/NEU.0000000000001447.

Courville, C. B. 1944. Some notes on the history of injury to the skull and brain. *Bull LA Neurol Society* 9:1–16.

Courville, C. B. 1967. *Injuries of the Skull and Brain as Described in the Myths, Ledgends and Folk Tales of the World*. New York: Vantage Press.

da Carpi, B. 1535. *Tractatus Perutilis et Completus de Fractura Cranei*. Bologna: JB Pederzanus.

Denny-Brown, D. and W. R. Russell. 1941. Experimental cerebral concussion. *Brain* 64:93–163.

Dunn, I. F., G. Dunn, and A. L. Day. 2006. Neurosurgeons and their contributions to modern-day athletics: Richard C. Schneider Memorial Lecture. *Neurosurg Focus* 21 (4):E1.

Ebell, M. H., J. Siwek, B. D. Weiss, S. H. Woolf, J. Susman, B. Ewigman, and M. Bowman. 2004. Strength of recommendation taxonomy (SORT): A patient-centered approach to grading evidence in the medical literature. *J Am Board Fam Pract* 17 (1):59–67.

Echemendia, R. J., G. L. Iverson, M. McCrea, D. K. Broshek, G. A. Gioia, S. W. Sautter, S. N. Macciocchi, and W. B. Barr. 2012. Role of neuropsychologists in the evaluation and management of sport-related concussion: An inter-organization position statement. *Arch Clin Neuropsychol* 27 (1):119–122. doi: 10.1093/arclin/acr077.

Gennarelli, T. A. 1982. Cerebral concussion and diffuse brain injuries. In *Athletic Injuries of the Head, Nneck and Face.*, edited by J. S. Torg, pp. 93–104. Philadelphia, PA: Lea & Febiger.

Gersoff, W. 1991. Head and neck injuries. In *Sports Medicine: The School Age Athlete*, edited by B. Reider. Philadelphia, PA: W B Saunders.

Giza, C. C., J. S. Kutcher, S. Ashwal, J. Barth, T. S. Getchius, G. A. Gioia, G. S. Gronseth et al. 2013. Summary of evidence-based guideline update: Evaluation and management of concussion in sports: Report of the guideline development subcommittee of the American academy of neurology. *Neurology*. doi: 10.1212/WNL.0b013e31828d57dd.

Guskiewicz, K. M., S. L. Bruce, R. C. Cantu, M. S. Ferrara, J. P. Kelly, M. McCrea, M. Putukian, and T. C. McLeod. 2004. Recommendations on management of sport-related concussion: Summary of the national Athletic Trainers' Association position statement. *Neurosurgery* 55 (4):891–895; discussion 896.

Guyatt, G. H., A. D. Oxman, H. J. Schunemann, P. Tugwell, and A. Knottnerus. 2011. GRADE guidelines: A new series of articles in the journal of clinical epidemiology. *J Clin Epidemiol* 64 (4):380–382. doi: 10.1016/j.jclinepi.2010.09.011.

Halstead, M. E., K. D. Walter, Medicine Council on Sports, and Fitness. 2010. American academy of pediatrics. Clinical report—sport-related concussion in children and adolescents. *Pediatrics* 126 (3):597–615. doi: 10.1542/peds.2010-2005.

Harmon, K. G., J. Drezner, M. Gammons, K. Guskiewicz, M. Halstead, S. Herring, J. Kutcher, A. Pana, M. Putukian, and W. Roberts. 2013. American medical society for sports medicine position statement: Concussion in sport. *Clin J Sport Med* 23 (1):1–18. doi: 10.1097/JSM.0b013e31827f5f93.

Herring, S. A., R. C. Cantu, K. M. Guskiewicz, M. Putukian, W. B. Kibler, J. A. Bergfeld, L. A. Boyajian-O'Neill, R. R. Franks, P. A. Indelicato, and Medicine American college of sports. 2011. Concussion (mild traumatic brain injury) and the team physician: A consensus statement—2011 update. *Med Sci Sports Exerc* 43 (12):2412–2422. doi: 10.1249/MSS.0b013e3182342e64.

Herring, S. A., J. Bergfeld, A. Boland, L. A. Boyajian-O'Neill, R. Cantu, E. Hershman, P. Indelicato, R. Jaffe, W. B. Kibler, D. B. McKeag, R. Pallay, and M. Putukian. 2006. Concussion (mild traumatic brain injury) and the team physician: A consensus statement. *Med Sci Sports Exerc* 38 (2):395–399. doi: 10.1249/01.mss.0000202025.48774.31 00005768-200602000-00029 [pii].

Hugenholtz, H. and M. T. Richard. 1982. Return to athletic competition following concussion. *Can Med Assoc J* 127 (9):827–829.

Johnston, K. M., P. McCrory, N. G. Mohtadi, and W. H. Meeuwisse. 2001. Evidence based review of sport-related concussion—Clinical science. *Clin J Sport Med* 11:150–160.

Kelly, J. P., J. S. Nichols, C. M. Filley, K. O. Lillehei, D. Rubinstein, and B. K. Kleinschmidt-DeMasters. 1991. Concussion in sports. Guidelines for the prevention of catastrophic outcome. *Jama* 266 (20):2867–2869.

Kelly, J. P. and J. H. Rosenberg. 1998. The development of guidelines for the management of concussion in sports. *J Head Trauma Rehabil* 13 (2):53–65.

Kolb, J. 1989. Cerebral concussion. *Sports Training, Medicine and Rehabilitation* 1:165–171.

Kulund, D. N. 1982. Athletic injuries to the head, neck and face. In *The Injured Athlete*, edited by D. N. Kulund, pp. 225–257. Philadelphia, PA: J B Lippincott.

Lanfrancus. 1565. *A Most Excellent and Learned Worke of Chirurgery Called Chirurgia Por va Lanfranci*. London, UK: T Marshe.

Langlois, J. A., W. Rutland-Brown, and M. M. Wald. 2006. The epidemiology and impact of traumatic brain injury: A brief overview. *J Head Trauma Rehabil* 21 (5):375–378. doi: 00001199-200609000-00001 [pii].

Langlois, J. A. and R. W. Sattin. 2005. Traumatic brain injury in the United States: Research and programs of the centers for disease control and prevention (CDC). *J Head Trauma Rehabil* 20 (3):187–188. doi: 00001199-200505000-00001 [pii].

Maroon, J. C., C. Mathyssek, and J. Bost. 2014. Cerebral concussion: A historical perspective. *Prog Neurol Surg* 28:1–13. doi: 10.1159/000358746.

Maroon, J. C., P. B. Steele, and R. Berlin. 1980. Football head and neck injuries--an update. *Clin Neurosurg* 27:414–429.

McCrory P., N. Feddermann-Demont, J. Dvorak, J. D. Cassidy, A. S. McIntosh , P. E. Vos, R. Echemendia, W. Meeuwisse, and A. A. Tarnutzer. 2017a. What is the definition of consussion: A systematic review. *Br J Sports Med* 51 (12):969–977.

McCrory, P., K. Johnston, W. Meeuwisse, M. Aubry, R. Cantu, J. Dvorak, T. Graf-Baumann, J. Kelly, M. Lovell, and P. Schamasch. 2005. Summary and agreement statement of the 2nd international conference on concussion in sport, Prague, 2004. *Br J Sports Med* 39 (4):196–204. doi: 10.1136/bjsm.2005.018614.

McCrory, P., W. Meeuwisse, J. Dvorak, M. Aubry, J. Bailes, S. Broglio, R. C. Cantu et al. 2017b. Consensus statement on concussion in sport-the 5th international conference on concussion in sport held in Berlin, October 2016. *Br J Sports Med*. doi: 10.1136/bjsports-2017-097699.

McCrory, P., W. H. Meeuwisse, M. Aubry, B. Cantu, J. Dvorak, R. J. Echemendia, L. Engebretsen et al. 2013. Consensus statement on concussion in sport: The 4th international conference on concussion in sport held in Zurich, November 2012. *Br J Sports Med* 47 (5):250–258. doi: 10.1136/bjsports-2013-092313.

McCrory, P., W. Meeuwisse, K. Johnston, J. Dvorak, M. Aubry, M. Molloy, and R. Cantu. 2009. Consensus statement on concussion in sport: The 3rd international conference on concussion in sport held in Zurich, November 2008. *Br J Sports Med* 43 (1):i76–i90. doi: 10.1136/bjsm.2009.058248.

McCrory, P. R., and S. F. Berkovic. 2001. Concussion: The history of clinical and pathophysiological concepts and misconceptions. *Neurology* 57 (12):2283–2289.

Meeuwisse, W. H., K. J. Schneider, J. Dvorak, O. T. Omu, C. F. Finch, K. A. Hayden, and P. McCrory. 2017. The Berlin 2016 process: A summary of methodology for the 5th international consensus conference on concussion in sport. *Br J Sports Med*. doi: 10.1136/bjsports-2017-097569.

Miller, J. J. 2011. *The Big Scrum: How Teddy Roosevelt Saved Football*. New York: Harper Perennial.

Moreau, W. J., D. C. Nabhan, C. Roecker, M. N. Kimura, A. Klein, B. Guimard, K. Pierce et al. 2015. The American chiropractic board of sports physicians position statement on pre-participation examinations: An expert consensus. *J Chiropr Med* 14 (3):176–182. doi: 10.1016/j.jcm.2015.08.004.

NCAA. 2014. Guideline 2I: Sport related concussion, *2014–15 Sports Medicine Handbook*, pp. 56–65. Indianapolis, IN: NCAA. http://www.ncaa.org/sites/default/files/SMH_Guideline_21_20160217.pdf (accessed July 8, 2017).

Nelson, W. E., J. A. Jane, and J. H. Gieck. 1984. Minor head injury in sports: A new system of classification and management. *Phys Sportsmed* 12:103–107.

Ommaya, A., S. D. Rockoff, and M. Baldwin. 1964. Experimental concussion. *J Neurosurg* 21:241–265.

Ommaya, A. K. and T. A. Gennarelli. 1974. Cerebral concussion and traumatic unconsciousness. Correlation of experimental and clinical observations of blunt head injuries. *Brain* 97 (4):633–654.

Ommaya, A. K. 1990. Biomechanical aspects of head injuries in sports. In *Sports Neurology*, edited by B. Jordan, P. Tsaris, and R. Warren. Rockville, MD: Aspen Publishers.

Ommaya, A. K. and T. A. Gennarelli. 1975. Experimental head injury. In *Henadbook of Clinical Neurology*, edited by P. J. Vincken and D. W. Bruyn, pp. 67–90. Amsterdam, North-Holland: Elsevier.

Parkinson, D. 1977. Concussion. *Mayo Clin Proc* 52:492–499.

Pearce, J. M. 2007. Observations on concussion. A review. *Eur Neurol* 59 (3–4):113–119.

Polin, R. S., W. M. Alves, and J. A. Jane. 1996. Sports and head injuries. In *Neurology and Trauma*, edited by R. W. Evans, pp. 166–185. Philadelphia, PA: WB Saunders and Co.

Rhazes, A. 1497. *Opera Medica Varia*. Venice, Italy: Bonetus Locctellus.

Roberts, W. 1992. Who plays? Who sits? Managing concussion on the sidelines. *Phys Sportsmed* 20:66–72.

Ruff, R. M. and P. Jurica. 1999. In search of a unified definition for mild traumatic brain injury. *Brain Inj* 13 (12):943–952.

Russell, W. R. 1932. Cerebral involvement in head injury. A study based on the examination of two hundred cases. *Brain* 55:549–603.

Russell, W. R. 1971. *The Traumatic Amnesias*. New York: Oxford University Press.

Saal, J. A. 1991. Common American football injuries. *Sports Med* 12:132–147.

Schneider, R. C. 1973. *Head and Neck Injuries in Football: Mechanisms, Treatment and Prevention*. Baltimore, MD: Williams and Wilkins.

Smith, A. M., M. J. Stuart, D. W. Dodick, W. O. Roberts, P. W. Alford, A. B. Ashare, M. Aubrey et al. 2015. Ice hockey summit II: Zero tolerance for head hits and fighting. *PM R* 7 (3):283–295. doi: 10.1016/j.pmrj.2015.02.002.

Smith, A. M., M. J. Stuart, R. M. Greenwald, B. W. Benson, D. W. Dodick, C. Emery, J. T. Finnoff, J. P. Mihalik, W. O. Roberts, C. A. Sullivan, and W. H. Meeuwisse. 2011. Proceedings from the ice Hockey summit on concussion: A call to action. *PM R* 3 (7):605–612. doi: 10.1016/j.pmrj.2011.05.013.

Stone, J. L., V. Patel, and J. E. Bailes. 2014. The history of neurosurgical treatment of sports concussion. *Neurosurgery* 75 (4):S3–S23. doi: 10.1227/NEU.0000000000000488.

Torg, J. F. ed. 1991. *Athletic Injuries to the Head, Neck and Face*. 2nd ed. St Louis, MO: Mosby Year Book.

Turner, M. 1998. *Concussion and Head Injuries in Horse Racing*. London, UK: The Jockey Club Conference on head injury in sport.

Wilberger, J. E. and J. C. Maroon. 1989. Head injuries in athletes. *Clin Sports Med* 8:1–9.

*chapter three*

---

# Concussion incidence, risk factors, and prevention
## What is the scope of the problem?

*Amanda Black, Paul Eliason, Declan Patton, and Carolyn Emery*

## Contents

## Concussion incidence: How common is concussion?

Concussion and the consequences of concussion are a significant public health burden, gaining increased attention in the media over the past decade. Estimating how common concussion is across sports is challenging because of the heterogeneity and methodological limitations of the available studies. Different definitions of concussion (see Chapter 2), different methods of concussion identification (e.g., self-report, medically diagnosed), different settings (e.g., emergency room, sport medicine clinic, family physician office, field), lack of consideration for athlete participation hours, and athlete characteristics can contribute to different estimates of injury risk.

Studies that examine concussion burden commonly take one of three forms: (1) community-based cohort studies using prospective surveillance that record the number of concussions and exposure hours over a period of time; (2) hospital-based cohort studies that record the number of concussions and use population and sport-specific participation estimates or consider the proportion of people sustaining concussions that visit the hospital relative to other injuries; and (3) cross-sectional studies examine self-reported history of concussion. Although all three study designs provide information about how common concussions are, the most valuable studies are community-based cohort studies using validated injury surveillance that allow us to understand the risk of concussion relative to the amount of time that the players are exposed to risk and take into account key risk factors that affect risk (e.g., age, level of play, previous history of concussion/injury, sex).

It is important to recognize that concussion rates vary based on what denominator is selected. Depending on the data collected, estimates are presented relative to player-hours exposed (P-H), athlete exposure (AE; one athlete participating in one session), per number of athletes, or as a proportion of all injuries. Concussion identification has been largely dependent on our ability to detect this injury, and the methods used have changed over time. Therefore, it is important to note that this chapter will summarize the evidence available regarding sport concussion incidence estimates since 2005.

Table 3.1 provides an overview of the ranges of risk estimates of concussion in different sports by age and sex. The highest competition concussion incidence rates were found in primarily contact or collisions sports including American football, Australian football league, ice hockey, rugby, lacrosse, soccer, and wrestling. Concussion represented the highest proportion of all injuries in ice hockey representing between 7.9% and 66% of all injuries seen in the sport depending on sex and age group. The appendix summarizes a complete list of the estimates from different studies by country and sport.

## Sport-specific considerations, prevalence, and risk factors: What are the risk and severity of concussion in my sport?

### American football

American football is a play-by-play collision sport with very fast and physical elements. It is primarily played professionally in North America, but several other countries have professional leagues, and many more have amateur competitions. Injury rate data have been collected primarily in the United States through the National Collegiate Athletics Association (NCAA) surveillance system, the high school reporting injury surveillance system, and through the support of community leagues. Game concussion incidence rates range between 2.01 and 6.61 concussions per 1000 AE, and concussions represent between 4% and 21% of all injuries seen in the sport (Hootman et al. 2007; Shankar et al. 2007;

*Table 3.1* Risk of concussion in different sports by age and sex where available

| Sport and ages/sex (M = male, F = female, U = unspecified) | Competition incidence[a] | Training incidence[a] | Overall incidence[a] | Proportion of all injuries (ED = seen in emergency department) |
|---|---|---|---|---|
| **American football** | | | | |
| Professional (M) | 6.61(AE) | — | — | — |
| Collegiate (M) | 3.01–4.35(AE) | 0.42–0.82(AE) | 0.37–1.41(AE) | 8%–21% |
| High school (M) | 1.55–2.01(AE) | 0.21–0.66(AE) | 0.47–0.92(AE) | 4%–12% |
| Youth (M) | 2.38–6.16(AE) | 0.24–0.59(AE) | 0.61–1.76(AE) | 9.6% |
| **Australian football league** | | | | |
| Professional (M) | 1.3–5.6(P-H) | — | — | — |
| **Baseball** | | | | |
| Professional (M) | — | — | 0.42(AE) | — |
| Collegiate (M/U) | 0.12–0.26(AE) | 0.03–0.07(AE) | 0.07–0.12(AE) | 2.5%–3.3% |
| High school (M/U) | 0.08–0.11(AE) | 0.01–0.03(AE) | 0.04–0.06(AE) | 3%–5.5% |
| **Basketball** | | | | |
| Professional (M) | 0.2(AE) | — | — | 0.8% |
| Professional (F) | 0.6(AE) | — | — | 1.8% |
| Collegiate (M) | 0.32–0.61(AE) | 0.12–0.34(AE) | 0.16–0.39(AE) | 3.2%–4% |
| Collegiate (F) | 0.85–1.09(AE) | 0.12–0.44(AE) | 0.22–0.60(AE) | 4.7%–7% |
| High school (M) | 0.11–0.39(AE) | 0.06(AE) | 0.07–0.24(AE) | 3%–10% |
| High school (F) | 0.55–0.60(AE) | 0.06(AE) | 0.16–0.37(AE) | 3.3%–19% |
| **Cheerleading** | | | | |
| All Star (U) | — | — | — | 1.4% |
| Collegiate (U) | — | — | — | 12.5% |
| High school (U) | 0.12(AE) | 0.14(AE) | 0.06–0.14(AE) | 5.7%–20.7% |
| **Field hockey** | | | | |
| Collegiate (F) | 0.52–1.11(AE) | 0.09–0.18(AE) | 0.18–0.40(AE) | 3.4%–9.4% |
| High school (F) | 0.41(AE) | 0.14(AE) | 0.03–0.22(AE) | 12% |

*(Continued)*

*Table 3.1 (Continued)* Risk of concussion in different sports by age and sex where available

| Sport and ages/sex (M = male, F = female, U = unspecified) | Competition incidence[a] | Training incidence[a] | Overall incidence[a] | Proportion of all injuries (ED = seen in emergency department) |
|---|---|---|---|---|
| **Gymnastics** | | | | |
| Collegiate (F) | 0.48(AE) | 0.24(AE) | 0.16–0.27(AE) | 2.3% |
| High school (F) | 0.24(AE) | 0.03(AE) | 0.07–0.08(AE) | 3%–3.4% |
| Youth (U-ages: 6–17) | – | – | – | 1.7%(ED) |
| **Ice hockey** | | | | |
| Professional (M) | 1.8(P-H) | – | – | – |
| Collegiate (M) | 2.07–2.49(AE) | 0.16–0.25(AE) | 0.41–0.79(AE) | 7.9% |
| Collegiate (F) | 1.78–2.01(AE) | 0.29–0.30(AE) | 0.66–0.91(AE) | 18.3% |
| High school (M) | 1.46–1.67(AE) | 0.11–0.15(AE) | 0.54–0.64(AE) | 21%–28% |
| Youth (U-ages: 12–18) | 2.46(AE) | 1.17(AE) | 2.46(AE) | – |
| Midget (U-ages: 15–17) | – | – | 0.82(P-H) | 13% |
| Bantam (U-ages: 13–14) | 0.79(P-H) | – | 0.53–0.97(P-H) | 20%–23% |
| Peewee[b] (U-ages: 11–12) | 1.47–2.73(P-H) | – | 0.81–1.72(P-H) | 25%–66% |
| Peewee (U-ages: 11–12) | 0.39–1.82(P-H) | – | 0.28–0.64(P-H) | 25%–57% |
| Atom (U-ages: 9–10) | – | – | 0.24(P-H) | 13% |
| **Lacrosse** | | | | |
| Collegiate (M) | 0.93–2.30(AE) | 0.20–0.24(AE) | 0.26–0.54(AE) | 5.6% |
| Collegiate (F) | 0.25–1.50(AE) | 0.15–0.26(AE) | 0.25–0.52(AE) | 4.6%–9.8% |
| High school (M) | 1.04(AE) | 0.11(AE) | 0.30–0.40(AE) | 17% |
| High school (F) | 0.86(AE) | 0.13(AE) | 0.20–0.35(AE) | 21% |
| **Rugby union** | | | | |
| Professional (M) | 0.17–13.8 (P-H) | – | – | – |
| Professional (F) | – | – | – | – |
| Semi-Professional (M) | 2.9–8.4(P-H) | – | – | – |

*(Continued)*

Table 3.1 (*Continued*) Risk of concussion in different sports by age and sex where available

| Sport and ages/sex (M = male, F = female, U = unspecified) | Competition incidence[a] | Training incidence[a] | Overall incidence[a] | Proportion of all injuries (ED = seen in emergency department) |
|---|---|---|---|---|
| Amateur (M) | 8.7–11.0(P-H) | – | – | – |
| Collegiate (M) | 2.2(P-H) | 0.40(P-H) | – | 8.7%–20.0% |
| Collegiate (F) | 1.6(P-H) | 0.30(P-H) | – | 15% |
| Youth (M-ages 7–18) | 0.0–12.7(P-H) | – | – | 16.1% |
| Youth (F) | – | – | – | 14.3% |
| **Soccer** | | | | |
| Professional (M) | 1.06(P-H) | – | 0.06(P-H) | 0.1%–9% |
| Professional (F) | 2.56(P-H) | – | – | – |
| Collegiate (M) | 0.97–1.80(AE) | 0.17–0.24(AE) | 0.28–0.49(AE) | 3.9%–5% |
| Collegiate (F) | 0.97–1.94(AE) | 0.21–0.25(AE) | 0.41–0.65(AE) | 5.3%–7% |
| High school (M) | 0.59(AE) | 0.04(AE) | 0.22–0.28(AE) | 9.3–9.5 |
| High school (F) | 0.79(AE) | 0.09(AE) | 0.36–0.45(AE) | 12.2%–15% |
| Middle school (F) | 5.3(AE) | 0.2(AE) | 1.20(AE) | – |
| **Softball** | | | | |
| Collegiate (F/U) | 0.37–0.56(AE) | 0.07–0.17(AE) | 0.14–0.33 | 4.3% |
| High school (F/U) | 0.04–0.29(AE) | 0.07–0.09(AE) | 0.07–9.16 | 5.5%–13% |
| **Volleyball** | | | | |
| Collegiate (F) | 0.13–0.56(AE) | 0.18–0.27(AE) | 0.09–0.36(AE) | 2.1%–6.4% |
| High school (F) | 0.05–0.11(AE) | 0.04–0.05(AE) | 0.05–0.20(AE) | 3%–8% |
| **Wrestling** | | | | |
| Collegiate (M/U) | 1.0–5.5(AE) | 0.35–0.57(AE) | 0.35–1.09(AE) | 3.3%–5.8% |
| High school (M/U) | 0.32–0.48(AE) | 0.10–0.13(AE) | 0.15–0.57(AE) | 5.4%–10% |

[a] Incidence is reported by adult/youth, male/female, and level of play as the number of injuries per 1000 hours of training and competition (P-H) or per 1000 athlete exposure (AE).

[b] Peewee players participating in a league where body checking is permitted.

Badgeley et al. 2013; Kontos et al. 2013; Dompier et al. 2015; Zuckerman et al. 2015; Nathanson et al. 2016; Willigenburg et al. 2016). Between 1997 and 2008, the rate of concussion in high-school football has been increasing annually by an average of 8% (Lincoln et al. 2011). It should be noted that the rate of concussion is substantially higher in games than practice across all levels (Kontos et al. 2013; Dompier et al. 2015; Zuckerman et al. 2015; Willigenburg et al. 2016).

In American football, helmets are compulsory, in addition to shoulder, hip, and knee pads, with many other optional forms of padding (Goodell 2015). The tackle and block phases are responsible for approximately two-thirds of concussions sustained by high school (Badgeley et al. 2013; Kerr et al. 2014) and collegiate (Zuckerman et al. 2012) football players and over three quarters of concussions sustained by professionals (Casson et al. 2010). Helmet-to-helmet contact is a common mechanism for concussion in American football, which is responsible for 45% of concussions at the youth level (Kontos et al. 2013) and over half of all concussions at the high school (Meehan 3rd et al. 2010) and collegiate (Delaney et al. 2014) levels.

The National Football League (NFL) is continually implementing rule changes in an attempt to protect players from impacts that may cause concussion (Casson et al. 2010). In 2013, a class action by more than 4500 retired American football players resolved concussion litigation against the NFL (Alternative Dispute Resolution Center 2013). Almost US$800 million was contributed by the NFL to provide medical and other benefits, as well as compensation, to qualifying injured players or their families. A recent pilot study in collegiate football players investigating a helmetless-tackling intervention found that players participating in helmetless-tackling drills during training experienced a 28% reduction in head impact frequency per athletic exposure over a single season (Swartz et al. 2015).

## Australian football

Australian football is a fast, kicking, and running game played professionally throughout Australia, in addition to amateur level competitions in other countries (Australian Football League 2016a). The Australian Football League (AFL) has commissioned an annual injury surveillance report since 1992 and, in 1996, was the first professional sporting body to publically release surveillance injury data (Orchard et al. 2013). Between 2000 and 2009, the concussion incidence rate in professional level AFL has ranged between 5.5 and 13 concussions per 1000 player hours (Gibbs et al. 2009; Makdissi et al. 2009; Austalian Football League Research Board Australian Football League Medical Officers' Association 2011). During the 2014 AFL season, there were approximately 1.3 new concussions per club, which were higher than previous years: 2011–2013, 1.0 new concussions per club; 2008–2010, 0.5 new concussions per club; and 2002–2004, 0.4 new concussions per club (Orchard et al. 2014).

AFL rules do not promote head contact. The tackle laws in Australian football require the tackling player to hold the ball carrier below the shoulders and above the knees (Australian Football League 2016b). However, video analysis of head injuries occurring in professional AFL has reported that direct head impact during collision or contesting ball possession is still responsible for a large proportion of concussions (McIntosh et al. 2000).

## Baseball

Based on data from the National High School Athletics Participation Survey and the NCAA Sports Sponsorship and Participation Rates Report, approximately 487,000 high-school men, 1200 high-school women, and 34,000 collegiate men played baseball in the United States during the 2014–2015 season (National Collegiate Athletic Association 2015;

The National Federation of State High School Associations 2015). Relative to other sports, the incidence of concussion in baseball is relatively small and accounts for approximately 1%–5% of all injuries at the high-school level and 2.5% at the collegiate level (Gessel et al. 2007; Dick et al. 2007d; Hootman et al. 2007; Lincoln et al. 2011; Marar et al. 2012). Although the range of concussion rates across studies suggests the concussion rate at the collegiate level may be higher than at the high-school level, the difference is not statistically significant (Gessel et al. 2007). Both collegiate and high-school athletes sustained a higher rate of concussions in games than practices (Dick et al. 2007a; Gessel et al. 2007; Castile et al. 2012; Marar et al. 2012). Between 1998 and 2008, the rate of concussion in high-school baseball has been increasing annually by an average of 14% (Lincoln et al. 2011).

The mechanism of concussions in amateur baseball typically includes head contact with the pitched ball or fielding a batted ball (Gessel et al. 2007; Marar et al. 2012), whereas at the professional level, contact between players and fielding a batted ball were the most common mechanisms of concussion (Green et al. 2015). This is supported by Cantu & Mueller (2009) who suggest the top three reasons for catastrophic injury in high school and collegiate baseball are related to the athlete being hit by either a thrown or batted ball, the athlete colliding with a teammate while chasing a fly ball, or the athlete using a head first slide technique and makes contact with their head and the opposing players' lower body or the base (Cantu and Mueller 2009). At the professional level, catchers were more likely to incur a concussion than any other position (Green et al. 2015), which may be due to collisions with runners at home plate (Rosenbaum and Davis 2014).

## Basketball

Basketball is a popular sport played around the world. Although the most common injury in basketball is ankle sprain injury, concussions have been reported to represent between 1.8% and 19% of all injuries sustained in basketball (Dick et al. 2007c; Borowski et al. 2008; Rechel et al. 2008; Pappas et al. 2011; Marar et al. 2012; Fridman et al. 2013). Over the last decade, concussion rates in basketball have increased significantly at all competitive levels from high school to professional players in the NBA (Rosenthal et al. 2014; Padaki et al. 2016). Basketball accounted for 115/4745 sport-related concussion hospitalizations in Victoria, Australia between 2002 and 2011 (Finch et al. 2013). Furthermore, concussions from basketball made up 9.2% of all sport-related concussions in youth ages 8–19 in the United States (Bakhos et al. 2010). The majority of studies have found that female basketball players have a higher rate of concussion than male basketball players (Marar et al. 2012; Rosenthal et al. 2014; Zuckerman et al. 2015).

The most common mechanism of concussion in basketball is player contact while either defending, rebounding, or general play (Borowski et al. 2008; Marar et al. 2012; Zuckerman et al. 2015). Unfortunately, primary prevention strategies in basketball have not been successful. For example, Labella et al. (2002) examined the use of mouth guards as a preventive measure for concussion in Division 1 college basketball teams. Although they found mouth guard users had lower rates of dental injuries, there were no significant differences in concussion rates between mouth guard users and nonusers (RR = 0.63 95%CI: 0.12–2.02).

## Cheerleading

Cheerleading is a dynamic and complex sport combining dance, gymnastics, and individual as well as group stunts. Despite the popularity across North America, injury surveillance data on cheerleading injuries are limited and only available from the United

States. Strains/sprains, fractures, and contusions are the most common injuries sustained by cheerleaders (Jacobson et al. 2012). However, concussions represent between 3.5% and 20.7% of all injuries in high-school cheerleading, 12.5% of all injuries in collegiate cheerleading, and 3.5% of cheerleading injuries seen at emergency departments among ages 5–17 (Shields and Smith 2006; Shields et al. 2009; Meehan et al. 2011a; Marar et al. 2012). The most common activity associated with concussions is stunts with a triple base (i.e., toss, lift) (Marar et al. 2012). In a study examining injury risk in high-school cheerleading, 45% of concussions occurred when there was no spotter (Marar et al. 2012).

Different types of cheerleading teams are at different risk of concussion. Shields et al. 2009 examined stunt-related injuries among cheerleaders participating in five different types of cheerleading teams. They reported that cheerleaders on collegiate teams were more likely to sustain a stunt-related concussion than cheerleaders on all-star or high-school teams. Stunt-related concussions were more likely to occur in training sessions than competitions. Finally, fifty percent of stunt-related concussions result in time lost equal to or greater than seven days (Shields et al. 2009).

## Field hockey

Field hockey is played recreationally by men and women around the world. Data on concussion in field hockey from outside North America or in a male population are minimal and limited to tournament style of play. During the 2008 and 2012 summer Olympics games, only 1 concussion was identified among all male and female field hockey athletes (Junge et al. 2009; Engebretsen et al. 2013) though, during the 2009 Men's Junior World Cup, there were 5 concussions reported over 58 matches with 3 concussions resulting in the player being removed from the game (Mukherjee 2012). The majority of available prospective concussion research has been conducted in the high-school and collegiate settings in North America where women primarily play the sport. Concussion incidence rates among female field hockey players range between 0.03 and 0.22 per 1000 AE in high school and between 0.18 and 0.40 at the collegiate level (Lincoln et al. 2011; Marar et al. 2012; Kriz et al. 2015).

The most common mechanism of concussions in women's field hockey is player to player contact (Dick et al. 2007d). This contact could occur while handling the ball, running, or stick contact during general play (Zuckerman et al. 2015). In a report of high-school concussions in field hockey, 35.3% of concussions were sustained by midfielders, 29.4% were sustained by defenders, and 21.6% were sustained by forwards (Marar et al. 2012). Between 1998 and 2008, the rate of concussion among women's high-school field hockey has been increasing annually by an average of 20% (Lincoln et al. 2011). In a study examining 15 sport-related concussions in women's collegiate field hockey, players reported on average 5.93 symptoms following concussion, and 20% resulted in players taking greater than 28 days to return to sport (Wasserman et al. 2015).

Despite more equipment being required for ice hockey than field hockey, concussions are more prevalent among ice hockey players when compared with field hockey players (Yard and Comstock 2006). Although some field hockey players may choose to wear mouth guards and/or eyewear, facial protective equipment is not mandatory for all players. In 2011, the National Federation of State High School Associations (NFHS) implemented a mandate that required all high-school field hockey players to wear protective eyewear in sanctioned competitions (Kriz et al. 2012). This rule change resulted in a 69% reduction in the number of eye injuries and did not affect the rate of concussion (IRR = 0.77 [95%CI:0.58-1.02]) (Kriz et al. 2015).

One suggested strategy to reduce head injuries in field hockey is the removal of the penalty corner. In an editorial by John Batten, it is argued that penalty corners hold the potential risk of serious head injury, and it is suggested that, instead, infringements within the defensive area be penalized by power plays. This is a system currently used by International Super Series Hockey (Batten et al. 2016).

## Gymnastics

Gymnastics is a sport where each individual element presents its own unique risk. However, these details are not typically captured in concussion surveillance data, and the majority of evidence focuses on female athletes. Although strains and sprains represent the majority of injuries seen in gymnastics, the concussion incidence rate is reportedly between 0.07 and 0.08 per 1000 AE among high-school athletes (Meehan et al. 2011b; Marar et al. 2012) and 0.16–0.27 among collegiate athletes (Hootman et al. 2007; Zuckerman et al. 2015). Concussions are more likely to occur in competitions than in practice. Marar et al. (2012) reported that concussions occurred 8.5 times more often in competition than in practice.

Common mechanisms resulting in concussion in women's gymnastics are surface contact during floor routing or uneven bars and contact with the balance beam (Zuckerman et al. 2015). Therefore, it is recommended that a coach monitors spot athletes during these activities, especially when learning new routines. A study including 96 female gymnasts from competitive levels 4 to 10 (ages 7–17) reported a lifetime occurrence of concussion in 30.2% (O'Kane et al. 2011). Although concussion prevention strategies have not been evaluated in gymnastics, recommended injury prevention strategies include making sure that the equipment is in good condition (e.g., padded floors, secured mats under apparatus), using a safety harness for learning difficult moves, and insisting on spotters when learning a new routine.

## Ice hockey

The sport of ice hockey is one of the most popular sports in the world and continues to grow in popularity globally (International Ice Hockey Federation 2015). Canada leads the world in registration numbers with over 550,000 male and 87,000 female players (Hockey Canada 2015). The next largest country in participation is the United States with over 530,000 total players (USA Hockey 2016).

Historically, ice hockey has had the highest concussion incidence rate in male high-school team sports (Koh et al. 2003), although a recent study found that it was second only to American football (Marar et al. 2012). Regardless, concussion is the most common specific injury type for youth ice hockey players (Koh et al. 2003; Emery and Meeuwisse 2006). Concussion accounts for 25%–66% of all injuries in Pee Wee (11–12 years old) players playing with body checking, and 25%–57% in a league not allowing body checking (Emery and Meeuwisse 2006; Emery et al. 2010b; Black et al. 2016). In addition, an American study found that concussions accounted for 22.2% of total injuries, the greatest proportion among 20 high-school sports (Marar et al. 2012).

Risk of concussion was identified as being consistently higher in games than practices (Emery et al. 2010a), with one study finding concussions were 13 times more likely to occur during game play (Marar et al. 2012). In a recent systematic review which included a meta-analysis, body checking was identified as a consistent risk factor for all game-related injuries (summary rate ratio: 2.45%; 95% CI 1.7–3.6) and concussion (summary odds ratio: 1.71%; 95% CI 1.2–2.44) (Emery et al. 2010a). In addition, those with a history of concussion are at an increased risk of incurring a future concussion (Emery and Meeuwisse 2006; Emery et al. 2010a; Emery et al. 2010b; Emery et al. 2011; Black et al. 2016). Players that are lighter in body weight may also be at an increased risk of injury (Emery et al. 2010b).

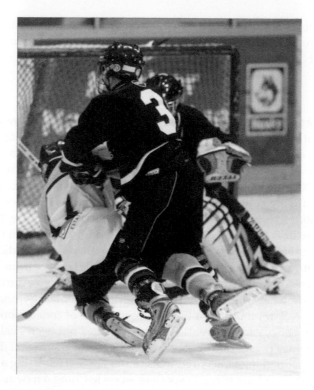

***Figure 3.1*** An example of body checking in youth ice hockey.

Other risk factors for injury in youth may also exist such as age, level of play, and player position, yet the research remains inconclusive (Emery et al. 2010a).

   With body checking being the single most consistent risk factor for injury in ice hockey, policy implications regarding delaying body checking to older age groups and only allowing body checking in the most elite levels of play should be considered (Emery et al. 2010b; Brenner et al. 2014; Kontos et al. 2016). Other strategies for the prevention of injury in ice hockey include proper rule enforcement and education of players concerning the risk of injury related to rule violation (Cantu and Mueller 2009), as well as educating the proper techniques to give and receive legal body check (Figure 3.1).

## Lacrosse

Over the 2014–2015 season, there were 13,165 male and 10,994 female collegiate lacrosse players participating in the National Collegiate Athletics Association (NCAA) (National Collegiate Athletic Association 2015) as well as 193,235 (male: 108,450, female: 84,785) high-school lacrosse players (The National Federation of State High School Associations 2015). Concussion has been identified as one of top three game injuries at the collegiate level (Putukian et al. 2014). Concussion incidence rates for games and practices combined range between 0.26–0.54 and 0.25–0.52 concussions per 1000 AE among collegiate males and females, respectively, and concussions make up between 4.6% and 9.8% of all injuries. Although high-school lacrosse players have reported slightly lower rates of concussion than collegiate athletes, concussions represent a higher proportion of injuries seen in high-school lacrosse (Lincoln et al. 2007, 2011; Marar et al. 2012). In a study investigating high-school lacrosse injuries in the United states between 2008 and 2010, concussions represented 17% and 21% of the injuries sustained among boys and girls, respectively (Marar et al. 2012). Between 1998 and 2008, the rate of concussion among high-school lacrosse increased annually by an average of 17% and 14% for boys and girls, respectively (Lincoln et al. 2011). In a study examining 51 and 55 sport-related concussions in men and women collegiate lacrosse, players reported on average 5.12 and 5.69 symptoms following concussion (Wasserman et al. 2015).

In men's lacrosse, the most common mechanisms of concussion are player contact during general play and when chasing a loose ball (Lincoln et al. 2007; Zuckerman et al. 2015). In a study exploring lacrosse injuries from 1988 to 2004, nearly 80% of concussion injuries were due to contact with another player (Dick et al. 2007b), whereas in women's lacrosse, the most common mechanism is when a player is defending either through player contact or stick contact (Lincoln et al. 2007; Zuckerman et al. 2015).

There are differences between the rules in the men's and women's lacrosse game specially surrounding equipment and contact. The men's game is a high-speed, contact game that has mandatory hard shell helmets, facemasks, mouth guards, gloves, and padding for the upper body (Lincoln et al. 2007). Aggressive stick checking and body checking are legal strategies (Putukian et al. 2014). But the women's game only allows incidental contact and women were only required to wear mouth guards up until 2005 when U.S. lacrosse also made protective eyewear mandatory. The introduction of helmets in women's lacrosse is controversial. Hard shell helmets are not permitted and although some players choose to wear soft protective headgear, U.S. lacrosse has not made it mandatory (Putukian et al. 2014).

## Mixed martial arts

Mixed martial arts (MMA) has seen a surge in popularity in both North America and internationally (Smith 2010; Sanchez Garcia and Malcolm 2010) and, in some areas, has become more popular than boxing. Despite its popularity, MMA has been heavily criticized by many medical communities as being too violent and dangerous, and posing a significant risk of brain injury (Canadian Medical Association 2013; American Medical Association, n.d.; British Medical Association 2007; Australian Medical Association 2013). However, the research examining the injuries sustained during MMA, particularly concussion, remains limited. One difficulty in determining the incidence of concussion in MMA is the classification of either a knockout (KO) or a technical knockout (TKO) as a concussion. The United Fighting League (UFC) defines a KO as occurring when a fighter is knocked down and either unconscious, disoriented, or unable to intelligently defend himself (Discover UFC), and a TKO occurring when a referee stops a fight when a fighter is unable to defend themselves intelligently (Discover UFC). In professional MMA, the rate of knockouts ranges from 15.4 to 64 per 1000 athlete exposures (Buse 2006; Ngai et al. 2008; Hutchison et al. 2014).

A systematic review and meta-analysis on injuries in MMA found that the head was the most commonly injured anatomical region (66.8%–78.0%), whereas concussion accounted for 3.8%–20.4% of all injuries (Lystad et al. 2014). Studies have found that the incidence of KO in professional MMA ranged from 15.4 to 64 per 1000 AE (Buse 2006; Ngai et al. 2008; Hutchison et al. 2014). Using video analysis techniques, one study identified that all KOs in their sample were due to impact with the head, and over 50% were due to a strike to the mandible (Hutchison et al. 2014). Hutchison et al. (2014) found that 90% of TKOs were due to direct and repetitive strikes to the head leading to defenselessness of the fighter. Although diagnosis of concussion in cases of TKO was not certain, the combination of KO and TKO secondary to repetitive head strikes was 159 per 1000 AE and may suggest a more liberal estimate of the incidence of brain injury in MMA (Hutchison et al. 2014).

The prevention of head injuries due to KO and TKO in MMA is difficult to be implemented in a sport that promotes and awards victory and financial bonuses for such match outcomes (e.g., *knockout of the night* is a bonus awarded to the fighter with the most impressive KO/TKO) (Hutchison et al. 2014). Although MMA fighters are required to wear gloves, one study found that similar make of glove did not reduce the accelerations that may produce brain injury, and may actually protect the attackers hands more than the defenders head (Schwartz et al. 1986). Because fighters can sustain further strikes to the head after sustaining a KO and before the referee can intervene (Hutchison et al. 2014). Hutchison et al. (2014) recommends policies and practices to reduce continuing head trauma after a KO. The authors propose a rule similar to boxing where a fighter is stopped for a count of 10 seconds after a knockdown to assess for identification of brain injury, which also eliminates further strikes after KO (Hutchison et al. 2014). Further recommendations include training of referees to better identify defenceless fighters and those that have lost consciousness and stop the fight immediately, and a uniform cross-jurisdictional injury database for all fighters to prevent premature return to sport after a brain injury (Hutchison et al. 2014).

## Rodeo

Participation rates in North American rodeo are difficult to ascertain as no comprehensive registry exists. One study obtained registration numbers from twelve rodeo associations including most of the largest rodeo associations in North America and estimated that approximately 33,000 rodeo participants competed in 2009 (Butterwick et al. 2011). The National high school athletics participation survey reported approximately 135 men and 139 women participated in American high school rodeo over 2014–2015 (The National Federation of State High School Associations 2015).

There is a paucity of research that has investigated the incidence of concussion in rodeo. Only one study was identified that estimated the incidence rate of 3.4/1000 competition exposures (Butterwick et al. 2011). However, caution should be given to this estimate as the data were collected from 1995 to 1999 and may be an underestimate of more current rates. Historically, concussions accounted for between 11% and 13.9% of all injuries in bull riding and bareback riding, respectively (Butterwick et al. 2002; Butterwick and Meeuwisse 2003). However, more recent report found that concussions were the most common major injury and represented 55.8% of all major injuries during the 2001–2005 rodeo seasons (Mobile Sport Medicine System 2005).

Of all the events in rodeo, bull riding has accounted for the majority of injuries representing approximately 50% of the total injuries in all events (Mobile Sport Medicine System 2005). Between 1996 and 2005, bull riders were more likely to sustain injuries to their head and face, usually due to colliding with the head or horns of the bull (Mobile Sport Medicine System 2005). Although there is limited research that has investigated the use of protective head gear in bull riding, the authors and signatories of the agreement statement from the 1st International Rodeo Research and Clinical Care Conference agree that the risks of bull riding without head protection far outweigh the risks of bull riding with head protection (Butterwick et al. 2005).

## Rugby league

Rugby league is a code of football, which evolved from rugby union in the late nineteenth century as a professional sport for lower class citizens and is a popular sport in Australia, New Zealand, and England.

As with rugby union, the tackle phase of play in rugby league has been identified as having the highest concussion risk (Norton and Wilson 1995; Gissane et al. 2003; Gabbett and Domrow 2005; King et al. 2010), and one study reported that concussions occurred in 40% of all illegal tackles (Hinton-Bayre et al. 2004). Until recently, the tackle laws in rugby league did not require the tackler to lead with the arms but could instead lead with the shoulder, which is known as a *shoulder charge*. At the end of 2012, the Australian Rugby League Commission (ARLC) outlawed the shoulder charge, which was supported by the Rugby League International Federation (RLIF) and applied to all international competition from 2013 onwards (National Rugby League 2012). In New Zealand, the *shoulder charge* has been outlawed in domestic competition since 1995 (New Zealand Rugby League 2012).

Few studies have reported the incidence of concussion during rugby league training. No concussions were reported during a prospective study of training injuries to rugby league players from a professional club over the 2008 season (Gabbett and Godbolt 2010). During the 2009 National Rugby League (NRL) season, concussion comprised 6.1% of all injuries during competitive matches but only 1.4% of all training injuries. Concussion incidence rates in adult male rugby league have been found to vary with player position: 5.0–6.9 and 1.9–30.7 concussions per 1000 player hours for forwards and backs, respectively (Gabbett 2005b; O'Connor 2009; King and Clark 2012; Orr and Cheng 2015). In a comparison of limited and unlimited interchange, incidence rates are 5.1 and 3.0 concussions per 1000 player-hours, respectively (Gabbett 2005).

## Rugby sevens

Rugby sevens is a variation of rugby union, in which seven players per side compete shorter game times with modified rules on a full-sized rugby field (World Rugby 2016b). Although developed in Scotland during the late nineteenth century, rugby sevens has only grown in popularity during the last few decades and several international competitions now exist, such as the World Rugby Sevens Series and Rugby World Cup Sevens. Rugby sevens has been contested at the Commonwealth Games since 1998 and had its debut as an Olympic sport in Rio 2016.

As with rugby union, the tackle phase of play in rugby sevens has been identified as having the highest concussion risk, during which approximately 63%–71% and 62% of all concussions are sustained for males (Fuller et al. 2015; Lopez et al. 2016) and females (Lopez et al. 2016), respectively. For both males and females, backs are more likely to sustain concussions compared with forwards and the incidence of concussion at the elite level is nearly threefold that of the nonelite levels (Lopez et al. 2016). Rugby league also has a sevens variant (Australian Rugby League 2015), for which a concussion incidence of 6.5 per 1000 player hours has been reported for amateur and semiprofessional male players (King et al. 2006).

## Rugby union

Rugby union originated in England and was traditionally played throughout the United Kingdom, Ireland, Australia, New Zealand, and South Africa. In 2015, there were 7.73 million rugby union players from over 100 countries (World Rugby 2016a).

For youth rugby union players, McIntosh et al. (2005, 2009b, 2010) found that concussion incidence tended to increase with age. Concussions during competition matches have a significantly higher incidence than training (Gardner et al. 2014), which have been reported as 0.0–0.1, 0.3 and 0.4 per 1000 player hours for professional male (Brooks 2005; Holtzhausen et al. 2006; Kemp et al. 2008; Fuller et al. 2008; Fuller et al. 2013), collegiate male, and collegiate female players (Kerr et al. 2008), respectively. Some studies have investigated concussion incidence for the different playing positions of professional male rugby union players: 2.0–8.8 and 2.1–6.7 concussions per 1000 player-hours for forwards and backs, respectively (Brooks et al. 2005; Kemp et al. 2008; Fuller et al. 2008; Fuller et al. 2013; Fuller et al. 2015).

The tackle phase of play in rugby union has been identified as having the highest concussion risk (Hendricks and Lambert 2010; Whitehouse et al. 2016), during which between half and two-thirds of all concussions are sustained to the tackler, ball carrier, and/or support players (Bird et al. 1998; Collins et al. 2008; Kemp et al. 2008; Fuller et al. 2015). The rugby tackle must be carried out below shoulder level with the arms wrapping around the ball carrier player. This technique removes the danger of leading with the shoulder; however, it requires the head to be located close to the hips, thighs, and knees of the ball carrier, all of which have the potential to cause head injury. World Rugby allows soft-shelled padded headgear to be worn during rugby union matches (World Rugby 2015); however, laboratory and field studies have demonstrated that commercially available headgear is currently ineffective in reducing the risk of concussion (Patton and McIntosh 2016).

## Soccer

Soccer, which is also known as football or association football, is commonly referred to as the *world's game* as it is the most popular sport in the world with 265 million players (Federation Internationale de Football Association 2007). During open play, opposing players may come into contact with each other while competing for the ball; however, the objective is to play the ball, and intentional collisions are not allowed.

Concussion in soccer is most commonly caused by player-to-player contact (Andersen et al. 2004; Pickett et al. 2005; Fuller et al. 2005), with the highest concussion risk event being identified as the aerial challenge (Powell and Barber-Foss 1999; Kirkendall et al. 2001; Kirkendall and Garrett 2001; Fuller et al. 2005; Delaney et al. 2014). An aerial challenge occurs when two opposing team members jump into the air and both attempt to play the ball with their heads. Head-to-head contact and being struck by the upper extremity of an opponent are reportedly responsible for most concussions sustained during aerial challenges (Boden et al. 1998; Fuller et al. 2005), with head-to-head having the highest risk of concussion (Withnall et al. 2005). Elbow-to-head contact is another common cause of head injuries and concussion in soccer (Figure 3.2) (Boden et al. 1998; Andersen et al. 2004; Fuller et al. 2005).

It is generally accepted that there is not enough force in a single heading impact to cause concussion (Boden et al. 1998; Barr and Beusenberg 2001; McCrory 2003; Andersen et al. 2004). However, the effects of cumulative minor head impacts from heading is uncertain (Niedfeldt 1991; Asken and Schwartz 1998; Baroff 1998; Kirkendall et al. 2001; Kirkendall and Garrett 2001; McCrory 2003; Levy et al. 2012; Punnoose 2012), with retrospective studies suggesting an association between heading and cognitive impairment (Tysvaer and Storli 1981; Tysvaer and Løchen 1991; Tysvaer 1992; Matser et al. 2001; Witol and Webbe 2003; Lipton et al. 2013), but prospective studies find no association between heading and cognitive impairment in both youth (Janda et al. 2002; Pickett et al. 2005; Rutherford et al. 2005; Kaminski et al. 2008; Kontos et al. 2011) and adult (Barnes et al. 1998; Putukian et al. 2000; Guskiewicz et al. 2002; Broglio et al. 2004; Mangus et al. 2004; Schmitt et al. 2004; Straume-Naesheim et al. 2005; Zetterberg et al. 2006) players. Concussions from ball-to-head impacts, where the ball comes off a players boot and strikes the head of another player, have been reported (Boden et al. 1998; Andersen et al. 2004; Fuller et al. 2005).

Interestingly, several studies have consistently reported higher concussion incidence rates for females than those for males in soccer (Gessel et al. 2007; Hootman et al. 2007;

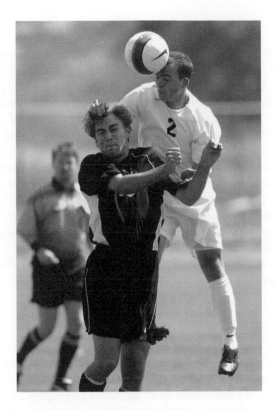

***Figure 3.2*** Elbow-to-head contact during an aerial challenge in soccer.

Comstock et al. 2015; Zuckerman et al. 2015; Covassin et al. 2016). However, some people have argued that this could be due to differences in concussion symptom reporting affecting identification (Covassin and Elbin 2011).

## *Softball*

Relative to baseball, there is slightly less participation in softball in the United States with approximately 1,500 high-school men, 374,000 high-school women, and 19,600 collegiate women who played either fast or slow pitch during the 2014–2015 season (National Collegiate Athletic Association 2015; The National Federation of State High School Associations 2015). Although softball and baseball have different rules and equipment, the sports have similar methods of play. At both the high-school and collegiate level, softball had a higher rate of concussion than baseball (Gessel et al. 2007; Hootman et al. 2007; Lincoln et al. 2011; Castile et al. 2012; Marar et al. 2012). In addition to the differing rates, the mechanism of concussion also seems to differ with a greater proportion of amateur baseball players' concussions caused by being hit by the pitch than softball players (Gessel et al. 2007; Marar et al. 2012).

Suggestions to prevent catastrophic injury in baseball, which may also be applicable to softball and aid in the prevention of concussions, include making batting helmet use mandatory for both practice and game situations with proper helmet fitting, the use of protective screens during batting practice, teaching strategies to avoid contact when multiple players are chasing a fly ball, and teaching the proper skills and technique for head first slide (Cantu and Mueller 2009). Major League Baseball has also introduced rules to reduce the number of injuries caused by collisions at home plate (Office of the Comissioner of Baseball 2015).

## Volleyball

Approximately 500,000 men and 5.5 million women play volleyball in high school and 15,000 men and 200,000 women play volleyball at a university level (Daneshvar et al. 2011). Although volleyball is typically considered a noncontact sport with a limited risk of concussion, concussions do still occur. In women's high-school volleyball, the concussion rate reportedly ranges between 0.05 and 0.17 concussions per 1000 AE (Rosenthal et al. 2014; Reeser et al. 2015). At the collegiate level, the rate is higher ranging from 0.2 to 0.36 concussions per 1000 AE (Reeser et al. 2015; Zuckerman et al. 2015). The majority of studies have not reported concussions in male volleyball because of low numbers. Concussions are most likely to occur during defensive digging and common mechanisms include ball contact, surface contact, and then player contact (Marar et al. 2012; Zuckerman et al. 2015). In a high-school sample, concussion in boys' volleyball was primarily a result of player-to-player contact (Marar et al. 2012) whereas in females, player-playing surface contact and player–ball contact resulted in a greater proportion of concussions (Marar et al. 2012). The risk associated with position was reported by Marar et al. (2012) where the outside hitter and setter positions sustained over half of the concussions in a high-school sample.

## Wrestling

Wrestling is one of the top 10 (ranked 6) most popular sports programs for boys in the National Federation of State High School Association (The National Federation of State High School Associations 2015). Although the popularity of wrestling among female athletes has increased since its introduction in the 2004 Olympics, available data on female wrestlers are limited. Wrestling is a sport that dictates absolute respect for one's opponent and although wrestlers are supposed to be in control at all times during throwing and takedowns, concussions and other injuries do occur. Concussion represents between 3% and 10% of all injuries in wrestling with and incidence rate between 0.15 and 0.57 per 1000 AE among high-school wrestlers and 0.25–1.09 per 1000 AE among collegiate wrestlers (Yard et al. 2007; Gessel et al. 2007; Hootman et al. 2007; Rechel et al. 2008; Lincoln et al. 2011; Castile et al. 2012; Marar et al. 2012; Rosenthal et al. 2014; Zuckerman et al. 2015). Concussions are most likely to occur during competition, and the most common activities leading to concussions were takedowns (42.6%) and sparring (21.9%) in a sample of high-school students (Marar et al. 2012).

## Key risk factors—how do I identify athletes at risk?

Identifying risk factors is important to help understand which athletes are more likely to be injured and what prevention strategies can be implemented to reduce risk. Risk factors can be broadly categorized as intrinsic (factors that are internal to the athlete) and extrinsic (factors that are outside of the body). Although all risk factors provide valuable information, modifiable risk factors (factors you can change) provide the greatest opportunity for injury prevention. Currently there is very limited evidence on many of the proposed risk factors, and the data are conflicting. However, being aware how position, level, specific mechanisms, weather, weight, fitness, or preseason symptoms may affect risk, may assist with the identification or prevention of concussion. As the previous section describes sport-specific risk factors, Table 3.2 describes the evidence of purported risk factors. The only risk factors with strong evidence are a previous history of concussion, playing in a game versus a practice, and exposure to contact (body checking).

*Table 3.2* Intrinsic and extrinsic risk factors for concussion in different sports

| Risk factor | Relative risk[a] | Evidence[b] | Comments |
|---|---|---|---|
| **Intrinsic risk factors** | | | |
| History of concussion (Abrahams et al. 2014) | | | |
| Increased risk with previous concussions | 1.65–6.60x | ++ | Studies examined ice hockey, football, soccer, rugby union, and NCAA athletes. Only three out of thirteen studies identified (Delaney et al. 2000, 2001, 2002) found that previous concussion had no effect on risk and the studies were of moderate to low quality. |
| Age (Abrahams et al. 2014) | | | |
| Younger cohort increased risk | 1.21–1.89x | ± | Studies that found increased risk for younger cohort compared: high school versus college football players, middle versus high school taekwondo athletes and youth ice skaters less than six years versus greater than six years old. Included high to moderate quality studies. |
| Older cohort increased risk | 1.52–4.01x | | Studies that found increased risk for older cohort examined collegiate versus high school, football 12–17 versus 6–11, youth soccer players 15–18 versus <15 years, cheerleaders collegiate versus younger, ice hockey players, rugby players adult versus high school, lacrosse players, and youth athletes (10–14 and 15–18 versus 5–10 years). Three studies out of the 14 studies in youth ice hockey, rugby, and lacrosse found no effect of age on risk. |
| Sex (Abrahams et al. 2014) | | | |
| Male at increased risk | 1.61–2.99x | ± | Studies that found an increased risk in males (4/23) examined: High-school lacrosse, alpine sports, youth football, junior high athletics. Studies were primarily moderate quality with one high quality study. Studies that found females were at increased risk (10/23) examined: high-school soccer, basketball, softball and baseball players, high-school athletes, professional basketball players, collegiate athletes, adolescent soccer players, collegiate soccer players, and wheelchair baseball players. Nine of the 23 studies found no effect of sex on risk among taekwondo, rugby, soccer, high school, and lacrosse athletes. |
| Female at increased risk | 1.5–3.00x | | |

*(Continued)*

*Table 3.2 (Continued)* Intrinsic and extrinsic risk factors for concussion in different sports

| Risk factor | Relative risk[a] | Evidence[b] | Comments |
| --- | --- | --- | --- |
| Genetics (Abrahams et al. 2014) Increased risk with *TT APOE* genotype | 2.70x | ± | One of the three studies identified found an increased risk of concussion with football and soccer players that had the *TT APOE* genotype and concussion history. The remaining studies in collegiate athletes found no effect of having the APOE E4 allele or rare APOE allele. |
| Neck strength (Collins et al. 2014) Increased risk with weaker neck strength | NA | ± | A study including 6704 soccer, basketball, and lacrosse high-school athletes found that for every pound increase in neck strength, the odds of concussion decreased 5%. |
| Playing position (Abrahams et al. 2014; Black et al. 2016) Inconsistent risk differences between positions | NA | ± | Six studies identified no effect of playing position in football, hockey and rugby, whereas two studies have found being a goalie to be protective in hockey and one study found that quarterbacks are at an increased risk in football when compared with other positions. |
| Level of play (Abrahams et al. 2014) Increased risk with lower division levels | 1.4–2.3x | ± | Of the six studies identified in football, ice hockey and rugby league, two studies found that lower playing level is associated with increased risk, and four studies found no effect of level of play on risk. |
| Baseline Symptoms (Schneider et al. 2013) Increased risk associated with preseason reports of headache, neck pain or dizziness | NA | ± | In a study including 175 concussions in youth ice hockey, symptom reporting was associated with a 1.47x increase of concussion risk for headache, 1.67x increase with neck pain, and a 3.11x increased risk of dizziness. |

(*Continued*)

*Table 3.2 (Continued)* Intrinsic and extrinsic risk factors for concussion in different sports

| Risk factor | Relative risk[a] | Evidence[b] | Comments |
|---|---|---|---|
| **Weight or BMI** (Abrahams et al. 2014) | | | |
| Increased risk with low weight or low BMI | NA | ± | Two studies identified, one in rugby and one in ice hockey players reported that lower 25% weight and lower BMI are associated with an increased risk of concussion. But both were moderate quality studies. |
| **Fitness level** (Abrahams et al. 2014) | | | |
| Increased risk with less training | NA | ± | Two studies were identified. One study in community rugby players reported a hazard ratio of 1.48 associated with less training, whereas the other study reported no effect on risk in high-school football players. |
| **Extrinsic risk factors** | | | |
| **Game versus Practice** (Abrahams et al. 2014) | | | |
| Increased risk with games | 2–205x | ++ | The risk of concussion was identified as greater in games than practices in all 30 studies identified and across sports. |
| **Environment** (Abrahams et al. 2014) | | | |
| Grass versus Artificial turf | NA | ± | Three studies were identified in soccer. Two studies found no significant difference between the two surfaces and one study found a slight reduction in concussion risk on artificial turf. |
| **Match Period** (Abrahams et al. 2014) | | | |
| Mixed results about when players are more at risk | NA | ± | Two studies were identified. One study found a greater risk of concussion in the 2nd versus 3rd period of hockey, whereas the other study found no differences in the 1st versus 2nd half in rugby. |
| **Body Checking** (Emery et al. 2010; Hagel et al. 2006; Macpherson, Rothman, and Howard 2006; Black et al. 2016) | | | |
| Increased risk with body checking leagues | 2.83–3.88x | ++ | Body checking has been identified as a significant risk factor for concussion in youth ice hockey. Body checking experience has not been identified as protective. |

[a]  Relative risk indicates the increased risk of injury to an individual with this risk factor relative to an individual who does not have this characteristic. A relative risk of 1.2x means that the risk of injury is 20% higher for an individual with this characteristic. NA: Not available.

[b]  Evidence indicates the level of scientific evidence for this factor being a risk factor for concussion: ++ convincing evidence from high-quality studies with consistent results; ± evidence from lesser quality studies or mixed results; 0 expert opinion or hypothesis without scientific evidence.

## Sport-concussion prevention: What can be done to prevent concussions?

Preventing concussions can be understood across the full spectrum of care. This spectrum consists of primary prevention (preventing the initial occurrence), secondary prevention (early detection), and tertiary prevention (full recovery and prevention of second occurrence). Primary prevention of concussions is challenging because the evidence to support purported prevention strategies has methodological limitations or is still theoretical. These commonly promoted strategies include properly fitting equipment (e.g., helmets, mouthguards, headgear), rules and rule enforcement, improving coaching techniques, contact restriction, improving neck strength, and promoting respect and fair play (Cantu 1992; Smith et al. 2009; Emery et al. 2010b; Navarro 2011; Benson et al. 2013). Table 3.3 presents a summary of some of the proposed prevention strategies that are often discussed.

## Does protective equipment work?

Typically, sport-governing bodies have rules and regulations outlining the use of protective equipment including helmets, headgear, and mouthguards. Although helmets protect against catastrophic focal head injuries, headgear can reduce superficial facial wounds (Jako 2002; Jákó 2009; Zazryn et al. 2009), and mouthguards protect against oral injuries (Labella et al. 2002; Quarrie et al. 2005; Cohenca et al. 2007; Tanaka et al. 2014), this equipment is not completely effective at preventing concussions from occurring (Benson et al. 2009; Benson et al. 2013). Studies examining helmet fit, design, and age have reported a reduction of concussion symptoms and symptom duration associated with appropriate helmet fit (Greenhill et al. 2016), a reduction of concussion risk associated with a helmet that has thicker padding over the zygoma and mandible (Riddell revolution helmet) when compared with other helmets (Collins et al. 2006; Rowson et al. 2014), and no difference between helmets that are different ages (McGuine et al. 2014). Adding either full or half face shields to a helmet has not been shown to affect concussion risk (Benson et al. 2002;

*Table 3.3* Summary of the proposed prevention strategies

| Primary prevention (preventing the initial occurrence) | Secondary prevention (early detection) | Tertiary prevention (full recovery and prevention of second occurrence) |
| --- | --- | --- |
| Helmets | Education | Vestibular rehabilitation |
| Headgear | Policies | Ocular rehabilitation |
| Mouthguards | | Return to play protocols |
| Rule changes | | |
| Technique education | | |
| Contact restriction neck strengthening | | |
| Nutrition | | |
| Encouraging safe play | | |
| Vision training | | |

Stuart et al. 2002). Biomechanical studies suggest that helmets may reduce forces applied to the brain, but there is no laboratory test or current standards that evaluate a helmet's capability to prevent a concussion from occurring because the force needed to sustain a concussion is still not well defined (Crisco and Greenwald 2013; Benson et al. 2013).

Evidence that examines the effectiveness of headgear in the prevention of concussion is inconsistent. Randomized controlled trials in rugby have found no protective effect (McIntosh et al. 2009; McIntosh and McCrory 2001), whereas some prospective studies and cross-sectional studies in soccer and rugby have found a 43%–62% reduction in risk (Kemp et al. 2008; Delaney et al. 2008; Hollis et al. 2009). The argument against the use of headgear in sport is that wearing it encourages athletes to take more risks and increases aggressive play. In a survey of 122 male rugby players, 42.2% reported that they would be more aggressive during running or tackling if they were wearing headgear (Menger et al. 2016). However, this did not translate to an increased risk of concussion in the randomized controlled trials (McIntosh et al. 2009; McIntosh and McCrory 2001).

There are three common types of mouthguards: (1) custom-fabricated made by dental professionals; (2) form-fitted, boil, and bite made by athlete biting the mouthguard; and (3) stock, bought directly over the counter (Tuna and Ozel 2014). The goal of a mouthguard is to dissipate the force between the upper and lower teeth and act as a shock absorber (Farrington et al. 2012; Tuna and Ozel 2014). This can assist with reducing forces to the head with blows to the jaw. The evidence on the effectiveness of mouthguards in preventing concussion is inconclusive. There is some evidence to suggest that custom-fit mouthguards may offer an advantage over other mouthguards. But, currently studies are limited by small sample size, improper selection of comparison group, and poor identification of concussion. The potential of mouthguards to reduce the risks of concussions that result from blows to the jaw, and the proven effectiveness to reduce dental injuries in contact sports supports the use of mouthguards as an injury prevention strategy but further research is needed.

## Rule changes and rule enforcement

Changing the rules in sport can be a challenging but effective means of reducing concussion. The key to an effective rule change is monitoring what mechanisms or environmental factors place an athlete at risk and then what rules can be put in place or mechanisms eliminated to reduce that risk. A recent example of an effective rule change is Hockey Canada's decision to delay body checking until Bantam (ages 13–14). Multiple surveillance studies using both community surveillance and emergency room data identified body checking as a consistent risk factor for injury and concussion in youth ice hockey (Emery and Meeuwisse 2006; Hagel et al. 2006; Warsh et al. 2009; Emery et al. 2010b; Black et al. 2016). Studies comparing provinces where body checking was allowed at the Pee Wee (ages 11–12) level to provinces where it was not permitted reported a 2.8 to 4-fold increased risk of concussion associated with playing Pee Wee in a body checking league (Emery et al. 2010b; Black et al. 2016). Furthermore, not having experience with body checking at the Pee Wee level did not significantly increase a players' injury risk in Bantam when they were allowed to body check (Emery et al. 2011). The removal of body checking at the Pee Wee level resulted in a reduction of concussions when the same city was compared before and after the change (Emery et al. 2016).

Stricter enforcement of rules that sanction players for head contact have yielded mixed results when it comes to concussion prevention. In 2010, the Football Association of Norway and Norwegian Professional League Association decided to implement stricter rule enforcement by referees (Bjørneboe et al. 2013). The changes included giving an automatic red card for two-foot tackles, tackles with excessive force, and intentional high elbows (Bjørneboe et al. 2013). Comprehensive referee training and a media release to the public that explicitly outlined the changes accompanied the rule enforcement decision. When they compared video of soccer games the year after the rule enforcement was implemented to games a year before the changes, they found a 19% reduction in the number of hits to the head. The reduction in exposure to head contact could possibly reduce concussions over time. However, the study was limited by a low number of concussion incidents. On the other hand, when Hockey Canada decided to implement a zero tolerance for head contact rule where players would be penalized by referees for any contact to the head, it did not decrease concussion risk or head contacts (Krolikowski et al. 2017). Although it is possible that the lack of protective effect might have been due to the increasing rates of concussion across all sports when the historical cohort study took place, it may also be that referee enforcement was not enough to modify the hockey players behaviors, or the enforcement was not consistent.

Understanding how to implement a rule change that will be effective at reducing concussions in sport begins with understanding the mechanisms of concussion for that sport. The rule change should aim to eliminate or reduce exposure to that mechanism. Implementation should include the organization, referees, parents, coaches, and players.

## Coaching, neck strength, training, nutrition, and encouraging safe behaviors

Coaching strategies, vision training, neck strengthening, nutrition, encouraging safe behavior, and education campaigns promoting certain techniques (e.g., Respect on ice and USA Hockey's, *Heads up don't duck*) (USA Hockey HQ 2012) have been postulated as injury prevention strategies. However, the evidence in support of these strategies is sparse, inconsistent, or nonexistent at this time (Benson et al. 2013).

Coach education about proper tackling techniques, equipment fitting, and strategies to reduce contact in football combined with limiting contact in practice shows promise as a prevention strategy (Cobb et al. 2013; Kerr et al. 2015; Swartz et al. 2015). When concussion rates were compared between teams with coaches who were both exposed to the Head's Up Football program education and restricted contact in practice to teams who did not do the program or contact restriction, an 82% reduction of concussion in practice was reported (Kerr et al. 2015). Another study compared football players exposed to 5 minutes of tackling training without helmets during practice to players who did not get the training and found a reduction in game head impact frequency for the players exposed (Swartz et al. 2015). Limiting contact in practice and teaching appropriate techniques for collisions are strategies that can be used in many contact sports. Although the results of these three studies of coaching strategies are promising, more research is needed.

Overall neck strength has been identified as a predictor of concussion, with one study reporting that within a high-school sample for every one-pound increase in neck strength, the odds of concussion decrease by five percent (Collins et al. 2014). This has led many to suggest that if you strengthen the neck, you can reduce your risk of concussion. Although training cervical musculature has been associated with increases in neck strength, no evidence has examined the effects of a neck strengthening program on concussion risk (Benson et al. 2013).

One new strategy that has been proposed to reduce the rate of concussion is vision training. As part of the University of Cincinati football program, the team conducted vision enhancement training during the preseason using Nike strobe glasses and tracking drills. Clark et al. (2015) monitored concussion incidence over four seasons of training and compared the incidence rate with the rate over the previous four seasons. The study found a significant reduction in concussion incidence. However, further research is needed to see if these results are consistent across different teams, or sports.

The possibility of nutritional interventions as a possible strategy for concussion prevention is still in its infancy. Omega-3 fatty acids, curcumin, resvestrol, melatonin, creatine, Vitamins C, D and E, and S. baicalensis are purported interventions for concussion prevention and management, but most have not been tested in human trials (Ashbaugh and McGrew 2016). High-dose docosahexanoic acid (DHA) supplementation has been shown to reduce markers of axonal damage in varsity football players (Oliver et al. 2016) and reduce the damage inflicted to traumatic brain injury mouse models (Mills et al. 2011), but whether DHA has the ability to prevent concussions is still not clear.

Encouraging safe behaviors and respect is a commonly promoted strategy for injury prevention that can be used across all sports. Fair-Play rules reward teams for not committing fouls or disrespecting other athletes. While endorsed by some recreational leagues, the effect of programs on injury has only been examined in one study that found a reduction in overall injuries but was unable to detect a difference in concussion specifically due to a limited sample size (Roberts et al. 1996). There is evidence, however, to suggest it can affect player behavior. A Hockey Education Program in Minnesota, with Fair Play, reduced potentially dangerous infractions by 30% when compared with standard practice rules (Roberts, Brust, and Leonard 1999; Smith et al. 2009).

## Secondary prevention: Policy and concussion education

Trainers, parents, players, and coaches all play a role in identifying and ensuring proper management of concussion (Denke 2008; Echlin 2010; Adler 2011). Poor symptom recognition or lack of concussion awareness can contribute to unrecognized concussions that increase the risk continuing to play with a concussion and prolong recovery or make the injury worse. Policy on concussion management and education has been proposed as a method for increasing appropriate concussion management. In 2009, Washington state adopted legislation (the Lystedt Law) that outlined how concussion should be managed and promoted education for coaches, parents, and players. Similar legislation was adopted across the United States. One evaluation of the implementation of concussion legislation reported that since adopting the legislation, there have been increases in visits to the emergency department for concussions, which has been attributed to more individuals seeking care following concussion (Mackenzie et al. 2015).

Although raising awareness through education and policy is important to assist with identification of concussion, the beliefs of parents, players, and coaches can affect whether or not they choose to respond appropriately (Glanz and Bishop 2010). These beliefs can include, but are not limited to, the perception of risks of negative outcomes associated with a given behavioral response (e.g., player reporting symptoms), expectation of what will happen if they perform the desired behavior and perceived confidence in their ability to perform the behavior (Murgraff et al. 2003). Education that is not theory based and does not consider how to address the beliefs that underlie player behavior may lead to the opposite of intended effects. For example, a study of adolescent male junior ice hockey players found that providing publically available concussion education that is designed to increase awareness but not address beliefs that underlie behavior can actually decrease a player's intentions to report their symptoms to an adult (Kroshus et al. 2014). This lack of reporting can contribute to undiagnosed concussions. On the other hand, when a group of coaches received access to a theory-driven course designed to address the beliefs that underlie behavior, the intervention group demonstrated a greater increase in behavioral intention to remove an athlete than the group of coach who just received safety information to read (Glang et al. 2010). When deciding how to use education or legislation to assist with concussion secondary prevention or primary prevention, it is essential to first understand the beliefs and motivations of the population you are educating.

### *Tertiary prevention: Return to sport and prevention of second occurrence*

Safe return to play protocols, vestibular rehabilitation, and ocular rehabilitation have all been identified as methods to assist with return to sport and reducing the risk of a second occurrence. These topics will be covered in depth in Chapters 8, 14, and 15.

## Conclusion

Concussions have become a major health problem in sport. Although concussion can occur in any sport, the incidence is highest in collision and/or contact sports including American football, Australian football league, ice hockey, rugby, lacrosse, soccer, and wrestling. Sport characteristics, games when compared with practices, and a previous history of concussion are consistent risk factors. Finally, although primary prevention is difficult, identifying the mechanisms of injury and potential rule modification that can limit exposure to that mechanism have been identified as successful concussion risk reduction strategies.

## *Appendix: Concussion rates across sport, level of play, and country*

**American football**

| Study | Year(s) | Country | Sex (M-male, F-female, U-unspecified) | Level | Concussion incidence | | | |
|---|---|---|---|---|---|---|---|---|
| | | | | | Incidence proportion | 1000 P–H | 1000 A–E | % All injuries |
| Nathanson et al. (2016) | 2012/2013–2013/2014 | United States | M | Professional | – | – | G: 6.61 | – |
| Willigenburg et al. (2016) | 2012/2013–2014/2015 | United States | M | Collegiate | – | – | G: 4.35 P: 0.82 O: 1.04 | 21.00% |
| Dompier et al. (2015) | 2012/2013–2013/2014 | United States | M | Youth | – | – | G: 2.38 P: 0.59 O: 0.99 | 9.60% |
| | | | | High school | – | – | G: 2.01 P: 0.66 O: 0.92 | 4.00% |
| | | | | Collegiate | – | – | G: 3.74 P: 0.53 O: 0.83 | 8.00% |
| Tietze et al. (2015) | 2012 | United States | M | Collegiate | – | – | O: 1.41 | – |
| Zuckerman et al. (2015) | 2009/2010–2013/2014 | United States | M | Collegiate | – | – | G: 3.01 P: 0.42 O: 0.67 | – |
| Badgeley et al. (2013) | Not reported | United States | M | High school | – | – | – | 12.50% |
| Kontos et al. (2013) | 2011 | United States | M | Youth | – | – | G: 6.16 P: 0.24 O: 1.76 | – |
| Lincoln et al. (2011) | 1997/1988–2007/2008 | United States | M | High school | – | – | O: 0.60 | – |
| Bakhos et al. (2010) | 2001–2005 | United States | M & F | Youth (Ages 7–11) | 0.08% | – | – | – |
| | | | | Youth (Ages 12–17) | 0.27% | – | – | – |

*(Continued)*

| Study | Year(s) | Country | Sex (M-male, F-female, U-unspecified) | Level | Incidence proportion | 1000 P–H | 1000 A–E | % All injuries |
|---|---|---|---|---|---|---|---|---|
| Gessel et al. (2007) | 2005/2006 | United States | M | High school | – | – | G: 1.55 / P: 0.21 / O: 0.47 | 10.5%[a] |
| | | | | Collegiate | – | – | G: 3.02 / P: 0.39 / O: 0.61 | 7.0%[a] |
| Hootman et al. (2007) | 1988/1989–2003/2004 | United States | M | Collegiate | – | – | O: 0.37 | 6.00% |
| Shankar et al. (2007) | 2005/2006 | United States | M | High school | – | – | – | 12.00% |
| | | | | Collegiate | – | – | – | 14.00% |
| **Australian football** | | | | | | | | |
| AFL Research Board and AFL Medical Officers' Association (2011) | Not reported | Australia | M | Professional | – | G:5.5 | – | – |
| Gibbs et al. (2009) | 2000–2009 | Australia | M | Professional | – | G:13 | – | – |
| Makdissi et al. (2009) | 2000–2003 | Australia | M | Professional | – | G:5.6 | – | – |
| **Baseball** | | | | | | | | |
| Covassin et al. (2016) | 2004/2005–2008/2009 | United States | M | Collegiate | – | – | G: 0.26 / P: 0.05 / O: 0.12 | – |
| Green et al. (2015) | 2011/2012 | North America | M | Professional | – | – | O: 0.42 | – |
| Zuckerman et al. (2015) | 2009/2010–2013/2014 | United States | M | Collegiate | – | – | G: 0.12 / P: 0.07 / O: 0.09 | – |
| Castile et al. (2012) | 2005–2010 | United States | U | High school | – | – | G: 0.077 / P: 0.014 / O: 0.037 | – |

*(Continued)*

| Study | Year(s) | Country | Sex (M-male, F-female, U-unspecified) | Level | Concussion incidence | | | |
|---|---|---|---|---|---|---|---|---|
| | | | | | Incidence proportion | 1000 P–H | 1000 A–E | % All injuries |
| Marar et al. (2012) | 2008–2010 | United States | M | High school | – | – | G: 0.11<br>P: 0.01<br>O: 0.05 | –<br>5.5%[a]<br>– |
| Lincoln et al. (2011) | 1997/1988–2007–2008 | United States | M | High school | – | – | O: 0.06 | – |
| Bakhos et al. (2010) | 2001–2005 | United States | U | Ages 7–11<br>Ages 12–17 | 0.01%<br>0.03% | –<br>– | –<br>– | –<br>– |
| Dick et al. (2007) | 1988/1999–2003–2004 | United States | M | Collegiate | – | – | G: 0.19<br>P: 0.03 | 3.30%<br>1.60% |
| Gessel et al. (2007) | 2005/2006 | United States | U | High school | – | – | G: 0.08<br>P: 0.03<br>O: 0.05 | 3%[a] |
| | | | U | Collegiate | – | – | G: 0.23<br>P: 0.03<br>O: 0.09 | 2.5%[a] |
| Hootman et al. (2007) | 1988/1999–2003/2004 | United States | M | Collegiate | – | – | O: 0.07 | 2.50% |

[a] Data estimated based on figures within studies.

| Study | Year(s) | Country | Sex (M-male, F-female, U-unspecified) | Level | Concussion incidence | | | |
|---|---|---|---|---|---|---|---|---|
| | | | | | Incidence proportion | 1000 P–H | 1000 A–E | % All injuries |
| **Basketball** | | | | | | | | |
| Black et al. (2016) | 2008/2009–2010/2011 | Canada | M | Collegiate | 27.59% | – | – | – |
| | | | F | Collegiate | 15.79% | – | – | – |
| Covassin et al. (2016) | 2004/2005–2008/2009 | United States | M | Collegiate | – | – | G: 0.61 P: 0.27 O: 0.33 | – |
| | | | F | Collegiate | – | – | G: 0.97 P: 0.33 O: 0.47 | – |
| Zuckerman et al. (2015) | 2009/2010–2013/2014 | United States | M | Collegiate | – | – | G: 0.56 P: 0.34 O: 0.39 | – |
| | | | F | Collegiate | – | – | G: 1.09 P: 0.44 O: 0.60 | – |
| Rosenthal et al. (2014) | 2005/2006 | United States | M | High school | – | – | O: 0.07 | – |
| Rosenthal et al. (2014) | 2011/2012 | United States | M | High school | – | – | O: 0.24 | – |
| Rosenthal et al. (2014) | 2005/2006 | United States | F | High school | – | – | O: 0.22 | – |
| Rosenthal et al. (2014) | 2011/2012 | United States | F | High school | – | – | O: 0.37 | – |
| Liraz et al. (2013) | 2007/2008–2009/2010 | Canada | M | 5–19 years | – | – | – | ED: 2.3% |
| | | | F | 5–19 years | – | – | – | ED: 2.1% |

*(Continued)*

| Study | Year(s) | Country | Sex (M-male, F-female, U-unspecified) | Level | Concussion incidence | | | |
|---|---|---|---|---|---|---|---|---|
| | | | | | Incidence proportion | 1000 P–H | 1000 A–E | % All injuries |
| Marar et al. (2012) | 2008/2009–2009/2010 | United States | M | High school | – | – | G: 0.39 / P: 0.06 / O: 0.16 | 10%[b] |
| | | | F | High school | – | – | G: 0.55 / P: 0.06 / O: 0.21 | 13%[b] |
| Lincoln et al. (2011) | 1997/1998–2007/2008 | United States | M | High school | – | – | O: 0.10 | – |
| | | | F | High school | – | – | O: 0.16 | – |
| Pappas et al. (2011) | 2000–2006 | United States | M & F | Ages 7–17 | – | – | – | ED: 1.8% |
| Bakhos et al. (2010) | 2001–2005 | United States | M & F | Ages 7–11 | 0.01% | – | – | – |
| | | | | Ages 12–17 | 0.04% | – | – | – |
| Borowski et al. (2008) | 2005/2006–2006/2007 | United States | M | High school | – | – | – | G: 6% / P: 3% |
| | | | F | High school | – | – | – | G: 14% / P: 5% |
| Rechel et al. (2008) | 2005/2006 | United States | M | High school | – | – | – | G: 3.7% / P: 3.4% |
| | | | F | High school | – | – | – | G: 19.0% / P: 3.3% |
| Dick et al. (2007) | 1988–1989–2003–2004 | United States | M | Collegiate | – | – | G: 0.32 / P: 0.12 | G: 3.6% / P: 3.0% |

*(Continued)*

| Study | Year(s) | Country | Sex (M-male, F-female, U-unspecified) | Level | Incidence proportion | 1000 P—H | 1000 A—E | % All injuries |
|---|---|---|---|---|---|---|---|---|
| | | | | | | | **Concussion incidence** | |
| Gessel et al. (2007) | 2005/2006 | United States | M | High school | – | – | G: 0.11 / P: 0.06 / O: 0.07 | 4%[b] |
| | | | | Collegiate | – | – | G: 0.45 / P: 0.22 / O: 0.27 | 4%[b] |
| | | | F | High school | – | – | G: 0.60 / P: 0.06 / O: 0.21 | 12%[b] |
| | | | | Collegiate | – | – | G: 0.85 / P: 0.31 / O: 0.43 | 7%[b] |
| Hootman et al. (2007) | 1988/1999–2003/2004 | United States | M | Collegiate | – | – | O: 0.16 | O: 3.2% |
| | | | F | Collegiate | – | – | O: 0.22 | O: 4.7% |
| Deitch et al. (2006) | NBA:1996–2002 | United States | M | Professional | – | – | G: 0.2 | G: 1.0 / O: 0.8% |
| | WNBA: 1997–2002 | | F | Professional | – | – | G: 0.6 | G: 2.4% / O: 1.8% |
| **Cheerleading** | | | | | | | | |
| Marar et al. (2012) | 2008/2009–2009/2010 | United States | F | High school | – | – | G: 0.12 / P: 0.14 / O: 0.14 | O: 20.3% |
| Lincoln et al. (2011) | 1997/1998–2007/2008 | United States | F | High school | – | – | O: 0.06 | – |
| Meehan III (2011) | 2009–2010 | United States | F | High school | – | – | O: 0.12 | O: 20.7% |

*(Continued)*

| Study | Year(s) | Country | Sex (M-male, F-female, U-unspecified) | Level | Concussion incidence | | | |
|---|---|---|---|---|---|---|---|---|
| | | | | | Incidence proportion | 1000 P–H | 1000 A–E | % All injuries |
| Shields et al. (2009) | 2006–2007 | United States | U | All Star | – | – | – | O: 1.4% |
| | | | | Collegiate | – | – | – | O: 12.5% |
| | | | | High school | – | – | – | O: 5.7% |
| Shields and Smith (2006) | 1990–2002 | United States | U | Ages 5–18 | – | – | – | ED: 3.5% |
| **Field hockey** | | | | | | | | |
| Black et al. (2016) | 2008/2009–2010/2011 | Canada | F | Collegiate | 17.86% | – | – | – |
| Gardner et al. (2015) | 2004/2005–2008/2009 | United States | F | Collegiate | – | – | O: 0.40 | – |
| Kriz et al. (2015) | 2009–2013 | United States | F | High school | – | – | MPE: O: 0.03 No MPE: O: 0.08 | – |
| Zuckerman et al. (2015) | 2009/2010–2013/2014 | United States | F | Collegiate | – | – | G: 1.11 P: 0.18 O: 0.40 | – |
| Marar et al. (2012) | 2008/2009–2009/2010 | United States | F | High school | – | – | G: 0.41 P: 0.14 O: 0.22 | O: 12%[b] |
| Lincoln et al. (2011) | 1997/1998–2007/2008 | United States | F | High school | – | – | O: 0.10 | – |
| Hootman et al. (2007) | 1988/1999–2003/2004 | United States | F | Collegiate | – | – | O: 0.18 | O: 3.9% |
| Dick et al. (2007) | 1988/1999–2003/2003 | United States | F | Collegiate | – | – | G: 0.52 P: 0.09 | G: 9.4% P: 3.4% |

MPE: Mandatory Protective Eyewear

b  Estimated based on Graph.

| Study | Year(s) | Country | Sex (M-male, F-female, U-unspecified) | Level | Concussion incidence | | | |
|---|---|---|---|---|---|---|---|---|
| | | | | | Incidence proportion | 1000 P–H | 1000 A–E | % All injuries |
| **Gymnastics** | | | | | | | | |
| Zuckerman et al. (2015) | 2009/2010–2013/2014 | United States | F | Collegiate | – | – | G: 0.483 P: 0.243 O: 0.265 | – |
| Marar et al. (2012) | 2008/2009–2009/2010 | United States | F | High school | – | – | G: 0.24 P: 0.03 O: 0.07 | 3%[c] |
| Meehan III et al. (2011) | 2009–2010 | United States | F | High school | – | – | O: 0.08 | 3.40% |
| Singh et al. (2008) | 1990–2005 | United States | M+F | Ages 6–17 | – | – | – | ED: 1.7% |
| Hootman et al. (2007) | 1988/1999–2003/2004 | United States | F | Collegiate | – | – | O: 0.16 | 2.30% |
| **Ice hockey** | | | | | | | | |
| Black et al. (2016) | 2011–2012 | Canada | M+F | Pee Wee | 0.07 | G: 2.73 O: 1.72 | G: – | G: 66% O: 64% |
| | | | | Pee Wee[v] | 0.021 | G: 1.82 O: 0.64 | G: – | G: 57% O: 58% |
| Covassin et al. (2016) | 2004/2005–2008/2009 | United States | M | Collegiate | – | – | G: 2.07 P: 0.16 O: 0.59 | – |
| | | | F | Collegiate | – | – | G: 1.78 P: 0.29 O: 0.66 | – |
| Kontos et al. (2016) | 2012/2013–2013/2014 | United States | M+F | Youth (12–18) | 0.0–93 | – | G: 2.46 P: 1.17 O: 1.58 | – |
| | | | | Youth (12–14) | – | – | O: 2.84 | – |
| | | | | Youth (15–18) | – | – | O: 1.18 | – |

*(Continued)*

| Study | Year(s) | Country | Sex (M-male, F-female, U-unspecified) | Level | Concussion incidence | | | |
|---|---|---|---|---|---|---|---|---|
| | | | | | Incidence proportion | 1000 P–H | 1000 A–E | % All injuries |
| Matic et al. (2015) | 2008/2009–2012/2013 | United States | M | High school | – | – | G: 1.67 P: 0.15 O: 0.64 | G: 30% P: 21% O: 28% |
| Zuckerman et al. (2015) | 2009/2010–2013/2014 | United States | M | Collegiate | – | – | G: 2.49 P: 0.25 O: 0.79 | – |
| | | | F | Collegiate | – | – | G: 2.01 P: 0.30 O: 0.75 | – |
| Marar et al. (2012) | 2008–2010 | United States | M | High school | – | – | G: 1.46 P: 0.11 O: 0.54 | O: 22.2% |
| Benson et al. (2011) | 1997/1998–2003–2004 | North America | M | Professional | – | G: 1.8 | – | – |
| Emery et al. (2011) | 2008–2009 | Canada | M+F | Bantam[T] | 0.051 | G: 0.79 O: 0.53 | – | G: 20% O: 19% |
| | | | | Bantam[U] | 0.05 | G: 0.91 O: 0.57 | – | G: 20% O: 20% |
| Bakhos et al. (2010) | 2001–2005 | United States | M+F | Ages 7–11 | 0.10% | – | – | – |
| | | | | Ages 12–17 | 0.29% | – | – | – |

*(Continued)*

| Study | Year(s) | Country | Sex (M-male, F-female, U-unspecified) | Level | Concussion incidence | | | |
|---|---|---|---|---|---|---|---|---|
| | | | | | Incidence proportion | 1000 P–H | 1000 A–E | % All injuries |
| Emery et al. (2010) | 2007–2008 | Canada | M+F | Pee Wee | 0.07 | G: 1.47<br>O: 0.91 | –<br>– | G: 35%<br>O: 32% |
| | | | | Pee Wee[v] | 0.021 | G: 0.39<br>O: 0.28 | –<br>– | G: 29%<br>O: 25% |
| Hootman et al. (2007) | 1988/1999–2003/2004 | United States | M | Collegiate | – | – | O: 0.41 | 7.90% |
| | 2001/2002–2003/2004 | United States | F | Collegiate | – | – | O: 0.91 | 18.30% |
| Emery and Meeuwisse (2006) | 2004–2005 | Canada | M+F | Atom[v] | – | O: 0.24 | – | O: 21% |
| | | | | Pee Wee | – | O: 0.81 | – | O: 25% |
| | | | | Bantam | – | O: 0.97 | – | O: 23% |
| | | | | Midget | – | O: 0.82 | – | O: 13% |

[v] Delineates age groups that played without body checking
[T] With previous body checking experience
[U] Without previous body checking experience
[c] Atom (9/10 years), Pee Wee (11/12), Bantam (13/14), Midget (15/16).

| Study | Year(s) | Country | Sex (M-male, F-female, U-unspecified) | Level | Incidence proportion | 1000 P–H | 1000 A–E | % All injuries |
|---|---|---|---|---|---|---|---|---|
| **Lacrosse** | | | | | | | | |
| Covassin et al. (2016) | 2004/2005–2008/2009 | United States | M | Collegiate | – | – | G: 2.30<br>P: 0.24<br>O: 0.54 | – |
| | | | F | Collegiate | – | – | G: 1.50<br>P: 0.26<br>O: 0.50 | – |
| Zuckerman et al. (2015) | 2009/2010–2013/2014 | United States | M | Collegiate | – | – | G: 0.931<br>P: 0.195<br>O: 0.318 | – |
| | | | F | Collegiate | – | – | G: 1.308<br>P: 0.330<br>O: 0.521 | – |
| Liraz et al. (2013) | 2007/2008–2009/2010 | Canada | M | 5–19 years | – | – | – | ED: 4.1% |
| | | | F | 5–19 years | – | – | – | ED: 2.7% |
| Marar et al. (2012) | 2008/2009–2009/2010 | United States | M | High school | – | – | G: 1.04<br>P: 0.11<br>O: 0.40 | 17%[d] |
| | | | F | High school | – | – | G: 0.86<br>P: 0.13<br>O: 0.35 | 21%[d] |
| Lincoln et al. (2011) | 1997/1998–2007/2008 | United States | M | High school | – | – | O: 0.30 | – |
| | | | F | High school | – | – | O: 0.20 | – |

*(Continued)*

| Study | Year(s) | Country | Sex (M-male, F-female, U-unspecified) | Level | Concussion incidence | | | |
|---|---|---|---|---|---|---|---|---|
| | | | | | Incidence proportion | 1000 P—H | 1000 A—E | % All injuries |
| Dick et al. (2007) | 1988/1989–2003/2004 | United States | F | Collegiate | – | – | G: 0.70 P: 0.15 | G: 9.8% P: 4.6% |
| Hootman et al. (2007) | 1988/1999–2003/2004 | United States | M | Collegiate | – | – | O: 0.26 | O: 5.6% |
| | | | F | Collegiate | – | – | O: 0.25 | O: 6.3% |
| Lincoln et al. (2007) | 2000/2001–2003/2004 | United States | M | Collegiate | | | O: 0.37 | |
| | | | F | Collegiate | | | O: 0.32 | |
| | | | M | High school | | | O: 0.28 | |
| | | | F | High school | | | O: 0.21 | |
| **Mixed martial arts** | | | | | | | | |
| Hutchison et al. (2014) | 2006–2012 | Undeclared | M | Professional | 0.213 | – | KO: 64 TKO: 95 O: 159 | – |
| Ngai et al. (2008) | 2002–2007 | Undeclared | U | Professional | – | – | KO: 15.4 | – |
| Buse (2006) | 1993–2003 | Undeclared | M | Professional | – | – | KO: 48.3 | – |

KO stands for knockout and TKO stands for technical knockout.

| Study | Year(s) | Country | Sex (M-male, F-female, U-unspecified) | Level | Incidence proportion | 1000 P–H | 1000 A–E | % All injuries |
|---|---|---|---|---|---|---|---|---|
| **Rugby league** | | | | | | | | |
| Gabbett (2005) | 2000–2003 | Australia | M | Semi-professional | – | 3 | – | – |
| King (2006) | 2005 | New Zealand | M | U16 | – | 4.3 | – | – |
| | | | | U18 | – | 18.5 | – | – |
| King et al. (2007) | 2005 | New Zealand | F | Professional | – | 6.1 | – | 2.00% |
| Gabbett (2008) | 2003–2006 | Australia | M | U19 | – | 4.6 | – | – |
| King et al. (2009) | 2006 | New Zealand | M | Amateur | – | 27.2 | – | 3.90% |
| | 2008 | New Zealand | M | Amateur | – | 12.9 | – | 4.80% |
| O'Connor (2009) | 2008 | Australia | M | Professional | – | 2.5 | – | – |
| | 2009 | Australia | M | Professional | – | 4.3 | – | 6.10% |
| King et al. (2012) | 2008–2010 | New Zealand | M | Amateur | – | 19.3 | – | – |
| King et al. (2012) | 2011 | New Zealand | M | Amateur | – | 12.1 | – | – |
| Savage et al. (2013) | 1998–2012 | Australia | M | Professional | – | 28.3 | – | – |
| Orr et al. (2016) | 2012 | Australia | M | U16, U18 | – | 4.8 | – | 7.30% |
| **Rugby sevens** | | | | | | | | |
| Fuller et al. (2010) | 2008/2009 | International | M | Elite | – | 2 | – | – |
| Fuller et al. (2015) | 2008/2009–2012/2013 | International | M | Elite | – | 8.3 | – | – |
| Lopez et al. (2016) | 2010 | United States | M+F | Amateur | – | 8.1 | – | 14.60% |
| Lopez et al. (2016) | 2010–2013 | United States | M | Nonelite, elite | – | 7.6 | – | – |
| | | | F | Nonelite, elite | – | 8.1 | – | – |
| | | | M+F | Nonelite | – | 6.4 | – | – |
| | | | | Elite | – | 18.3 | – | – |
| **Rugby union** | | | | | | | | |
| Willigenburg et al. (2016) | 2012–2014 | United States | M | Collegiate | – | – | 2.5 | 16% |

*(Continued)*

| Study | Year(s) | Country | Sex (M-male, F-female, U-unspecified) | Level | Incidence proportion | 1000 P–H | 1000 A–E | % All injuries |
|---|---|---|---|---|---|---|---|---|
| Fuller et al. (2015) | 2007/2008–2010/2011 | England | M | Professional | – | 4.6 | – | – |
| | 2007, 2011 | International | M | Professional | – | 5.2 | – | – |
| | 2008, 2010–2013 | International | M | U20 | – | 3.7 | – | – |
| | 2012, 2013 | Pacific Islands | M | Professional | – | 5.4 | – | – |
| McFie et al. (2015) | 2011–2014 | South Africa | M | U13 | – | 8.3 | – | 10.90% |
| Moore et al. (2015) | 2012–2014 | Wales | M | Professional | – | 13.8 | – | – |
| | | | | U16 | – | 9.1 | – | 19.00% |
| | | | | U18 | – | 5.5 | – | 10.70% |
| Willigenburg et al. (2014) | 2012–2014 | United States | M | Collegiate | – | – | 2.57 | 20% |
| Fuller et al. (2013) | 2011 | International | M | Professional | – | 7.8 | – | – |
| King et al. (2013) | 2012 | New Zealand | M | Amateur | – | 2.3 | – | – |
| Peck et al. (2013) | 2006/2007–2010/2011 | United States | M | Collegiate | – | – | 0.33 | 8.70% |
| | | | F | Collegiate | – | – | 0.44 | 15.00% |
| Roberts et al. (2013) | 2009/2010–2011/2012 | England | M | Amateur, Semiprofessional | – | 1.2 | – | 7.00% |
| Chalmers et al. (2012) | 2004 | New Zealand | M | U13–U18, amateur | – | – | – | 7.80% |
| Haseler et al. (2010) | 2008/2009 | England | M | U9–17 | – | 1.8 | – | – |
| Nicol et al. (2010) | 2008/2009 | Scotland | M | U11–U18 | – | 10.8 | – | – |
| Taylor et al. (2011) | 2010 | International | F | Professional | – | – | – | 10.30% |
| McIntosh et al. (2010) | 2002–2007 | Australia | M | Amateur | 6.1% | 1.6 | – | 10.8% |
| | | | | U9–U10 | – | 3.8 | – | – |
| Hollis et al. (2009) | 2005–2007 | Australia | M | Amateur | – | 8.7 | – | – |
| | | | | Semiprofessional | – | 8.4 | – | – |
| Schneiders et al. (2009) | 2002 | New Zealand | M | Semiprofessional | – | 2.9 | – | 5.50% |
| Collins et al. (2008) | 2005–2006 | United States | M | High school | – | – | – | O: 16.1% |
| | | | F | High school | – | – | – | O: 14.3% |

*(Continued)*

| Study | Year(s) | Country | Sex (M-male, F-female, U-unspecified) | Level | Concussion incidence | | | |
|---|---|---|---|---|---|---|---|---|
| | | | | | Incidence proportion | 1000 P–H | 1000 A–E | % All injuries |
| Fuller et al. (2008) | 2007 | International | M | Professional | – | G: 2.6 | – | – |
| Kemp et al. (2008) | 2002/2003–2004/2005 | England | M | Professional | – | G: 4.1 P: 0.02 | – | 4.30% |
| Kerr et al. (2008) | 2005/2006 | United States | M | Collegiate | – | G: 2.16 P: 0.37 | – | 12.80% |
| | | | F | Collegiate | – | G: 1.58 P: 0.30 | – | 5.30% |
| Schick et al. (2008) | 2006 | International | F | Professional | – | O: 0.56 | – | O: 6.2% |
| Holtzhausen et al. (2006) | 1999 | South Africa | M | Professional | – | G: 0.17 | – | O: 1.6% |
| Best et al. (2005) | 2003 | International | M | Professional | – | – | – | G: 2.1% |
| Brooks et al. (2005) | 2002/2003–2003/2004 | England | M | Professional | – | G: 4.4 | – | – |
| **Soccer** | | | | | | | | |
| Covassin et al. (2016) | 2004/2005–2008/2009 | United States | M | Collegiate | – | – | G: 1.32 P: 0.17 O: 0.42 | – |
| | | | F | Collegiate | – | – | G: 1.89 P: 0.24 O: 0.65 | – |
| Comstock et al. (2015) | 2005/2006–2013/2014 | United States | M | High school | – | – | O: 0.28 | – |
| | | | F | High school | – | – | O: 0.45 | – |
| Zuckerman et al. (2015) | 2009/2010–2013/2014 | United States | M | Collegiate | – | – | G: 0.97 P: 0.18 O: 0.34 | – |
| | | | F | Collegiate | – | – | G: 1.94 P: 0.21 O: 0.63 | – |

*(Continued)*

| Study | Year(s) | Country | Sex (M-male, F-female, U-unspecified) | Level | Concussion incidence | | | |
|---|---|---|---|---|---|---|---|---|
| | | | | | Incidence proportion | 1000 P—H | 1000 A—E | % All injuries |
| Nordstrom et al. (2014) | 2001/2002–2011/2012 | Europe | M | Professional | – | – | – | O: 9% |
| O'Kane et al. (2014) | 2008–2012 | United States | F | Middle school | – | – | G: 5.3; P: 0.2; O: 1.20 | – |
| Nilsson et al. (2013) | 2001/2002–2009/2010 | Europe | M | Professional | – | O: 0.06 | – | – |
| Ekstrand et al. (2011) | 2001–2008 | Europe | M | Professional | – | O: 0.06 | – | O: 0.10% |
| Yard et al. (2008) | 2005–2007 | United States | M | High school | – | – | – | O: 9.3% |
| | | | F | High school | – | – | – | O: 12.2% |
| Gessel et al. (2007) | 2005/2006 | United States | M | High school | – | – | G: 0.59; P: 0.04; O: 0.22 | O: 9.5%d |
| | | | | Collegiate | – | – | G: 1.38; P: 0.24; O: 0.49 | O: 5%d |
| | | | F | High school | – | – | G: 0.97; P: 0.09; O: 0.36 | O: 15%d |
| | | | | Collegiate | – | – | G: 1.80; P: 0.25; O: 0.63 | O: 7%d |
| Hootman et al. (2007) | 1988/1989–2003/2004 | United States | M | Collegiate | – | – | O: 0.28 | O: 3.9% |
| | | | F | Collegiate | – | – | O: 0.41 | O: 5.3% |
| Fuller et al. (2005) | 1998–2004 | International | M | Professional | – | G: 1.06 | – | – |
| | | | F | Professional | – | G: 2.56 | – | – |

*(Continued)*

| Study | Year(s) | Country | Sex (M-male, F-female, U-unspecified) | Level | Concussion incidence | | | |
|---|---|---|---|---|---|---|---|---|
| | | | | | Incidence proportion | 1000 P–H | 1000 A–E | % All injuries |
| **Softball** | | | | | | | | |
| Covassin et al. (2016) | 2004/2005–2008/2009 | United States | F | Collegiate | – | – | G: 0.37 P: 0.14 O: 0.23 | – |
| Zuckerman et al. (2015) | 2009/2010–2013/2014 | United States | F | Collegiate | – | – | G: 0.56 P: 0.17 O: 0.33 | – |
| Castile et al. (2012) | 2005–2010 | United States | U | High school | – | – | G: 0.147 P: 0.074 O: 0.099 | – |
| Marar et al. (2012) | 2008–2010 | United States | F | High school | – | – | G: 0.29 P: 0.09 O: 0.16 | 13%[d] |
| Lincoln et al. (2011) | 1997/1988–2007–2008 | United States | F | High school | – | – | O: 0.11 | – |
| Gessel et al. (2007) | 2005/2006 | United States | U | High school | – | – | G: 0.04 P: 0.09 O: 0.07 | 5.5%[d] |
| | | | U | Collegiate | – | – | G: 0.37 P: 0.07 O: 0.19 | 4%[d] |
| Hootman et al. (2007) | 1988/1999–2003/2004 | United States | F | Collegiate | – | – | O: 0.14 | 4.30% |
| **Volleyball** | | | | | | | | |
| Black et al. (2016) | 2008/2009–2010/2011 | Canada | M | Collegiate | 15.38% | – | – | – |
| | | | F | Collegiate | 10.00% | – | – | – |
| Zuckerman et al. (2015) | 2009/2010–2013/2014 | United States | F | Collegiate | – | – | G: 0.557 P: 0.269 O: 0.357 | – |

*(Continued)*

| Study | Year(s) | Country | Sex (M-male, F-female, U-unspecified) | Level | Concussion incidence | | | |
|---|---|---|---|---|---|---|---|---|
| | | | | | Incidence proportion | 1000 P—H | 1000 A—E | % All injuries |
| Rosenthal et al. (2014) | 2005/2006 | United States | F | High school | – | – | O: 0.05 | – |
| Rosenthal et al. (2014) | 2011/2012 | United States | F | High school | – | – | O: 0.17 | – |
| Reeser et al. (2015) | 2005/2006 | United States | F | Collegiate | – | – | G: 0.25 | G: 6.4% |
| | | | | | | | P: 0.18 | P: 4.4% |
| | 2008/2009 | States | | | | | O: 0.2 | O: 4.8% |
| | | | F | High school | | | G: 0.11 | G: 7.9% |
| | | | | | | | P: 0.04 | P: 3% |
| | | | | | | | O: 0.06 | O: 8% |
| Liraz et al. (2013) | 2007/2008–2009/2010 | Canada | M | 5–19 years | – | – | | ED: 1.4% |
| | | | F | 5–19 years | – | – | | ED: 2.1% |
| Castile et al. (2012) | 2005–2010 | United States | U | High school | – | – | G: 0.10 | – |
| | | | | | | | P: 0.04 | |
| | | | | | | | O: 0.06 | |
| Marar et al. (2012) | 2008/2009–2009/2010 | United States | F | High school | – | – | G: 0.10 | 6%[a] |
| | | | | | | | P: 0.05 | |
| | | | | | | | O: 0.06 | |
| Rechel et al. (2008) | 2005/2006 | United States | F | High school | – | – | – | G: 1.5% |
| | | | | | | | | P: 4.2% |
| Gessel et al. (2007) | 2005/2006 | United States | U | High school | – | – | G: 0.05 | O: 3%[d] |
| | | | | | | | P: 0.05 | |
| | | | | | | | O: 0.05 | |
| | | | U | Collegiate | | | G: 0.13 | O: 3.5%[d] |
| | | | | | | | P: 0.21 | |
| | | | | | | | O: 0.18 | |
| Hootman et al. (2007) | 1988/1999–2003/2004 | United States | F | Collegiate | – | – | O: 0.09 | 2.10% |

*(Continued)*

## Wrestling

| Study | Year(s) | Country | Sex (M-male, F-female, U-unspecified) | Level | Incidence proportion | 1000 P–H | 1000 A–E | % All injuries |
|---|---|---|---|---|---|---|---|---|
| Zuckerman et al. (2015) | 2009/2010–2013/2014 | United States | M | Collegiate | – | – | G: 5.55 / P: 0.57 / O: 1.09 | – |
| Rosenthal et al. (2014) | 2005/2006 | United States | M | High school | – | – | O: 0.17 | – |
| Rosenthal et al. (2014) | 2011/2012 | United States | M | High school | – | – | O: 0.57 | – |
| Castile et al. (2012) | 2005–2010 | United States | U | High school | – | – | G: 0.32 / P: 0.10 / O: 0.15 | – |
| Marar et al. (2012) | 2008/2009–2009/2010 | United States | M | High school | – | – | G: 0.48 / P: 0.13 / O: 0.22 | O: 10%[d] |
| Lincoln et al. (2011) | 1997/1998–2007/2008 | United States | M | High school | – | – | O: 0.17 | – |
| Yard et al. (2008) | 2005/2006 | United States | M | High school | – | – | – | O: 5.4% |
|  |  |  | M | Collegiate | – | – | – | O: 5.8% |
| Rechel et al. (2008) | 2005/2006 | United States | M | High school | – | – | – | G: 6.3% / P: 5.6% |
| Gessel et al. (2007) | 2005/2006 | United States | U | High school | – | – | G: 0.32 / P: 0.13 / O: 0.18 | O: 5.5%[d] |
|  |  |  | U | Collegiate | – | – | G: 1.00 / P: 0.35 / O: 0.42 | O: 4.5%[d] |
| Pappas (2007) | 2002–2005 | United States | M+F | All ages | – | – | – | ED: 3.0% |
| Hootman et al. (2007) | 1988/1999–2003/2004 | United States | M | Collegiate | – | – | O: 0.25 | O: 3.3% |

[d] Estimated based on graph.

## References

Abrahams, S., S. Mc Fie, J. Patricios, M. Posthumus, and A. V. September. 2014. Risk factors for sports concussion: An evidence-based systematic review. *British Journal of Sports Medicine* 48 (2): 91–97. doi:10.1136/bjsports-2013-092734.

Adler, R. H. 2011. Youth sports and concussions: Preventing preventable brain injuries. One client, one cause, and a new law. *Physical Medicine and Rehabilitation Clinics of North America* 22 (4): 721–728, ix. doi:10.1016/j.pmr.2011.08.010.

Alternative Dispute Resolution Center. 2013. *NFL, Retired Players Resolve Concussion Litigation; Court Apointed Mediator Hails "Historic" Agreement*. Newport Beach, CA.

American Medical Association. n.d. H-470.965 Ultimate and extreme fighting. Accessed April 1, 2016. https://www.ama-assn.org/ssl3/ecomm/PolicyFinderForm.pl?site=www.ama-assn.org&uri=/resources/html/PolicyFinder/policyfiles/HnE/H-470.965.HTM.

Andersen, T. E., A. Arnason, L. Engebretsen, and R. Bahr. 2004. Mechanisms of head injuries in elite football. *British Journal of Sports Medicine* 38 (6): 690–696. doi:10.1136/bjsm.2003.009357.

Ashbaugh, A. and C. McGrew. 2016. The role of nutritional supplements in sports concussion treatment. *Current Sports Medicine Reports* 15 (1): 16–19. doi:10.1249/JSR.0000000000000219.

Asken, M. J. and R. C. Schwartz. 1998. Heading the ball in soccer: What's the risk of brain injury? *The Physician and Sportsmedicine* 26 (11): 37–44. doi:10.3810/psm.1998.11.1190.

Australian Football League Research Board Australian Football League Medical Officers' Association. 2011. *The Management of Concussion in Australian Football*. AFL Research Board. Docklands, VIC, Australia.

Australian Football League. 2016a. *About the AFL*. Docklands, VIC, Australia.

Australian Football League. 2016b. *Laws of Australian Football*. Docklands, VIC, Australia.

Australian Medical Association. 2013. Mixed martial arts must be banned. Accessed April 1, 2016. http://www.amawa.com.au/mixed-martial-arts-must-be-banned-ama-wa/.

Australian Rugby League. 2015. Laws of rugby league sevens (7's). Accessed April 1, 2016. http://www.group2refereesassociation.com/Web%20Docs/ARL%20Laws%20of%20Rugby%20League%20Sevens%20(7s).pdf.

Badgeley, M. A., N. M. McIlvain, E. E. Yard, S. K. Fields, and R. D. Comstock. 2013. Epidemiology of 10,000 high school football injuries: Patterns of injury by position played. *Journal of Physical Activity & Health* 10 (2): 160–69.

Bakhos, L. L., G. R. Lockhart, R. Myers, and J. G. Linakis. 2010. Emergency department visits for concussion in young child athletes. *Pediatrics* 126 (3): e550–e556. doi:10.1542/peds.2009-3101.

Barnes, B. C., L. Cooper, D. T. Kirkendall, T. P. McDermott, B. D. Jordan, and W. E. Garrett. 1998. Concussion history in elite male and female soccer players. *The American Journal of Sports Medicine* 26 (3): 433–38. doi:10.1177/03635465980260031601.

Baroff, G. S. 1998. Is heading a soccer ball injurious to brain function? *The Journal of Head Trauma Rehabilitation* 13 (2): 45–52.

Barr, C. and M. Beusenberg. 2001. Probability of concussion from single heading events in football. *British Journal of Sports Medicine* 35: 367–77.

Batten, J., A. J. White, and E. Anderson. 2016. Preventing penalty corner injuries and head trauma in field hockey: Time to consider the power play? *British Journal of Sports Medicine*, bjsports-2016-096201. doi:10.1136/bjsports-2016-096201.

Benson, B. W., G. M. Hamilton, W. H. Meeuwisse, P. McCrory, and J. Dvorak. 2009. Is protective equipment useful in preventing concussion? A systematic review of the literature. *British Journal of Sports Medicine* 43 (1): i56–i67. doi:10.1136/bjsm.2009.058271.

Benson, B. W., A. S. McIntosh, D. Maddocks, S. A. Herring, M. Raftery, and J. Dvorák. 2013. What are the most effective risk-reduction strategies in sport concussion? *British Journal of Sports Medicine* 47 (5): 321–326. doi:10.1136/bjsports-2013-092216.

Benson, B. W., M. S. Rose, and W. H. Meeuwisse. 2002. The impact of face shield use on concussions in ice hockey: A multivariate analysis. *British Journal of Sports Medicine* 36 (1): 27–32. doi:10.1136/bjsm.36.1.27.

Bird, Y. N., A. E. Waller, S. W. Marshall, J. C. Alsop, D. J. Chalmers, and D. F. Gerrard. 1998. The New Zealand rugby injury and performance project: V. epidemiology of a season of rugby injury. *British Journal of Sports Medicine* 32 (4): 319–325. doi:10.1136/bjsm.32.4.319.

Bjørneboe, J., R. Bahr, J. Dvorak, and T. E. Andersen. 2013. Lower incidence of arm-to-head contact incidents with stricter interpretation of the laws of the game in norwegian male professional football. *British Journal of Sports Medicine* 47 (8): 508–514.

Black, A. M., A. K. Macpherson, B. E. Hagel, M. A Romiti, L. Palacios-Derflingher, J. Kang, W. H. Meeuwisse, and C. A. Emery. 2016. Policy change eliminating body checking in non-elite ice hockey leads to a threefold reduction in injury and concussion risk in 11- and 12-Year-Old players. *British Journal of Sports Medicine* 50 (1): 55–61. doi:10.1136/bjsports-2015-095103.

Boden, B. P., D. T. Kirkendall, and W. E. Garrett. 1998. Concussion incidence in elite college soccer players. *The American Journal of Sports Medicine* 26 (2): 238–241.

Borowski, L. A., E. E. Yard, S. K. Fields, R. D. Comstock, L. A. Borowski, E. E. Yard, and S. K. Fields. 2008. The epidemiology of US high school basketball injuries, 2005–2007. *American Journal of Sports Medicine* 36 (12): 2328–2335. doi:10.1177/0363546508322893.

Brenner, J. S., A. Brooks, R. A. Demorest, M. E. Halstead, A. K. Weiss Kelly, C. G. Koutures, C. R. LaBella, et al. 2014. Reducing injury risk from body checking in boys' youth ice hockey. *Pediatrics* 133 (6): 1151–1157. doi:10.1542/peds.2014-0692.

British Medical Association. 2007. Ban ultimate fighting as well as boxing, says BMA. http://web.bma.org.uk/pressrel.nsf/wlu/SGOY-76QEY8?OpenDocument.

Broglio, S. P., K. M. Guskiewicz, T. C. Sell, and S. M. Lephart. 2004. No acute changes in postural control after soccer heading. *British Journal of Sports Medicine* 38 (5). England: 561–567. doi:10.1136/bjsm.2003.004887.

Brooks, J. H. M. 2005. Epidemiology of injuries in english professional rugby union: Part 2 training injuries. *British Journal of Sports Medicine* 39 (10): 767–775. doi:10.1136/bjsm.2005.018408.

Brooks, J. H. M., C. W. Fuller, S. P. T. Kemp, and D. B. Reddin. 2005. Epidemiology of injuries in english professional rugby union: Part 1 match injuries. *British Journal of Sports Medicine* 39 (10): 757–766. doi:10.1136/bjsm.2005.018135.

Buse, G J. 2006. No Holds Barred Sport Fighting: A 10 Year Review of Mixed Martial Arts Competition. *British Journal of Sports Medicine* 40 (2): 169–72. doi:10.1136/bjsm.2005.021295.

Butterwick, D. J., B. Hagel, D. S. Nelson, M. R. LeFave, and W. H. Meeuwisse. 2002. Epidemiologic analysis of injury in five years of canadian professional rodeo. *The American Journal of Sports Medicine* 30 (2): 193–198.

Butterwick, D. J., M. A. Brandenburg, D. M. Andrews, K. Brett, H. Bugg, K. J. Carlyle, T. R. Freeman III, et al. 2005. Agreement statement from the 1st international rodeo research and clinical care conference, calgary, Alberta, Canada (July 7–9, 2004). *Clinical Journal of Sport Medicine* 15 (3): 192–95.

Butterwick, D. J., M. R. Lafave, B. H. F. Lau, and T. Freeman. 2011. Rodeo catastrophic injuries and registry: Initial retrospective and prospective report. *Clinical Journal of Sport Medicine* 21 (3): 243–248.

Butterwick, D. H. J. and W. H. H. Meeuwisse. 2003. Bull riding injuries in professional rodeo: Data for prevention and care. *Physician and Sportsmedicine* 31 (6): 37–41.

Canadian Medical Association. 2013. *Canadian Medical Association Submision on Bill S-209, An Act to Amend the Criminal Code*. Vasa, Ottawa, Ont.

Cantu, R. C. 1992. Cerebral concussion in sport. Management and prevention. *Sports Medicine* 14 (1): 64–74.

Cantu, R. C. and F. O. Mueller. 2009. The prevention of catastrophic head and spine injuries in high school and college sports. *British Journal of Sports Medicine* 43 (13): 981–986.

Casson, I. R., D. C. Viano, J. W. Powell, and E. J. Pellman. 2010. Twelve years of national football league concussion data. *Sports Health* 2 (6): 471–483. doi:10.1177/1941738110383963.

Castile, L., C. L. Collins, N. M. McIlvain, and R. Dawn Comstock. 2012. The epidemiology of new versus recurrent sports concussions among high school athletes, 2005–2010. *British Journal of Sports Medicine* 46 (8): 603–610.

Clark, J. F., P. Graman, J. K. Ellis, R. E. Mangine, J. T. Rauch, B. Bixenmann, K. A. Hasselfeld, J. G. Divine, A. J. Colosimo, and G. D. Meyer. 2015. An exploratory study of the potential effects of vision training on concussion incidence in football. *Optometry & Visual Performance* 3 (2): 116–125.

Cobb, B. R., J. E. Urban, E. M. Davenport, S. Rowson, S. M. Duma, J. A. Maldjian, C. T. Whitlow, A. K. Powers, and J. D. Stitzel. 2013. Head impact exposure in youth football: Elementary school ages 9–12 years and the effect of practice structure. *Annals of Biomedical Engineering* 41 (12): 2463–2473. doi:10.1007/s10439-013-0867-6.

Cohenca, N., R. A. Roges, and R. Roges. 2007. The incidence and severity of dental trauma in intercollegiate athletes. *Journal of the American Dental Association (1939)* 138 (8): 1121–1126.

Collins, C. L., E. N. Fletcher, S. K. Fields, L. Kluchurosky, M. K. Rohrkemper, R. D. Comstock, and R. C. Cantu. 2014. Neck strength: A protective factor reducing risk for concussion in high school sports. *The Journal of Primary Prevention* 35 (5): 309–319. doi:10.1007/s10935-014-0355-2.

Collins, C. L., L. J. Micheli, E. E. Yard, R. D. Comstock, C. L. Collins, L. J. Micheli, and E. E. Yard. 2008. Injuries sustained by high school rugby players in the United States, 2005–2006. *Archives of Pediatrics and Adolescent Medicine* 162 (1): 49–54. doi:10.1001/archpediatrics.2007.1.

Collins, M., M. R. Lovell, G. L. Iverson, T. Ide, and J. Maroon. 2006. Examining concussion rates and return to play in high school football players wearing newer helmet technology: A three-year prospective cohort study. *Neurosurgery* 58 (2): 275–286. doi:10.1227/01.NEU.0000200441.92742.46.

Comstock, R. D., D. W. Currie, L. A. Pierpoint, J. A. Grubenhoff, and S. K. Fields. 2015. An evidence-based discussion of heading the ball and concussions in high school soccer. *JAMA Pediatrics* 169 (9): 830–837. doi:10.1001/jamapediatrics.2015.1062.

Covassin, T. and R. J. Elbin. 2011. The female athlete: The role of gender in the assessment and management of sport-related concussion. *Clinics in Sports Medicine* 30 (1): 125–131, x. doi:10.1016/j.csm.2010.08.001.

Covassin, T., R. Moran, and R. J. Elbin. 2016. Sex differences in reported concussion injury rates and time loss from participation: An update of the national collegiate athletic association injury surveillance program from 2004–2005 through 2008–2009. *Journal of Athletic Training* 51 (3): 189–194. doi:10.4085/1062-6050-51.3.05.

Crisco, J. J. and R. M. Greenwald. 2013. Let's get the head further out of the game: A proposal for reducing brain injuries in helmeted contact sports. *Current Sports Medicine Reports* 10 (1): 7–9. doi:10.1249/JSR.0b013e318205e063.

Daneshvar, D. H., C. J. Nowinski, A. C. McKee, R. C. Cantu, Daneshvar D.H., Nowinski C.J., Mckee A.C., et al. 2011. The epidemiology of sport-related concussion. *Clinics in Sports Medicine* 30 (1): 1–17. doi:10.1016/j.csm.2010.08.006.

Delaney, J. S., A. Al-Kashmiri, and J. A. Correa. 2014. Mechanisms of injury for concussions in university football, ice hockey, and Soccer. *Clinical Journal of Sport Medicine: Official Journal of the Canadian Academy of Sport Medicine* 24 (3): 233–237. doi:10.1097/JSM.0000000000000017.

Delaney, J. S., A. Al-Kashmiri, R. Drummond, and J. A. Correa. 2008. The effect of protective headgear on head injuries and concussions in adolescent football (Soccer) players. *British Journal of Sports Medicine* 42 (2): 110–115; discussion 115. doi:10.1136/bjsm.2007.037689.

Delaney, J. S., V. J. Lacroix, C. Gagne, and J. Antoniou. 2001. Concussions among university football and soccer players: A pilot study. *Clinical Journal of Sport Medicine* 11 (4): 234–240. doi:10.1097/00042752-200110000-00005.

Delaney, J. S., V. J. Lacroix, S. Leclerc, and K. M. Johnston. 2000. Concussions during the 1997 Canadian football league season. *Clinical Journal of Sport Medicine: Official Journal of the Canadian Academy of Sport Medicine* 10 (1): 9–14.

Delaney, J. S., V. J. Lacroix, S. Leclerc, and K. M. Johnston. 2002. Concussions among university football and soccer players. *Clinical Journal of Sport Medicine: Official Journal of the Canadian Academy of Sport Medicine* 12 (6): 331–338. doi:10.1097/00042752-200211000-00003.

Denke, N. J. 2008. Brain injury in sports. *Journal of Emergency Nursing* 34 (4): 363–364. doi:10.1016/j.jen.2008.04.013.

Dick, R., J. Hertel, J. Agel, J. Grossman, and S. W. Marshall. 2007c. Descriptive epidemiology of collegiate men's basketball injuries: National collegiate athletic association injury surveillance system, 1988–1989 through 2003–2004. *Journal of Athletic Training* 42 (2): 194–201.

Dick, R., J. M. Hootman, J. Agel, L. Vela, S. W. Marshall, and R. Messina. 2007d. Descriptive epidemiology of collegiate women's field hockey injuries: National collegiate athletic association injury surveillance system, 1988–1989 through 2002–2003. *Journal of Athletic Training* 42 (2): 211–220.

Dick, R., W. A. Romani, J. Agel, J. G. Case, and S. W. Marshall. 2007b. Descriptive epidemiology of collegiate men's lacrosse injuries: National collegiate athletic association injury surveillance system, 1988–1989 through 2003–2004. *Journal of Athletic Training* 42 (2): 255–261.

Dick, R., E. L. Sauers, J. Agel, G. Keuter, S. W. Marshall, K. McCarty, and E. McFarland. 2007a. Descriptive epidemiology of collegiate men's baseball injuries: National collegiate athletic association injury surveillance system, 1988–1989 through 2003–2004. *Journal of Athletic Training* 42 (2): 183–93.

Discover UFC. n.d. Championship UF. Rules and Regulations. http://www.ufc.ca/discover/sport/rules-and-regulations (accessed April 1, 2016).

Discover UFC. n.d. Ways to win. http://www.ufc.ca/discover/sport/ways-to-win (accessed April 1, 2016).

Dompier, T. P., Z. Y. Kerr, S. W. Marshall, B. Hainline, E. M. Snook, R. Hayden, and J. E. Simon. 2015. Incidence of concussion during practice and games in youth, high school, and collegiate American football players. *JAMA Pediatrics* 169 (7): 659. doi:10.1001/jamapediatrics.2015.0210.

Echlin, P. S. 2010. Concussion education, identification, and treatment within a prospective study of physician-observed junior ice hockey concussions: Social context of this scientific intervention. *Neurosurgical Focus* 29 (5): E7. doi:10.3171/2010.10.FOCUS10222.

Emery, C. A., A. M. Black, L. Palacios-Derflingher, K. J. Schneider, and B. E. Hagel. 2016. The risk of injury associated with body checking among pee wee ice hockey players: An evaluation of hockey Canada's national body checking policy change (Abstract). *Clinical Journal of Sport Medicine* 26 (3): e95–e96.

Emery, C. A., B. Hagel, M. Decloe, and M. Carly. 2010a. Risk factors for injury and severe injury in youth ice hockey: A systematic review of the literature. *Injury Prevention: Journal of the International Society for Child and Adolescent Injury Prevention* 16 (2): 113–118. doi:10.1136/ip.2009.022764.

Emery, C. A., J. Kang, I. Shrier, C. Goulet, B. E. Hagel, B. W. Benson, A. Nettel-Aguirre, J. R. McAllister, G. M. Hamilton, and W. H. Meeuwisse. 2010b. Risk of injury associated with body checking among youth ice hockey players. *JAMA* 303 (22): 2265–2272. doi:10.1001/jama.2010.755.

Emery, C., J. Kang, I. Shrier, C. Goulet, B. Hagel, B. Benson, A. Nettel-Aguirre, J. McAllister, and W. Meeuwisse. 2011. Risk of injury associated with bodychecking experience among youth hockey players. *Canadian Medical Association Journal* 183 (11): 1249–1256. doi:10.1503/cmaj.101540.

Emery, C. A. and W. H. Meeuwisse. 2006. Injury rates, risk factors, and mechanisms of injury in minor hockey. *The American Journal of Sports Medicine* 34 (12): 1960–1969. doi:10.1177/0363546506290061.

Engebretsen, L., K. Steffen, J. Manuel Alonso, M. Aubry, J. Dvorak, A. Junge, W. Meeuwisse, M. Mountjoy, P. Renström, and M. Wilkinson. 2013. Sports injuries and illnesses during the London summer olympic games 2012. *British Journal of Sports Medicine* 44 (11): 772–780. doi:10.1136/bjsm.2010.076992.

Farrington, T., G. Onambele-Pearson, R. L. Taylor, P. Earl, and K. Winwood. 2012. A review of facial protective equipment use in sport and the impact on injury incidence. *The British Journal of Oral & Maxillofacial Surgery* 50 (3): 233–238. doi:10.1016/j.bjoms.2010.11.020.

Federation Internationale de Football Association (FIFA). 2007. Big count 2006: Statistical summary report by gender/category/region. http://www.fifa.com/media/news/y=2007/m=5/news=fifa-big-count-2006-270-million-people-active-football-529882.html (accessed April 1, 2016).

Finch, C., A. Clapperton, and P. McCrory. 2013. Increasing incidence of hospitalisation for sport-related concussion in VA, Australia. *Medical Journal of Australia* 198 (May): 427–430. doi:10.5694/mja12.11217.

Fridman, L., J. L. Fraser-Thomas, S. R. McFaull, and A. K. Macpherson. 2013. Epidemiology of sports-related injuries in children and youth presenting to canadian emergency departments from 2007–2010. *BMC Sports Science, Medicine and Rehabilitation* 5: 30. doi:10.1186/2052-1847-5-30.

Fuller, C. W., A. Junge, J. Dvorak, C. W. Fuller, A. Junge, and J. Dvorak. 2005. A six year prospective study of the incidence and causes of head and neck injuries in international football. *British Journal of Sports Medicine* 39 (1): i3–i9. doi:10.1136/bjsm.2005.018937.

Fuller, C. W., F. Laborde, R. J. Leather, and M. G. Molloy. 2008. International rugby board rugby world cup 2007 injury surveillance study. *British Journal of Sports Medicine* 42 (6): 452–459. doi:10.1136/bjsm.2008.047035.

Fuller, C. W., K. Sheerin, and S. Targett. 2013. Rugby world cup 2011: International rugby board injury surveillance study. *British Journal of Sports Medicine* 47 (18): 1184–1191. doi:10.1136/bjsports-2012-091155.

Fuller, C. W., A. Taylor, and M. Raftery. 2015. Epidemiology of concussion in men's elite rugby-7s (Sevens World Series) and rugby-15s (Rugby World Cup, Junior World Championship and Rugby Trophy, Pacific Nations Cup and English Premiership). *British Journal of Sports Medicine* 49 (7): 478–483. doi:10.1136/bjsports-2013-093381.

Gabbett, T. J. 2005a. Influence of the limited interchange rule on injury rates in sub-elite rugby league players. *Journal of Science and Medicine in Sport/Sports Medicine Australia* 8 (1): 111–1115.

Gabbett, T. J. 2005b. Influence of playing position on the site, nature, and cause of rugby league injuries. *Journal of Strength and Conditioning Research/National Strength & Conditioning Association* 19 (4): 749–755. doi:10.1519/R-16504.1.

Gabbett, T. J. 2008. Incidence of injury in junior Rugby league players over four competitive seasons. *Journal of Science and Medicine in Sport* 11 (3): 323–328.

Gabbett, T. J. and N. Domrow. 2005. Risk factors for injury in subelite rugby league players. *The American Journal of Sports Medicine* 33 (3): 428–434. doi:10.1177/0363546504268407.

Gabbett, T. J. and R. J. B. Godbolt. 2010. Training injuries in professional rugby league. *Journal of Strength and Conditioning Research/National Strength & Conditioning Association* 24 (7): 1948–1953. doi:10.1519/JSC.0b013e3181ddad65.

Gardner, A. J., G. L. Iverson, W. H. Williams, S. Baker, and P. Stanwell. 2014. A systematic review and meta-analysis of concussion in rugby union. *Sports Medicine* 44 (12): 1717–1731. doi:10.1007/s40279-014-0233-3.

Gessel, L. M., S. K. Fields, C. L. Collins, R. W. Dick, R. Dawn Comstock. 2007. Concussions among United States high school and collegiate athletes. *Journal of Athletic Training* 42 (4): 495–503.

Gibbs, N., D. Bates, and M. Watsford. 2009. Concussion management in a professional senior AFl team over 10 years: Assessing re-injury and performance. In *Annual Scientific Conference of the Australian College of Sports Physicians*, 1–3. Surfers Paradise, QLD, Australia.

Gissane, C., D. Jennings, K. Kerr, and J. White. 2003. Injury rates in rugby league football: Impact of change in playing season. *The American Journal of Sports Medicine* 31 (6): 954–958.

Glang, A., M. C. Koester, S. V. Beaver, J. E. Clay, and K. A. McLaughlin. 2010. Online training in sports concussion for youth sports coaches. *International Journal of Sports Science & Coaching* 5 (1): 1–12. doi:10.1260/1747-9541.5.1.1.

Glanz, K. and D. B. Bishop. 2010. The role of behavioral science theory in development and implementation of public health interventions. *Annual Review of Public Health* 31 (January): 399–418. doi:10.1146/annurev.publhealth.012809.103604.

Goodell, R. 2015. Official playing rules of the national football league. *National Football League*, p. 20.

Green, G. A., K. M. Pollack, J. D.'Angelo, M. S. Schickendantz, R. Caplinger, K. Weber, A. Valadka, et al. 2015. Mild traumatic brain injury in major and minor league baseball players. *The American Journal of Sports Medicine* 43 (5): 1118–1126. doi:10.1177/0363546514568089.

Greenhill, D. A., P. Navo, H. Zhao, J. Torg, R. Dawn Comstock, and B. P. Boden. 2016. Inadequate helmet fit increases concussion severity in American high school football players. *Sports Health* 8 (3): 238–243. doi:10.1177/1941738116639027.

Guskiewicz, K. M., S. W. Marshall, S. P. Broglio, R. C. Cantu, and D. T. Kirkendall. 2002. No evidence of impaired neurocognitive performance in collegiate soccer players. *The American Journal of Sports Medicine* 30 (2): 157–162.

Hagel, B. E., J. Marko, D. Dryden, A. B. Couperthwaite, J. Sommerfeldt, and B. H. Rowe. 2006. Effect of bodychecking on injury rates among minor ice hockey players. *CMAJ* 175 (2): 155–160. doi:10.1503/cmaj.051531.

Hendricks, S. and M. Lambert. 2010. Tackling in rugby: Coaching strategies for effective technique and injury prevention. *International Journal of Sports Science & Coaching* 5 (1): 117–135.

Hinton-Bayre, A. D., G. Geffen, and P. Friis. 2004. Presentation and mechanisms of concussion in professional rugby league football. *Journal of Science & Medicine in Sport* 7 (3): 400–404. doi:10.1016/S1440-2440(04)80035-5.

Hockey Canada. 2015. 2014–2015 Annual Report. www.hockeycanada.ca.

Hollis, S. J., M. R. Stevenson, A. S. McIntosh, E. Arthur Shores, M. W. Collins, and C. B. Taylor. 2009. Incidence, risk, and protective factors of mild traumatic brain injury in a cohort of Australian nonprofessional male rugby players. *The American Journal of Sports Medicine* 37 (12): 2328–2333. doi:10.1177/0363546509341032.

Holtzhausen, L. J., M. P. Schwellnus, I. Jakoet, and A. L. Pretorius. 2006. The incidence and nature of injuries in South African rugby players in the rugby super 12 competition. *South African Medical Journal = Suid-Afrikaanse Tydskrif Vir Geneeskunde* 96 (12): 1260–1265.

Hootman, J. M., R. Dick, and J. Agel. 2007. Epidemiology of collegiate injuries for 15 sports: Summary and recommendations for injury prevention initiatives. *Journal of Athletic Training* 42 (2): 311–319.

Hutchison, M. G., D. W. Lawrence, M. D. Cusimano, and T. A. Schweizer. 2014. Head trauma in mixed martial arts. *The American Journal of Sports Medicine* 42 (6): 1352–1358. doi:10.1177/0363546514526151.

International Ice Hockey Federation. 2015. Survey of players. http://www.iihf.com/iihf-home/the-iihf/survey-of-players/.

Jacobson, N. A., L. G. Morawa, and C. A. Bir. 2012. Epidemiology of cheerleading injuries presenting to NEISS hospitals from 2002 to 2007. *The Journal of Trauma and Acute Care Surgery* 72 (2): 521–526. doi:10.1097/TA.0b013e31823f5fe3.

Jákó, P. 2002. Safety measures in amateur boxing. *British Journal of Sports Medicine* 36 (6): 394–395. doi:10.1136/bjsm.36.6.394.

Jákó, P. 2009. Boxing. In *Combat Sports Medicine*, edited by W. A. Kordi, N. Maffuli, N. Wroble, R.R. Wallace. Springer, London, UK.

Janda, D. H., C. A. Bir, and A. L. Cheney. 2002. An evaluation of the cumulative concussive effect of soccer heading in the youth population. *Injury Control and Safety Promotion* 9: 25–31 ST–An evaluation of the cumulative concus. doi: 10.1076/icsp.9.1.25.3324

Junge, A., L. Engebretsen, M. L. Mountjoy, J. M. Alonso, P. A. F. H. Renström, M. J. Aubry, and J. Dvorak. 2009. Sports injuries during the summer olympic games 2008. *The American Journal of Sports Medicine* 37 (11): 2165–2172. doi:10.1177/0363546509339357.

Kaminski, T. W., E. S. Cousino, and J. J. Glutting. 2008. Examining the relationship between purposeful heading in soccer and computerized neuropsychological test performance. *Research Quarterly for Exercise & Sport* 79 (2): 235–244. doi:10.1080/02701367.2008.10599486.

Kemp, S. P. T., Z. Hudson, J. H. M. Brooks, and C. W. Fuller. 2008. The epidemiology of head injuries in english professional rugby union. *Clinical Journal of Sport Medicine: Official Journal of the Canadian Academy of Sport Medicine* 18 (3): 227–234. doi:10.1097/JSM.0b013e31816a1c9a.

Kerr, H. A., C. Curtis, L. J. Micheli, M. S. Kocher, D. Zurakowski, S. P. T. Kemp, and J. H. M. Brooks. 2008. Collegiate rugby union injury patterns in New England: A prospective cohort study. *British Journal of Sports Medicine* 42 (7): 595–603. doi:10.1136/bjsm.2007.035881.

Kerr, Z. Y., C. L. Collins, J. P. Mihalik, S. W. Marshall, K. M. Guskiewicz, and R. Dawn Comstock. 2014. Impact locations and concussion outcomes in high school football player-to-player collisions. *Pediatrics* 134 (3): 489–496. doi:10.1542/peds.2014-0770.

Kerr, Z. Y., S. Yeargin, T. C. Valovich McLeod, V. C. Nittoli, J. Mensch, T. Dodge, R. Hayden, and T. P Dompier. 2015. Comprehensive coach education and practice contact restriction guidelines result in lower injury rates in youth American football. *Orthopaedic Journal of Sports Medicine* 3 (7). doi:10.1177/2325967115594578.

King, D. and T. Clark. 2012. Injuries in amateur representative rugby league over three years. *New Zealand Journal of Sports Medicine* 39 (2): 48–51.

King, D. A., T. J. Gabbett, C. Dreyer, and D. F. Gerrard. 2006. Incidence of injuries in the New Zealand national rugby league sevens tournament. *Journal of Science and Medicine in Sport/ Sports Medicine Australia* 9 (1–2): 110–118. doi:10.1016/j.jsams.2005.09.001.

King, D. A., P. A. Hume, P. D. Milburn, and D. Guttenbeil. 2010. Match and training injuries in rugby league: A review of published studies. *Sports Medicine (Auckland, N.Z.)* 40 (2): 163–178. doi:10.2165/11319740-000000000-00000.

Kirkendall, D. T. and W. E. Garrett. 2001. Heading in soccer: Integral skill or grounds for cognitive dysfunction? *Journal of Athletic Training* 36 (3): 328–333.

Kirkendall, D. T., S. E. Jordan, and W. E. Garrett. 2001. Heading and head injuries in soccer. *Sports Medicine (Auckland, N.Z.)* 31 (5): 369–386.

Koh, J. O., J. D. Cassidy, and E. J. Watkinson. 2003. Incidence of concussion in contact sports: A systematic review of the evidence. *Brain Injury* 17 (10): 901–917. doi:10.1080/0269905031000088869.

Kontos, A. P., A. Dolese, R. J. Elbin, T. Covassin, and B. L. Warren. 2011. Relationship of soccer heading to computerized neurocognitive performance and symptoms among female and male youth soccer players. *Brain Injury* 25 (12): 1234–1241. doi:10.3109/02699052.2011.608209.

Kontos, A. P., R. J. Elbin, V. C. Fazio-Sumrock, S. Burkhart, H. Swindell, J. Maroon, and M. W. Collins. 2013. Incidence of sports-related concussion among youth football players aged 8–12 Years. *The Journal of Pediatrics* 163 (3): 717–720. doi:10.1016/j.jpeds.2013.04.011.

Kontos, A. P., R. J. Elbin, A. Sufrinko, S. Dakan, K. Bookwalter, A. Price, W. P. Meehan, and M. W. Collins. 2016. Incidence of concussion in youth ice hockey players. *Pediatrics* 137 (2): 1–6. doi:10.1542/peds.2015-1633.

Kriz, P. K., R. David Zurakowski, J. L. Almquist, J. Reynolds, D. Ruggieri, C. L. Collins, P. A. D'Hemecourt, et al. 2015. Eye protection and risk of eye injuries in high school field hockey. *Pediatrics* 136 (3): 521–527. doi:10.1542/peds.2015-0216.

Kriz, P. K., R. Dawn Comstock, D. Zurakowski, J. L. Almquist, C. L. Collins, and P. A. D'Hemecourt. 2012. Effectiveness of protective eyewear in reducing eye injuries among high school field hockey players. *Pediatrics* 130 (6): 1069–1075.

Krolikowski, M., A. M. Black, L. Palacios-Derflingher, T. A. Blake, K. J. Schneider, and C. A. Emery. 2017. The effect of the "Zero tolerance for head contact" rule change on the risk of concussions in youth ice hockey players. *The American Journal of Sport Medicine* 45 (2): 468–473. doi:10.1177/0363546516669701.

Kroshus, E., D. H. Daneshvar, C. M. Baugh, C. J. Nowinski, and R. C. Cantu. 2014. NCAA concussion education in ice hockey: An ineffective mandate. *British Journal of Sports Medicine* 48 (2): 135–140. doi:10.1136/bjsports-2013-092498.

Labella, C. R., B. W. Smith, A. Sigurdsson. 2002. Effect of mouthguards on dental injuries and concussions in college basketball. *Medicine and Science in Sports and Exercise* 34 (1): 41–44. doi:10.1097/00005768-200201000-00007.

Levy, M. L., A. S. Kasasbeh, L. C. Baird, C. Amene, J. Skeen, and L. Marshall. 2012. Concussions in soccer: A current understanding. *World Neurosurgery* 78 (5): 535–544. doi:10.1016/j.wneu.2011.10.032.

Lincoln, A. E., S. V. Caswell, J. L. Almquist, R. E. Dunn, J. B. Norris, and R. Y. Hinton. 2011. Trends in concussion incidence in high school sports: A prospective 11-year study. *The American Journal of Sports Medicine* 39 (5): 958–963. doi:10.1177/0363546510392326.

Lincoln, A. E., R. Y Hinton, J. L. Almquist, S. L. Lager, and R. W. Dick. 2007. Head, face, and eye injuries in scholastic and collegiate lacrosse: A 4-Year prospective study. *The American Journal of Sports Medicine* 35 (2): 207–215. doi:10.1177/0363546506293900.

Lipton, M. L., N. Kim, M. E. Zimmerman, M. Kim, W. F. Stewart, C. A. Branch, and R. B. Lipton. 2013. Soccer heading is associated with white matter microstructural and cognitive abnormalities. *Radiology* 268 (3): 850–857. doi:10.1148/radiol.13130545.

Lopez, V., R. Ma, M. G. Weinstein, R. C. Cantu, L. S. D. Myers, N. S. Nadkar, C. Victoria, and A. A. Allen. 2016. Concussive injuries in rugby-7s: An American experience and current review. *Medicine and Science in Sports and Exercise* 48 (7): 1320–1330. doi:10.1249/MSS.0000000000000892.

Lystad, R. P., K. Gregory, and J. Wilson. 2014. The epidemiology of injuries in mixed martial arts: A systematic review and meta-analysis. *Orthopaedic Journal of Sports Medicine* 2 (1): 2325967113518492. doi:10.1177/2325967113518492.

Mackenzie, B., P. Vivier, S. Reinert, J. Machan, C. Kelley, and E. Jacobs. 2015. Impact of a state concussion law on pediatric emergency department visits. *Pediatric Emergency Care* 31 (1): 25–30. doi:10.1097/PEC.0000000000000325.

Makdissi, M., P. McCrory, A. Ugoni, D. Darby, and P. Brukner. 2009. A prospective study of postconcussive outcomes after return to play in Australian football. *The American Journal of Sports Medicine* 37 (5): 877–883. doi:10.1177/0363546508328118.

Mangus, B. C., H. W. Wallmann, and M. Ledford. 2004. Analysis of postural stability in collegiate soccer players before and after an acute bout of heading multiple soccer balls. *Sports Biomechanics/International Society of Biomechanics in Sports* 3 (2): 209–220. doi:10.1080/14763140408522841.

Marar, M., N. M. McIlvain, S. K. Fields, and R. Dawn Comstock. 2012. Epidemiology of concussions among United States high school athletes in 20 sports. *The American Journal of Sports Medicine* 40 (4): 747–755. doi:10.1177/0363546511435626.

Matser, J. T., A. G. H. Kessels, M. D. Lezak, and J. Troost. 2001. A dose-response relation of headers and concussions with cognitive impairment in professional soccer players a dose-response relation of headers and concussions with cognitive impairment in professional soccer players. *Journal of Clinical and Experimental Neuropsychology* 23 (6): 770–774. doi:10.1076/jcen.23.6.770.1029.

McCrory, P. R. 2003. Brain injury and heading in soccer. *BMJ (Clinical Research Ed.)* 327 (7411): 351–352. doi:10.1136/bmj.327.7411.351.

McGuine, T. A., S. Hetzel, M. McCrea, and M. Alison Brooks. 2014. Protective equipment and player characteristics associated with the incidence of sport-related concussion in high school football players: A multifactorial prospective study. *The American Journal of Sports Medicine* 42 (10): 2470–2478. doi:10.1177/0363546514541926.

McIntosh, A. S., P. McCrory, and J. Comerford. 2000. The dynamics of concussive head impacts in rugby and Australian rules football. *Medicine and Science in Sports and Exercise* 32 (12): 1980–1984. doi:10.1097/00005768-200012000-00002.

McIntosh, A. S. and P. McCrory. 2001. Effectiveness of headgear in a pilot study of under 15 rugby Union football. *British Journal of Sports Medicine* 35 (3): 167–169. doi:10.1136/bjsm.35.3.167.

McIntosh, A. S., P. McCrory, C. F. Finch, J. P. Best, D. J. Chalmers, and R. Wolfe. 2009a. Does padded headgear prevent head injury in rugby Union football? *Medicine and Science in Sports and Exercise* 41 (2): 306–313. doi:10.1249/MSS.0b013e3181864bee.

McIntosh, A. S., P. R. McCrory, and J. P. Best. 2005. *Rugby Headgear Study: Final Report*. UNSW, Australia.

McIntosh, A. S. and R. Dutfield. 2010. *Rugby Pathways: Final Report*. Kensington, NSW, Australia.

McIntosh, A. S., T. N. Savage, and R. Dutfield. 2009b. *Rugby Union Injury Surveillance Study: Final Report for 2008 Season*. UNSW, Australia.

Meehan 3rd, W. P., P. Hemecourt, R. D. Comstock. 2010. High school concussions in the 2008–2009 academic year: Mechanism, symptoms, and management. *The American Journal of Sports Medicine* 38 (12): 2405–2409. doi:10.1177/0363546510376737.

Meehan, W. P., A. M. Taylor, and M. Proctor. 2011a. The pediatric athlete: Younger athletes with sport-related concussion. *Clinics in Sports Medicine* 30 (1): 133–144. doi:10.1016/j.csm.2010.08.004.

Meehan, W. P., P. D'Hemecourt, C. L. Collins, and R. Dawn Comstock. 2011b. Assessment and management of sport-related concussions in United States high schools. *The American Journal of Sports Medicine* 39 (11): 2304–2310. doi:10.1177/0363546511423503.

Menger, R., A. Menger, and A. Nanda. 2016. Rugby headgear and concussion prevention: Misconceptions could increase aggressive play. *Neurosurgical Focus* 40 (4): E12. doi:10.3171/2016.1.FOCUS15615.

Mills, J. D., J. E. Bailes, C. L. Sedney, H. Hutchins, and B. Sears. 2011. Omega-3 fatty acid supplementation and reduction of traumatic axonal injury in a rodent head injury model. *Journal of Neurosurgery* 114 (1): 77–84. doi:10.3171/2010.5.JNS08914.

Mobile Sport Medicine System. 2005. Mobile sport medicine system 25 year injury study. studylib.net/doc/7713989/25-year-injury-study---mobile-sports-medicine-systems.

Mukherjee, S. 2012. Head and face injuries during the men's field hockey junior world cup 2009. *The American Journal of Sports Medicine* 40 (3): 686–690. doi:10.1177/0363546511426697.

Murgraff, V., M. R. McDermott, and J. Walsh. 2003. Self-efficacy and behavioral enactment: The application of schwarzer's health action process approach to the prediction of low-risk, single-occasion drinking. *Journal of Applied Social Psychology* 33 (2): 339–361. doi:10.1111/j.1559-1816.2003.tb01900.x.

Nathanson, J. T., J. G. Connolly, F. Yuk, A. Gometz, J. Rasouli, M. Lovell, and T. Choudhri. 2016. Concussion incidence in professional football: Position-specific analysis with use of a novel metric. *Orthopaedic Journal of Sports Medicine* 4 (1). doi:10.1177/2325967115622621.

National Collegiate Athletic Association. 2015. Student-Athlete Participation 1981-82-2014-15 NCAA Sports Sponsorship and Participation Rates Report. https://www.ncaa.org/.

National Rugby League. 2012. RLIF bans shoulder charge. http://www.nrl.com (accessed May, 2016).

Navarro, R. R. 2011. Protective equipment and the prevention of concussion—What is the evidence? *Current Sports Medicine Reports* 10 (1): 27–31. doi:10.1249/JSR.0b013e318205e072.

New Zealand Rugby League. 2012. NZRL supports ruling on shoulder charges. www.nzrl.co.nz.

Ngai, K. M., F. Levy, and E. B. Hsu. 2008. Injury trends in sanctioned mixed martial arts competition: A 5-year review from 2002 to 2007. *British Journal of Sports Medicine* 42 (8): 686–689. doi:10.1136/bjsm.2007.044891.

Niedfeldt, M. W. 1991. Head injuries, heading, and the use of headgear in soccer. *Current Sports Medicine Reports* 10 (6): 324–329. doi:10.1249/JSR.0b013e318237be53.

Norton, R. and M. Wilson. 1995. Rugby league injuries and patterns. *New Zealand Journal of Sports Medicine* 33: 428–434.

O'Connor, D. 2009. NRL surveillance report 2009 season. Sydney University, Camperdown, Australia.

O'Kane, J. W., M. R. Levy, K. E. Pietila, D. J. Caine, and M. A. Schiff. 2011. Survey of injuries in seattle area levels 4–10 female club gymnasts. *Clinical Journal of Sport Medicine* 21 (6): 486–492. doi:10.1097/JSM.0b013e31822e89a8.

O'Kane, J. W., A. Spieker, M. R. Levy, M. Neradilek, N. L. Polissar, M. A. Schiff, et al. 2014. Concussion among female middle-school soccer players'. *JAMA Pediatrics* 258. Doi:10.1001/jamapediatrics.2013.4518.

Office of the Comissioner of Baseball. 2015. Official Baseball Rules. http://mlb.mlb.com/mlb/downloads/y2015/official_baseball_rules.pdf (accessed April 1, 2016).

Oliver, J. M., M. T. Jones, K. Michele Kirk, D. A. Gable, J. T. Repshas, T. A. Johnson, U. Andréasson, N. Norgren, K. Blennow, and H. Zetterberg. 2016. Effect of docosahexaenoic acid on a biomarker of head trauma in American football. *Medicine and Science in Sports and Exercise*, 48 (6): 974–982.doi:10.1249/MSS.0000000000000875.

Orchard, J., H. Seward, and J. Orchard. 2013. 2012 AFL Injury Report, pp. 1–26. Australian Football League, Docklands, Australia.

Orchard, J., H. Seward, and J. Orchard. 2014. AFL injury report. *AFL Reports*, pp. 1–26. Australian Football League, Docklands, Australia.

Orr, R. and H. L. Cheng. 2015. Incidence and characteristics of injuries in elite Australian junior rugby league players. *Journal of Science and Medicine in Sport* 19 (3): 212–217. doi:10.1016/j.jsams.2015.03.007.

Padaki, A. S., B. J. Cole, and C. S. Ahmad. 2016. Concussion incidence and return-to-play time in national basketball association players: Results from 2006 to 2014. *The American Journal of Sports Medicine* 44 (9): 2263–2268. doi:10.1177/0363546516634679.

Pappas, E., B. T. Zazulak, E. E. Yard, and T. E. Hewett. 2011. The epidemiology of pediatric basketball injuries presenting to U.S. emergency departments: 2000–2006. *Sports Health* 3 (4): 331–335.

Patton, D. A. and A. S. McIntosh. 2016. Considerations for the performance requirements and technical specifications of soft-shell padded headgear. *Proceedings of the Institution of Mechanical Engineers, Part P: Journal of Sports Engineering and Technology* 230 (1): 29–42. doi:10.1177/1754337115615482.

Pickett, W., S. Streight, K. Simpson, and R. J. Brison. 2005. Head injuries in youth soccer players presenting to the emergency department. *British Journal of Sports Medicine* 39 (4): 226–231. doi:10.1136/bjsm.2004.013169.

Powell, J. W. and K. D. Barber-Foss. 1999. Traumatic brain injury in high school athletes. *Journal of the American Medical Association* 282 (10): 958–963. doi:http://dx.doi.org/10.1001/jama.282.10.958.

Punnoose, A. R. 2012. Study raises concerns about "heading" in soccer, but jury is still out on risks. *JAMA* 307 (10): 1012–1114. doi:10.1001/jama.2012.231.

Putukian, M., R. J. Echemendia, and S. Mackin. 2000. The acute neuropsychological effects of heading in soccer: A pilot study. *Clinical Journal of Sport Medicine: Official Journal of the Canadian Academy of Sport Medicine* 10 (2): 104–109. doi:10.1097/00042752-200004000-00004.

Putukian, M., A. E. Lincoln, J. J. Crisco, M. Putukian, and A. E. Lincoln. 2014. Sports-specific issues in men's and women's lacrosse. *Current Sports Medicine Reports* 13 (5) 334–340. doi:10.1249/JSR.0000000000000092.

Quarrie, K. L., S. M. Gianotti, D. J. Chalmers, and W. G. Hopkins. 2005. An evaluation of mouthguard requirements and dental injuries in New Zealand rugby Union. *British Journal of Sports Medicine* 39 (9): 650–651. doi:10.1136/bjsm.2004.016022.

Rechel, J. A., E. E. Yard, and R. Dawn Comstock. 2008. An epidemiologic comparison of high school sports injuries sustained in practice and competition. *Journal of Athletic Training* 43 (2): 197–204.

Reeser, J. C., A. Gregory, R. L. Berg, and R. D. Comstock. 2015. A comparison of women's collegiate and girls' high school volleyball injury data collected prospectively over a 4-year period. *Sports Health: A Multidisciplinary Approach* 7 (6): 504–510. doi:10.1177/1941738115600143.

Roberts, W. O., J. D. Brust, and B. Leonard. 1999. Youth ice hockey tournament injuries: Rates and patterns compared to season play. *Medicine and Science in Sports and Exercise* 31 (1): 46–51. doi:http://dx.doi.org/10.1097/00005768-199901000-00009.

Roberts, W. O., J. D. Brust, B. Leonard, and B. J. Hebert. 1996. Fair-play rules and injury reduction in ice hockey. *Archives of Pediatrics and Adolescent Medicine* 150 (2): 140–145.

Rosenbaum, D. and S. Davis. 2014. Injury risk due to collisions in major league baseball. *International Journal of Sports Medicine* 35 (8): 704–707. doi:10.1055/s-0033-1363253.

Rosenthal, J. A., R. E. Foraker, C. L. Collins, and R. Dawn Comstock. 2014. National high school athlete concussion rates from 2005–2006 to 2011–2012. *The American Journal of Sports Medicine* 42 (7): 1710–1715. doi:10.1177/0363546514530091.

Rowson, S., S. M. Duma, R. M. Greenwald, J. G. Beckwith, J. J. Chu, K. M. Guskiewicz, J. P. Mihalik, et al. 2014. Can helmet design reduce the risk of concussion in football? *J Neurosurg* 120 (4): 919–922. doi:10.3171/2014.1.JNS13916.

Rutherford, A., R. Stephens, D. Potter, and G. Fernie. 2005. Neuropsychological impairment as a consequence of football (Soccer) play and football heading: Preliminary analyses and report on university footballers. *Journal of Clinical and Experimental Neuropsychology* 27 (3): 299–319. doi:10.1080/13803390490515504.

Sanchez Garcia, R. and D. Malcolm. 2010. Decivilizing, civilizing or informalizing? the international development of mixed martial arts. *International Review for the Sociology of Sport* 45 (1): 39–58. doi:10.1177/1012690209352392.

Schmitt, D. M., J. Hertel, T. A. Evans, L. C. Olmsted, and M. Putukian. 2004. Effect of an acute bout of soccer heading on postural control and self-reported concussion symptoms. *International Journal of Sports Medicine* 25 (5): 326–331. doi:http://dx.doi.org/10.1055/s-2004-819941.

Schneider, K. J., W. H. Meeuwisse, J. Kang, G. M. Schneider, and C. A. Emery. 2013. Preseason reports of neck pain, dizziness, and headache as risk factors for concussion in male youth ice hockey players. *Clinical Journal of Sport Medicine: Official Journal of the Canadian Academy of Sport Medicine* 23 (4): 267–272. doi:10.1097/JSM.0b013e318281f09f.

Schwartz, M. L., A. R. Hudson, G. R. Fernie, K. Hayashi, and A. A. Coleclough. 1986. Biomechanical study of full-contact karate contrasted with boxing. *Journal of Neurosurgery* 64 (2): 248–252. doi:10.3171/jns.1986.64.2.0248.

Shankar, P. R., S. K. Fields, C. L. Collins, R. W. Dick, and R. Dawn Comstock. 2007. Epidemiology of high school and collegiate football injuries in the United States, 2005–2006. JOUR. *The American Journal of Sports Medicine* 35 (8): 1295–1303. doi:10.1177/0363546507299745.

Shields, B. J., S. A. Fernandez, and G. A. Smith. 2009. Epidemiology of cheerleading stunt-related injuries in the United States. *Journal of Athletic Training* 44 (6): 586–594. doi:10.4085/1062-6050-44.6.586.

Shields, B. J. and G. A. Smith. 2006. Cheerleading-related injuries to children 5 to 18 years of age: United States, 1990–2002. *Pediatrics* 117 (1): 122–129. doi:10.1542/peds.2005-1139.

Smith, J. T. 2010. Fighting for regulation: Mixed martial arts legislation in the United States. *Drake Law Review* 58 (2009–2010): 617–655.

Smith, A. M., M. Jorgenson, M. C. Sorenson, D. Margenau, A. A. Link, M. MacMillan, M. J. Stuart, R. Greenwald, A. Ashare, and S. W. Dean. 2009. Hockey education program (HEP): A statewide measure of fair play, skill development, and coaching excellence. *Journal of ASTM International* 6 (4): 101857. doi:10.1520/JAI101857.

Straume-Naesheim, T. M., T. E. Andersen, J. Dvorak, and R. Bahr. 2005. Effects of heading exposure and previous concussions on neuropsychological performance among norwegian elite footballers. *British Journal of Sports Medicine* 39 (1): i70–i77. doi:10.1136/bjsm.2005.019646.

Stuart, M. J., A. M. Smith, S. A. Malo-Ortiguera, T. L. Fischer, and D. R. Larson. 2002. A comparison of facial protection and the incidence of head, neck, and facial injuries in junior a hockey players. A function of individual playing time. *The American Journal of Sports Medicine* 30 (1): 39–44.

Swartz, E. E., S. P. Broglio, S. B. Cook, R. C. Cantu, M. S. Ferrara, K. M. Guskiewicz, and J. L. Myers. 2015. Early results of a helmetless-tackling intervention to decrease head impacts in football players. *Journal of Athletic Training* 50 (12): 1219–1222. doi:10.4085/1062-6050-51.1.06.

Tanaka, Y., Y. Maeda, T.-C. Yang, T. Ando, Y. Tauchi, and H. Miyanaga. 2014. Prevention of orofacial injury via the use of mouthguards among young male rugby players. *International Journal of Sports Medicine* 36 (3): 254–261. doi:10.1055/s-0034-1390498.

Taylor, A. E., C. W. Fuller, and M. G. Molloy. 2011. Injury surveillance during the 2010 IRB Women's Rugby World Cup. *British Journal of Sports Medicine* 45 (15): 1243–1245.

The National Federation of State High School Associations. 2015. *2014–2015 High School Athletics Participation Survey.* http://www.nfhs.org/ParticipationStatics/PDF/2014-15_Participation_Survey_Results.pdf (accessed April 1, 2016).

Tietze, D. C., J. Borchers, B. D. Roewer, and T. E. Hewett. 2015. A prospective, longitudinal analysis of division 1 collegiate football injuries. *Clinical Journal of Sport Medicine* 23 (2): 148.

Tuna, E. B. and E. Ozel. 2014. Factors affecting sports-related orofacial injuries and the importance of mouthguards. *Sports Medicine (Auckland, N.Z.)* 44 (6): 777–783. doi:10.1007/s40279-014-0167-9.

Tysvaer, A. T. 1992. Head and neck injuries in soccer: Impact of minor trauma. *Sports Medicine.* 14 (13): 200–213.

Tysvaer, A. T. and E. A. Løchen. 1991. Soccer injuries to the brain. A neuropsychologic study of former soccer players. *The American Journal of Sports Medicine* 19 (1): 56–60. doi:10.1177/036354659101900109.

Tysvaer, A. T. and O. Storli. 1981. Association football injuries to the brain. A preliminary report. *British Journal of Sports Medicine* 15 (3): 163–166. doi:10.1136/bjsm.15.3.163.

USA Hockey HQ. 2012. Heads up, don't duck safety video. *YouTube.* https://www.youtube.com/watch?v=rwu4mwkEMaQ.

USA Hockey. 2016. Membership statistics. *2015.* Accessed April 13. http://www.usahockey.com/page/show/839306-membership-statistics.

Warsh, J. M., S. A. Constantin, A. Howard, and A. Macpherson. 2009. A systematic review of the association between body checking and injury in youth ice hockey. *Clinical Journal of Sport Medicine: Official Journal of the Canadian Academy of Sport Medicine* 19 (2): 134–144. doi:10.1097/JSM.0b013e3181987783.

Wasserman, E. B., Z. Y. Kerr, S. L. Zuckerman, and T. Covassin. 2015. Epidemiology of sports-related concussions in national collegiate athletic association athletes from 2009 to 2010 to 2013 to 2014: Symptom prevalence, symptom resolution time, and return-to-play time. *The American Journal of Sports Medicine* 44 (1): 226–233. doi:10.1177/0363546515610537.

Whitehouse, T., R. Orr, E. Fitzgerald, S. Harries, and C. P. McLellan. 2016. The epidemiology of injuries in Australian professional rugby Union 2014 super rugby competition. *Orthopaedic Journal of Sports Medicine* 4 (3): 2325967116634075. doi:10.1177/2325967116634075.

Willigenburg, N. W., J. R. Borchers, R. Quincy, C. C. Kaeding, and T. E. Hewett. 2016. Comparison of injuries in American collegiate football and club rugby: A prospective cohort study. *The American Journal of Sports Medicine* 44 (3): 753–760. doi:10.1177/0363546515622389.

Withnall, C., N. Shewchenko, R. Gittens, and J. Dvorak. 2005. Biomechanical investigation of head impacts in football. *British Journal of Sports Medicine* 39 (1): i49–i57. doi:10.1136/bjsm.2005.019182.

Witol, A. D. and F. M. Webbe. 2003. Soccer heading frequency predicts neuropsychological deficits. *Archives of Clinical Neuropsychology: The Official Journal of the National Academy of Neuropsychologists* 18 (4): 397–417. doi:10.1016/S0887-6177(02)00151-8.

World Rugby. 2015. *Regulation 12. Schedule 1. Specifications Relating to Players' Dress. Law 4 - Players' Clothing.* Dublin, Ireland.

World Rugby. 2016a. *Player Number.* Dublin, Ireland.

World Rugby. 2016b. *Rugby Sevens.* Dublin, Ireland.

Yard, E. E., C. L. Collins, R. W. Dick, and R. Dawn Comstock. 2007. An epidemiologic comparison of high school and college wrestling injuries. *The American Journal of Sports Medicine* 36 (1): 57–64. doi:10.1177/0363546507307507.

Yard, E. E. and R. D. Comstock. 2006. Injuries sustained by pediatric ice hockey, lacrosse, and field hockey athletes presenting to United States emergency departments, 1990–2003. JOUR. *Journal of Athletic Training* 41 (4): 441–449.

Zazryn, T. R., P. R. McCrory, and P. A. Cameron. 2009. Injury rates and risk factors in competitive professional boxing. *Clinical Journal of Sport Medicine* 19 (1): 20–25. doi:10.1097/JSM.0b013e31818f1582.

Zetterberg, H., M. A. Hietala, M. Jonsson, N. Andreasen, E. Styrud, I. Karlsson, A. Edman, et al. 2006. Neurochemical aftermath of amateur boxing. *Archives of Neurology* 63 (9): 1277–1280. doi:10.1001/archneur.63.9.1277.

Zuckerman, S. L., Z. Y. Kerr, A. Yengo-Kahn, E. Wasserman, T. Covassin, and G. S. Solomon. 2015. Epidemiology of sports-related concussion in NCAA athletes from 2009–2010 to 2013–2014. *The American Journal of Sports Medicine* 43 (11): 2654–2662. doi:10.1177/0363546515599634.

Zuckerman, S. L., Y. M. Lee, M. J. Odom, G. S. Solomon, J. A. Forbes, and A. K. Sills. 2012. Recovery from sports-related concussion: Days to return to neurocognitive baseline in adolescents versus young adults. *Surgical Neurology International* 3: 130. doi:10.4103/2152-7806.102945.

## *Additional helpful resources*

Concussion Awareness Training tool, http://www.cattonline.com
Parachute Canada's concussion App, http://www.parachutecanada.org/concussion/whattodo
Consensus Guidelines, http://bjsm.bmj.com/content/51/11/838
Stop Sports Injuries, http://www.stopsportsinjuries.org

# chapter four

## Biomechanics of sports concussion
### How do sport concussions happen?

*Blaine Hoshizaki, Anna Oeur, Andrew Post, David Koncan,*
*Marshall Kendall, Clara Karton, and Philippe Rousseau*

### Contents

Defining the relationship between an event and injury appears straightforward with conventional wisdom following that the harder the impact, the more severe the injury. This relationship holds when one considers low-energy impacts to the head are a common everyday occurrence whereas very high-energy impacts can result in death. However, concussions are not described by either very low- or very high-energy impacts to the head but land somewhere in the middle. Brain tissue trauma resulting from a concussive impact is followed by acute cellular changes described by indiscriminant presynaptic release of neurotransmitters that activate postsynaptic receptors (Giza and Hovda, 2001; Prins et al., 2013). This initial response is followed by a prolonged glucose metabolic depression that can last up to ten days. Concussions are diagnosed using a wide range of signs and symptoms including but not limited to decreased cognitive function, improper balance, speech, vision, muscle coordination, memory, and inappropriate behavior. Events resulting in concussive injuries are varied and not easily described by simple head impact dynamics. Over the years, the search for a means of capturing useful dynamic measures to predict the severity of the resulting concussion has proven elusive. Initially, concussion was primarily defined by loss of consciousness following a direct impact to the head. This was followed by describing the relationship between intracranial pressure and loss of consciousness and ultimately the search for an algorithm employing dynamic response variables to predict the risk and severity of a concussion. More recently finite element models of the brain and skull have been employed to calculate a host of mechanical variables describing tissue response of the brain to loading. Research efforts attempting to correlate event characteristics and the risk of concussion injury has important implications in setting policy, and rule changes to govern safety in sport and to establish performance parameters to certify safety equipment.

The brain is structurally and functionally heterogeneous in its organization with a high degree of complex interconnectivity and interindividual variability. This creates an unpredictable relationship between the mechanical force and symptom diagnosed injury. Although concussions are diagnosed using changes in behavior and symptoms, these injury characteristics are often inconsistent in their presentation. This relatively broad, varied, and inconsistent list of characteristics describing a concussion reflects a complex injury. It is also important to note that the symptoms can arise from structures not involving brain tissue including the inner ear, optic nerve, and muscle and neck strain. Studies undertaken to find out how severe an impact needs to be before it results in a concussion cannot be done using human subjects. To establish head injury tolerance curves, data are collected by a variety of indirect means including film analysis, instrumented helmets, event reconstructions using an anthropomorphic test device (ATD), and computer models. Each method of data collection has advantages and disadvantages and needs to be interpreted in accordance with these characteristics.

The following topics will be covered: the first describes the relationship among impact characteristics and the resulting dynamic response of the head and associated maximum principal strain (MPS). Initial concerns involving head injuries in sport primarily focussed on managing severe injuries. This resulted in the advent of helmets and other environmental cushioning materials to decrease the magnitude of the impact decreasing the risk of traumatic brain injuries but did little in managing concussive injuries. Understanding the effect of material dampening on event duration and injury risk for concussion is instrumental in describing the risk associated with sport injury events. The third topic will describe the use of finite element models to obtain brain tissue information defining the relationship between the head impact and resulting tissue trauma. Concussion events include falls, collisions, projectiles, and punches with each impact representing unique characteristics that influence injury risk for concussion. The explanation of how these characteristics interact to create risk will be covered in the fourth section. Concussion can be described as a transient event with no lingering symptoms or a permanent condition with serious disabilities. Unfortunately, the capacity to predict the risk for either outcome using biomechanical characteristics is further complicated by the wide ranging individual profiles that include a history of concussions, migraine headaches, and depression. Although concussive injuries lie between no recorded symptoms and death following a head impact, the continuum of brain trauma and resulting injury is not well defined. Concussion will be discussed in the fifth section in terms of its contribution to the risk of all neurological disorders associated with brain trauma. Finally, there are a number of methods used to measure brain trauma associated with sport, each with their benefits and limitations. This will be discussed in the sixth and final sections of the chapter.

## Head injury predictors

Head injury biomechanics is used to establish relationships between mechanical parameters of the impact event and injury outcome to predict the risk of head injury for known loads. In the literature, head acceleration is a dynamic response measure of the input force and is associated with injury severity or probability where higher magnitudes of acceleration are associated with unfavorable outcomes (Newman et al., 2000a). Historically, relationships between head injury and linear acceleration were established from experiments involving cadaver drop tests inducing skull fracture, and pressure pulses delivered to exposed animal brains. Notably, the work by Gurdjian et al. (1954) and Lissner et al. (1960)

was used to create the widely referenced Wayne state tolerance curve (WSTC), a plot illustrating the relationship between average linear acceleration and duration and tolerance for concussion. Head injury indices including the Gadd severity index (GSI; Equation 4.1) and head injury criterion (HIC) are formulations based on information contained in the WSTC. In 1966, Gadd plotted the WSTC on logarithmic paper and formulated the following equation:

$$GSI = \int_0^t a(t)^{2.5} dt \tag{4.1}$$

where:
    $a$ is the acceleration
    $t$ is the impact duration (Gadd, 1966)

The exponent was taken from the slope of the line from the log plot. GSI is used by the National Operating Committee on Standards for Athletic Equipment (NOCSAE) where a value of 1200 SI was set as a pass/fail criterion for American football helmets. In 1971, Versace modified the GSI and proposed the head injury criterion (HIC; Equation 4.2) (Versace, 1971).

$$HIC = \left[ \frac{1}{t_2 - t_1} \int_{t_1}^{t_2} a(t)dt \right]^{2.5} (t_2 - t_1) \tag{4.2}$$

HIC is similar to GSI, but "$t_1$" and "$t_2$" specify the time duration of the acceleration pulse with which to maximize the HIC value. Incorporating time limits into the indices was necessary to avoid unrealistically high GSI values for longer duration accelerations that did not correspond to reasonable levels of injury risk (Versace, 1971). The time specifications for HIC can be set between 15 and 36 ms depending on its use in evaluating motorcycle crash helmets or interior vehicle safety systems (Versace, 1971). However, head injury indices developed for high-energy loading scenarios like car crashes, may not be appropriate for evaluating protective capacity of sports equipment subject to environments governed by lower impact energies. An HIC value of 1000 correlated with an 18% risk of sustaining traumatic brain injuries such as skull fracture or subdural hematoma and was used to specify protective design measures where a threat to life was the primary concern (Gadd, 1966; Versace, 1971; Backaitis, 1981; Prasad and Mertz, 1985; Hutchinson et al., 1998). It has been recommended that a lower value of HIC (<1000) be used to reflect milder brain injuries like concussion, because HIC 1000 was not meant to predict the risk for mild brain injuries but as a coarse severity measure for fatal versus nonfatal injuries within crash environments (Newman et al., 2000a).

    A common criticism of these injury indices is that they neglect other factors contributing to concussion risk including impact direction and angular motion (Ommaya and Hirsch, 1971; Gennarelli et al., 1982; Patton et al., 2012). Newman et al. (2000b) proposed a more complex injury criteria based on the concept that the rate of kinetic energy, or power transferred to the head, plays an important role in the ensuing brain injury. The head impact power Equation 4.2 was formulated using both linear and angular accelerations of the head and incorporates weighted coefficients to take into account directional sensitivity or tolerance to injury (Newman et al., 2000b).

$$HIP = C_1 a_x \int a_x dt + C_2 a_y \int a_y dt + C_3 a_z \int a_z dt + C_4 \propto_x \int \propto_x dt + C_5 \propto_y \int \propto_y dt + C_6 \propto_z \int \propto_z dt \quad (4.3)$$

The "$C_{1-3}$" coefficients correspond to the mass of the human head in the three primary directions: "$C_{4-6}$" to the moments of inertia, "$a$" is linear acceleration, and "$\propto$" is angular acceleration (Newman et al., 2000b). Newman et al. (2000a) constructed probability risk curves for concussion based on reconstructions of concussions in American football and evaluated the ability of commonly used head injury criteria to reflect the risk of sustaining a concussion statistically. He concluded that HIP was a better predictor of concussion than HIC, and with further refinements of HIP coefficients, these criteria had the potential to correlate better with concussion than existing injury criteria (Newman et al., 2000a).

In sport, there are a number of different types of impact events that result in a concussion (Daneshvar et al., 2011; Hutchison et al., 2013). Body collisions are common causes for concussion in contact sports like American football and elite ice hockey but, in cheerleading falls, are the leading cause of injury (Pellman et al., 2003; Daneshvar et al., 2011; Hutchison et al., 2013). Each event type can be described using four variables: velocity, mass, compliance, and location. Impact variables play a role in the nature of energy transferred to the head in terms of the direction, magnitude, duration, and rate of linear and angular acceleration and therefore injury risk. Impact mass is related to the weight of the striking object or person contacting the head. Impact compliance describes the overall stiffness of an impact where adding compliance to the head, that is, wearing a helmet, decreases the magnitude of head acceleration by elongating the duration of the acceleration pulse (Newman, 2002; Hoshizaki and Brien, 2004). Impact location, defined by the site and angle, describes where, on the head, the impact occurred and determines the direction of head and brain motion in space.

Gurdjian et al. (1964) investigated the effects of velocity and compliance (bare head versus helmeted condition) on peak linear acceleration of an instrumented cadaver (Lissner et al., 1960; Gurdjian et al., 1964). Overall, an increase in impact velocity resulted in an increase in linear acceleration. The effect of compliance was observed when comparing the results between the unprotected and helmeted conditions. The addition of the helmet shifted the velocity-acceleration relationship, where higher velocities were required to maintain the same levels of peak acceleration when compared with the bare head condition (Gurdjian et al., 1964).

Karton et al. (2014) investigated the effects of impact striking masses between 4 and 14 kg representative of a low-mass punch to a high-mass shoulder collision in sport. Overall, striking mass had a positive relationship with peak linear and angular acceleration, where an increase in mass caused an increase in response. Gimbel and Hoshizaki (2008) also studied the complex interactions between velocity, compliance, and mass by impacting different densities of expanded polystyrene (EPS) foam, typical of materials used in bike helmets, with masses ranging from 3.6 to 5.6 kg, representative of the mass of a child's head to that of an adult head (Gimbel and Hoshizaki, 2008). In general, the heavier mass (5.6 kg) caused material failure of the foams, resulting in a spike in peak linear acceleration at lower impact velocities where higher velocities were required to bottom out the foams at the low mass (Gimbel and Hoshizaki, 2008).

In experimental animal research, impact location and loading direction affected the duration of unconsciousness in concussed subhuman primates (Gennarelli et al., 1982, 1987; Hodgson et al., 1983). These researchers investigated impact and nonimpact loading inputs in the primary directions on primates: anterior–posterior, medial–lateral, and oblique (midpoint between the front and side locations). These studies support the notion that medial–lateral loading produces the highest severities of injury (Gennarelli et al., 1982; Hodgson et al., 1983). Recent research conducted by Walsh et al. (2011) explored the effect of impact location and angle on headform dynamic response, testing 5 common locations about the headform and 4 different impact angles, resulting in 20 unique conditions. Impacts to the front and side had the highest linear accelerations, but side and rear impacts had the highest angular accelerations (Walsh et al., 2011). In addition, noncentric conditions, where the impact vector is aligned outside the center of gravity of the head, are an important factor in creating relatively high angular acceleration in comparison with center of gravity hits (Walsh et al., 2011).

Within the context of predicting concussion risk, impact velocity, compliance, mass, and location influence head dynamic response. In some cases, their effects can be easily predicted, that is, velocity increases response, compliance decreases response, by increasing the duration of that response (Newman, 2002; Hoshizaki and Brien, 2004).

Researchers have proposed that head dynamic response criteria are too imprecise of a measure for brain injuries like concussion, where tissue stresses and strains are better representations of local tissue trauma causing injury (Ommaya et al., 1966; King et al., 2003). Finite element (FE) models of the human brain in head impact investigations use the full acceleration time histories of both linear and angular acceleration in the three axes of motion for an individual impact event and calculate resulting tissue stresses and strains from the loading inputs. The FE model takes into consideration other aspects of the acceleration loading curve in addition to peak magnitude, such as curve shape, duration, slope, and time to peak (Figure 4.1).

The effect of acceleration-loading patterns on FE results was investigated by Post et al. (2012) and Yoganandan et al. (2008). Post et al. (2012a) conducted a study comparing acceleration curves with a slow rise at the beginning and a high peak toward the end of the curve result in comparatively higher values of stress and strain than those with a high peak at the beginning followed by a slow descent. Yoganandan et al. (2008) examined the effects of mono- and bi-phasic angular acceleration and deceleration pulses on brain tissue strain. These types of pulses represent the motions where the head is quickly accelerated and then decelerated (Yoganandan et al., 2008). They reported that a single head acceleration or deceleration pulse produced similar levels of strain, and that bi-phasic pulses

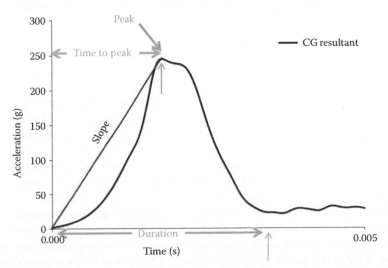

*Figure 4.1* Peak, slope, time to peak, and duration–acceleration curve characteristics.

(acceleration then deceleration or vice versa) resulted in unique patterns of strains where longer pauses between acceleration and deceleration increased strain values (Yoganandan et al., 2008). These studies demonstrate that the full kinematic description is important in creating stress and strain in the brain as calculated from FEA.

Impact velocity, mass, compliance, and location influence levels of peak head acceleration; however, the interaction of these variables contributes to the challenge with predicting risk. These variables influence the peak magnitudes of acceleration as well as the shape and duration of the loading curve. Acceleration-loading characteristics and type of acceleration have been demonstrated to influence levels of stress and brain tissue strain from FE analyses.

## Impact compliance in sport and risk of concussion

Brain tissue strain results from a combination of linear and rotational accelerations from an impact to the head (Zhang et al., 2004). Although the peak magnitude of these variables are important in terms of injury and head protection (Willinger and Baumgartner, 2003; Zhang et al., 2004; Kleiven, 2007), other aspects of this acceleration loading curve have an effect on brain tissue strain and its relationship to concussion (Yoganandan et al., 2008; Post et al., 2012). Recently there has been a focus on the effects of longer duration acceleration pulses on the brain tissue, in particular rotational acceleration pulses, as rotational motion is an important factor in the mechanisms of concussion (Kleiven, 2005; Kimpara and Iwamoto, 2011; Forero Rueda et al., 2011). In sporting environments, the duration/compliance of an impact is determined by the surface stiffness of an impact. The less compliant the impact, the shorter duration the linear and rotational acceleration curves. For example, an unhelmeted head impact for a person falling to low compliance concrete is typically around 5 ms in duration (Doorly and Gilchrist, 2006; Post et al., 2015a, 2015b). A high compliance (soft) system is represented in ice hockey where a padded shoulder hits a helmeted head (Rousseau and Hoshizaki, 2015). The padding on both sides of the striking/struck equation such as those in ice hockey results in long duration accelerations of 20–30 ms (Rousseau, 2014; Rousseau and Hoshizaki, 2015).

The relationship between magnitude and duration of a head contact event has been studied since the early 1950s, though its impact in current sporting environments is only beginning to be realized. The original magnitude/duration research was conducted primarily by Gurdjian et al. (1953, 1954) who, through impacts to canines, demonstrated a link between acceleration and severe brain injury and concussion where short duration events resulted in traumatic brain injury and the longer events concussion symptoms. From these data, Gurdjian et al. (1953, 1954) developed the Wayne state tolerance curve, which is a linear acceleration curve that showed a theoretical relationship between magnitude and duration of event and human tolerance to head injury. Van Lierde (2005) developed a similar curve for rotational acceleration and duration, the Brain injury curve leven (BICLE), from reconstructions of bicycle head injuries. A similar plot can be created from human brain injury reconstruction data from the literature using anthropometric dummies (Figure 4.2). Similar to the WSTC and BICLE, the magnitudes required to cause brain injury was shown to decrease as the duration of event (impact) increased.

The underlying mechanics of the magnitude–duration of event relationship was investigated by several authors. Gennarelli (1983) found that short-term accelerations resulted in subdural hematoma (SDH), with longer accelerations resulting in diffuse axonal injury (DAI). Research by Willinger et al. (1992), Kleiven (2005), and more recently Stemper et al. (2015) using mathematical, finite element, and animal models supported the conclusions

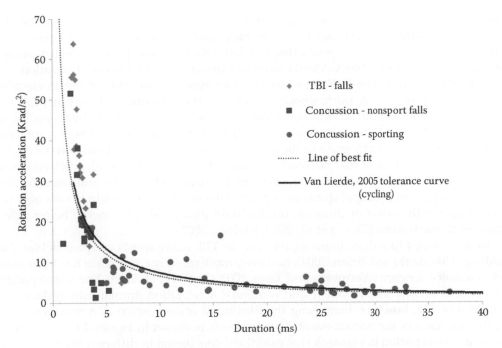

*Figure 4.2* Plotted rotational acceleration versus duration for reconstructions (Rousseau, 2014; Post, 2015a, 2015b; Kendall, 2016) of brain injury events using a Hybrid III headform.

of Gennarelli (1983) and Gurdjian et al. (1953, 1954). This relationship was suggested by Gilchrist (2003) to be a manifestation of the mechanical properties of viscoelastic properties of the brain tissues, where damage would incur at lower magnitudes with extended durations of strain loading, with the brain being less resistant to rotationally induced shearing as the duration of the event increases.

When considering risk of injury, it is important to understand that the duration of the event will have an effect on the amount of brain tissue strain. Protective equipment for athletes in sport reduces the risk of traumatic brain injury by lowering the magnitude of the event by lengthening the duration and absorbing energy. With the potential risk posed from longer impact durations in terms of concussion, this research has implications for future helmet designs and rules governing athlete behaviors. This relationship is important for the development and interpretation of the variables currently used to quantify risk of an impact in sport.

When helmets were first developed, peak linear acceleration was a commonly used metric in design as it had been shown to be correlated with pressure in the brain that was associated with the mechanisms of TBI (Thomas et al., 1966). Further investigations involving the safety performance of the helmets demonstrated that peak linear acceleration was not highly correlated to TBI which led to the development of integrations of the acceleration time curve: GSI and HIC (Gadd, 1966; Versace, 1971). The combination of using a linear acceleration-based metric has reduced the incidence of TBI but not concussion. Rotational acceleration has been identified as the primary mechanism of tissue deformation, playing an important role in diffuse white-matter injuries such as concussion (Holbourn, 1943; Kleiven, 2005). The proposed rotational injury risk variables for concussion include peak rotational acceleration, peak rotational velocity, GAMBIT, and HIP (Newman, 1986; Newman et al., 2000a). Using peak rotational magnitudes such as acceleration and/or velocity are limited as they do not account for the effect of the event duration on the brain tissue. The GAMBIT and HIP are more complex metrics that incorporate the use of rotational acceleration in terms of predicting risk but have not been applied in injury analysis (Newman et al., 2000b). The GAMBIT does not incorporate the effects of duration in its determination of risk. The HIP does introduce an aspect of duration of the accelerations into its calculation of risk but without considering the relationship between peak rotational acceleration and duration as shown in Figure 4.1. HIP lacks predictive capacity, and as a result, HIP has not been widely used in brain injury research. Without a rotational tolerance curve, the effectiveness of these types of predictive calculations is reduced. One commonly used measure that currently incorporates the effect of peak acceleration and duration on brain injury risk is maximum principal strain obtained by finite element modeling. As maximum principal strain incorporates the loading of the brain tissues over time accounting for the effect of duration on the brain injury risk, this metric better reflects localized tissue trauma (Zhang et al., 2004; Kleiven, 2007).

In an attempt to reduce brain injury risk for TBI, many sports adopted helmets and padding (Hoshizaki and Brien, 2004); however, more recently concussion has been identified as a major concern (Wennberg and Tator, 2003; Casson et al., 2010). The added padding reduced the magnitudes of linear and rotational acceleration dramatically reducing the incidence of TBI, however, increasing the likelihood of concussion as a result of extending the duration of the impact event. This trade-off is shown in Figure 4.1, as well as the risk of injury reported in research that examined concussion in different types of padded environments (Table 4.1). It has also been argued that the increased protection provided by padding caused athletes to play more aggressively creating an environment where the athletes do not feel the hit (Hedlund, 2000; Hagel and Meeuwisse, 2004). Extending the duration of the event and creating an environment where athletes feel free to impact the opponent in the head contributed to the incidence of concussion in padded sports.

The present helmet certification testing for ice hockey and football are based upon impacts to hard noncompliant surfaces (CSA 2015; NOCSAE 2014). These surfaces do not reflect the most common concussion mechanism event within sport, and the resulting helmets are not designed to manage the lower magnitude longer duration events that increase brain tissue strain associated with concussion.

Risk of brain injury in sport is affected by the magnitude and the duration of the accelerations incurred by the brain tissues. As increased padding is added through helmets and body pads, the dynamic response magnitudes that reflect the risk of a concussion are reduced.

*Table 4.1* Rotational acceleration thresholds for concussion from the literature where duration was reported

| Threshold for 50% risk of concussion (rad/s²) | Approximate duration | Event | Reference |
|---|---|---|---|
| 8020 | 10–15 ms | Australian rules football | Fréchède and McIntosh (2009) |
| 5900 | 15 ms | American football—helmet to helmet | Zhang et al. (2004) |
| 3100 | 20–30 ms | Ice hockey—Shoulder to head | Rousseau (2014) |

## Using finite element models to predict concussive risk

Finite element (FE) models of the brain are created using medical images (CT and MRI), rendering sliced images into a representation of the human head made up of thousands of elements meshed together. These models are used to investigate tissue responses from forces transmitted to the brain during head impacts in sports. Finite element models can be used to interpret the unique dynamic response characteristics of different sports environments, that is, body-to-head, head-to-head, and head to various ground surfaces by incorporating the material characteristics of the brain to assess how impact conditions influence the tissue response.

A number of brain FE models have been developed and published in the literature for use in brain injury research topics such as concussion, traumatic brain injury, and car crash analyses (Willinger et al., 1999; Zhang et al., 2001b; Kleiven and von Holst, 2002; Horgan and Gilchrist, 2004; Takhounts et al., 2008; McAllister et al., 2011). For each tissue that is represented in the model, material properties are assigned based on mechanical tissue investigations (Fallenstein et al., 1969; Shuck and Advani, 1972; McElhaney et al., 1973; Mendis et al., 1995; Donnelly and Medige, 1997; Thibault and Margulies, 1998; Prange and Margulies, 2002; Gefen et al., 2003; Nicolle et al., 2004; Chatelin et al., 2012). Viscoelasticity is an important characteristic of brain tissue resulting in time-varying stiffness, based on the loading rate and duration that the tissue is under load. Brain tissue subjected to longer duration loading is more compliant and at risk of larger strains (Mendis et al., 1995). Finite element models employ dynamic response characteristics (acceleration magnitude, impact duration, impact location, direction) and output the mechanical tissue response. Subtle differences in loading curves are interpreted by the model; differences that may not be captured by dynamic response variables such as peak linear or peak rotational acceleration. These models can include all aspects of the loading curve and quantify the effect on tissue response, making them an important tool in concussion research.

Finite element models are usually constructed using either medical images of an individual or an averaged set of images of a number of individuals. Averaged or general models can be criticized for not representing specific individuals. However, they are helpful as a consistent measurement tool to investigate the subtleties of impact dynamics leading to concussion. Models based on a single person can be used both as a general model and as a patient-specific model. If used as a general model, there will be limitations because it does not necessarily represent a population's average size and geometry. One drawback of patient-specific models is a larger variance in output metrics as a result of every model having a slightly different construction. Patient-specific models offer the ability to ask different questions, more specific to the individual but more difficult to apply to a general population. General models do not necessarily represent any individual but will have less variance in output measures, allowing for investigations applied to the general population. Many efforts have been made to create models with characteristics more representative of a larger population, including modifying shape characteristics to reflect an averaged shape (Takhounts et al., 2008), as well as introducing axonal tract directional response based on DTI imaging (Giordano and Kleiven, 2014; Sahoo et al., 2014). Model improvements such as axonal tract implementation have not significantly altered the response (Giordano and Kleiven, 2014). These characteristics are helpful to increase the anatomical accuracy and allow for more precise investigations.

Finite element models can output many tissue response measures for analysis (stress, strain, pressure, and strain rate); however, few metrics have been validated against cadaveric tests. At present, cadaveric data have been used to validate: intracranial pressure from pressure sensors inserted into the skull (Nahum et al., 1977; Trosseille et al., 1992); relative brain/skull motion from tracking of neutral density targets implanted into the brain of cadavers using high-speed X-rays (Hardy et al., 2001, 2007); and skull stiffness from skull compressions (Nyquist et al., 1986; Yoganandan et al., 1995; Loyd, 2011). Many models use inertial loads from accelerometer recordings distant from the impact site, assuming a rigid skull definition making skull deformation validations unnecessary.

Concussion is described as a rotationally induced strain-based injury (Holbourn, 1943; Ommaya and Gennarelli, 1974; King et al., 2003; Kleiven, 2007; Post and Hoshizaki, 2015) making neutral density target tracking data (Hardy et al., 2001, 2007) the most appropriate validation method as it relates to the relative tissue motion under load. Although intracranial pressure is a commonly used metric to validate models, it is seldom used to measure concussive injuries as it is correlated with linear acceleration (Zhang et al., 2001; King et al., 2003) and has been reported to contribute little to causing brain motion and strain (Hardy et al., 2001; Kleiven, 2007).

Cadaveric validation data are valuable, but they have not kept up pace with finite element model development. For investigations involving concussions, it is important to recognize that metrics used to predict risk of injury are often unable to be validated against cadaveric data. As a result, caution should be exercised when interpreting output metrics as they are representations of tissue response and not exact measures. Model improvements such as axonal tracts with directional responses provide a tool for understanding more complex questions of brain tissue response, and how it relates to risk of concussion. Although the axonal tract response has not yet been validated, their implementation has not negatively affected the model validation (Giordano and Kleiven, 2014) allowing for more anatomically precise representations of tissue response.

Part of the difficulty in predicting risk of concussion over the last several decades has been the evolving definition of a concussion. Historically, concussion was primarily associated with loss of consciousness. Currently, concussion is diagnosed based on the presence of a variety of symptoms with no visible damage on medical images. The symptoms are thought to be the result of physiological cascades following impact (Giza and Hovda, 2001; Hovda, 2014). As a result, research aiming to find a tissue-level threshold for causing concussion has used animal and brain tissue tests designed to elicit a measured physiological response, without causing mechanical injury. A summary of the proposed tissue-related FE metrics associated concussion are presented in Table 4.2.

The above metrics have been employed to calculate risk of concussive injury using logistic regression of concussive and noninjury events. The events driving these regressions were primarily drawn from American football head-to-head impacts and have been used for a variety of FE models (King et al., 2003; Willinger and Baumgartner, 2003; Zhang et al., 2004; Kleiven, 2007). Table 4.3 presents a summary of proposed metric values associated with a 50% risk of concussion from different FE models. Model response will differ based on their size, geometry, mesh density, and material property selection influencing output metric values (Kleiven and Hardy, 2002; Kleiven, 2007; Ji et al., 2014). Values are typically similar across models but cannot be compared as being equal (Figure 4.3).

The large range and standard deviations of MPS values shown in Figure 4.3 can be partially attributed to the variability present with humans. An additional challenge in predicting concussive risk is the sporting environment that people are exposed to, and how changes in impact characteristics contribute to risk of injury. Different sports such as soccer, American football, rugby, and ice hockey are unique in the way the game is played as well as the type of protective equipment that is worn. This results in different impact events (falls, collisions, and projectiles) which then result in different magnitudes

***Table 4.2*** Sources and rationale for use of finite element model metrics in predicting concussion

| Metric | Rationale | Test method | Sources |
|---|---|---|---|
| Maximum principal strain (MPS) | Functional disturbances observed without mechanical damage | Squid axon stretch Guinea pig optic nerve stretch | Galbraith et al. (1993), Bain and Meaney (2000) |
| Strain rate | Strain rate dependent physiological responses | Single axon stretch Strain of cultured cells | Galbraith et al. (1993), LaPlaca et al. (1997) |
| Product of strain and strain rate | Incorporates both strain and strain rate, both of which elicit physiological responses | Ferret impacts | Viano and Lövsund (1999) |
| Von Mises stress | Stress distribution correlated well with observed neurological lesions from a motorcycle accident | Accident reconstruction –modeling | Kang et al. (1997) |
| Cumulative strain damage measure (CSDM) | Quantifies the volume of the brain experiencing strain above a certain level Hypothesized to be associated with diffuse axonal injury | Finite element modeling—simulated event | Bandak and Eppinger (1994) |

***Table 4.3*** Published 50% risk of concussive injury based on several finite element model output metrics. The most common FE metric presented in studies of concussion is MPS. A 50% risk of concussion corresponds with MPS values between 0.19 and 0.26 (Table 4.2). From real-world reconstructions of concussive events shown in Figure 4.1, MPS results consistently above 0.19 demonstrating a significant risk of concussive injury. Even though cases are drawn from a variety of sources and types of events, MPS consistently identifies risk of concussive injury

| Metric value | Metric predicting risk | Location | Source |
|---|---|---|---|
| 0.21 | Maximum principal strain | Corpus callosum | Kleiven (2007) |
| 0.26 | Maximum principal strain | Grey matter | Kleiven (2007) |
| 0.19 | Maximum principal strain | Grey matter | Zhang et al. (2004) |
| 48.5 $s^{-1}$ | Strain rate | Grey matter | Kleiven (2007) |
| 60 $s^{-1}$ | Strain rate | Brain | King et al. (2003) |
| 10.1 $s^{-1}$ | Product of strain and strain rate | Grey matter | Kleiven (2007) |
| 19 $s^{-1}$ | Product of strain and strain rate | Brain | King et al. (2003) |
| 8.4 kPa | Von mises stress | Corpus callosum | Kleiven (2007) |
| 18 kPa[a] | Von mises stress | Brain | Willinger and Baumgartner (2003) |
| 0.47 | CSDM (0.10)[b] | White matter | Kleiven (2007) |
| 0.40[c] | CSDM (0.25) | | Takhounts et al. (2013) |

[a] The value presented by the author corresponds to *moderate neurological lesions*, not solely concussion
[b] CSDM measure based on principal logarithmic strain, not MPS
[c] Threshold as stated by the author refers to AIS3+ injury—stated as a severe concussion, 1–6 hrs unconsciousness

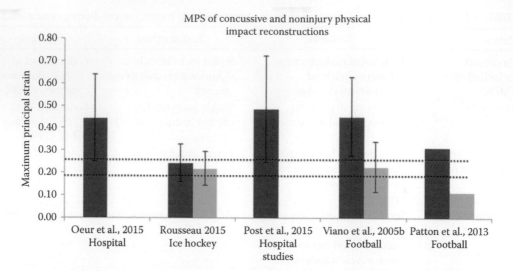

***Figure 4.3*** Maximum principal strain values from reconstructions of concussive events (red) and noninjurious head impacts (green) from various types of events. Dotted black lines represent the range of published MPS values corresponding to 50% risk of concussion.

of accelerations, impact durations, and strain responses in the brain (Kendall et al., 2012; Kendall, 2016), leading to difficulty in predicting injury across different sports.

As improvements in finite element models continue, more precise investigations of the tissue response to impact will be possible. By using a tool that interprets the unique characteristics of impacts across different events as well as the characteristics of brain tissue, complex interactions of impact characteristics can be quantified and compared with a single metric. MPS shows promise in predicting concussion across different types of impact events.

## The relationship between injury events and concussion risk

Concussions have been described as the most common injuries sustained by athletes across all levels of play and age groups in ice hockey (Kelly et al., 1991; Cantu, 1996; Pashby et al., 2001; Goodman et al., 2001; Marchie and Cusimano, 2003; Flik et al., 2005; Agel et al., 2007). How these injuries occur can be quite different depending on the conditions of the impact event within a particular sport (Kendall, 2016). The complexity of the impact events creating the risks associated with concussive injuries makes it difficult to predict injuries.

Recent studies investigating the incidence of concussion in professional ice hockey identified player-to-player collisions (80%–87%) as the most common injury event. This was followed by falls to the ice (8%–12%) and fighting/projectile/other which accounted for the remainder of the injuries (Hutchison et al., 2013; Cantu, 1996; Powell, 1998). Whether it is a fall in sports or a fall outside of sport activity, the impact event leading to the concussion has a significant effect on the kinematics of the head. Each of these impact events is distinct from one another in mass, impact velocity, compliance, and impact location. Collisions commonly experienced in sports typically involve a shoulder or elbow impact to the head (Cusimano et al., 2011; Emery et al., 2010; Hagel et al., 2006; Honey, 1998; Hutchison et al., 2013). Previous research described the striking mass of collision type events to be approximately 12 kg (Rousseau et al., 2015). This mass, coupled with highly compliant protective

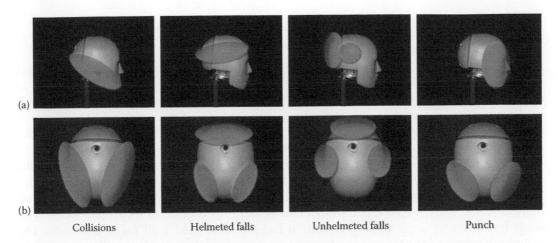

| Collisions | Helmeted falls | Unhelmeted falls | Punch |

*Figure 4.4*  Right side (a) and top view (b) of common impact regions for four different impact events (Collision, Falls [helmeted and unhelmeted], and Punch).

equipment (shoulder pads and elbow pads) and mid impact velocities describe the collision impact events as a mid-high mass (12 kg) + mid velocity (6.5 m/s) + high compliance type impact. Impact locations for these impacts tend to occur to the front-side region of the head (Figure 4.4).

Falls tend to involve the highest striking mass among the impact events due to the head impacting an *immovable* surface (i.e., the ground). The impact velocities are usually related to the individuals' height whereas the impact surfaces can vary depending on the activity and if a helmet is worn. This type of impact event would be described by high mass (immovable), low velocity (3.5–4.5 m/s) impacts with the compliance for the helmeted impacts classified as mid-high compliance, and unhelmeted falls having a low compliance. The most common impact locations vary between these two impact conditions where the helmeted fall injuries primarily occur in the rear and front boss regions of the head due primarily to collision activities in sports creating high-speed impacts to the ground where the player cannot break a fall to protect themselves, whereas unhelmeted falls tend to involve impact to the rear location of the head, likely due to the inability to break the fall after a slip on ice or falling backwards (Figure 4.4). Ice hockey is also unique in that the rules permit fighting at the junior and professional levels which also increase the likelihood of concussive injuries (Donaldson et al., 2013). Other contact sports, such as boxing and mixed martial arts (MMA), are environments with increased concussive injury risk to the athletes. These punch impact events would be characterized by low mass + mid-high velocity as described in previous research by Walilko et al. (2005). Compliance for this type of impact event would be described as mid-level compliance due to human deformability and protective MMA gloves worn by the fighters. Impact locations for punches are primarily to the front and side regions of the head because combatants are facing each other (Figure 4.4). Projectiles are also a source of concussive injury, although less frequent, in sports like ice hockey, baseball, and lacrosse (Gessel et al., 2007). Projectile injuries involve very high velocities (17–27 m/s) coupled with low-mass objects (less than 0.5 kg). Given the low compliance of the projectiles, such as a hockey puck, lacrosse ball, or baseball, these are described as a low mass (>0.5 kg) + high velocity (<15 m/s) + low compliance event. The impact location for projectile events can be highly variable depending on the situation at the time of the injury, that is, battling with a defenseman in front of the net (side or rear of head) versus a batter in baseball facing a 90 mph pitch and unable to get out of the way (front boss region of the head).

Each of these concussive injury events is described by unique combinations of impact parameters (mass, velocity, and compliance). The variance of these parameters specific to each of the impact event creates important differences in linear and rotational dynamic loading curves (Figure 4.5). It is, therefore, important to understand how the different combinations of these parameters influence the strain fields within the brain and ultimately how they influence the risks associated with the concussive injury risk.

Researchers have attempted to describe and quantify brain injury using algorithms involving kinematic parameters (HIC, GAMBIT, and GSI, HIP). Helmet certification standards (ASTM, CSA, and ISO) employ peak linear acceleration to determine helmet performance. While early research has shown that peak linear acceleration correlates well with skull fracture and intracranial pressure, it has not correlated well for concussions. The use of a single peak linear acceleration value or an algorithm employing linear response

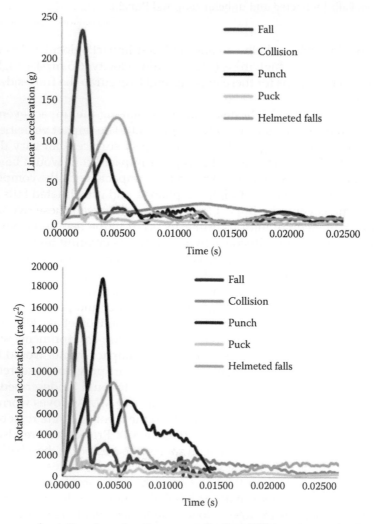

*Figure 4.5*  Linear and rotational acceleration curves for five different concussive impact events.

*Table 4.4* Kinematic and MPS values from different concussive injury impact events

| Concussive injury impact event | Impact duration (s) | Peak linear acc. (g) | Peak angular acc. (rad/s²) | MPS | HIC | GSI |
|---|---|---|---|---|---|---|
| Collisions | 0.025 | 29.5 | 3221 | 0.32 | 30.9 | 32.6 |
| | (0.003) | (9.6) | (1379) | (0.12) | (21.2) | (29.4) |
| Falls (helmeted) | 0.014 | 113.7 | 7783 | 0.51 | 337.5 | 664.0 |
| | (0.003) | (48.5) | (2957) | (0.14) | (245.8) | (606.0) |
| Falls (unhelmeted) | 0.004 | 291.9 | 18,631 | 0.55 | 153.5 | 1587.6 |
| | (0.001) | (84.1) | (5745) | (0.13) | (95.9) | (1003.4) |
| Punches | 0.007 | 75.4 | 12,228 | 0.50 | 31.9 | 98.9 |
| | (0.001) | (30.4) | (5344) | (0.16) | (24.0) | (85.3) |
| [a]Projectile | 0.002 | 111.1 | 10,800 | 0.19 | 6 | 76 |
| | | (5.0) | (1,100) | (0.01) | | |

[a]  Data from Rousseau, P., Analysis of concussion metrics of real-world and noninjurious elbow and shoulder to head collisions in ice hockey (PhD dissertation), Ottawa, Canada: University of Ottawa, 2014—Protective capacity of ice hockey player helmets again puck impacts—DOI:10.1520/STP155220120159.

characteristics is not sufficient to define risk for concussive impact events. This is evident in the data presented in Table 4.4, where a wide range of values for peak linear, peak angular, HIC, and GSI values across four concussive injury events can be observed. Although all the injury events in this dataset were confirmed concussions, the dynamic response variables in this table do not indicate what has been reported as high risk for concussive injury. Maximal principal strain values for each of the different concussive injury events were, however, consistent with reported values for a 50% risk of concussive injury.

Concussive injury risk thresholds for GSI were developed to compare impacts with different acceleration–time curves as they relate to the proposed concussive injury risks. GSI values of 24, 291, and 559 were associated with a 5%, 50%, and 95% risk for concussion, respectively (Newman, 2002). Based on these threshold values, only the helmeted and unhelmeted falls would be above a 50% risk for concussive injury. For the HIC calculation, a tolerance value for the HIC calculation was set to 1000 for life threatening head injuries; however, thresholds for concussive injury were estimated to be between 150 and 400 (Prasad and Mertz, 1985). Once again, only the helmeted and unhelmeted falls present greater than a 50% risk for concussive injury. Considering that the algorithms for the GSI and HIC calculation come from cadaveric and animal head drop tests, it is not surprising that these metrics successfully identified as high risk for concussion for similar fall impact events (helmeted and unhelmeted). On the other hand, these metrics did not demonstrate a risk to concussion for the remaining impact events. These findings highlight the challenge of using a single dynamic response metric to predict injury risk for the various impact events that can lead to concussion.

Peak acceleration values are often used to determine concussive injury risk; however, a recent study revealed that each event may be characterized by a combination of completely different dynamic response variables dependant on the specific event characteristics (Kendall, 2016). This study reported that peak linear acceleration was not influential in characterizing concussive injury in impact events with the exception of collisions. More specifically, each injury event was primarily characterized by a unique dynamic response variable; for example; punch events were characterized by resultant angular velocity whereas unhelmeted falls were characterized by directional peak linear and angular acceleration and pulse durations. Although peak dynamic response variables were unable to consistently identify high risk for concussive injury, MPS reported 50% risk for concussive injury across all injury events. Although MPS seems to be a good indicator for concussive injury, this variable is not easily measured. Concussive risk thresholds are event specific and need to be established for each type of concussive injury event. The use of current single dynamic response parameters to assess concussive injury risk may not be appropriate for the numerous types of impact events resulting in concussion. In addition, it is important to understand how the different impact parameters influence injury risk during each event and how they relate to one another.

## Tissue trauma and brain injury

Neurological injuries sustained from head impacts do not always exhibit signs or symptoms indicating neurocognitive dysfunction with concussion only partially predicted by the trauma load. Traumatic brain injury may not be appropriately classified as a dichotomy (injury versus no injury) but rather a series of injuries each with a unique mechanism. This paradigm will be described in the context of the head/brain's response to head contact as successive cumulative stages represented by three grades from the lowest to highest strain levels: (1) molecular changes (trauma induced protein changes), (2) metabolic alterations (concussion), (3) and structural damage (severe injury). There is increased documentation of the long-term consequences of low-magnitude head impacts that present no immediate consequences but increase one's risk for the second impact syndrome and have the potential to present serious progressive neurodegeneration. This supports the notion that repetitive concussion and trauma-induced protein changes (TIPC) as well as high-energy injuries lead to psychiatric disorders and cognitive deficits. Trauma-induced brain injuries are complex representing a variety of mechanisms and types of injuries with overlapping and inconsistent symptoms. Molecular changes to cellular protein, metabolic response to changes in the semipermeable membrane, damage to white matter, vascular structures, and skull fracture all interfere with the functions of the brain.

Grade-III head injuries represent the most severe, causing immediate and detectible structural damage as the materials composing the human skull/brain complex are unable to deal with high level of stress created by the impact and fail. Traumatic, life-threatening injury mechanisms within sport are often the result of high-energy impacts, such as in motor racing, cycling, and ski-snowboard accidents. These events typically involve falling onto a hard or low compliant surface such as concrete or ice resulting in high magnitude, short-duration accelerations (Depreitere et al., 2004; Post et al., 2012a; Post, 2013). As one can imagine, these injuries are easily identified and require immediate medical attention. Crash helmets were originally designed for use in these applications; however, with concerns of serious injury and death in American football, helmet use and safety standards graduated into the contact sporting realm (P. D. Halstead et al., pers. comm., 2004; Newman, 2005). Following the implementation of mandatory use of helmets within contact sports, catastrophic outcomes became rare transferring concern to concussion and TIPC (Bailes and Cantu, 2001).

Despite the absence of macroscopic damage, axonal brain tissue strains causing a grade-II head injury may be present and reveal themselves through clinical symptoms reflecting a temporary functional disturbance, defined as a concussion. It has been well documented that without evidence of damage, the metabolic functioning of neuronal cell is altered following impacts of concussive injury levels (Katayama et al., 1990; Giza and Hovda, 2001). This temporary neuronal dysfunction expresses in the form of ionic shifts, altered metabolism, impaired connectivity, and/or changes in neurotransmission (Julian and Goldman, 1962; Takahashi et al., 1981; Hubschmann and Korhauser, 1983; Katayama et al., 1990; Giza and Hovda, 2001). An increased demand for energy coupled with a reduced cerebral blood flow leads to a discrepancy between supply and demand for glucose putting the brain in a state of cellular energy crisis (Yuan et al., 1998; Giza and Hovda, 2001). This response contributes to the signs and symptoms that we recognize as concussion. Clinical symptoms, however, may not solely be the product of axonal strains but may arise from other parts of the neurons, the vasculature, or a multitude of anatomical structures within the brain/skull complex and may not involve brain tissue (Gennarelli, 2015). Consequently, concussive level impacts resulting in metabolic shifts yet lacking symptoms may go undiagnosed. The way we presently rely on observable symptoms as a way to monitor recovery may not be prudent as axonal degeneration and functional impairment could be present and remain despite cognitive recovery (Creed et al., 2011). Therefore, current means of defining and diagnosing concussions through the presence of symptoms are likely providing an incomplete representation of brain trauma exposure and risk to recurrent injury. Furthermore, impacts that do not present with signs and symptoms may be contributing to TIPC, grade-I injuries, with the potential to lead to structural injury and degeneration of neurons (Omalu et al., 2005; McKee et al., 2009, 2013). Neurological disorders are closely associated with activities involving direct impacts to the head. Under particular conditions, unstable proteins miss fold or unfold preventing them from forming into their biochemically functional native form. These toxic conformations have the ability to form aggregates creating neurofibrillary tangles and neuropil threads leading to neural cell degeneration (Stefani and Dobson, 2003; McKee et al., 2013). Further amplifying the process, these toxic configurations have the ability to interact with nearby native proteins that catalyze their transition into a similar toxic state. There is considerable evidence that shows patients who have suffered a single moderate to severe traumatic brain injury are at an increased risk of developing cognitive impairments from progressive and psychiatric disorders (Masel and DeWitt, 2010). Today, there is growing evidence suggesting that neural tissues experiencing repetitive head impacts and, showing no immediate consequences, have the potential to manifest into a progressive disease causing serious disability (Omalu et al., 2005; McKee et al., 2009, 2013). Neurological consequences of repetitive head impacts date back to 1928 when Martland was the first to describe similar risks and neuropsychiatric sequelae from chronic exposure to repeat brain trauma Martland (1928). He termed this *punch drunk* as a way to describe the symptoms that were being demonstrated by boxers who had sustained multiple hits to the head. A number of published reports on the risks of repeat impact within boxing are followed (Millspaugh, 1937; Brandenburg and Hallervorden, 1954; Courville, 1962; Roberts, 1969; Corsellis et al., 1973; Mendez, 1995). It was not until a little over a decade ago when a similar neuropathology was observed upon autopsy of a retired National Football League player (Omalu et al., 2005), which is now widely known as chronic traumatic encephalopathy or CTE. CTE resulting from trauma-induced protein changes (TIPC) has now been observed in boxing, BMX cycling, American football, ice hockey, and rugby. Particularly, those who have or are participating in contact sports and activities where head trauma has a repetitive nature are the greatest risk (Bieniek et al., 2015; Kondo et al., 2015). Kondo and researchers (2015) have shown similar durations of elevated levels of pathogenic *cis* phosphorylated tau protein in a repeat trauma model to one of a single severe traumatic event. What this indicates is that lower magnitude brain trauma, if repetitive, may show similar pathological outcomes to one traumatic event, suggesting that there may be a similar neurological risk associated with the cumulative effect of trauma to neural tissues (Kondo et al., 2015).

There may be a risk in relying on the presence of symptoms as a way of identifying the point at which brain trauma becomes dangerous and risks to grade-I and II head injury are present. Yuen and colleagues (2009) used cell cultures to show that a 5% strain was the minimum level of injury required to induce a calcium influx and interestingly observed a significant increase in calcium when two subthreshold injuries were repeated within 24 hrs. Considering that one who has sustained a grade-II injury becomes more susceptible to repeat injury (Cantu, 1998), and that subsequent injuries are often more severe, it may be postulated that as the brain is initially injured and in a state of energy crises, a lower magnitude impact could potentially have a similar injurious effect, potentially involving cell death (Giza and Hovda, 2001; Guskiewicz et al., 2003). If a second insult is experienced during the window of vulnerability, that of decreased cerebral metabolic rate of glucose, the degree of depressive state increases and prolongs the duration of recovery (DeFord et al., 2002; Creeley et al., 2004; Longhi et al., 2005; Friess et al., 2009; Prins et al., 2013).

A relationship between head trauma and long-term disability has been documented, although the amount of energy that is required to cause grade-I injury is very much still speculation. However, as low as 5%–15% brain strain levels have been associated with functional impairment of signal transmission in the absence of structural damage (Bain and Meaney, 2000; Singh et al., 2006; Elkin and Morrison, 2007; Yuen et al., 2009; Zanetti et al., 2013). Reconstructions of head impacts with no reported symptoms experienced by American football lineman during game play show 20–30 g head accelerations with strain values of 9%–11% (Zanetti et al., 2013). As these athletes are experiencing conceivable estimates of upwards of 1000 head impacts over one season (Bazarian et al., 2014; Schnebel et al., 2007; Crisco et al., 2010, 2011), the cumulative effect of TIPC must be considered.

As CTE is often not evident until many years post-trauma, research has focused, in part, on ways to identify axonal damage immediately following trauma even in the absence of cognitive signs and symptoms. The physiological response to trauma may be detectable within blood and cerebrospinal fluid (CSF) in the form of elevated levels of biological makers that, overtime, may lead to an accumulation of protein tangles and neurofil aggregates (Petzold et al., 2008; Shahani and Brandt, 2002). Elevated levels of neurofilament light protein and total-tau (T-tau) have been measured in athletes participating in contact sports such as boxing and ice hockey. These observations were made in the blood and CSF of athletes sustaining head impacts resulting in concussion as well as those not presenting with symptoms. Interestingly, axonal biomarkers remained elevated for longer durations in knock-out boxers vs both no knock-out boxers and concussed ice hockey players (Zetterberg et al., 2006; Neselius et al., 2012, 2015; Shahim et al., 2014). These findings suggest that trauma frequency and/or time interval may be contributing to long-term damage, and that damage can be detected in the absence of concussive levels magnitudes.

Using symptoms to characterize risks to CTE has not been informative in measuring overall trauma exposure associated with neurodegeneration associated with repetitive TIPC. Research involving trauma exposure has indicated that in addition to the magnitude of the impact, the frequency of the trauma and time interval between impacts to the head may interact to create risks of chronic neurodegeneration (Koerte et al., 2012; McKee et al., 2013; Bazarian et al., 2014; Banks et al., 2014; Bernick et al., 2015; Oliver et al., 2016; Montenigro et al., 2016). Similar reports have also supported this relationship using diffusion tensor imaging (DTI) and functional magnetic resonance imaging (fMRI) measures following asymptomatic head trauma (Cubon et al., 2011; Bazarian et al., 2012, 2014; Breedlove et al., 2012; Koerte et al., 2012; Talavage et al., 2014). Significant relationships have been reported between neurophysiological changes detected by fMRI and the number of head hits experienced (Breedlove et al., 2012). Moreover, changes in DTI measures worsened in athletes who experienced a higher number of impacts exceeding an estimated rotational acceleration threshold (Bazarian et al., 2014). Using biomarker methodologies, Oliver and researchers (2016) compared serum levels of neurofilament light polypeptide (NFL) in American football players at 4 measurement points over the course of one season. Starting athletes experienced significant increases in serum neurofilament light protein levels throughout the season compared with both nonstarters and controls, where changes coincided with an increase in intensity and hours of contact. Characterized as a tauopathy disease, research on how CTE manifests itself has postulated a similar mechanism to a number of other neurodegenerative diseases (Iliff et al., 2012, 2013; Jessen et al., 2015). It has been proposed that the accumulation of disrupted protein in CTE cases may result as the brain's ability to clear waste from the brain parenchyma is overwhelmed and/or compromised ultimately leading to cell degeneration. Furthermore, as levels of tau protein remain elevated within a chronic state and accumulation of perivascular tau takes place, blood–brain barrier dysfunction results, potentially exacerbating pathology (Blair et al., 2015). This is supported by consistent findings indicating the role of length of athletic career and overall amount of exposure to head trauma as significant contributors of behavioral and cognitive abnormalities (McKee et al., 2013; Banks et al., 2014; Bernick et al., 2015; Stamm et al., 2015; Montenigro et al., 2016).

A variety of mechanisms and types of trauma-induced brain injuries exist, and what we presently define as a concussion injury represents a level of trauma eliciting functional disturbances in the absence of gross structural damage. However, impacts of lower magnitudes of neuronal tissue trauma as evidenced through changes in cellular proteins are putting athletes at risk long term. The molecular changes caused by trauma are the precursor for suffering neurocognitive deficits consistent with neurological degenerative diseases later in life. This is amplified by trauma that causes physiological response. Knowing this, brain trauma risk assessment cannot be limited to concussion and severe traumatic injuries, because they are not the only cause of long-term brain degeneration; TIPC should also be considered and biomarkers should be tracked when attempting to evaluate the brain-injury risk associated with a given sport. Consideration of cumulative brain trauma exposure is warranted when dealing with the long-term brain health of athletes and sports participants.

## Measuring brain trauma in sport

Measuring the head's response to insult and establishing tolerance limits for the neuronal tissues within the human head are the two primary objectives set by impact scientists. Direct measurement of brain tissue deformation would be useful in predicting concussion; yet the methods to do so are invasive and cannot be used with human subjects. Thus, most of the research is concentrated on identifying relatively simple injury metrics to predict concussion risk. Kinematic parameters do not describe all injury mechanisms associated with concussion; however, they provide information to be useful in predicting and prevention of concussion. Laboratory reconstructions of impacts enable the study of impact characteristics to isolate their influence on injury risk. For these reasons, the following methodologies are currently used to assess the safety of equipment and play environments based on the assumption that a decrease in one parameter results in a decrease in all other parameters.

The moral and ethical challenges associated with the use of human subjects can be resolved by reconstructing real-world collisions in laboratory. Multiple cameras, documented athlete information, injuries diagnosed by physicians, and recovery time in professional sports provide an opportunity to obtain good head injury data. The first step when attempting to reconstruct an event post-hoc is video analysis. This step provides valuable information to reconstruct an event in laboratory using physical models or computer simulations. To reconstruct a head impact, the following parameters need to be determined: (a) velocity, (b) orientation, (c) location, (d) effective mass, and (e) compliance. Impact velocity can be calculated using the distance and time from video recordings of the event. Distance can be measured once the video coordinates are transformed into real-world coordinates. This process can be challenging when using a noncalibrated camera yet can be achieved using known distances visible in the field of the camera to convert pixels to meters. Anatomical features, standard equipment size, and field markings have all been used to calibrate the field of view (McIntoshet al., 2000; Pellman et al., 2003; Rousseau, 2014). Impact location and direction are obtained using close-ups of the impact as well as by doing a qualitative comparison of the kinematic reaction between the struck head form and the game footage.

Effective mass and compliance of an event cannot be calculated using video footage; they can, however, be estimated once the nature of the object coming into contact with the head is identified. Falls can be easily replicated in laboratory once the characteristics of the material forming the playing surface (e.g., turf, loose soil, ice) are known. Impacts caused by a projectile can also be replicated by propelling the same object (e.g., baseball, hockey puck) toward the head surrogate. Player-to-player collisions on the other hand are complex events that require a more profound analysis. The effective striking mass of a player coming into contact with another player's head is a product of the mass of the body part coming into contact with the head as well as the additional muscular and inertial forces applied by the striking athlete. Athletes involved in contact sports are taught to anticipate a collision and position themselves by flexing their knees, leaning forward, keeping their feet shoulder-width apart, and driving their legs through the collision. Thus, athletes can manipulate their effective impact mass and each sport-specific striking techniques must be analyzed in laboratory with the help of skilled participants (Viano et al., 2005; Walilko et al. 2005a; Withnall et al., 2005; Rousseau and Hoshizaki, 2015).

The second step in recreating the event involves obtaining five impact characteristics from the video. This can be done using surrogate human bodies or computer simulations. For example, Hybrid III anthropometric test devices were used to reconstruct impacts in American football, ice hockey, and soccer (Pellman et al., 2003; Withnall et al., 2005; Rousseau, 2014) because the hybrid III head form can be outfitted with accelerometers which record the three-dimensional linear and angular acceleration of the head following an impact at a high sampling rate (20 kHz) (Padgaonkar et al., 1975). This is an important feature because head impacts typically last between 3 and 40 ms (Pellman et al., 2003; Rousseau, 2014; Rousseau and Hoshizaki, 2015) and impulse features such as peak and event duration can be lost at lower sampling rates. The hybrid III head surrogate is typically used for the reconstruction of direct impacts despite being developed to mimic the motion of the human head following an impulse to the body during a car accident (i.e., an indirect impact). This preference could be explained by the device's reliability and robustness. Although the low compliance of the bare steel head form may amplify peak acceleration and reduce the impulse time of unprotected head impacts, this effect is most likely mitigated by the increase in compliance present in a body-to-head collision to a helmeted head such as those commonly seen in American football or ice hockey.

Computer simulations using numerical models have also been used to measure the motion of the head upon impact. Mathematical dynamic models (MADYMO), a rigid-body model, were used to recreate rugby and Australian rules football collisions (Fréchède and McIntosh, 2009). Computer simulations are valuable when reconstructing complex events because the rigid-body models can be used to reproduce the relative motion of each player before and after impact. Furthermore, the mass and inertia of each body segment can be adjusted to match the known anthropometry of the athletes involved in the collision. Computer models are often preferred because they are less time consuming than physical reconstructions. Unfortunately, computer simulations do not reliably replicate the complex interactions that exist between the five impact parameters, more notably, the influence of compliance. Most contact sports are played with equipment of varying mass and compliance. Although they can be easily included in physical reconstructions, they need to be digitized with their precise mechanical properties defined when performing a computer simulation. Basic characteristics such as mass and size can be digitized but the equipment's interaction with velocity, location, orientation, and effective mass is often undefined making it extremely challenging to accurately digitize.

Reconstructions conducted using surrogate head forms or computer models provide researchers with the ability to measure the dynamic response of the cranium; yet it is important to remember that the measured acceleration is a reflection of the tools used by impact biomechanics researchers and cannot be readily generalized to the human population until an adequate validation protocol is established. Nevertheless, surrogate head forms can be an appropriate tool to evaluate safety of helmets and other protective devices (e.g., playground structures) where reliability and reproducibility are valued over validity. Numerical reconstructions also provide data concerning head motion, often at a lower operating cost and can be used for complex events.

In efforts to manage the potential negative long-term effects of repeated impacts sustained during sport, a number of head impact sensor technologies have been developed to assist coaches and parents in monitoring the amount of brain trauma sustained by athletes (Crisco et al., 2010; Oeur et al., 2014). Information obtained from head impact sensor technologies can provide measures of brain trauma for athletes over the course of a game or season of play and support informed decisions about managing accumulated brain trauma. Although the potential benefits of head/helmet sensors are attractive, it is important to recognize the systems have not been fully validated. To be effective, head impact sensors need to be tested using scientifically rigorous test protocols to ensure that they provide accurate information and report reliable information.

While the potential benefits of using in-game sensors are undeniable, their limitations are numerous and the systems used in American football or ice hockey helmets have not yet been sufficiently validated to be used for advanced biomechanical analyses. The systems were validated for impacts through the center of gravity of a hybrid III head form at low velocity (Gwin et al., 2006) despite the fact that most head collisions occur at high velocity and the impact vectors are typically not in line with the center of gravity of the athlete's head (Pellman et al., 2003; Rousseau, 2014). This is concerning because it is common for the helmet and the head to decouple when hit off axis at high velocity, resulting in erroneous data (Allison et al., 2014; Jadishke et al., 2013). Moreover, the systems measured head acceleration at a sampling rate of 1000 Hz and filtered using a 400 Hz low-pass filter, both of which are below the 10,000 Hz collection rate and 1650 Hz low-pass filter recommended by the industry (SAE, 2007). Using such a low collection rate and filter to capture acceleration during direct impacts to a helmeted head prevents researchers from obtaining accurate impulse peaks and durations. This is problematic because impulse characteristics are used to drive finite element models; inaccurate input data will invariably lead to inaccurate concussion risk assessments.

Although in-game measurement tools are not yet adequate for concussion prediction, they are useful for tracking the number and frequency of head impacts. As discussed earlier in this chapter, brain tissue is sensitive to low disturbances and a high frequency of them may lead to the early onset of neurological dysfunction.

Predicting brain tissue deformation is challenging because the brain is an organic, viscoelastic structure highly dependent on the magnitude, rate, location, and orientation of an applied stress. Thus, it is critical to measure and report accurately the entirety of the impulse created by a direct impact to the head using a reliable methodology. The emergence of sophisticated brain models provides an opportunity to study the mechanism of traumatic brain injuries. Although these models can calculate the brain tissue's response to an impact, three-dimensional acceleration curves are required as input. Physical reconstructions and computer simulations can provide the necessary dynamic response that best approximates a real-world event. In-game data measurements are not yet able to provide the data necessary to drive a finite element brain model, yet the instruments can provide valuable data concerning impact count and frequency. Considering that brain injuries are complex in nature and cannot easily be measured or predicted, there cannot be a consensus on which method is best to measure the trauma resulting from an impact. Laboratory reconstructions are reliable and reproducible, which make them appropriate methods to measure the acceleration curve magnitude and shape of real-world collisions whereas in-game data devices allow for the measurement of impact count and frequency in real-world conditions. A combination of both methods will most likely be necessary to finally understand how to predict the occurrence of a brain injury.

The emergence of sophisticated brain models provides an opportunity to study the mechanism of traumatic brain injuries. Although these models calculate the brain tissue's response to an impact, three-dimensional acceleration curves are required as input. Physical reconstructions and computer simulations provide the necessary dynamic response that best approximates a real-world event. In-game data measurements are not yet able to provide the quality of data necessary to drive a finite element brain model, yet the instruments can provide valuable data concerning impact count and frequency. Considering that brain injuries are complex and not easily be measured or predicted, there is no consensus on which method is best to measure the severity of an impact. Laboratory reconstructions are reliable and reproducible which makes them appropriate methods to measure the magnitude and curve shape of real-world collisions while in-game data devices allow for the measurement of impact count and frequency in real-world conditions. A combination of both methods will most likely be necessary to finally understand and predict brain injuries in sport.

## Conclusion

Head trauma in sport has been described as causing transient concussions, persistent concussions, traumatic brain injuries, skull fractures, and more recently neurological disorders including chronic traumatic encephalopathy. Sport is, by definition, an artificial endeavor governed by rules designed to maintain fair play and safety. Understanding the biomechanical characteristics of an impact event and its relationship for predicting brain injury involves defining accurate and reliable predictors. Recent research describing the relationship between the visco-elastic properties of brain tissue and duration of the impact event contributes to a better understanding and prediction of brain injury risk. Whether the injury event involves a fall, collision, punch, or a projectile defines biomechanical impact characteristics that are important in predicting the risk for brain tissue injury. Understanding the relationship between injury and brain tissue trauma is not fully described by the signs and symptoms associated with concussions and requires a better understanding of the effect of brain tissue trauma at molecular and cellular levels on neurological injury. Finally, a number of methods for measuring impact characteristics are available with each data measurement system having both benefits and limitations. No system is without limitations, and the resulting data have to be treated within the limitations of the system. As well, each system does provide valuable information contributing to better understanding the relationship between the impact event and risk of injury. This continued search to better define the association between event characteristics and the risk of concussion injury has important implications in setting policy to govern safety in sport, establish performance parameters to certify safety equipment including helmets and sport surfaces, and create safe rules of play for sporting activities. Understanding the relationship between characteristics that describe head impacts and how they contribute the risk of concussion injuries is essential to this endeavor.

## *References*

Agel, J., Dompier, T. P., Dick, R., and Marshall, S.W. (2007). Descriptive epidemiology of collegiate men's ice hockey injuries: National Collegiate Athletic Association injury surveillance system, 1988-1989 through 2003-2004. *Journal of Athletic Training*, 42(2), 241–248.

Allison, M. A., Kang, Y. S., Bolte, J. H., Maltese, M. R., and Arbogast, K. B. (2014). Validation of a helmet-based system to measure head impact biomechanics in ice hockey. *Medicine and Science in Sports and Exercise*, 46(1), 115–123.

Backaitis, S. H. (1981). The head injury criterion. In *Head and Neck Injury Criteria: A Consensus Workshop* (pp. 175–177). Washington, DC: US Department of Transportation.

Bailes, J. E. and Cantu, R. C. (2001). Head injury in athletes. *Neurosurgery*, 48(1), 26–45.

Bain, A. C. and Meaney, D. F. (2000). Tissue-level thresholds for axonal damage in an experimental model of central nervous system white matter injury. *Journal of Biomechanical Engineering*, 122(6), 615–622.

Bandak, F. A. and Eppinger, R. H. (1994). A three-dimensional finite element analysis of the human brain under combined rotational and translational accelerations. In *Proceedings of the 38th Stapp Car Crash Conference* (Vol. 38, pp. 145–163), Warrendale, PA.

Banks, S. J., Mayer, B., Obuchowski, N., Shin, W., Lowe, M., and Phillips, M. (2014). Impulsiveness in professional fighters. *The Journal of Neuropsychiatry and Clinical Neuroscience*, 26(1), 44–50.

Bazarian, J. J., Zhu, T., Blyth, B., Borrino, A., and Zhong, J. (2012). Subject-specific changes in brain white matter on diffusion tensor imaging after sports-related concussion. *Magnetic Resonance Imaging*, 30(2), 171–180.

Bazarian, J. J., Zhu, T., Zhong, J., Janigro, D., Rozen, E., Roberts, A., Javien, H., Merchant-Borna, K., Abar, B., and Blackman, E. G. (2014). Persistent, long-term cerebral white matter changes after sports-related repetitive head impacts. *PLoS ONE*, 9(4), e94734.

Bernick, C., Banks, S. J., Shin, W., Obuchowski, N., Butler, S., Noback, M., Phillips, M., Lowe, M., Jones, S., and Modic, M. (2015). Repeated head trauma is associated with smaller thalamic volumes and slower processing speed: The professional fighters' brain health study. *British Journal of Sports Medicine*, 49(15), 1007–1011.

Bieniek, K. F., Ross, O. A., Cormier, K. A., Walton, R. L., Soto-Ortolaza, A., Johnston, A. E., DeSaro, P., Boylan, K. B., Graff-Radford, N. R., Wszolek, Z. K., and Rademakers, R. (2015). Chronic traumatic encephalopathy pathology in a neurodegenerative disorders brain bank. *Acta Neuropathologica*, 130(6), 877–889.

Blair, L. J., Frauen, H. D., Zhang, B. O., Nordhues, B. A., Bijan, S., Lin, Y. C., Zamudio, F., Hernandez, L. D., Sabbagh, J. J., Selenica, M. L. B., and Dickey, C. A. (2015). Tau depletion prevents progressive blood-brain barrier damage in a mouse model of tauopathy. *Acta Neuropathologica Communications*, 3(1), 1–22.

Brandenburg, W. and Hallervorden, J. (1954). Dementia pugilistica with anatomical findings. *Virchows Archiv für pathologische Anatomie und Physiologie und für klinische Medizin*, 325(6), 680–709.

Breedlove, E. L., Robinson, M., Talavage, T. M., Morigaki, K. E., Yoruk, U., O'Keefe, K., King, J., Leverenz, L. J., Gilger, J. W., and Nauman, E.A. (2012). Biomechanical correlates of symptomatic and asymptomatic neurophysiological impairment in high school football. *Journal of Biomechanics*, 45(7), 1265–1272.

Cantu, R. C. (1992). Cerebral concussion in sport. *Sports Medicine*, 14(1), 64–74.

Cantu, R. C. (1996). Head injuries in sport. *British Journal of Sports Medicine*, 30(4), 289–296.

Cantu, R. C. (1998). Second-impact syndrome. *Clinics in Sports Medicine*, 17(1), 37–44.

Casson, I. R., Viano, D. C., Powell, J. W., and Pellman, E. J. (2010). Twelve years of national football league concussion data. *Sports Health: A Multidisciplinary Approach*, 2(6), 471–483.

Chatelin, S., Vappou, J., Roth, S., Raul, J. S., and Willinger, R. (2012). Towards child versus adult brain mechanical properties. *Journal of the Mechanical Behaviour of Biomedical Materials*, 6, 166–173.

Corsellis, J. A., Bruton, C. J., and Freeman-Browne, D. (1973). The aftermath of boxing. *Psychological Medecine*, 3(3), 270–303.

Courville, C. B. (1962). Punch drunk, its pathogenesis and pathology on the basis of a verified case. *Bulletin of the Los Angel Neurological Society*, 27, 160–168.

Creed, J. A., Wozniak, D. F., Bayly, P. V., Oley, J. W., and Lewis, L. M. (2011). Concussive brain trauma in the mouse results in acute cognitive and sustained impairment of axonal function. *Journal of Neurotrauma*, 28(4), 547–563.

Creeley, C. E., Wozniak, D. F., Bayly, P. V., Olney, J. W., and Lewis, L. M. (2004). Multiple episodes of mild traumatic brain injury result in impaired cognitive performance in mice. *Academic Emergency Medicine*, 11(8), 809–819.

Crisco, J. J., Fiore, R., Beckwith, J. G., Chu, J. J., Brolinson, P. G., Duma, S., McAllister, T. W., Duhaime, A.-C., and Greenwald, R. M. (2010). Frequency and location of head impact exposures in individual collegiate football players, *Journal of Athletic Training*, 45(6), 549–559.

Crisco, J. J., Wilcox, B. J., Beckwith, J. G., Chu, J. J., Duhaine, A.-C., Rowson, S., Duma, S. M., Maerlender, A. C., McAllister, T. W., and Greenwald, R. M. (2011). Head impact exposure in collegiate football players. *Journal of Biomechanics*, 44(15), 2673–2678.

CSA. (2015). *Ice Hockey Helmets* (Z262.1-15). Toronto, Canada: Canadian Standard Association.

Cubon, V. A., Putukian, M., Boyer, C., and Dettwiler, A. (2011). A diffusion tensor imaging study on the white matter skeleton in individuals with sports-related concussion. *Journal of Neurotrauma*, 28(2), 189–201.

Daneshvar, D. H., Nowinski, C. J., McKee, A. C., and Cantu, R. C. (2011). The epidemiology of sport-related concussion. *Clinics in Sports Medicine*, 30(1), 1–17.

DeFord, S. M., Wilson, M. S., Rice, A. C., Clausen, T., Rice, L. K., Barabnova, A., Bullock, R., and Hamm, R. J. (2002). Repeated mild brain injuries result in cognitive impairment in B6C3F1 mice. *Journal of Neurotrauma*, 19(4), 427–438.

Depreitere, B., Lierde, C. V., Maene, S., Plets, C., Vander Sloten, J., Van Audekercke, R., Van der Perre, G., and Goffin, J. (2004). Bicycle-related head injury: A study of 86 cases. *Accident Analysis & Prevention*, 36(4), 561–567.

Donnelly, B. R. and Medige, J. (1997). Shear properties of human brain tissue. *Journal of Biomechanical Engineering*, 119(4), 423–432.

Doorly, M. C. and Gilchrist, M. D. (2006). The use of accident reconstruction for the analysis of traumatic brain injury due to head impacts arising from falls. *Computer Methods in Biomechanics and Biomedical Engineering*, 9(6), 371–377.

Elkin, B. S. and Morrison III, B. (2007). Region-specific tolerance criteria for the living brain. *Stapp Car Crash Journal*, 51, 127–138.

Fallenstein, G. T., Hulce, V. D., and Melvin, J. W. (1969). Dynamic mechanical properties of human brain tissue. *Journal of Biomechanics*, 2(3), 217–226.

Flik, K., Lyman, S., and Marx, R. G. (2005). American collegiate men's ice hockey: An analysis of injuries. *American Journal of Sports Medicine*, 33(2), 183–187.

Forero Rueda, M. A., Cui, L., and Gilchrist, M. D. (2011). Finite element modelling of equestrian helmet impacts exposes the need to address rotational kinematics in future helmet designs. *Computer Methods in Biomechanics and Biomedical Engineering*, 14(12), 1021–1031.

Fréchède, B. and McIntosh, A. (2009). Numerical reconstruction of real-life concussive football impacts. *Medicine and Science in Sports and Exercise*, 41(2), 390–398.

Friess, S. H., Ichord, R. N., Ralston, J., Ryall, K., Helfaer, M. A., Smith, C., and Margulies, S. S. (2009). Repeated traumatic brain injury affects composite cognitive function in piglets. *Journal of Neurotrauma*, 26(7), 1111–1121.

Gadd, C.W. (1966). Use of a weighted impulse criterion for estimating injury hazard. SAE Technical Paper 660793. doi: 10.4271/660793.

Galbraith, J. A., Thibault, L. E., and Matteson, D. R. (1993). Mechanical and electrical responses of the squid axon to simple elongation. *Journal of Biomechanical Engineering*, 115(1), 13–22.

Gefen, A., Gefen, N., Zhu, Q., Raghupathi, R., and Margulies, S. S. (2003). Age-dependent changes in material properties of the brain and braincase of the rat. *Journal of Neurotrauma*, 20(11), 1163–1177.

Gennarelli, T. A. (1983). Head injury in man and experimental animals: Clinical aspects. *Acta Neurochirurgica, Suppl*, 32, 1–13.

Gennarelli, T. A. (2015). The Centripetal theory of concussion (CTC) revisited after 40 years and a proposed new symptomcentric concept of the concussions. In *Proceedings of IRCOBI Conference* (No. IRC-15-02). Zurich, Switzerland: International Research Council on the Biomechanics of Impact.

Gennarelli, T. A., Thibault, L. E., Adams, J. H., Graham, D. I., Thompson, C. J., and Marcincin, R. P. (1982). Diffuse axonal injury and traumatic coma in the primate. *Annals of Neurology*, 12(6), 564–574.

Gennarelli, T., Thibault, L. E., Tomei, G., Wiser, R., Graham, D., and Adams, J. (1987). Directional dependence of axonal brain injury due to centroidal and non-centroidal acceleration. In *Proceedings of the 31st Stapp Car Crash Conference* (No. 872197). Zurich, Switzerland: International Research Council on the Biomechanics of Impact.

Gessel, L. M., Fields, S. K., Collins, C. L., Dick, R. W., and Comstock, R. D. (2007). Concussions among United States high school and collegiate athletes. *Journal of Athletic Training*, 42(4), 495–503.

Gilchrist, M. (2003). Modelling and accident reconstruction of head impact injuries. *Key Engineering Materials*, 245, 417–432.

Gimbel, G. M. and Hoshizaki, T. B. (2008). Compressive properties of helmet materials subjected to dynamic impact loading of various energies. *European Journal of Sport Science*, 8(6), 341–349.

Giordano, C. and Kleiven, S. (2014). Connecting fractional anisotropy from medical images with mechanical anisotropy of a hyperviscoelastic fibre-reinforced constitutive model for brain tissue. *Journal of the Royal Society Interface*, 11(91), 20130914.

Giza, C. and Hovda, D. (2001). The neurometabolic cascade of concussion. *Journal of Athletic Training*, 36(3), 228–235.

Goodman, D., Gaetz, M., and Meichenbaum, D. (2001). Concussions in hockey: There is cause for concern. *Medicine and Science in Sports and Exercise*, 33(12), 2004–2009.

Gurdjian, E. S., Hodgson, V. R., Hardy, W. G., Patrick, L. M., and Lissner, H. R. (1964). Evaluation of the protective characteristics of helmets in sports. *The Journal of Trauma*, 4(3), 309–324.

Gurdjian, E. S., Lissner, H. R., Latimer, F. R., Haddad, B. F., and Webster, J. E. (1953). Quantitative determination of acceleration and intracranial pressure in experimental head injury: Preliminary report. *Neurology*, 3(6), 417–423.

Gurdjian, E. S., Lissner, H. R., Webster, J. E., Latimer, F. R., and Haddad, B. F. (1954). Studies on experimental concussion: Relation of physiologic effect to time duration of intracranial pressure increase at impact. *Neurology*, 4(9), 674–681.

Guskiewicz, K. M., McCrea, M., Marshall, S. W., Cantu, R. C., Randolph, C., Barr, W., Onate, J. A., and Kelly, J. P. (2003). Cumulative effects associated with recurrent concussion in collegiate football players. *Journal of the American Medical Association*, 290(19), 2549–2555.

Gwin, J. T., Chu, J. J., and Greenwald, R. M. (2006). Head impact telemetry system for measurement of head acceleration in ice hockey. *Journal of Biomechanics*, 39, S153.

Hagel, B. and Meeuwisse, W. (2004). Risk compensation: A "side effect" of sports injury prevention. *Clinical Journal of Sports Medicine*, 14(4), 193–196.

Hagel, B. E., Marko, J., Dryden, D., Couperthwaite, A. B., Sommerfeldt, J., et al. (2006). Effect of body-checking on injury rates among minor ice hockey players. *Canadian Medical Association Journal*, 175, 155–60.

Hardy, W. N., Foster, C. D., Mason, M. J., Yang, K. H., King, A. I., and Tashman, S. (2001). Investigation of head injury mechanisms using neutral density technology and high-speed biplanar x-ray. *Stapp Car Crash Journal*, 45, 337–368.

Hardy, W. N., Mason, M. J., Foster, C. D., Shah, C. S., Kopacz, J. M., Yang, K. H., King, A. I., Bishop, J., Bey, M., Anderst, W., and Tashman, S. (2007). A Study of the response of the human cadaver head to impact. *Stapp Car Crash Journal*, 51, 17–80.

Hedlund, J. (2000). Risky business: Safety regulations, risk compensation, and individual behavior. *Injury Prevention*, 6(2), 82–90.

Hodgson, V. R., Thomas, L. M., and Khalil, T. B. (1983). The role of impact location in reversible cerebral concussion. SAE Technical Paper 831618. doi: 10.4271/831618.

Holbourn, A. H. S. (1943). Mechanics of head injuries. *The Lancet*, 242(6267), 438–441.

Honey, C. R. (1998). Brain injury in ice hockey. *Clinical Journal of Sports Medicine*, 8, 43–46.

Horgan, T. J. and Gilchrist, M. D. (2004). Influence of FE model variability in predicting brain motion and intracranial pressure changes in head impact simulations. *International Journal of Crashworthiness*, 9(4), 401–418.

Hoshizaki, T. B. and Brien, S. E. (2004). The science and design of head protection in sport. *Neurosurgery*, 55(4), 956–967.

Hubschmann, O. R. and Korhauser, D. (1983). Effects of intraparenchymal hemorrhage on extracellular potassium in experimental head trauma. *Journal of Neurosurgery*, 59(2), 289–293.

Hutchinson, J., Kaiser, M. J., and Lankarani, H. M. (1998). The head injury criterion (HIC) functional. *Applied Mathematics and Computation*, 96(1), 1–16.

Hutchison, M. G., Comper, P., Meeuwisse, W. H., and Echemendia, R. J. (2013). A systematic video analysis of national hockey league (NHL) concussions, part I: Who, when, where and what? *British Journal of Sports Medicine*, 49, 547–551.

Iliff, J. J., Lee, H., Yu, M., Feng, T., Logan, J., Nedergaard, M., and Benveniste, H. (2013). Brain-wide pathway for waste clearance captured by contrast-enhanced MRI. *The Journal of Clinical Investigation*, 123(3), 1299–1309.

Iliff, J. J., Wang, M., Liao, Y., Plogg, B. A., Peng, W., Gundersen, G. A., Benveniste, H., Vates, G. E., Deane, R., Goldman, S. A., and Nagelhus, E. A. (2012). A paravascular pathway facilitates CSF flow through the brain parenchyma and the clearance of interstitial solutes, including amyloid β. *Science translational medicine*, 4(147), 147ra111.

Jadischke, R., Viano, D. C., Dau, N., King, A. I., and McCarthy, J. (2013). On the accuracy of the head impact telemetry (HIT) system used in football helmets. *Journal of Biomechanics*, 46(13), 2310–2315.

Jessen, N. A., Munk, A. S. F., Lundgaard, I., and Nedergaard, M. (2015). The glymphatic system: A beginner's guide. *Neurochemical Research*, 40(12), 2583–2599.

Ji, S. G., H., Bolander, R. P., Beckwith, J. G., Ford, J. C. McAllister, T. W. et al. (2014). Parametric comparisons of intracranial mechanical responses from three validated finite element models of the human head. *Annals of Biomedical Engineering*, 42(1), 11–24.

Julian, F. and Goldman, D. (1962). The effects of mechanical stimulation on some electrical properties of axons. *The Journal of general physiology*, 46(2), 297–313.

Kang, H. S. Willinger, R., Diaw, B. M., and Chinn, B. (1997). Validation of a 3D anatomic human head model and replication of head impact in motorcycle accident by finite element modeling. In *Proceedings of the 41st Stapp Car Crash Conference* (pp. 329–338), Orlando, FL.

Karton, C., Hoshizaki, T. B., and Gilchrist, M. D. (2014). The influence of impactor mass on the dynamic response of the Hybrid III headform and brain tissue deformation. In *Mechanism of Concussion in Sport*, Atlanta, GA.

Katayama, Y., Becker, D. P., Tamura, T., and Hovda, D. A. (1990). Massive increase in extracellular potassium and the indiscriminate release of glutamate following concussive brain injury. *Journal of Neurosurgery*, 73(6), 889–900.

Kelly, J. P., Nichols, J. S., Filley, C. M., Lillehei, K. O., Rubinstein, D., and Kleinschmidt-DeMasters, B. K. (1991). Concussion in sports. Guidelines for the prevention of catastrophic outcome. *Journal of the American Medical Association*, 266(20), 2867–2869.

Kendall, M. (2016). Comparison and characterization of different concussive brain injury events (PhD dissertation), Ottawa, Canada: University of Ottawa.

Kendall, M., Post, A., Rousseau, P., Oeur, A., Gilchrist, M. D., and Hoshizaki, T. B. (2012). A comparison of dynamic impact response and brain deformation metrics within the cerebrum of head impact reconstructions representing three mechanisms of head injury in ice hockey. In *Proceedings of theInternational Research Council on the Biomechanics of Injury Conference* (Vol. 40, pp. 430–440).

Kimpara, H. and Iwamoto, M. (2011). Mild traumatic brain injury predictors based on angular accelerations during impacts. *Annals of Biomedical Engineering*, 40(1), 114–126.

King, A. I., Yang, K. H., Zhang, L., Hardy, W. N., and Viano, D. C. (2003). Is head injury caused by linear or angular acceleration? In *Proceedings of theInternational Research Council on the Biomechanics of Injury Conference* (Vol. 31), Lisbon, Portugal.

Kleiven, S. (2005). Influence of direction and duration of impacts to the human head evaluated using the finite element method. In *Proceedings of theInternational Research Council on the Biomechanics of Injury Conference* (Vol. 33, pp. 41–58), Prague, Czech Republic.

Kleiven, S. (2007). Predictors for traumatic brain injuries evaluated through accident reconstructions. *Stapp Car Crash Journal*, 51, 81–114.

Kleiven, S. and Hardy, W. N. (2002). Correlation of an fe model of the human head with local brain motion—Consequences for injury prediction. *Stapp Car Crash Journal*, 46, 123.

Kleiven, S. and von Holst, H. (2002). Consequences of head size following trauma to the human head. *Journal of Biomechanics*, 35(2), 153–160.Koerte, I. K., Kaufmann, D., Hartl, E., Bouix, S., Pasternak, O., Kubicki, M., Rauscher, A., Li, D. K., Dadachanji, S. B., Taunton, J. A., and Forwell, L. A. (2012). A prospective study of physician-observed concussion during a varsity university hockey season: White matter integrity in ice hockey players. Part 3 of 4. *Neurosurgical Focus*, 33(6), E3.

Kondo, A., Shahpasand, K., Mannix, R., Qiu, J., Moncaster, J., Chen, C. H., Yao, Y., Lin, Y. M., Driver, J. A., Sun, Y., and Wei, S. (2015). Antibody against early driver of neurodegeneration cis P-tau blocks brain injury and tauopathy. *Nature*, 523(7561), 431–436.

LaPlaca, M. C., Lee, V. M., and Thibault, L. E. (1997). An in vitro model of traumatic neuronal injury: Loading rate-dependent changes in acute cytosolic calcium and lactate dehydrogenase release. *Journal of Neurotrauma*, 14(6), 355–368.

Lissner, H. R., Lebow, M., and Evans, F. G. (1960). Experimental studies on the relation between acceleration and intracranial pressure changes in man. *Surgery, Gynecology & Obstetrics*, 111, 329–338.

Longhi, L., Saatman, K. E., Fujimoto, S., Raghunpathi, R., Meaney, D. F., Davis, J., McMillan, A., Conte, V., Laurer, H. L., Stein, S., and Stocchetti, N. (2005). Temporal window of vulnerability to repetitive experimental concussive brain injury. *Neurosurgery* 56, 364–374.

Loyd, A. M. (2011). Studies of the human head from neonate to adult: An inertial, geometrical and structural analysis with comparisons to the ATD head (PhD Dissertation), Duke University, Durham NC.

Marchie, A. and Cusimano, M. D. (2003). Bodychecking and concussions in ice hockey: Should our youth pay the price? *Canadian Medical Association Journal*, 169(2), 124–128.

Martland, H. S. (1928). Punch drunk. *Journal of the American Medical Association*, 91(15), 1103–1107.

Masel, B. E. and DeWitt, D. S. (2010). Traumatic brain injury: A disease process, not an event. *Journal of Neurotrauma*, 27(8), 1529–1540.

McAllister, T. W., Ford, J. C., Ji, S., Beckwith, J. G., Flashman, L. A., Paulsen, K. D., and Greenwald, R. M. (2011). Maximum principal strain and strain rate associated with concussion diagnosis correlates with changes in corpus callosum white matter indices. *Annals of Biomedical Engineering*, 40(1), 127–140.

McElhaney, J. H., Melvin, J. W., Roberts, V. L., and Portnoy, H. D. (1973). Dynamic characteristics of the tissues of the head. In R. M. Kenedi (Ed.), *Perspectives in Biomedical Engineering* (pp. 215–222). London, UK: Macmillan Press Ltd.

McIntosh, A. S., McCrory, P., and Comerford, J. (2000). The dynamics of concussive head impacts in rugby and Australian rules football. *Medicine and Science in Sports and Exercise*, 32(12), 1980–1984.

McKee, A. C., Cantu, R. C., Nowinski, C. J., Hedley-Whyte, E. T., Gavett, B. E., Budson, A. E., Santini, V. E., Lee, H. S., Kubilus, C. A., and Stern, R. A. (2009). Chronic traumatic encephalopathy in athletes: Progressive tauopathy after repetitive head injury. *Journal of Neuropathology & Experimental Neurology*, 68(7), 709–735.

McKee, A. C., Stern, R. A., Nowinski, C. J., Stein, T. D., Alvarez, V. E., Daneshvar, D. H., Lee, H. S., Hall, G., Wojtowicz, S. M., Baugh, C. M. and Riley, D. O. (2013). The spectrum of disease in chronic traumatic encephalopathy. *Brain*, 136(1), 43–64.Mendez, M. F. (1995). The neuropsychiatric aspects of boxing. *The International Journal of Psychiatry in Medicine*, 25(3), 249–262.

Mendis, K. K., Stalnaker, R. L., and Advani, S. H. (1995). A constitutive relationship for large deformation finite element modeling of brain tissue. *Journal of Biomechanical Engineering*, 117(3), 279–285.

Millspaugh, J. A. (1937). Dementia pugilistica. *United States Naval Medical Bulletin*, 35, 297–303.

Montenigro, P. H., Alosco, M. L., Martin, B. M., Daneshvar, D. H., Mez, J., Chaisson, C., Nowinski, C. J., Au, R., McKee, A. C., Cantu, R. C., and McClean, M. (2016). Cumulative head impact exposure predicts later-life depression, apathy, executive dysfunction, and cognitive impairment in former high school and college football players. *Journal of Neurotrauma*. doi: 10.1089/neu.2016.

Nahum, A. M., Smith, R., and Ward, C. (1977). Intracranial pressure dynamics during head impact. In *Proceedings of the 21st Stapp Car Crash Conference* (No. 770922), Warrendale, PA.

Neselius, S., Brisby, H., Granholm, F., Zetterberg, H., and Blennow, K. (2015). Monitoring concussion in a knocked-out boxer by CSF biomarker analysis. *Knee Surgery, Sports Traumatology, Arthroscopy*, 23(9), 2536–2539.

Neselius, S., Brisby, H., Theodorsson, A., Blennow, K., Zetterberg, H., and Marcusson, J. (2012). CSF—biomarkers in Olympic boxing: Diagnosis and effects of repetitive head trauma. *PLoS ONE*, 7(4), e33606.

Newman, J. (1986). A generalized acceleration model for brain injury threshold (GAMBIT). *Proceedings of theInternational Research Council on the Biomechanics of Injury Conference* (Vol. 14, pp. 121–131), Bron, France.

Newman, J. A. (2002). Biomechanics of head trauma: Head protection. In A. Nahum and J. Melvin (Eds.), *Accidental Injury* (pp. 303–323). New York: Springer.

Newman, J. A. (2005). The biomechanics of head trauma and the development of the modern helmet: How far have we really come? In *Proceedings of theInternational Research Council on the Biomechanics of Injury Conference* (Vol. 33), Prague, Czech Republic.

Newman, J., Barr, C., Beusenberg, M., Fournier, E., Shewchenko, N., Welbourne, E., and Withnall, C. (2000a). A new biomechanical assessment of mild traumatic brain injury. Part 2: Results and conclusions. In *Proceedings of theInternational Research Council on the Biomechanics of Injury Conference* (Vol. 28, pp. 223–233), Montpellier, France.

Newman, J. A., Shewchenko, N., and Welbourne, E. (2000b). A proposed new biomechanical head injury assessment function—The maximum power index. *Stapp Car Crash J*, 44, 215–247.

Nicolle, S., Lounis, M., and Willinger, R. (2004). Shear properties of brain tissue over a frequency range relevant for automotive impact situations: New experimental results. *Stapp Car Crash Journal*, 48, 239–258.

NOCSAE (2014). *Standard Performance Specification for Newly Manufactured Football Helmets (ND002-14)*. Overland Park, KS: National Operating Committee on Standards for Athletic Equipment.

Nyquist, G. W., Cavanaugh, J. M., Goldberg, S. J., and King, A. I. (1986). Facial impact tolerance and response. SAE Technical Paper 861896.

Oeur, R. A., Karton, C., and Hoshizaki, T. B. (2014). *Impact Frequency Validation of Head Impact Sensor Technology for Use in Sport*. Tsukuba, Japan: 34th International Society of Biomechanics in Sport.

Oeur, R. A., Karton, C., Post, A., Rousseau, P., Hoshizaki, T. B., Marshall, S., Brien, S. E., Smith, A., Cusimano, M. D., and Gilchrist, M. D. (2015). A comparison of head dynamic response and brain tissue stress and strain using accident reconstructions for concussion, concussion with persistent postconcussive symptoms, and subdural hematoma. *Journal of Neurosurgery*, 123(2), 415–422.

Oliver, J. M., Jones, M. T., Kirk, K. M., Gable, D. A., Repshas, J. T., Johnson, T., Andreasson, U., Norgren, N., Blennow, K., and Zetterberg, H. (2016). Serum neurofilament light in American football athletes over the course of a season. *Journal of Neurotrauma*, ahead of print. doi: 10.1089/neu.2015.4295.

Omalu, B. I., DeKosky, S. T., Minister, R. L., Kamboh, M. I., Hamilton, R. L., and Wecht, C. H. (2005). Chronic traumatic encephalopathy in a national football league player. *Neurosurgery*, 57(1), 128–134.

Ommaya, A. K. and Gennarelli, T. A. (1974). Cerebral concussion and traumatic unconsciousness: Correlation of experimental and clinical observations on blunt head injuries. *Brain*, 97(1), 633–654.

Ommaya, A. K, and Hirsch, A. E. (1971). Tolerances for cerebral concussion from head impact and whiplash in primates. *Journal of Biomechanics*, 4(1), 13–21.

Ommaya, A. K., Hirsch, A. E., Flamm, E. S., and Mahone, R. H. (1966). Cerebral concussion in the monkey: An experimental model. *Science*, 153(3732), 211–212.Padgaonkar, A. J., Krieger, K. W., and King, A. I. (1975). Measurement of angular acceleration of a rigid body using linear accelerometers. *Journal of Applied Mechanics*, 42(3), 552–556.

Pashby, T., Carson, J. D., Ordogh, D., Johnston, K. M., Tator, C. H. and Mueller, F. O. (2001). Eliminate head-checking in ice hockey. *Clinical Journal of Sport Medicine*, 11(4), 211–213.

Patton, D. A., McIntosh, A. S., and Kleiven, S. (2013). The biomechanical determinants of concussion: Finite element simulations to investigate brain tissue deformations during sporting impacts to the unprotected head. *Journal of Applied Biomechanics*, 29(6), 721–730.

Patton, D. A., McIntosh, A. S., Kleiven, S., and Frechede, B. (2012). Injury data from unhelmeted football head impacts evaluated against critical strain tolerance curves. *Journal of Sports Engineering and Technology*, 226(3–4), 177–184.

Pellman, E. J., Viano, D. C., Tucker, A. M., Casson, I. R., and Waeckerle, J. F. (2003). Concussion in professional football: Reconstruction of game impacts and injuries. *Neurosurgery*, 53(4), 799–814.

Petzold, A., Michel, P., Stock, M., and Schluep, M. (2008). Glial and axonal body fluid biomarkers are related to infarct volume, severity, and outcome. *Journal of Stroke and Cerebrovascular Diseases*, 17(4), 196–203.

Post, A. (2013). The influence of dynamic response characteristics on traumatic brain injury (PhD Dissertation), Ottawa, Canada: University of Ottawa.

Post, A., and Hoshizaki, T. B. (2015). Rotational acceleration, brain tissue strain, and the relationship to concussion. *Journal of Biomechanical Engineering*, 137(3), 030801.

Post, A., Hoshizaki, B., and Gilchrist, M. D. (2012a). Finite element analysis of the effect of loading curve shape on brain injury predictors. *Journal of Biomechanics*, 45(4), 679–683.

Post, A., Hoshizaki, T. B., Gilchrist, M. D., and Brien, S. (2012b). Analysis of the influence of independent variables used for reconstruction of a traumatic brain injury event. *Journal of Sports Engineering and Technology*, 226(3–4), 290–298.

Post, A., Hoshizaki, T. B., Gilchrist, M. D., Brien, S., Cusimano, M. D., and Marshall, S. (2015a). The dynamic response characteristics of traumatic brain injury. *Accident Analysis and Prevention*, 79, 33–40.

Post, A., Kendall, M., Koncan, D., Cournoyer, J., Hoshizaki, T. B., Gilchrist, M. D., Brien, S., Cusimano, M. D., and Marshall, S. (2015b). Characterization of persistent concussive syndrome through injury reconstruction and finite element modelling. *Journal of the Mechanical Behavior of Biomedical Materials*, 41, 325–335.

Powell, J. W. (1998). The evolution of ice hockey related injuries in the NHL. In N. Biasca, W-D. Montag, C. Gerber (Eds.) *Safety in Ice Hockey: IIHF International Symposium on Medicine and Science in Ice Hockey on the occasion of the 8th Ice Hockey World Championship*, pp. 19–25. Zurich: IIHF.

Prange, M. T. and Margulies, S. S. (2002). Regional, directional, and age-dependent properties of the brain undergoing large deformation. *Journal of Biomechanical Engineering*, 124(2), 244–252.

Prasad, P. and Mertz, H. J. (1985). The position of the United States delegation to the ISO working group 6 on the use of HIC in the automotive environment.*SAE Transactions*, 94, 106–116.

Prins, M. L., Alexander, D., Giza, C. C., and Hovda, D. A. (2013). Repeated mild traumatic brain injury: Mechanisms of cerebral vulnerability. *Journal of Neurotrauma*, 30(1), 30–38.

Roberts, A. H. (1969). *Brain Damage in Boxers*. London, UK: Pitman Publishing.

Rousseau, P. (2014). Analysis of concussion metrics of real-world and non-injurious elbow and shoulder to head collisions in ice hockey (PhD dissertation), Ottawa, Canada: University of Ottawa.

Rousseau, P., and Hoshizaki, T. B. (2015). Defining the effective impact mass of elbow and shoulder strikes in ice hockey. *Sports Biomechanics*, 14(1), 57–67.

Rousseau, P., Hoshizaki, T. B., and Gilchrist, M. D. (2014), For ASTM F-08: Protective capacity of ice hockey player helmets against puck impacts. In A. Ashare and M. Ziejewski (Eds.) *Mechanism of Concussion in Sports, STP 1552*. West Conshohocken, PA: ASTM International.

SAE (Society of Automotive Engineers International). (2007). Instrumentation for impact test–part 1–electronic instrumentation, SAE International Surface Vehicle Recommended Practice, Standard J211-1.

Sahoo, D., Deck, C., and Willinger, R. (2014). Development and validation of an advanced anisotropic visco-hyperelastic human brain FE model. *Journal of the Mechanical Behaviour of Biomedical Materials*, 33, 24–42.

Schnebel, B., Gwin, J. T., Anderson, S., and Gatlin, R. (2007). In vivo study of head impacts in football: A comparison of national collegiate athletic association division I versus high school impacts. *Neurosurgery*, 60(3), 490–495.

Shahani, N. and Brandt, R. (2002). Functions and malfunctions of the tau proteins. *Cellular and Molecular Life Sciences*, 59(10), 1668–1680.

Shahim, P., Tegner, Y., Wilson, D. H., Randall, J., and Skillback, T. (2014). Blood biomarkers for brain injury in concussed professional ice hockey players. *JAMA Neurology*, 71(6), 684–692.

Shuck, L. Z. and Advani, S. H. (1972). Rheological response of human brain tissue in shear. *Journal of Basic Engineering*, 94(4), 905–911.

Singh, A., Lu, Y., Chen, C., Kallakuri, S., and Cavanaugh, J. M. (2006). A new model of traumatic axonal injury to determine the effects of strain and displacement rates. *Stapp Car Crash Journal*, 50, 601–623.

Stamm, J. M., Koerte, I. K., Muehlmann, M., Pasternak, O., Bourlas, A. P., et al. 2015. Age of first exposure to football is associated with altered corpus callosum white matter microstructure in former professional football players. *Journal of Neurotrauma*, 32(22), 1768–1776.

Stefani, M. and Dobson, C. M. (2003). Protein aggregation and aggregate toxicity: New insights into protein folding, misfolding diseases and biological evolution. *Journal of molecular medicine*, 81(11), 678–699.

Stemper, B. D., Shah, A. S., Pintar, F. A., McCrea, M., Kurpad, S. N., Glavaski-Joksimovic, A., Olsen, C., and Budde, M. D. (2015). Head rotational acceleration characteristics influence behavioral and diffusion tensor imaging outcomes following concussion. *Annals of Biomedical Engineering*, 43(5), 1071–1088.

Takahashi, H., Manaka, S., and Sano, K. (1981). Changes in extracellular potassium concentration in cortex and brain stem during the acute phase of experimental closed head injury. *Journal of Neurosurgery*, 5(5), 708–717.

Takhounts, E. G., Craig, M. J., Moorhouse, K., McFadden, J., and Hasija, V. (2013). Development of brain injury criteria (BrIC). *Stapp Car Crash Journal*, 57, 243–266.

Takhounts, E. G., Ridella, S. A., Hasija, V., Tannous, R. E., Campbell, J. Q., Malone, D., Danelson, K., Stitzel, J., Rowson, S., and Duma, S. (2008). Investigation of traumatic brain injuries using next generation of simulated injury monitor (SIMon) Finite Element Head Model. *Stapp Car Crash Journal*, 52, 1–31.

Talavage, T. M., Nauman, E. A., Breedlove, E. L., Yoruk, U., Dye, A. E., Morigaki, K. E., Feuer, H., and Leverenz, L. J. (2014). Functionally-detected cognitive impairment in high school football players without clinically-diagnosed concussion. *Journal of Neurotrauma*, 31(4), 327–338.

Thibault, K. and Margulies, S. S. (1998). Age-dependent material properties of the porcine cerebrum: Effect on pediatric inertial head injury criteria. *Journal of Biomechanics*, 31(12), 1119–1126.

Thomas, L. M., Roberts, V. L., and Gurdjian, E. S. (1966). Experimental intracranial pressure gradients in the human skull. *Journal of Neurology, Neurosurgery and Psychiatry*, 29(5), 404–411.

Trosseille, X., Tarriere, C., Lavaste, F., Guillon, F., and Domont, A. (1992). Development of a FEM of the human head according to a specific test protocol. In *Proceedings of the 36th Stapp Car Crash Conference* (Vol. 36, pp. 261–280). Warrandale, PA: Stapp.

Van Lierde, C. (2005). Biomechanics of head injury—Damage criteria for skull and brain lesions (PhD Dissertation), K.U. Leuven, Belgium.

Versace, J. (1971). A review of the severity index. In *Proceedings of the 15th STAPP Car Crash Conference* (Vol. 15, pp. 43-69), Warrendale, PA.

Viano, D. C., Casson, I. R., Pellman, E. J., Bir, C. A., Zhang, L., Sherman, D. C., and Boitano, M. A. (2005a). Concussion in professional football: Comparison with boxing head impacts: Part 10. *Neurosurgery*, 57(6), 1154–1172.

Viano, D. C., Casson, I. R., Pellman, E. J., Zhang, L., King, A. I., and Yang, K. H. (2005b). Concussion in professional football: Brain responses by finite element analysis: Part 9. *Neurosurgery*, 57(5), 891–915.

Viano, D. C. and Lovsund, P. (1999). Biomechanics of brain and spinal-cord injury: Analysis of neuropathologic and neurophysiologic experiments. *Journal of Crash Prevention and Injury Control*, 1(1), 35–43.Walilko, T. J., Viano, D. C., and Bir, C. A. (2005), Biomechanics of the head for Olympic boxer punches to the face, *British Journal of Sports Medicine*, 39(10), 710–719.

Walsh, E. S., Rousseau, P., and Hoshizaki, T. B. (2011). The influence of impact location and angle on the dynamic impact response of a Hybrid III headform. *Sports Engineering*, 13(3), 135–143.

Wennberg, R., and Tator, C. (2003). National hockey league reported concussions, 1986–1987 to 2001–2002. *The Canadian Journal of Neurological Sciences*, 30(3), 206–209.

Willinger, R., and Baumgartner, D. (2003). Human head tolerance limits to specific injury mechanisms. *International Journal of Crashworthiness*, 8(6), 605–617.

Willinger, R., Kang, H. S., and Diaw, B. M. (1999). Développement et validation d'un modèle mécanique de la tête humaine. *Comptes Rendus de l'Académie des Sciences—Series IIB—Mechanics-Physics-Astronomy*, 327(1), 125–131.

Willinger, R., Ryan, G. A., McLean, A. J., and Kopp, C. M. (1992). Mechanisms of brain injury related to mathematical modeling and epidemiological data. *Accident Analysis and Prevention*, 26(6), 767–779.

Withnall, C., Shewchenko, N., Gittens, R., and Dvorak, J. (2005). Biomechanical investigation of head impacts in football. *British Journal of Sports Medicine*, 39(suppl 1), i49–i57.

Yoganandan, N., Li, J., Zhang, J., Pintar, F. A., and Gennarelli, T. A. (2008). Influence of angular acceleration-deceleration pulse shapes on regional brain strains. *Journal of Biomechanics*, 41(10), 2253–2262.

Yoganandan, N., Pintar, F. A., Sances Jr., A., Walsh, P. R., Ewing, C. L., Thomas, D. J., and Snyder, R. G. (1995). Biomechanics of skull fracture. *Journal of Neurotrauma*, 12(4), 659–668.

Yuan, X. Q., Prough, D. S., Smith, T. L., and DeWitt, D. S. (1998). The effects of traumatic brain injury on regional cerebral blood flow in rats. *Journal of Neurotrauma*, 5(4), 289–301.

Yuen, T. J., Browne, K. D., Iwata, A., and Smith, D. H. (2009). Sodium channelopathy induced by mild axonal trauma worsens outcome after a repeat injury. *Journal of Neuroscience Research*, 87(16), 3620–3625.

Zanetti, K., Post, A., Karton, C., Kendall, M., Hoshizaki, T. B., and Gilchrist, M. D. 2013. Identifying risk profiles for three player positions in American football using physical and finite element modeling reconstructions. *Proceedings of IRCOBI*, Gothenburg, Sweden.

Zetterberg, H., Hietala, M. A., Jonsson, M., Andreasen, N., Styrud, E., Karlsson, I., Edman, Å., Popa, C., Rasulzada, A., Wahlund, L. O., and Mehta, P. D. (2006). Neurochemical aftermath of amateur boxing. *Archives of Neurology*, 63(9), 1277–1280.Zhang, L., Yang, K., and King, A. (2001a). Biomechanics of neurotrauma. *Neurological Research*, 23(2–3), 144–156.

Zhang, L., Yang, K. H., Dwarampudi, R., Omori, K., Li, T., Chang, K., Hardy, W. N., Khalil, T. B., and King, A. I. (2001b). Recent advances in brain injury research: A new human head model development and validation. *Stapp Car Crash Journal*, 45, 369–394.

Zhang, L., Yang, K. H., and King, A. I. (2004). A proposed injury threshold for mild traumatic brain injury. *Journal of Biomechanical Engineering*, 126(2), 226–236.

*chapter five*

---

# Acute diagnosis of sports concussion
## How do we identify a concussion?

*Roger Zemek and Josh Stanley*

### Contents

## Diagnosis of concussion

Concussions across all age groups are commonly seen by first line health-care providers, including family and emergency medicine physicians. In the United States, approximately 300,000 sport-related concussions and an estimated 3.8 million recreation-related concussions occur annually (Halstead et al., 2010). Further, it is estimated that concussions make up approximately 1 in 220 pediatric emergency department (ED) visits in the United States (Faul et al., 2010; Meehan and Mannix, 2010), while in Canada, the incidence is thought to be even greater, composing 1 in 70 of ED visits (Langlois et al., 2006). In more recent years, there has been significant media attention directed toward the long-term effects of concussions including chronic traumatic encephalopathy (CTE) (Ban et al., 2016; Love and Solomon, 2014; McCrory et al., 2017). Despite the uncertain relationship between concussion and CTE, patients and families often express fear and anxiety related to potential consequences of the head injury (Love and Solomon, 2014; McCrory et al., 2013, 2017). However, not all head trauma produces traumatic brain injury (TBI) and may only result in superficial injuries, such as scalp hematoma. It is therefore critical for first line health-care providers to be able to accurately diagnose concussions and differentiate from more severe TBI or head injury without brain injury.

Upon presentation, the evaluation should begin with a detailed history of the injury and past medical history with risk factors (Choe and Giza, 2015; Halstead et al., 2010; McCrory et al., 2017; NSW Ministry of Health, 2011; Sabini and Reddy, 2010). One should enquire about the timing and mechanism of the injury, as well as the location of impact (Gioia and Collins, 2006; NSW Ministry of Health, 2011). It is important to ask details regarding specific characteristics associated with the injury, including anterograde and retrograde amnesia, loss of consciousness, seizures, and early signs post-injury such as slow response to and repetition of questions, forgetfulness, confusion, and being dazed or stunned (Gioia and Collins, 2006; NSW Ministry of Health, 2011). These features may indicate the need for further investigations such as head Computed Tomography (CT) imaging and/or the diagnosis of concussion (Gioia and Collins, 2006; Giza et al., 2013; Halstead et al., 2010; Jagoda et al., 2008; McCrory et al., 2017).

It is essential to elicit a detailed past medical history to determine risk factors and prior conditions that may exacerbate or mimic signs and symptoms of concussion. Clinicians should enquire about previous concussions and symptoms of concussions; specifically, the number of concussions, the duration of symptoms with each incident, and, in the case of multiple concussions, if less force resulted in injury (Gioia and Collins, 2006; McCrory et al., 2017). Sustaining multiple concussions or experiencing prolonged symptoms with successive concussions may influence patients' recovery, return to daily activities, the risk of potential complications, and the possibility of early retirement from sports (Cantu, 2003, 2009; McCrory et al., 2013). Physicians should ask about previous or concurrent injuries to the brain, head, face, or cervical spine (McCrory et al., 2017; NSW Ministry of Health, 2011), as this may also alter management (e.g., spinal cord stabilization in the case of suspected cervical spinal cord injury or loss of consciousness) (Halstead et al., 2010). Last, physicians should take note of concurrent or previous mental health and behavioral disorders such as depression, anxiety, sleep-disturbances, post-traumatic stress disorder (PTSD), learning disorders, and attention deficit hyperactivity disorder (ADHD) (McCrory et al., 2017; NSW Ministry of Health, 2011). Following TBI or concussion, patients may undergo changes in their mental health (Bailey et al., 2014; Halstead et al., 2010; Ilie et al., 2014; Jagoda et al., 2008; Johnston et al., 2004; McCrory et al., 2017; Meares et al., 2007; Motor Accidents Authority of NSW, 2008; Sabini and Reddy, 2010). Due to the overlap of signs and symptoms between mental health disorders and concussions (Table 5.1), it may be difficult to isolate these conditions (McAllister and Arciniegas, 2002; Mooney et al., 2005; Rose et al., 2015). Further, patients with preexisting psychiatric disorders, such as depression, may be at increased risk of acquiring a mental health disorder following injury (McAllister and Arciniegas, 2002).

Physicians should assess for signs and symptoms of concussions, which can be subcategorized as physical, cognitive, emotional, or sleep-related, and compare them to baseline functioning (see Table 5.1 for a more detailed list) (Gioia and Collins, 2006). It is important to ascertain the severity of symptoms, particularly in the first several days post-injury, as this has been found to be a significant and reliable predictor for slow recovery (McCrory et al., 2017). In addition, a physical examination should also be performed. Depending on the clinical setting and the scope of practice for the clinicians, the examination may

*Table 5.1* List of signs and symptoms of concussion

| Physical | Cognitive | Emotional | Sleep |
|---|---|---|---|
| **Headache** | Difficulty concentrating | Irritability | Drowsiness |
| **Nausea** | Difficulty remembering | Sadness | Hypersomnia |
| **Vomiting** | Feeling slowed down | Anxiety/nervousness | Insomnia-either |
| **Fatigue** | Feeling mentally foggy | More emotional | sleeping less than |
| **Blurred or double vision** | | | usual or difficulty |
| **Seeing stars or lights** | | | falling asleep |
| **Problems with balance** | | | |
| **Dizziness, Photophobia** | | | |
| **and Phonophobia** | | | |
| **Tinnitus** | | | |

*Source:*   Gioia, G. and Collins, M., Acute Concussion Evaluation (ACE): Physician/Clinician Office Version, 2006.

be more or less extensive. A detailed neurological examination, including Glasgow coma scale (GCS), mental status and cognition, cranial nerves, ocular and vestibular function, extremity tone, strength, and reflexes, sensory, gait, coordination and balance, is indicated as part concussion evaluation in order to assess for focal neurological deficits and rule out other brain injuries (Halstead et al., 2010; McCrory et al., 2017; Motor Accidents Authority of NSW, 2008; Sabini and Reddy, 2010). Specific tests include the standardized assessment of concussion (SAC), which is a cognitive assessment that tests orientation, immediate memory, concentration, and delayed recall (McCrea, 2001), a Maddocks Score that tests memory and attention (Maddocks et al., 1995), balance testing including tandem gait (Schneiders et al., 2010a, 2010b) or the Modified Balance Error Scoring System (BESS) testing (Guskiewicz, 2003), and coordination examination with finger-to-nose task (McCrory et al., 2013). Physicians should also perform a musculoskeletal examination and general inspection of the head (McCrory et al., 2013; Motor Accidents Authority of NSW, 2008). If any focal abnormalities are present, it is important that the patient is referred to the appropriate specialist and for potential imaging.

Within the adult and pediatric population, various validated tools can be used to assist physicians with this task, including the acute concussion evaluation (ACE) (Gioia and Collins, 2006; Gioia et al., 2008, 2009), the sports concussion assessment tool (SCAT)5 (Echemendia et al., 2017a) and Child-SCAT5 (Davis et al., 2017). A further comparison of these tools is outlined in Table 5.2.

When assessing patients for possible concussion, it is important to identify factors indicating more severe TBI, neurological deterioration and the need for further investigations, including obtaining a head CT scan (see Section "The need for head CT scan and other investigations"), and acute emergency management (Gioia et al., 2008; Giza et al., 2013; Halstead et al., 2010; Jagoda et al., 2008; Lee and Newberg, 2005). Worrisome signs and symptoms or *red flags* may include worsening or severe headaches, seizures, focal neurologic signs such as limb weakness or numbness, appearing drowsy and inability to be awakened, repeated vomiting, slurred speech, inability to recognize people and/or places, prolonged post-traumatic amnesia (i.e., greater than 24 hours), increased confusion or irritability, neck pain, unusual behavioral changes, and changes in state of consciousness (Gioia and Collins, 2006; Giza et al., 2013; Jagoda et al., 2008; Putukian et al., 2013). Concussion modifiers may also influence additional investigations, management, and sometimes can help predict if patients are at higher risk for persistent or prolonged symptoms (Table 5.3) (McCrory et al., 2013). With respect to the pediatric population, specific concussion modifiers and predictive factors will be discussed in Section "Prediction algorithm to provide accurate anticipatory guidance and to target high-risk pediatric and adult patients for early management".

Concussions are ultimately a clinical diagnosis and do not rely on abnormal findings on structural neuroimaging including CT scan and magnetic resonance imaging (MRI) (see Section "The need for head CT scan and other investigations") (Rose et al., 2015). Specifically, the diagnosis of concussions relies mainly on observed mechanism of injury and various physical, emotional, cognitive, sleep-related, and neurological signs and symptoms including balance impairment (McCrory et al., 2017; Piland et al., 2006). Due to the lack of diagnostic tests or markers to precisely diagnose a concussion (McCrory et al., 2017), controversy and a lack of consensus exist regarding exact diagnosis. While loss of consciousness was previously in the definition of concussion (Ropper and Gorson, 2007), or helped subcategorize concussions (Gioia and Collins, 2006; Gioia et al., 2008), more recent literature states that loss of consciousness may or may not be involved in concussion (Guskiewicz et al., 2000; McCrea et al., 2003; McCrory et al., 2017; Meehan et al., 2010). Additionally, the loss of consciousness neither indicates the severity of concussion

Table 5.2 Standardized tools for evaluation of suspected concussion

| | Acute concussion evaluation (ACE) (Gioia and Collins, 2006) | Sports concussion assessment tool (SCAT)5 (Echemendia et al., 2017a) | Child-SCAT5 (Davis et al., 2017) |
|---|---|---|---|
| Indicated age | Adults, children ≥3 years old | Adults, children ≥13 years old | Children 5–12 years old |
| Injury characterization | Yes | Yes | Yes |
| Sideline questionnaire | None | Maddocks Score | Incorporated into the Concussion Recognition Tool 5 (Echemendia et al., 2017b) |
| Symptoms checklist | Yes. Yes or No questionnaire. Includes worsening with physical or cognitive exertion and overall rating. Completed by patient or parent/caregiver. | Yes. Graded scale for symptoms severity. Includes worsening with physical or cognitive exertion and overall rating. Self-reporting, which should be done in resting state. | Yes. Graded scale for symptoms severity. Includes worsening with physical or cognitive exertion and an overall rating which is from 0 to 10 for the Child and from 0 to 100 for the Parent. Child reporting should be done in resting state. |
| Past medical history, including psychiatric and developmental | Yes. Personal and family history. | Yes. Personal and family history. | Yes. Personal and family history. |
| Cognitive examination | None | Standardized assessment of concussion (SAC) | Standardized Assessment of Concussion- Child version (SAC-C) |
| Physical examination | None | GCS, Rapid Neurologic Screen (RNS). RNS includes neck movement, ocular function, speech, reading ability, balance (Modified BESS testing including single leg stance, double leg stance and tandem gait), and coordination. | GCS. RNS includes neck movement, ocular function, speech, reading ability, balance (Modified BESS testing including, double leg, tandem gait and, for children 10–12, single leg stance), and coordination. |
| Assessment for Red Flags | Yes | Yes | Yes |

*Table 5.3* Concussion modifiers for adults

| Factor | Modifier |
| --- | --- |
| Symptoms | Number |
| | Duration (>10 days) |
| | Severity |
| Signs | Prolonged loss of consciousness (LOC; >1 minute), Amnesia[a] |
| Sequelae | Concussive convulsions |
| Temporal | Frequency- repeated concussions over time |
| | Timing- injuries close together in time |
| | Recent concussion or TBI |
| Threshold | Repeated concussions occurring with progressively less impact force or slower recovery after each successive concussion |
| Age | Child and adolescent (<18 years old) |
| Co and Premorbidities | Migraine, depression or other mental health disorder, ADHD, learning disability (LD), sleep disorder |
| Medication | Psychoactive drugs, anticoagulants |
| Behavior | Dangerous style of play |
| Sport | High risk activity |
| | Contact and collision sport |
| | High sporting level |

*Source:* McCrory, P. et al., *Br. J. Sports Med.*, 47, 250–258, 2013.

[a] Inconsistent evidence if loss of consciousness, retrograde, and anterograde amnesia are correlated with prolonged recovery and more significant short-term effects (McCrory et al., 2017).

(Leininger et al., 1990; Lovell et al., 1999) nor helps predict risk of persistent post-concussion symptoms (PPCS) (McCrory et al., 2017; Zemek et al., 2016). Further, the Mayo TBI classification system subdivides mild TBI into mild (probably) and symptomatic (possible) TBI based on the presence of post-traumatic amnesia, loss of consciousness, or skull fractures in addition to symptoms (Malec et al., 2007).

## The need for head CT scan and other investigations

When assessing patients for concussion, neuroimaging is often not indicated because concussions are thought to produce functional brain abnormalities, as opposed to a structural abnormalities, and thus cannot be seen on standard structural brain imaging (Lee and Newberg, 2005; McCrory et al., 2017; Rose et al., 2015; Sabini and Reddy, 2010). In particular, the pediatric concussion guidelines by the Ontario Neurotrauma Foundation (ONF) state that it is not necessary to utilize imaging for majority of children who have sustained a head injury (Zemek et al., 2014). However, in some adults and children, neuroimaging may be required in order to help rule out other acute, more serious and possibly life-threatening injuries, such as skull fractures and intracranial hemorrhage (Giza et al., 2013; Halstead et al., 2010; Hofman et al., 2000; Jagoda et al., 2008; McAllister et al., 2001; Ontario Neurotrauma Foundation, 2013; Sabini and Reddy, 2010). Head CT scan is main form of neuroimaging indicated to rule out such complications, as skull X-rays have been shown to have inadequate sensitivity, while MRI is more expensive and less readily available (Hofman et al., 2000; Lee and Newberg, 2005; McAllister et al., 2001; Sabini and Reddy, 2010). While the use of CT scan in children with head injury was previously more common, it has been decreasing dramatically; a recent Canadian multicenter cohort study found that of children presenting to the ED within 48 hours of head injury, only 3.1%–3.4% of children received CT imaging (Zemek et al., 2016). CT imaging does not come without risks, especially in the pediatric population. CT imaging exposes children to high doses of radiation, which may increase risk of lifetime cancer, is a costly resource that may be unnecessarily utilized, and may not always be accessible (Brenner and Hall, 2007; Pearce et al., 2012; Pickering et al., 2011). Therefore, there should be careful consideration utilizing head CT scans, particularly in the pediatric population.

In the adult population, two widely used and validated rules can be used to determine the need for neuroimaging in patients with minor head injury: the Canadian CT Head Rule (CCHR) (Stiell et al., 2001) and the New Orleans Criteria (NOC) (Haydel et al., 2000). According to these rules, CT scans are indicated in patients with minor head injury (in the case of the NOC, patients must also have a GCS of 15) if they meet any of the following criteria listed in Table 5.4.

Several studies have compared the CCHR and the NOC (Bouida et al., 2013; Kavalci et al., 2014; Smits et al., 2005; Stiell et al., 2005). In these studies, when used to predict the need for neurosurgical intervention and clinically important brain injuries, both rules demonstrated similarly high sensitivity (76.4%–100% for the CCHR and 82%–100% for the NOC) (Bouida et al., 2013; Kavalci et al., 2014; Smits et al., 2005; Stiell et al., 2005). While both studies did lack high specificity, the CCHR demonstrated greater specificity than the NOC (ranges of 37.2%–76.3% for CCHR and 3%–28% for NOC) (Bouida et al., 2013; Kavalci et al., 2014; Smits et al., 2005; Stiell et al., 2005). Further, majority of studies concluded that the CCHR has a greater potential to reduce CT imaging rates than the NOC (Bouida et al., 2013; Smits et al., 2005; Stiell et al., 2005).

For the pediatric population, several different guidelines exist regarding the use of CT imaging: Pediatric Emergency Care Applied Research Network (PECARN), Canadian

**Table 5.4** Guidelines for CT scan in adults

|  | Canadian CT head rule (Stiell et al., 2001) | New orleans criteria (Haydel et al., 2000) |
|---|---|---|
| Criteria | High Risk (for neurological intervention)<br><br>1. GCS score less than 15 at 2 hours after injury<br>2. Suspected or open or depressed skull fracture<br>3. Any sign of basal skull fracture (e.g., raccoon eyes, CSF otorrhea or rhinorrhea, Battle's sign, hemotympanum)<br>4. Two or more episodes of vomiting<br>5. Age 65 years or older medium risk (for brain injury on CT scan)<br>6. Amnesia before impact for 30 minutes or more<br>7. Dangerous mechanism of injury, including a pedestrian struck by a vehicle, occupant ejected from motor vehicle, fall from elevation greater than 3 feet or 5 stairs | 1. Headache<br>2. Vomiting<br>3. Age greater than 60 years old<br>4. Drug or alcohol intoxication<br>5. Persistent anterograde amnesia (deficits in short-term memory)<br>6. Visible trauma superior to the clavicle<br>7. Seizure |

*Source:*   Stiell, I.G. et al., *Lancet*, 357, 1391–1396, 2001; Haydel, M.J. et al., *N. Engl. J. Med.*, 343, 100–105, 2000.

Assessment of Tomography for Childhood Head injury (CATCH) and Children's Head Injury Algorithm for the Prediction of Important Clinical Events (CHALICE) (Dunning et al., 2006; Kuppermann et al., 2009; Osmond et al., 2010). As outlined in Table 5.5, each guideline utilizes different criteria to determine the need for CT.

When comparing these three clinical decision-making rules, one study found that while the CHALICE had the greatest overall specificity of 85%, the PECARN had a greater sensitivity of 100% and was the only one of the three with the ability to identify all clinically important traumatic brain injuries, including mortality related to TBI, neurosurgery requirements, intubation longer than 24 hours, and/or hospital admission more than two nights for TBI (Easter et al., 2014). Further, while physician practice was also found to have 100% sensitivity for identifying patients with clinically important TBI, the PECARN rule had superior specificity (62% vs. 50%) (Easter et al., 2014). Another study in the United Kingdom recommended the PECARN as the best clinical decision for children and infants with minor head injury because it had the largest size cohort, the highest sensitivity and acceptable specificity for clinically significant intracranial injury (Pickering et al., 2011). Lastly, the PECARN guidelines remain the only validated prediction rule of the three (Kuppermann et al., 2009).

While CT imaging is an acceptable and useful neuroimaging modality under certain circumstances, most other imaging technologies, including positron emission tomography (PET), diffusion tensor imaging, magnetic resonance spectroscopy, and functional connectivity, are not recommended except in research settings (McCrory et al., 2017; Rose et al., 2015; Sabini and Reddy, 2010). At the current moment, functional MRI (fMRI) is not generally used in the evaluation of concussion; however, some studies have found that fMRI exhibits activation patterns that are associated with the severity of symptoms and recovery in concussions (Chen et al., 2004a, 2004b, 2004c, 2007; Jantzen et al., 2004; Ptito et al., 2007). As concussions are believed to be functional damage as opposed to structural damage (Ptito et al., 2007; Sabini and Reddy, 2010), fMRI may offer further understanding to the underlying pathophysiology related to concussions (McCrory et al., 2013). The topic of neuroimaging and concussions is discussed in Chapter 20. Furthermore, while there is increasing research on concussion-related biomarkers, including Apolipoprotein E (ApoE), ApoE promoter, Tau polymerase, S-100 calcium binding protein B (S-100B), and glial fibrillary acidic protein (GFAP), that could have clinical utility in the future, at the present time, there is insufficient evidence and a lack of validation to support their use in the standard evaluation, diagnosis, and prognosis of concussions (Bressan and Babl, 2015; Broglio et al., 2014; Kristman et al., 2008; McCrory et al., 2017; Mondello et al., 2014; Papa et al., 2014; Terrell et al., 2008).

## Discharge planning

Once the diagnosis of concussion has been established, patients can be managed primarily in the outpatient setting. However, physicians must first ensure that patients can be safely discharged from the ED or other front-line health care settings. When considering discharge, it is prudent to observe patients for a period of time. For adults, it is recommended that patients be observed at least hourly for a minimum of 4 hours post time of injury (McCrory et al., 2013; Motor Accidents Authority of NSW, 2008; NSW Ministry of Health, 2011). For children, multiple observations for several hours following injury are required (McCrory et al., 2013). At this point, adult patient discharge for home observation can be considered if a patient has a GSC score of 15/15, no persistent post-traumatic amnesia, normal alertness, behavior and cognition, clinical improvement following observation, a

*Table 5.5* Guidelines for CT scan in children and adolescents

| | CATCH (Osmond et al., 2010) | PECARN (Kuppermann et al., 2009) | CHALICE (Dunning et al., 2006) |
|---|---|---|---|
| Indications for CT | Minor head injury: injury within the last 24 hours associated with witnessed loss of consciousness (LOC), definite amnesia, witnessed disorientation, persistent vomiting (>1 episode), or persistent irritability (in a child under 2 years old) in a patient with a GSC of 13–15. Patient must have minor head injury with any of the following: High Risk (need for neurosurgical intervention): GCS <15 at 2 hours post-injury, suspected open or depressed skull fracture, history of worsening headache, and/or irritability on examination. Medium Risk (brain injury on CT scan): any signs of basal skull fracture, large, boggy hematoma of the scalp, dangerous mechanism of injury. | 1. GCS = 14 or other signs of altered mental status or palpable skull fracture.    If criteria 1 not satisfied: must satisfy criteria 2 or 3 <br>2. GCS = occipital, parietal, or temporal scalp hematoma, history of LOC ≥5 seconds, severe mechanism of injury, or not acting normally per parent.    If yes to any of criteria 2: observation versus CT based on clinical factors including: physician experiences, multiple versus isolated findings, worsening symptoms/sign after ED observation, age <3 months, parental preference. <br>3. History of LOC, or history of vomiting, or severe mechanism of injury or severe headache.    If yes to any criteria 3: Observation versus CT based on clinical factors: physician experiences, multiple versus isolated findings, worsening symptoms/sign after ED observation, parental preference. | CT scan if any of the following present: <br>**History** <br>Witnessed loss of consciousness of >5 minutes duration. <br>History of amnesia (either anterograde or retrograde) of >5 minutes duration. <br>Abnormal drowsiness (defined as drowsiness in excess of that expected by the examining doctor). ≥3 vomiting episodes after head injury. <br>Suspicion of nonaccidental injury (NAI, defined as any suspicion of NAI by the examining doctor). <br>Seizure after head injury in a patient who has no history of epilepsy. <br>**Examination** <br>GCS < 14, or GCS <15 if <1 year old. <br>Suspicion of penetrating or depressed skull injury or tense fontanelle. <br>Signs of a basal skull fracture (evidence of blood or CSF from ear or nose, panda eyes, Battles sign, hemotympanum, facial crepitus, or serious facial injury). <br>Positive focal neurology (defined as any focal neurology, including motor, sensory, coordination, or reflex abnormality). |

*(Continued)*

*Table 5.5 (Continued)*  Guidelines for CT scan in children and adolescents

| CATCH (Osmond et al., 2010) | PECARN (Kuppermann et al., 2009) | CHALICE (Dunning et al., 2006) |
|---|---|---|
| | | Presence of bruise, swelling or laceration >5 centimeters if <1 year old. |
| | | **Mechanism** |
| | | High-speed road traffic accident either as pedestrian, cyclist or occupant (defined as accident with speed >40 m/h). |
| | | Fall of >3 meters in height. |
| | | High-speed injury from a projectile or an object. |
| | | If none present, the patient is at low risk of intracranial pathology. |

*Source:*   Dunning, J. et al., *Arch. Dis. Child.,* 91, 885–891, 2006; Kuppermann, N. et al., *Lancet,* 374, 1160–1170, 2009; Osmond, M.H. et al., *CMAJ,* 182, 341–348, 2010.

normal CT scan or no indication for CT scan, and no focal neurological deficits, neurological impairment, clinical suspicion of skull fracture, post-traumatic seizures or known drug or alcohol intoxication (Jagoda et al., 2008; Livingston et al., 2000; Motor Accidents Authority of NSW, 2008; NSW Ministry of Health, 2011; Vos et al., 2012). Elderly patients above the age of 65 with a known coagulopathy require clinical judgment for discharge due to the risk of delayed subdural hematoma and may need further clinical observation (Jagoda et al., 2008; Motor Accidents Authority of NSW, 2008; NSW Ministry of Health, 2011). Failure of any of these requirements may necessitate transportation to a hospital from an outpatient setting or hospital admission from the ED for prolonged observation. Previous studies have demonstrated that there is a low risk of complications, such as intracranial hematoma, in patients with GSC scores of 15, normal CT scans, and normal neurological examination (Af Geijerstam and Britton, 2005; Teasdale et al., 1990; Vos et al., 2012). Similarly, when determining if discharge is appropriate in the pediatric population, children or adolescents should have normal mental status, including alertness, behavior, and cognition, with improving symptoms, no clinical risk factors indicating the need for CT imaging (see Section "The need for head CT scan and other investigations" for clinical risk factors that support the use of CT imaging) or a normal CT scan if performed, and absence of clinical features that would indicate prolonged hospital observation, including worsening or persistent clinical symptoms, coagulopathy, multi-system injuries, or other comorbidities (Adams et al., 2001; Mitchell et al., 1994; Motor Accidents Authority of NSW, 2008; Teasdale et al., 1990; Vos et al., 2012; Zemek et al., 2014). Multiple studies have shown that children with isolated or minor head trauma, possessing many of these features, including a GCS of 15 and negative imaging findings, did not require neurosurgical intervention nor experience neurological complications, and could have likely been discharged without admission (Adams et al., 2001; Mitchell et al., 1994; Teasdale et al., 1990). A final consideration for discharge requires availability of an adult for monitoring at home, ability for a patient to return to a general practitioner or the ED if their condition deteriorates, and comprehension of discharge instructions by the patient and/or caregivers of pediatric patients (Motor Accidents Authority of NSW, 2008; Saunders et al., 1986).

At the time of discharge, verbal and written advice should be provided to the patients and, in the pediatric population, to their parents, caregivers and/or a reliable individual who takes responsibility to ensure instructions are followed by the patient (Motor Accidents Authority of NSW, 2008; Saunders et al., 1986; Waisman et al., 2005; Zemek et al., 2014). One study reviewing the ED discharge instructions from fifteen hospitals in Canada and the United States found that the instructions were often written at an inappropriately high grade-level or with vague wording (Fung et al., 2006). Therefore, discharge information should be written down in an appropriate language and at a reading level suitable for individuals of higher and lower educational backgrounds. Specific verbal and written advice on discharge will be discussed further in Chapter 7.

The final component of discharge in both pediatric and adult populations is to arrange and ensure adequate monitoring and follow up with their family physician or another health care specialist. For adult patients, if symptoms are resolving sufficiently within days, then follow up is only recommended as needed, while if symptoms persist, symptom-based multidisciplinary treatment may be considered with adequate follow up and reassessment in 4–6 weeks (Cifu et al., 2009; Ontario Neurotrauma Foundation, 2013). For children and adolescents, following the primary visit and discharge, health-care professionals should provide verbal and written information regarding the need for children/adolescents to be monitored daily, receive regular follow up with primary care or sports medicine physicians until their symptoms disappear, and, if patients have symptoms for

1 month following diagnosis, refer to specialized care (Babcock et al., 2013; Harvey and Bryant, 1998; McCrory et al., 2017; Ponsford et al., 2001; Sabini and Reddy, 2010; Swaine et al., 2008; Zemek et al., 2014).

## Prediction algorithm to provide accurate anticipatory guidance and to target high-risk pediatric and adult patients for early management

While many children experience symptom resolution within two weeks, approximately one-third suffer a combination of ongoing somatic, cognitive, psychological, and/or behavioral symptoms (Babcock et al., 2013; Barlow et al., 2011; Zemek et al., 2016). When symptoms persist beyond 28 days following concussion, the term PPCS is used (Ayr et al., 2009). However, a recent study set out to derive and validate a clinical risk score, based on certain factors, that could determine the likelihood of developing PPCS in children and youth following acute concussion (Zemek et al., 2016). Nine variables, including older age, female gender, prior history of concussions, history of migraine, answering questions slowly, having four or more errors on the BESS in tandem stance, headache, phonophobia, and fatigue, were incorporated into a PPCS risk score. The use of the PPCS risk score with physician clinical judgment was found to be superior at predicting PPCS for children presenting to the ED with concussion and head injury within the previous 48 hours compared to physician's clinical judgment alone (Zemek et al., 2016). However, external validation is required before this clinical risk score is applied in general practice outside the Pediatric ED setting.

While some studies have associated specific clinical factors, such as headaches at presentation and seizures post-injury, with persistent symptoms (Heidari et al., 2014), past research studies have not had great success in determining useful clinical predictors or models for PPCS, including in the adult population (Lange et al., 2013; Savola and Hillbom, 2003; Sheedy et al., 2006). Another recent study of children and adults attempted to establish a predictive clinical risk factor model for developing PPCS (Wojcik, 2014). Four clinical predictive factors of PPCS were incorporated into their model: past history of mTBI, history of anxiety, forgetfulness and/or poor memory, and photophobia. This model exhibited moderate robustness (AUC = 0.750), with a high negative predictive value (94.7%), moderate specificity (87.9%), and mild sensitivity (69.9%) (Wojcik, 2014). However, unlike in the other pediatric clinical risk score model previously mentioned, their model did not examine demographic information, such as age, gender, and mechanism of injury, as potential predictive factors (Wojcik, 2014), nor was this study validated.

More information on prognostic indications and predictors of persistent symptoms will be discussed in Chapter 6.

## References

Adams J, Frumiento C, Shatney-Leach L, and Vane DW (2001). Mandatory admission after isolated mild closed head injury in children: Is it necessary? *J. Pediatr. Surg. 36*, 119–121.

Af Geijerstam J-L and Britton M (2005). Mild head injury: Reliability of early computed tomographic findings in triage for admission. *Emerg. Med. J. 22*, 103–107.

Ayr LK, Yeates KO, Taylor HG, and Browne M (2009). Dimensions of postconcussive symptoms in children with mild traumatic brain injuries. *J. Int. Neuropsychol. Soc. 15*, 19–30.

Babcock L, Byczkowski T, Wade SL, Ho M, Mookerjee S, and Bazarian JJ (2013). Predicting postconcussion syndrome after mild traumatic brain injury in children and adolescents who present to the emergency department. *JAMA Pediatr. 167*, 156–161.

Bailey NW, Hoy KE, Maller JJ, Segrave RA, Thomson R, Williams N, Daskalakis ZJ, and Fitzgerald PB (2014). An exploratory analysis of go/nogo event-related potentials in major depression and depression following traumatic brain injury. *Psychiatry Res. - Neuroimaging 224*, 324–334.

Ban VS, Madden CJ, Bailes JE, Hunt Batjer H, and Lonser RR (2016). The science and questions surrounding chronic traumatic encephalopathy. *Neurosurg. Focus 40*, E15.

Barlow M, Schlabach D, Peiffer J, and Cook C (2011). Differences in change scores and the predictive validity of three commonly used measures following concussion in the middle school and high school aged population. *Int. J. Sports Phys. Ther. 6*, 150–157.

Bouida W, Marghli S, Souissi S, Ksibi H, Methammem M, Haguiga H, Khedher S, Boubaker H, Beltaief K, Grissa MH, et al. (2013). Prediction value of the Canadian CT head rule and the new orleans criteria for positive head CT scan and acute neurosurgical procedures in minor head trauma: A multicenter external validation study. *Ann. Emerg. Med. 61*, 521–527.

Brenner DJ and Hall EJ (2007). Computed tomography—An increasing source of radiation exposure. *N. Engl. J. Med. 357*, 2277–2284.

Bressan S and Babl FE (2015). Diagnosis and management of paediatric concussion. *J. Paediatr. Child Heal. 52*, 151–157.

Broglio SP, Cantu RC, Gioia GA, Guskiewicz KM, Kutcher J, Palm M, and McLeod TCV (2014). National athletic trainers' association position statement: Management of sport concussion. *J. Athl. Train. 49*, 245–265.

Cantu RC (2003). Recurrent athletic head injury: Risks and when to retire. *Clin. Sport. Med. 22*, 593–603.

Cantu RC (2009). When to disqualify an athlete after a concussion. *Curr. Sports Med. Rep. 8*, 6–7.

Chen JK, Johnston KM, Frey S, Petrides M, Worsley K, and Ptito A (2004a). Functional abnormalities in symptomatic concussed athletes: An fMRI study. *Neuroimage 22*, 68–82.

Chen JK, Johnston K, Collie A, McCrory P, and Ptito A (2004b). Behavioural and functional imaging outcomes in symptomatic concussed athletes measured with cogsport and functional MRI. *Br. J. Sports Med. 38*, 659.

Chen JK, Johnston KM, Collie A, McCrory P, and Ptito A (2004c). Association between symptoms severity, cogsport test results, and functional MRI activation in symptomatic concussed athletes. *Clin. J. Sport Med. 14*, 379.

Chen JK, Johnston KM, Collie A, McCrory P, and Ptito A (2007). A validation of the post concussion symptom scale in the assessment of complex concussion using cognitive testing and functional MRI. *J. Neurol. Neurosurg. Psychiatry 78*, 1231–1238.

Choe MC and Giza CC (2015). Diagnosis and management of acute concussion. *Semin. Neurol. 35*, 29–41.

Davis GA, Purcell L, Schneider KJ, Yeates KO, Gioia GA, Anderson V, Ellenbogen RG, Echemendia RJ, Makidissi M, Sills A, et al. (2017). The Child Sport Concussion Assessment Tool 5th Edition (Child SCAT5). *Br. J. Sports Med.* Published Online First: April 28, 2017. doi:10.1136/bjsports-2017-097492.

Cifu D, Hurley R, Peterson M, Cornis-Pop M, Rikli PA, Ruff RL, Scott SG, Sigford BJ, Silva KA, Tortorice K, et al. (2009). VA/DoD clinical practice guideline for management of concussion/mild traumatic brain injury. *J. Rehabil. Res. Dev. 46*, CP1–CP68.

Dunning J, Daly JP, Lomas J-P, Lecky F, Batchelor J, and Mackway-Jones K (2006). Derivation of the children's head injury algorithm for the prediction of important clinical events decision rule for head injury in children. *Arch. Dis. Child. 91*, 885–891.

Easter JS, Bakes K, Dhaliwal J, Miller M, Caruso E, and Haukoos JS (2014). Comparison of PECARN, CATCH, and CHALICE rules for children with minor head injury: A prospective cohort study. *Ann. Emerg. Med. 64*, 145–152.

Echemendia RJ, Meeuwisse W, McCrory P, Davis GA, Putukian M, Leddy J, Makidissi M, Sullivan SJ, Broglio SP, Raftery M, et al. (2017a). The Sport Concussion Assessment Tool 5th Edition (SCAT5). *Br. J. Sports Med.* Published Online First: April 28, 2017. doi:10.1136/bjsports-2017-097506.

Echemendia RJ, Meeuwisse W, McCrory P, Davis GA, Putukian M, Leddy J, Makidissi M, Sullivan SJ, Broglio SP, Raftery M, et al. (2017b). The Concussion Recognition Tool 5th Edition (CRT5). *Br. J. Sports Med.* Published Online First: April 28, 2017. doi:10.1136/bjsports-2017-097508.

Faul M, Xu L, Wald MM, and Coronado VG (2010). *Traumatic Brain Injury in the United States: Emergency Department Visits, Hospitalizations, and Deaths.* Centers for Disease Control and Prevention, National Center for Injury Prevention and Control, pp. 891–904.

Fung M, Willer B, Moreland D, and Leddy JJ (2006). A proposal for an evidenced-based emergency department discharge form for mild traumatic brain injury. *Brain Inj. 20,* 889–894.

Gioia G and Collins M (2006). Acute Concussion Evaluation (ACE): Physician/Clinician Office Version. Centers for Disease Control and Prevention. *Heads up: Brain injury in your practice: A tool kit for physicians.* http://www.cdc.gov/ncipc/tbi/Physicians_Tool_Kit.

Gioia GA, Collins M, and Isquith PK (2008). Improving identification and diagnosis of mild traumatic brain injury with evidence: Psychometric support for the acute concussion evaluation. *J. Head Trauma Rehabil. 23,* 230–242.

Gioia GA, Schneider JC, Vaughan CG, and Isquith PK (2009). Which symptom assessments and approaches are uniquely appropriate for paediatric concussion? *Br. J. Sports Med. 43*(Suppl 1), i13–i22.

Giza CC, Kutcher JS, Ashwal S, Barth J, Getchius TSD, Gioia GA, Gronseth GS, Guskiewicz K, Mandel S, Manley G, et al. (2013). Summary of evidence-based guideline update: Evaluation and management of concussion in sports: Report of the Guideline Development Subcommittee of the American Academy of Neurology. *Neurology 80,* 2250–2257.

Guskiewicz KM (2003). Assessment of postural stability following sport-related concussion. *Curr. Sports Med. Rep. 2,* 24–30.

Guskiewicz KM, Weaver NL, Padua DA, and Garrett WE (2000). Epidemiology of Concussion in Collegiate and High School Football Players. *Am. J. Sports Med. 28,* 643–650.

Halstead ME, Walter KD, and Council on Sports Medicine and Fitness (2010). American Academy of Pediatrics. Clinical report- sport-related concussion in children and adolescents. *Pediatrics 126,* 597–615.

Harvey A and Bryant R (1998). Acute stress disorder after mild traumatic brain injury. *J. Nerv. Ment. Dis. 186,* 333–337.

Haydel MJ, Preston CA, Mills TJ, Luber S, Blaudeau E, and DeBlieux PM (2000). Indications for computed tomography in patients with minor head injury. *N. Engl. J. Med. 343,* 100–105.

Heidari K, Asadollahi S, Jamshidian M, Abrishamchi SN, and Nouroozi M (2014). Prediction of neuropsychological outcome after mild traumatic brain injury using clinical parameters, serum S100B protein and findings on computed tomography. *Brain Inj. 29,* 33–40.

Hofman P, Nelemans P, Kemerink GJ, and Wilmink JT (2000). Value of radiological diagnosis of skull fracture in the management of mild head injury: Meta-analysis. *J. Neurol. Neurosurg. Psychiatry 68,* 416–422.

Ilie G, Mann RE, Boak A, Adlaf EM, Hamilton H, Asbridge M, Rehm J, and Cusimano MD (2014). Suicidality, bullying and other conduct and mental health correlates of traumatic brain injury in adolescents. *PLoS One 9,* 10–15.

Jagoda AS, Bazarian JJ, Bruns JJ, Cantrill S V, Gean AD, Howard PK, Ghajar J, Riggio S, Wright DW, Wears RL, et al. (2008). Clinical Policy: Neuroimaging and Decisionmaking in Adult Mild Traumatic Brain Injury in the Acute Setting. *Ann. Emerg. Med. 52,* 714–748.

Jantzen KJ, Anderson B, Steinberg FL, and Scott Kelso J (2004). A prospective functional MR imaging study of mild traumatic brain injury in college football players. *Am. J. Neuroradiol. 25,* 738–745.

Johnston KM, Bloom GA, Ramsay J, Kissick J, Montgomery D, Foley D, Chen J, and Ptito A (2004). Current concepts in concussion rehabilitation. *Curr. Sports Med. Rep. 3,* 316–323.

Kavalci C, Aksel G, Salt O, Yilmaz M, Demir A, Kavalci G, Akbuga Ozel B, Altinbilek E, Durdu T, Yel C, et al. (2014). Comparison of the Canadian CT head rule and the new orleans criteria in patients with minor head injury. *World J. Emerg. Surg. 9,* 31.

Kristman VL, Tator CH, Kreiger N, Richards D, Mainwaring L, Jaglal S, Tomlinson G, and Comper P (2008). Does the apolipoprotein epsilon 4 allele predispose varsity athletes to concussion? A prospective cohort study. *Clin. J. Sport Med. 18,* 322–328.

Kuppermann N, Holmes JF, Dayan PS, Hoyle JD, Atabaki SM, Holubkov R, Nadel FM, Monroe D, Stanley RM, Borgialli DA, et al. (2009). Identification of children at very low risk of clinically-important brain injuries after head trauma: A prospective cohort study. *Lancet 374,* 1160–1170.

Lange RT, Brickell TA, Ivins B, Vanderploeg RD, and French LM (2013). Variable, not always persistent, postconcussion symptoms after mild TBI in U.S. military service members: A five-year cross-sectional outcome study. *J. Neurotrauma 30*, 958–969.

Langlois JA, Rutland-Brown W, and Wald MM (2006). The epidemiology and impact of traumatic brain injury: A brief overview. *J. Head Trauma Rehabil. 21*, 375–378.

Lee B and Newberg A (2005). Neuroimaging in traumatic brain imaging. *NeuroRx 2*, 372–383.

Leininger BE, Gramling SE, Farrell AD, Kreutzer JS, and Peck EA (1990). Neuropsychological deficits in symptomatic minor head injury patients after concussion and mild concussion. *J. Neurol. Neurosurg. Psychiatry 53*, 293–296.

Livingston DH, Lavery RF, Passannante MR, Skurnick JH, Baker S, Fabian TC, Fry DE, and Malangoni MA (2000). Emergency department discharge of patients with a negative cranial computed tomography scan after minimal head injury. *Ann. Surg. 232*, 126–132.

Love S and Solomon GS (2014). Talking with parents of high school football players about chronic traumatic encephalopathy: A concise summary. *Am. J. Sports Med. XX*, 1–5.

Lovell MR, Iverson GL, Collins MW, McKeag DB, and Maroon J (1999). Does loss of consciousness predict neuropsychological decrements after concussion? *Clin. J. Sport Med. 9*, 193–198.

Maddocks DL, Dicker GD, and Saling MM (1995). The assessment of orientation following concussion in athletes. *Clin. J. Sport. Med. 5*, 32–35.

Malec JM, Brown AW, Leibson CL, Testa Flaada J, Mandrekar JN, Diehl NN, and Perkins PK (2007). The mayo classification system for traumatic brain injury severity. *J. Neurotrauma 24*, 1317–1424.

McAllister TW and Arciniegas D (2002). Evaluation and treatment of postconcussive symptoms. *NeuroRehabilitation 17*, 265–283.

McAllister TW, Sparling MB, Flashman LA, and Saykin AJ (2001). Neuroimaging findings in mild traumatic brain injury. *J. Clin. Exp. Neuropsychol. 23*, 775–791.

McCrea M (2001). Standardized mental status assessment of sports concussion. *Clin. J. Sport Med. 11*, 176–181.

McCrea M, Guskiewicz KM, Marshall SW, Barr W, Randolph C, Cantu RC, Onate JA, Kelly JP, Page P, Yang J, et al. (2003). Acute effects and recovery time following concussion in collegiate football players: The NCAA Concussion Study. *J. Am. Med. Assoc. 290*, 2556–2563.

McCrory P, Meeuwisse WH, Aubry M, Cantu B, Dvorák J, Echemendia RJ, Engebretsen L, Johnston K, Kutcher JS, Raftery M, et al. (2013). Consensus statement on concussion in sport: The 4th International Conference on Concussion in Sport held in Zurich, November 2012. *Br. J. Sports Med. 14*, e1–e13.

McCrory P, Meeuwisse W, Dvorak J, Aubry M, Bailes J, Broglio S, Cantu RC, Cassidy D, Echemendia RJ, Castellani RJ, et al. (2017). Consensus statement on concussion in sport-the 5th international conference on concussion in sport held in Berlin, October 2016. *Br. J. Sports Med.* Published Online First: April 26, 2017. doi:10.1136/bjsports-2017-097699.

Meares S, Shores E, Taylor A, Batchelor J, Bryant R, Baguley I, Chapman J, Gurka J, Dawson K, Capon L, et al. (2007). Mild traumatic brain injury does not predict acute postconcussion syndrome. *J. Neurol. Neurosurg. Psychiatry 79*, 300–306.

Meehan WP and Mannix R (2010). Pediatric concussions in United States emergency departments in the years 2002 to 2006. *J. Pediatr. 157*, 889–893.

Meehan WP, d'Hemecourt P, and Comstock RD (2010). High school concussions in the 2008-2009 academic year: Mechanism, symptoms, and management. *Am. J. Sports Med. 38*, 2405–2409.

Mitchell K, Fallat M, Raque G, Hardwick V, Groff D, and Nagaraj H (1994). Evaluation of minor head injury in children. *J. Pediatr. Surg. 29*, 851–854.

Mondello S, Schmid K, Berger RP, Kobiessy F, Italiano D, Jeromin A, Hayes RL, Tortella FC, and Buki A (2014). The challenge of mild traumatic brain injury: Role of biochemical markers in diagnosis of brain damage. *Med. Res. Rev. 34*, 503–531.

Mooney G, Speed J, and Sheppard S (2005). Factors related to recovery after mild traumatic brain injury. *Brain Inj. 19*, 975–987.

Motor Accidents Authority of NSW (2008). *Guidelines for Mild Traumatic Brain Injury Following Closed Head Injury*. Sydney, Australia.

NSW Ministry of Health (2011). *Adult Trauma Clinical Practice Guidelines: Initial Management of Closed Head Injury in Adults*. New South Wales.

Ontario Neurotrauma Foundation (2013). *Guidelines for Concussion/Mild Traumatic Brain Injury and Persistent Symptoms.* Toronto, Canada.

Osmond MH, Klassen TP, Wells GA, Correll R, Jarvis A, Joubert G, Bailey B, Chauvin-Kimoff L, Pusic M, McConnell D, et al. (2010). CATCH: A clinical decision rule for the use of computed tomography in children with minor head injury. *CMAJ 182*, 341–348.

Papa L, Ramia MM, Edwards D, Johnson BD, and Slobounov SM (2014). Systematic review of clinical studies examining biomarkers of brain Injury in athletes after sports-related concussion. *J. Neurotrauma 13*, 1–13.

Pearce MS, Salotti JA, Little MP, McHugh K, Lee C, Kim KP, Howe NL, Ronckers CM, Rajaraman P, Craft AW, et al. (2012). Radiation exposure from CT scans in childhood and subsequent risk of leukaemia and brain tumours: A retrospective cohort study. *Lancet 380*, 499–505.

Pickering A, Harnan S, Fitzgerald P, Pandor A, and Goodacre S (2011). Clinical decision rules for children with minor head injury: A systematic review. *Arch. Dis. Child. 96*, 414–421.

Piland SG, Moti RW, Guskiewicz KM, McCrea M, and Ferrara MS (2006). Structural validity of a self-report concussion-related symptom scale. *Med. Sci. Sports Exerc. 38*, 27–32.

Ponsford J, Willmott C, Rothwell A, Cameron P, Ayton G, Nelms R, Curran C, and Ng K (2001). Impact of early intervention on outcome after mild traumatic brain injury in children. *Pediatrics 108*, 1297–1303.

Ptito A, Chen J-K, and Johnston KM (2007). Contributions of functional magnetic resonance imaging (fMRI) to sport concussion evaluation. *NeuroRehabilitation 22*, 217–227.

Putukian M, Raftery M, Guskiewicz K, Herring S, Aubry M, Cantu RC, and Molloy M (2013). Onfield assessment of concussion in the adult athlete. *Br. J. Sports Med. 47*, 285–288.

Ropper AH and Gorson KC (2007). Concussion. *N. Engl. J. Med. 356*, 166–172.

Rose SC, Weber KD, Collen JB, and Heyer GL (2015). The diagnosis and management of concussion in children and adolescents. *Pediatr. Neurol. 53*, 108–118.

Sabini RC and Reddy CC (2010). Concussion management and treatment considerations in the adolescent population. *Phys. Sportsmed. 38*, 139–146.

Saunders CE, Cota R, and Barton CA (1986). Reliability of home observation for victims of mild closed-head injury. *Ann. Emerg. Med. 15*, 160–163.

Savola O and Hillbom M (2003). Early predictors of post-concussion symptoms in patients with mild head injury. *Eur. J. Neurol. 10*, 175–181.

Schneiders AG, Sullivan SJ, Kvarnström J, Olsson M, Ydén T, and Marshall S (2010a). The effect of footwear and sports-surface on dynamic neurological screening for sport-related concussion. *J. Sci. Med. Sport 13*, 382–386.

Schneiders AG, Sullivan SJ, Gray AR, Hammond-Tooke GD, and McCrory PR (2010b). Normative values for three clinical measures of motor performance used in the neurological assessment of sports concussion. *J. Sci. Med. Sport 13*, 196–201.

Sheedy J, Geffen G, Donnelly J, and Faux S (2006). Emergency department assessment of mild traumatic brain injury and prediction of post-concussion symptoms at one month post injury. *J. Clin. Exp. Neuropsychol. 28*, 755–772.

Smits M, Dippel D, de Haan G, Dekker H, Vos P, Kool D, Nederkoorn P, Hofman P, Twijnstra A, and Tanghe H (2005). External validation of the Canadian CT Head Rule and the New Orleans Criteria for CT scanning in patients with minor head injury. *JAMA 294*, 1519–1525.

Stiell IG, Wells GA, Vandemheen K, Clement C, Lesiuk H, Laupacis A, Douglas McKnight R, Verbeek R, Brison R, Cass D, et al. (2001). The Canadian CT Head Rule for patients with minor head injury. *Lancet 357*, 1391–1396.

Stiell IG, Clement CM, Rowe BH, Schull MJ, Brison R, Cass D, A Eisenhauer MA, Douglas McKnight R, Bandiera G, Holroyd B, et al. (2005). Comparison of the Canadian CT head rule and the New Orleans Criteria in patients with minor head injury. *JAMA 294*, 1511–1518.

Swaine BR, Gagnon I, Champagne F, Lefebvre H, Friedman D, Atkinson J, and Feldman D (2008). Identifying the specific needs of adolescents after a mild traumatic brain injury: A service provider perspective. *Brain Inj. 22*, 581–588.

Teasdale GM, Murray G, Anderson E, Mendelow AD, MacMillan R, Jennett B, and Brookes M (1990). Risks of acute traumatic intracranial haematoma in children and adults: Implications for managing head injuries. *BMJ 300*, 363–367.

Terrell TR, Bostick RM, Abramson R, Xie D, Barfield W, Cantu R, Stanek M, and Ewing T (2008). APOE, APOE promoter, and Tau genotypes and risk for concussion in college athletes. Clin. *J. Sport Med. 18*, 10–17.

Vos PE, Alekseenko Y, Battistin L, Ehler E, Gerstenbrand F, Muresanu DF, Potapov A, Stepan CA, Traubner P, Vecsei L, et al. (2012). Mild traumatic brain injury. *Eur. J. Neurol. 19*, 191–198.

Waisman Y, Siegal N, Siegal G, Amir L, Cohen H, and Mimouni M (2005). Role of diagnosis-specific information sheets in parents' understanding of emergency department discharge instructions. *Eur. J. Emerg. Med. 12*, 159–162.

Wojcik SM (2014). Predicting mild traumatic brain injury patients at risk of persistent symptoms in the Emergency Department. *Brain Inj. 28*, 422–430.

Zemek R, Duval S, DeMatteo C, Solomon B, Keightley M, and Osmond M (2014). *Guidelines for Diagnosing and Managing Pediatric Concussion*. Ontario Neurotrauma Foundation, Toronto, Canada.

Zemek R, Barrowman N, Freedman SB, Gravel J, Gagnon I, Mcgahern C, Aglipay M, Sangha G, Boutis K, Beer D, et al. (2016). Clinical risk score for persistent postconcussion symptoms among children with acute concussion in the ED. *JAMA 315*, 1014–1025.

*section two*

---

# Managing a concussion

*chapter six*

# Rest and recovery from concussion

## How should rest be used in concussion management?

*Noah D. Silverberg and Grant L. Iverson*

### Contents

## Introduction

Prescribing rest is one of the most common interventions for concussion. Rest is thought to have two primary objectives, to promote recovery and to prevent reinjury. In recent years, concerns have been raised about too much rest and activity restriction (Craton & Leslie, 2014; DiFazio, Silverberg, Kirkwood, Bernier, & Iverson, 2015; Silverberg & Iverson, 2013). After first providing a historical context, this chapter will outline the theoretical bases for the role of rest in concussion management, review evidence from the observational studies and clinical trials that contribute to our current understanding of the safety and efficacy of rest (and conversely, of activity resumption), summarize contemporary clinical practice recommendations that pertain to rest, and integrate these into practical recommendations for clinicians.

## Evolution of rest in traumatic brain injury care

Rest appears to have been the principle form of subacute treatment for traumatic brain injuries (TBIs) of all severities in the early twentieth century. By the 1920s, *a definite period of rest in bed* is described as an *old clinical maxim* for managing traumatic brain injury (TBI) (Trotter, 1924). Symonds (1928) specified that after the need for neurosurgical intervention has been ruled out, patients with a *major contusion* (loss of consciousness and extended period of post-traumatic amnesia) as well as those with relatively mild injuries (*minor contusion*) should rest in bed. Authors of this era urged not only physical rest with recumbence in bed but also mental rest, by restricting environmental stimulation, such as from loud noises, bright lights, and visitors (Symonds, 1928), and forbidding *mental work* (Pilkington, 1937). There was not universal agreement on the duration of rest. Some advised that the rest period should be proportionate to the severity of the injury (Trotter, 1924), whereas others advocated a minimum fixed duration, such as Watt's (1938) "firm belief that every patient who has been rendered unconsciousness requires a bed rest of at least three weeks" (p. 272). The protocol to *rest until asymptomatic* was also present in the early twentieth century literature. Symonds (1928) recommended that bed rest should continue until a patient's symptoms abate, and at that point, they should be encouraged to gradually reintroduce stimulation and return to their usual daily activities. Following this regimen was sufficient to achieve *complete* recovery in the majority of patients with minor contusion, Symonds wrote.

Following World War II, a trend emerged in medicine. Rest was critiqued as an ineffective and potentially dangerous treatment for conditions ranging from post-surgical recovery to psychiatric disorders (Allen, Glasziou, & Del Mar, 1999). Asher (1947) highlighted *The Dangers of Going to Bed* by describing the adverse effects of prolonged bed rest on the respiratory, circulatory, mulsculoskeletal, digestive, and nervous systems. He challenged the field to not assume the therapeutic benefits of bed rest and be mindful of its negative consequences. Around this time, several authors began to advocate for prompt hospital discharge and early mobilization for concussion (Jefferson, Cairns, Brain, & Gutmann, 1942; Meerloo, 1949; Russell, 1942; Voris, 1950). Meerloo (1949) acknowledged that the "classic therapy of absolute rest" has a role in concussion management, but warned that "too long a rest may cause a secondary neurotic syndrome" (p. 352). Similarly, Voris (1950) accepted that "rest is the best immediate treatment" but cautioned that "it must not be prolonged as then more is lost than gained" (p. 711). He was specifically concerned with iatrogenesis ("To keep such patients in bed is to suggest that they are more seriously injured…this may well become the basis for neurosis.") and physiological deconditioning (p. 710). Across the writings of this period, authors advocate that after a brief period of rest (up to a few days) patients should gradually reintroduce physically and mentally strenuous activity, short of aggravating symptoms (Jefferson et al., 1942; Russell, 1942), but "even at the cost of discomfort" (p. 711; Voris, 1950). Further, patients should attempt to return to work (Voris, 1950) or initiate active rehabilitation (Meerloo, 1949) within the first week after injury.

Departing from this trend, 50 years later, the first International Conference on Concussion in Sport held in Vienna in 2001 produced an agreement statement that summarized a protocol for athletes to return to sport after concussion (Aubry et al., 2002). *No activity, complete rest* until an athlete becomes asymptomatic was the first step in this protocol. The next edition of this agreement statement in 2005 reiterated the return to play protocol, beginning with complete rest (McCrory et al., 2005). It also highlighted rest as the *cornerstone of concussion management* but mentioned that most athletes are expected to recover within a few days, implying that rest usually need not extend beyond this timeframe (McCrory et al., 2005). The 2009 consensus statement introduced the importance of *cognitive rest*, particularly as it pertains to children limiting school work and extracurricular activities (e.g., text messaging and videogames) while still symptomatic (McCrory et al., 2009). The 2013 consensus statement recognized the ambiguity relating to the *rest until asymptomatic* recommendation and indicated that resting for the first 24–48 hours after a sport-related concussion *may be of benefit*, but acknowledged that the optimal duration of rest is not known (McCrory et al., 2013). The consensus statement from the 2016 International Conference on Concussion in Sport went further in retracting the *rest until asymptomatic* approach, instead recommending that after 24–48 hours of rest, "patients can be encouraged to become gradually and progressively more active while staying below their cognitive and physical symptom-exacerbation thresholds" (McCrory et al., 2017).

## Rationale for rest as treatment for concussion

There are three main reasons why rest might be beneficial following concussion. First, in the initial days following injury, injured athletes might be highly symptomatic, cognitively impaired, and they might have problems with dynamic balance (Broglio & Puetz, 2008). Their injured brain might be in a state of neurometabolic crisis (Barkhoudarian, Hovda, & Giza, 2011, 2016; Giza & Hovda, 2001). If so, then increased energy demand associated with physical exercise, for example, might hinder the restorative process. Exercise generally has positive neurobiological effects following induced TBI in rodents (Griesbach, 2011; Griesbach, Hovda, & Gomez-Pinilla, 2009; Mychasiuk, Hehar, Ma, Candy, & Esser, 2016). It is not clear whether exercise can impede recovery if offered too soon after injury (Griesbach, Hovda, Molteni, Wu, & Gomez-Pinilla, 2004; Mychasiuk et al., 2016). Second, athletes who sustain a second concussion in a single season might be at the greatest risk for doing so within the first 10 days following the initial injury (McCrea et al., 2009). The reasons for this are unclear, but it is possible that athletes' brains are more vulnerable to reinjury during this acute phase. Overlapping concussions might cause magnified pathophysiology. There is evidence in the animal literature that there is a temporal window of vulnerability in which a second injury results in magnified cognitive and behavioral deficits, greater levels of traumatic axonal injury, and other cellular pathophysiologies (Laurer et al., 2001; Longhi et al., 2005; Vagnozzi et al., 2007). Finally, rest might have indirect health benefits, although this has not been studied. Anecdotally, we have noted and heard from clinicians that some injured athletes, at the time of injury, might have chronic sleep insufficiency, life stress, and school stress—and resting following the injury might have some indirect benefits in those areas. Prolonged rest, however, might increase life and school stress and thus result in worse outcomes. This will be discussed in a later section.

## Evidence that rest facilitates recovery from concussion

The above-described benefits of rest are largely theoretical. We have learned from other health conditions that assumptions about the benefits of bed rest often do not hold up to scientific investigation (Allen et al., 1999). Fortunately, there is now a substantive body of evidence addressing the efficacy of rest for concussion. In one of the first empirical studies, Andreassen, Bach-Nielsen, Heckscher, and Lindberg (1957) reported a historical controlled study of patients admitted to the hospital with concussion. Concussion was operationally defined as having peri-injury amnesia and other post-concussion symptoms directly following head trauma, with a loss of consciousness not exceeding 30 minutes and no "neurological signs of focal brain injuries" (p. 241). The authors instituted a strict protocol of early mobilization and compared the rates of recovery in their cohort with those in previously published cohorts treated with lengthy bed rest. After resting in bed for 3–6 days, mobilization was encouraged, even for patients who had residual *minor complaints*. As long as increased activity did not exacerbate symptoms (which happened *rarely*), patients were "discharged immediately and advised to go back to work as soon as possible" (p. 242). Outcomes in the group with *mild concussion* (defined as having a loss of consciousness of no more than 30 minutes) were favorable: 90% returned to work within one month and 99% returned within 6 months, with 7%–8% reporting mild persistent symptoms. This was contrasted with earlier cohorts that had higher rates of persistent symptoms (35%–50%) following 2–3 weeks of bed rest. A randomized controlled trial by Relander et al. (1972) similarly reported benefits of early activation. They compared an active treatment group in which patients "were encouraged to get up as early as possible" and promptly received physical therapy to a usual care control group in which patients were "allowed to get up when they felt like it, but no special effort was made to make them get up" (p. 778; Relander et al., 1972). The active treatment group returned to work approximately twice as fast as the usual care group (mean 15–19 vs. 32–33 days). At one-year follow-up, the two groups contained a similar proportion of patients with chronic symptoms (32% vs. 40%).

There have been a number of observational designs over the last decade investigating the association between patient's level of activity after concussion and recovery. Majerske et al. (2008) retrospectively coded the activity level of 95 student athletes over the first month following a concussion. Student athletes who reported being the least active (no school or sports participation) and the most active (returned to school and sport) had relatively low neurocognitive performance relative to the groups with moderate activity levels. Symptoms were not significantly related to activity level. The authors hypothesized that the harmful effects of exertion may have explained why concussed athletes who were most active had poor neurocognitive outcomes. Since this report, several other observational studies have produced mixed findings. More cognitive activity (e.g., school attendance, homework, text messaging, video games, etc.) during the weeks after concussion has been shown to correlate with same-day symptom load (Makki et al., 2016) and longer symptom duration (Brown et al., 2014). However, student athletes who were specifically prescribed cognitive rest (extracted from chart review) did not recover faster than those who were not explicitly advised to avoid mental exertion (Corwin et al., 2014; Eisenberg, Andrea, Meehan, & Mannix, 2013; Gibson, Nigrovic, O'Brien, & Meehan, 2013). As well, students who adhered more closely to a sports medicine physician's advice to not participate in school and avoid using electronics tended to recover more slowly, defined by a longer time in treatment (Moor et al., 2015). Another study found no significant relationship between physical activity following sport-related concussion and symptom duration (Howell, Osternig, Van Donkelaar, Mayr, & Chou, 2013). Poor adherence to recommendations for physical rest was associated with faster recovery in one study (Moor et al., 2015). Finally, as part of the pan-Canadian Predicting Persistent Post-concussive Problems in Pediatrics (5P) study (N = 3063, 67.6% sport-related concussion), Grool et al. (2016) reported that, after matching on observed baseline characteristics, children who engaged in physical activity within the first week after presenting to an Emergency Department with concussion had a lower risk of persistent symptoms at one-month follow-up compared to children who were physically inactive for at least one week following concussion.

Rather than examine absolute activity levels over a period of days to weeks, some studies have investigated whether discrete bouts of activity influence the recovery trajectory. Hou et al. (2012) recruited adults from an Emergency Department and followed them in a prospective cohort design. A self-reported pattern of *all-or-nothing* behavior in which patients over-exerted themselves and then *crashed* with disabling fatigue (i.e., rested) was predictive of chronic symptoms at three-month follow-up. Silverberg et al. (2016) analyzed the activity diary and daily symptom ratings of youth with concussion over the first 10 days after visiting an Emergency Department. They operationalized *symptom spikes* as statistically reliable increases in post-concussion symptom reporting from one day to the next. Abrupt increases in mental activity, typically a return to full school days, were associated with an increased risk for a transient symptom spike, but not for impaired cognition or balance at the end of the 10-day observation period. Most symptom spikes were not preceded by high mental or physical activity. These findings suggest that symptom spikes cannot be avoided by rest. They also do not support the hypothesis that early cognitive or physical exertion slows recovery from concussion. Another study piloting objective measurement of activity with accelerometry in combination with a diary smartphone app found that higher symptom reporting was predicted by *lower* physical activity and *higher* cognitive activity on the same day and preceding two days (Wiebe et al., 2016). Like Silverberg et al. (2016), these authors found that irrespective of patients' activity levels most became asymptomatic by the end of the (two-week) observation period (Wiebe et al., 2016).

Several nonrandomized clinical trials have also contributed to this literature. Moser, Glatts, and Schatz (2012) described a cohort of 49 student athletes who were instructed to rest for a full week after their first concussion clinic visit. Specifically, they were given an extensive list of activities to avoid, including physical exercise, sports, school, homework, socializing, text messaging, shopping trips, reading, video games, and watching sports on television. On retesting one week later, the cohort performed better on cognitive testing and reported fewer post-concussion symptoms regardless of how recent their concussion was (1–7 vs. 8–30 vs. 31+ days prior to clinic visit). Limitations of this study included probable selection bias, conflation with other *active ingredients* in usual care, and a lack of control group, randomization, and systematic monitoring of adherence to prescribed rest. In a follow-up study, Moser, Schatz, Glenn, Kollias, and Iverson (2015) retrospectively studied 13 student athletes who underwent a post-injury assessment and were not instructed to rest or were not compliant with rest instructions, and then entered into the clinical protocol from Moser et al. (2012). These athletes showed greater improvement on cognitive testing and symptom reductions following a week of rest compared to the interval between their first post-injury assessment and the start of the rest protocol (mean = 25 days). In a historical controlled study, Buckley, Munkasy, and Clouse (2015) compared student athletes before versus after implementing a change in clinical practice. Student athletes seen before the change were not explicitly advised to rest. Following the change, every concussed student athlete was withheld from all school and sport activities for the remainder of the day and the day following their injury. To facilitate compliance, the sports medicine clinic provided documentation for class absences and team coaches were informed of the no-activity prescription. The group that was prescribed complete rest took longer to become symptom-free (5.2–3.9 days, on average) but there were no group differences on time to achieve baseline scores on cognition and balance testing.

To date, there have been two randomized controlled trials evaluating the efficacy of prescribing strict rest in prospective cohorts of patients seen in an Emergency Department. Adults in the strict rest group reported somewhat less intense post-concussion symptoms over the first few days post-injury, but the opposite trend was observed at the six month follow-up assessment, despite greater attrition in the no-rest group (de Kruijk, Leffers, Meerhoff, Rutten, & Twijnstra, 2002). Children prescribed strict rest for 5 days reported more symptoms over the 10-day observation period, taking on average 3 days longer than the usual care control group to achieve symptom resolution (Thomas, Apps, Hoffmann, McCrea, & Hammeke, 2015). The two groups performed similarly on measures of cognition and balance obtained at 3 and 10 days post-injury. Of note, compliance (as assessed through activity diaries) was modest in both of these studies, potentially weakening group differences in outcome.

Other randomized controlled trials have examined multifaceted behavioral treatments that included encouragement and/or clinical support to expediently resume preinjury activities (Bell et al., 2008; Matuseviciene, Borg, Stålnacke, Ulfarsson, & de Boussard, 2013; Mittenberg, Tremont, Zielinski, Fichera, & Rayls, 1996; Silverberg et al., 2013). Three found evidence favoring the treatment arm that included this intervention component versus usual care (Bell et al., 2008; Mittenberg et al., 1996; Silverberg et al., 2013) and a fourth found no significant group differences (Matuseviciene et al., 2013). In other words, these studies did not specifically address the efficacy of prescribed rest, but do suggest that interventions designed to promote prompt resumption of preinjury activities (i.e., the opposite of rest) may be beneficial for recovery, or at least are not harmful. We are not aware of any concussion studies that have evaluated the effectiveness of a stand-alone intervention that uses techniques with known efficacy for increasing life participation such as time-contingent progression for low back pain (increasing activity levels to quota rather than to tolerance; Lindström et al., 1992) or exposure hierarchies for anxiety disorders.

In summary, the best available evidence to date suggests that (1) rest does not accelerate recovery and (2) promptly resuming preinjury activities does not slow recovery. In fact, promptly resuming activities may be beneficial. The effects of vigorous (high intensity) physical activity within the first 48 hours of concussion are mostly unknown. Marsden et al. (2015) evaluated 12 amateur youth athletes with an exercise protocol within 72 hours of injury and found that mild-moderate exercise caused or exacerbated headaches, and these headaches were associated with alterations in intracranial velocities of cerebral perfusion. Based on the prevailing model of acute pathophysiology following injury (Barkhoudarian et al., 2016), animal models of exercise after TBI (Griesbach et al., 2004; Griesbach, 2011; but see Mychasiuk et al., 2016), and evidence from very early mobilization after stroke (AVERT Trial Collaboration group et al., 2015), vigorous physical activity within the first 48 hours of concussion should be avoided until further safety data are available.

## Possible harmful effects of rest and activity restriction

Rest, especially prolonged rest and activity restriction, might lead to physical deconditioning, exercise intolerance, maladaptive responses to vestibular symptoms, social isolation, life stress, and/or adverse psychological effects in some people. Bed rest results in physiologic changes after a relatively short period of time (Fortney, Schneider, & Greenleaf, 2011; Smorawinski et al., 2001). Deconditioning and exercise intolerance can begin after only 2–3 days of bed rest. Smorawinski and colleagues (2001) studied the effects of three days of bed rest on three groups of subjects: endurance-trained athletes, strength-trained athletes, and sedentary men. Three days of bed rest was associated with diminished work tolerance, aerobic capacity, and anaerobic threshold to the greatest extent in the endurance-trained men. Moreover, endurance trained athletes showed alterations in hormonal responses to exercise that were not shown by the other groups. One week of bed rest can substantially reduce skeletal muscle mass and lower whole-body insulin sensitivity (Dirks et al., 2016). Fourteen days of bed rest in young adults was associated with a low-grade systemic inflammatory response (i.e., increased serum visfatin, resistin, and adiponectin) (Jurdana et al., 2015).

An extended period of bed rest is contraindicated in a broad range of medical conditions, including stroke, low back injury, whiplash injury, and post-surgical recovery (Allen et al., 1999). Rest, combined with anxiety over symptoms, might lead some people with concussion to greatly restrict their movements and activities in such a way that perpetuates vestibular symptoms. One principle in vestibular therapy is that habituation exercises, such as repetitive head movements or eye movements in a manner that provokes symptoms, can be used to desensitize symptoms, leading to a gradual reduction in the intensity and duration of these symptoms (Gizzi, 1995; Tee & Chee, 2005).

In the general population, exercise training has beneficial cardiovascular effects in that it is associated with decreased resting and submaximal heart rate, and increased heart rate variability, total power, and high-frequency power (Carter, Banister, & Blaber, 2003). Prolonged rest and activity restriction might result in cardiovascular deconditioning. Some people who suffer from persistent symptoms following concussion develop intolerance for exercise (Kozlowski, Graham, Leddy, Devinney-Boymel, & Willer, 2013), and a supervised exercise program has been shown to reduce symptoms and improve functioning (Baker, Freitas, Leddy, Kozlowski, & Willer, 2012; Gagnon, Galli, Friedman, Grilli, & Iverson, 2009; Leddy et al., 2012).

Prolonged rest and activity restriction can result in social isolation, and social isolation can have adverse psychological effects. Separation from the ability to communicate with others by modern technology can cause distress in youth (Clayton, Leshner, & Almond, 2015). Students might miss a considerable amount of school; fall far behind in their classes, adding to their distress. Moreover, activity restriction (or a reduced capacity to participate in one's usual activities) following injury or illness is associated with depression (Lewinsohn, Hoberman, Teri, & Hautzinger, 1985; Walters & Williamson, 1999; Williamson, 2000). Activity restriction in adolescents who have chronic health problems appears to directly contribute to depression (Walters & Williamson, 1999).

Another potential concern is that strict advice to rest may engender maladaptive beliefs that negatively influence recovery from concussion. For example, warning patients that even routine activity such as text messaging could damage their brain implicitly communicates that they sustained a serious injury (Craton & Leslie, 2014), and this could contribute to anxiety and hypersensitivity to symptoms. Strong medical advice for prolonged rest and activity restriction could lead people to expect that they will have a slow recovery and contribute to the misattribution of all symptoms to the lingering effects of concussion versus other factors, such as life stress, school or work stress, mild depression, or anxiety. The *nocebo* effect, conceptualized as the causation of sickness by the expectations of sickness and by associated hyperarousal, can be related to prolonged symptoms after concussion (Vanderploeg, Belanger, & Kaufmann, 2014). If an individual views concussion as a serious injury that will produce lasting effects, it may in fact create or exacerbate the experience of symptoms after an injury. Indeed, there is evidence from multiple adult studies that people who expect to recover slowly or incompletely are more likely to have chronic symptoms (Cassidy, Boyle, & Carroll, 2014; Snell, Hay-Smith, Surgenor, & Siegert, 2013; Whittaker, Kemp, & House, 2007). Expectations, attributions, and other beliefs about symptoms can be strongly related to both the severity and the duration of symptoms in some people.

## Contemporary clinical practice recommendations for rest and return to activity

The American Medical Society for Sports Medicine position statement (Harmon et al., 2013) proposed that in the *early stages of a concussion recovery*, athletes should not engage in any physical or cognitively demanding activities that worsen their symptoms. They endorse the *rest until asymptomatic* guideline. The most recent iteration of the International Conference on Concussion in Sport consensus statement (McCrory et al., 2017) recommends that after resting for up to 48 hours, athletes should be encouraged to gradually increase their level of cognitive and physical activity at a pace that does not exacerbate their symptoms. The American Academy of Neurology practice parameter for sport-related concussion (Giza et al., 2013) highlights that return to activity with an elevated concussion risk should occur only once a qualified health professional has determined the concussion to be resolved, to prevent repeat concussion. This document does not otherwise address the role of rest in sport concussion management.

Children have been highlighted to require special consideration as it pertains to rest after concussion. The 4th International Conference on Concussion in Sport consensus statement (McCrory et al., 2013) contains a provision that the return to play protocol should be more conservative for children, and specifically, "It is appropriate to extend the amount of time of asymptomatic rest." DeMatteo et al. (2015a) developed pediatric specific recommendations that operationalize this period as one week. That is, children should rest until they become symptom free, and then continue resting for another week. However, they also caution clinicians to balance rest with the possible consequences of prolonged activity restriction, such as depression and deconditioning. Children who have been persistently symptomatic for beyond one month should consult with a physician about how to proceed, according to DeMatteo et al. (2015a). The 5th International Conference on Concussion in Sport consensus statement (McCrory et al., 2017), however, stated that additional rest time for children is not indicated. Rather, the timing of symptom-limited resumption of activity should be *similar to adults*.

Rest has not been favorably endorsed in recent clinical practice guidelines for nonsport concussion. The second edition of the Ontario Neurotrauma Foundation's Guidelines for Concussion/Mild Traumatic Brain Injury & Persistent Symptoms (2013) no longer advises rest in an unqualified manner. They encourage an initial period of rest to promote recovery, but specify that bed rest should not exceed three days and can be proceeded by a gradual return to activity *as tolerated*. The Department of Veterans Affairs and the Department of Defense Veterans (2009) guidelines for managing mild traumatic brain injury (MTBI) recommended *a period of rest* following concussion, but also that "should be encouraged to *expediently* return to normal activity" [emphasis added], suggesting that the period ought to be brief (VA/DoD, 2009). For individuals who have persistent symptoms, there is little guidance for how they might progress with their activities. The Progressive Return to Activity Following Acute Concussion/Mild TBI guideline produced by the Defense and Veterans Brain Injury Center (Ustün et al., 2014) more thoroughly operationalized the initial period of rest and subsequent stages of return to activity. Individuals who cannot progress to the next level within one week should be referred to a specialist. In the 2016 Department of Veterans Affairs and the Department of Defense Veterans guidelines for managing MTBI, recommendations to rest were altogether removed (VA/DoD, 2016).

## The knowledge-practice gap

Clinician surveys and chart reviews suggest that prescribing rest is one of the most common strategies for managing both sport-related concussions and concussions occurring in other settings. Most family physicians in the United States and Canada report routinely advising physical rest (76%–84%) (Lebrun et al., 2013). Rates of recommending cognitive rest have generally been lower and more variable across multiple studies and medical specialists (Arbogast et al., 2013; Lebrun et al., 2013; Stoller, Carson, Snow, Law, & Frémont, 2014; Zemek et al., 2015). There is also variability in how cognitive rest recommendations are implemented. Restricting television and computer screen time appears relatively common (70%–80%), but recommending complete cognitive rest by staying home from school, deferring schoolwork, and avoiding all forms of screen time may be much less common (Zemek et al., 2015).

Reflecting current clinical practice, virtually all patient education materials, on-line and in print, advocate for rest after concussion. For example, the Centers for Disease Control and Prevention materials (http://www.cdc.gov/headsup/pdfs/providers/facts_about_concussion_tbi-a.pdf) suggest that "rest is very important after a concussion because it helps the brain to heal." They also warn that exertion can *slow your recovery*. Similarly, WebMD.com (http://www.webmd.com/brain/tc/traumatic-brain-injury-concussion-overview?page=3) advises that "rest is the best way to recover from a concussion." Generic advice to *get plenty of rest* and more sleep is also included in the majority of Emergency Department written discharge instructions (Kempe, Sullivan, & Edmed, 2014; Kerr, Swann, & Pentland, 2007).

Studies investigating the clinical uptake of prescribed rest have universally concluded that this intervention is under-used and advocated for more aggressive knowledge translation efforts to increasingly incorporate prescribed rest into their routine care of patients with concussion (e.g., Arbogast et al., 2013; Lebrun et al., 2013; Stoller et al., 2014). This concern appears to be based on endorsement of the 2009 (or earlier) International Consensus on Concussion in Sport statement for use in all practice settings. However, when considering the most recent (2013/2017) version of this consensus statement, practice guidelines for nonsport concussion, and the accumulated empirical evidence reviewed earlier, we consider the knowledge-practice gap to be in the opposite direction. Clinicians should consider making only qualified time-limited recommendations to rest and include advice for how to go about returning to full activity.

## Recommendations for implementing rest and return to activity recommendations in clinical practice

The recommendations listed in this section represent an attempt to integrate the above-reviewed research evidence and consensus statements with our clinical experience.

1. *Define rest*: Patients' interpretations of advice to *rest* may range from complete recumbence in a dark bedroom to taking only brief breaks from a hectic schedule. When prescribing rest, clinicians are encouraged to specify what is meant by rest, such as reducing the frequency and intensity of their usual preinjury daily activities to a degree that minimizes symptoms. Specific activities that should be avoided or limited could be mentioned. It may also be helpful to communicate what rest is not, for example, *social isolation or sensory deprivation* (DeMatteo et al., 2015a) and explain that both physically and mentally demanding activities need to be curtailed in order to *rest the brain*.
2. *Communicate a timeline for rest*: Rest should not be prescribed for an indefinite period. The current evidence does not support that complete rest (e.g., no school, work, socializing, or physical activity or recreation) improves outcomes from concussion. Prescribing complete rest beyond 2–3 days should be weighed against the potential adverse effects of prolonged rest, described earlier. If applying the *rest until asymptomatic* criterion, clinicians should be mindful that it can be challenging to ascertain when an individual patient's concussion symptoms have fully resolved because post-concussion-like symptoms are common in healthy people (Iverson & Lange, 2003)

and they can be exacerbated by stress (Gouvier, Cubic, Jones, Brantley, & Cutlip, 1992), poor sleep (Silverberg, Berkner, Atkins, Zafonte, & Iverson, 2016), pain (Smith-seemiller, Fow, Kant, & Franzen, 2003), and other factors. Moreover, patients tend to misremember being relatively free of post-concussion-like symptoms prior to their concussion (Gunstad & Suhr, 2001).

3. *Negotiate a sequential return to activity*: Contemporary practice recommendations universally agree that youth should successfully reintegrate into school before attempting to return to sports. It may be prudent to delay return to activities that have an elevated risk for concussion and other injuries, such as collision sports or certain occupations and recreation activities, until the patient's cognition and balance have normalized. To be clear, we are not recommending activity restriction to promote recovery from the index injury, but rather to avoid reinjury while the brain is vulnerable.

4. *Operationalize the return to activity plan*: A gradual (vs. abrupt) return to preinjury activities may help to minimize the risk of symptom exacerbations (Silverberg et al., 2016). Activity-related symptom exacerbations might heighten anxiety and complicate a transition back to school or work in some people, so they should be avoided if possible. Because the threshold for provoking symptoms with exertion is not universal, the pace of activity progression should be individualized. For many patients, simple advice to gradually return to their usual activities *in a manner that does not significantly exacerbate symptoms* (McCrory et al., 2013; Ontario Neurotrauma Foundation, 2013) may suffice. For those with numerous residual symptoms or who are highly activity-intolerant or who are returning to very demanding roles, it may be helpful to collaboratively map out a detailed step-by-step plan for returning to a particular activity. In brief, the International Consensus on Concussion in Sport statement provides clear guidance for a stepwise return to competitive sport. The CanChild Return to School Guidelines for Children and Youth (DeMatteo et al., 2015b) is an excellent resource for planning staged academic reintegration. They describe intermediate stages to transition from rest to full school participation. Other resources for managing return to school following concussion are available (Echemendia et al., 2013; Gioia, 2014; Iverson & Gioia, 2016). The Defense Centers of Excellence (2015) Progressive Return to Activity Following Acute Concussion/Mild Traumatic Brain Injury guideline outlines a staged approach to returning to military service, including metrics for exertion intensity at each stage (Borg's Perceived Exertion scale) and advancement to the next stage of activity (based on the Neurobehavioral Symptom Inventory). Given the diversity of occupations and occupational demands, a plan for returning to work must be individually tailored. Extracting common principles from the previous consensus statements and guidelines, the plan should generally involve transitioning from rest to routine daily activities (e.g., going for a walk, reading for pleasure, housekeeping) to part-time work (potentially with modified duties or accommodations, such as rest breaks) to a full return to work. Progression can occur when a patient can tolerate a given activity intensity.

5. *Monitor adherence to the gradual return to activity plan*: It is clear from clinical trial data that adherence to activity restrictions tends to be modest. Strategies to promote adherence may include providing a clear rationale, creating a written plan, reviewing activity diaries, motivational interviewing, and enlisting cooperation from parents or other family members. In recovery from any injury, *setbacks* can be expected. Prior to initiating the return to activity plan, it may be helpful to caution patients

that symptomatic recovery may not follow a linear course and that symptom exacerbations are fairly common and usually transient (Silverberg et al., 2016). This may
help patients to get *back on track* if they progress too quickly. Some patients develop a
pattern of over-exertion followed by complete rest, and then over-exertion, etc. This
*boom and bust* cycle may be detrimental to recovery (Hou et al., 2012). Counseling to not
*overdo it*, when a patient feels relatively well, but rather adhering to the gradual return
to activity plan, may help avoid this maladaptive pattern, especially for patients with
*Type A* personality traits. Scheduling regular follow-up visits at key transition points
in the return to activity plan can help the clinician to monitor a patient's progress
and problem-solve as needed. Patients who do not attempt to increase their activity
as expected should be evaluated for a depressive, anxiety, and vestibular disorders,
because anhedonia, fear avoidance, or motion sensitivity may underlie their slow
progress. In patients who are highly activity-intolerant, physiological deconditioning, performance anxiety, migraines, and motion sensitivity should be considered as
possible explanations. These patients may require finer gradations in their stepwise
return to activity plan and potentially other interventions (e.g., migraine prophylax-
tic therapy, vestibular rehabilitation, and/or psychological therapy).

## Summary

Rest is perhaps the oldest and simplest medical treatment. Its rationale is intuitive and
its efficacy assumed. Over the first half of the twentieth century, rest gave way to early
mobilization in the treatment of concussion and other health conditions. Curiously, this
trend reversed into the early twenty-first century, as the *rest until asymptomatic* maxim
spread beyond sports medicine clinics to other health care settings, where recovery takes
(on average) weeks rather than days. The benefits of rest in the first few days following
injury remain unproven, but the pathophysiology of concussion supports this recommendation. The best available evidence now favors a gradual return to activity once a
patient has reached the subacute phase of recovery (48+ hours after injury), as tolerated.
Two recent systematic reviews in sport-related concussion arrived at this same conclusion,
for both children and adults (Davis et al., 2017; Schneider et al., 2017). Expert opinion has
also aligned in this direction over the past few years (Collins et al., 2016; McCrory et al.,
2017). Prescribing complete rest for subacute or post-acute concussion, like any other intervention, should be weighed against its possible adverse side effects. Patients who cannot
gradually resume activity require strategic clinical support or a referral to specialist care.

## References

Allen, C., Glasziou, P., & Del Mar, C. (1999). Bed rest: A potentially harmful treatment needing more
    careful evaluation. *The Lancet, 354*(9186), 1229–1233.
Andreassen, J., Bach-Nielsen, P., Heckscher, H., & Lindberg, O. (1957). Reassurance and brief bed rest
    in the treatment of concussion. *Acta Medica Scandinavica, CLVIII*, 239–248.
Arbogast, K. B., McGinley, A. D., Master, C. L., Grady, M. F., Robinson, R. L., & Zonfrillo, M. R. (2013).
    Cognitive rest and school-based recommendations following pediatric concussion: The need
    for primary care support tools. *Clinical Pediatrics, 52*, 397–402. doi:10.1177/0009922813478160
Asher, R. A. J. (1947). The dangers of going to bed. *British Medical Journal, 13*, 967–968.
Aubry, M., Cantu, R., Dvorak, J., Graf-Baumann, T., Johnston, K. M., Kelly, J., ... Schamasch, P. (2002).
    Summary and agreement statement of the 1st International Symposium on Concussion in
    Sport, Vienna 2001. *Clinical Journal of Sport Medicine, 12*(1), 6–11.

AVERT Trial Collaboration group, Bernhardt, J., Langhorne, P., Lindley, R. I., Thrift, A. G., Ellery, F., … Donnan, G. (2015). Efficacy and safety of very early mobilisation within 24 h of stroke onset (AVERT): A randomised controlled trial. *The Lancet, 386*(9988), 46–55. doi:10.1016/S0140-6736(15)60690-0.

Baker, J. G., Freitas, M. S., Leddy, J. J., Kozlowski, K. F., & Willer, B. S. (2012). Return to full functioning after graded exercise assessment and progressive exercise treatment of postconcussion syndrome. *Rehabilitation Research and Practice, 2012,* 705309. doi:10.1155/2012/705309.

Barkhoudarian, G., Hovda, D. A., & Giza, C. C. (2016). The molecular pathophysiology of concussive brain injury: An update. *Physical Medicine and Rehabilitation Clinics North America, 27*(2), 373–393.

Barkhoudarian, G., Hovda, D. A, & Giza, C. C. (2011). The molecular pathophysiology of concussive brain injury. *Clinics in Sports Medicine, 30*(1), 33–48. doi:10.1016/j.csm.2010.09.001.

Bell, K. R., Hoffman, J. M., Temkin, N. R., Powell, J. M., Fraser, R. T., Esselman, P. C., … Dikmen, S. (2008). The effect of telephone counselling on reducing post-traumatic symptoms after mild traumatic brain injury: A randomised trial. *Journal of Neurology, Neurosurgery & Psychiatry, 79*(11), 1275–1281. doi:10.1136/jnnp.2007.141762.

Broglio, S. P., & Puetz, T. W. (2008). The effect of sport concussion on neurocognitive function, self-report symptoms and postural control. *Sports Medicine, 38,* 53–67.

Brown, N. J., Mannix, R. C., O'Brien, M. J., Gostine, D., Collins, M. W., & Meehan, W. P. (2014). Effect of cognitive activity level on duration of post-concussion symptoms. *Pediatrics, 133*(2), e299–e304. doi:10.1542/peds.2013-2125.

Buckley, T., Munkasy, B., & Clouse, B. (2015). Acute cognitive and physical rest may not improve concussion recovery time. *Journal of Head Trauma Rehabilitation.*

Carter, J. B., Banister, E. W., & Blaber, A. P. (2003). The effect of age and gender on heart rate variability after endurance training. *Medicine and Science in Sports and Exercise, 35*(8), 1333–1340. doi:10.1249/01.MSS.0000079046.01763.8F.

Cassidy, J. D., Boyle, E., & Carroll, L. J. (2014). Population-based, inception cohort study of the incidence, course, and prognosis of mild traumatic brain injury after motor vehicle collisions. *Archives of Physical Medicine and Rehabilitation, 95*(3 Suppl), S278–S285. doi:10.1016/j.apmr.2013.08.295.

Clayton, R. B., Leshner, G., & Almond, A. (2015). The extended iSelf: The impact of iPhone separation on cognition, emotion, and physiology. *Journal of Computer-Mediated Communication, 20,* 119–135. doi:10.1111/jcc4.12109.

Collins, M. W., Kontos, A. P., Okonkwo, D. O., Almquist, J., Bailes, J., Barisa, M., … Zafonte, R. (2016). Statements of agreement from the targeted evaluation and active management (TEAM) approaches to treating concussion meeting held in Pittsburgh, October 15–16, 2015. *Neurosurgery, 79*(6), 1. doi:10.1227/NEU.0000000000001447.

Corwin, D. J., Zonfrillo, M. R., Master, C. L., Arbogast, K. B., Grady, M. F., Robinson, R. L., … Wiebe, D. J. (2014). Characteristics of prolonged concussion recovery in a pediatric subspecialty referral population. *Journal of Pediatrics, 165*(6), 1207–1215. doi:10.1016/j.jpeds.2014.08.034.

Craton, N., & Leslie, O. (2014). Is rest the best intervention for concussion? Lessons learned from the whiplash model. *Current Sports Medicine Reports, 13*(4), 201–204. doi:10.1249/JSR.0000000000000072.

Davis, G. A., Anderson, V., Babl, F. E., Gioia, G. A., Giza, C. C., Meehan, W., … Zemek, R. (2017). What is the difference in concussion management in children as compared with adults? A systematic review. *British Journal of Sports Medicine* 1–12. doi:10.1136/bjsports-2016-097415.

de Kruijk, J. R., Leffers, P., Meerhoff, S., Rutten, J., & Twijnstra, A. (2002). Effectiveness of bed rest after mild traumatic brain injury: A randomised trial of no versus six days of bed rest. *Journal of Neurology, Neurosurgery, and Psychiatry, 73*(2), 167–172.

DeMatteo, C., Stazyk, K., Giglia, L., Mahoney, W., Singh, S., Hollenberg, R., … Randall, S. (2015a). A balanced protocol for return to school for children and youth following concussive injury. *Clinical Pediatrics, 54,* 783–792. doi:10.1177/0009922814567305.

DeMatteo, C., Stazyk, K., Singh, S. K., Giglia, L., Hollenberg, R., Malcolmson, C. H., … McCauley, D. (2015b). Development of a conservative protocol to return children and youth to activity following concussive injury. *Clinical Pediatrics, 54*(2), 152–63. doi:10.1177/0009922814558256.

DiFazio, M., Silverberg, N. D., Kirkwood, M. W., Bernier, R., & Iverson, G. L. (2015). Prolonged Activity Restriction After Concussion: Are We Worsening Outcomes? *Clinical Pediatrics*. doi:10.1177/0009922815589914.

Dirks, M., Wall, B., van de Valk, B., Holloway, T., Holloway, G., Chabowski, A., ... van Loon, L. (2016). One week of bed rest leads to substantial muscle atrophy and induces whole-body insulin resistance in the absence of skeletal muscle lipid accumulation. *Diabetes, 65*, 2862–2875.

Echemendia, R. J., Iverson, G. L., McCrea, M., Macciocchi, S. N., Gioia, G. a, Putukian, M., & Comper, P. (2013). Advances in neuropsychological assessment of sport-related concussion. *British Journal of Sports Medicine, 47*(5), 294–298. doi:10.1136/bjsports-2013-092186.

Eisenberg, M. A., Andrea, J., Meehan, W., & Mannix, R. (2013). Time interval between concussions and symptom duration. *Pediatrics, 132*(1), 8–17. doi:10.1542/peds.2013-0432.

Fortney, S., Schneider, V., & Greenleaf, J. (2011). The physiology of bed rest. *Comprehensive Physiology*, Supp 14(889–939).

Ontario Neurotrauma Foundation (2013). *Guidelines for Concussion/Mild Traumatic Brain Injury & Persistent Symptoms*. Retrieved from http://onf.org/system/attachments/223/original/ONF_mTBI_Guidelines_2nd_Edition_COMPLETE.pdf

Gagnon, I., Galli, C., Friedman, D., Grilli, L., & Iverson, G. L. (2009). Active rehabilitation for children who are slow to recover following sport-related concussion. *Brain Injury, 23*(November), 956–964. doi:10.3109/02699050903373477.

Gibson, S., Nigrovic, L. E., O'Brien, M., & Meehan, W. P. (2013). The effect of recommending cognitive rest on recovery from sport-related concussion. *Brain Injury, 27*(7–8), 839–42. doi:10.3109/02699 052.2013.775494.

Gioia, G. A. (2014). Medical-school partnership in guiding return to school following mild traumatic brain injury in youth. *Journal of Child Neurology, 31*, 1–16. doi:10.1177/0883073814555604.

Giza, C. C., & Hovda, D. A. (2001). The Neurometabolic Cascade of Concussion. *Journal of Athletic Training, 36*(3), 228–235. Retrieved from http://www.pubmedcentral.nih.gov/articlerender.fcgi?artid=155411&tool=pmcentrez&rendertype=abstract

Giza, C. C., Kutcher, J. S., Ashwal, S., Barth, J., Getchius, T. S. D., Gioia, G. A, ... Zafonte, R. (2013). Summary of evidence-based guideline update: Evaluation and management of concussion in sports: Report of the Guideline Development Subcommittee of the American Academy of Neurology. *Neurology, 80*(24), 2250–2257. doi:10.1212/WNL.0b013e31828d57dd.

Gizzi, M. (1995). The efficacy of vestibular rehabilitation for patients with head trauma. *Journal of Head Trauma Rehabilitation, 10*(6), 60–77.

Gouvier, W. D., Cubic, B., Jones, G., Brantley, P., & Cutlip, Q. (1992). Postconcussion symptoms and daily stress in normal and head-injured college populations. *Archives of Clinical Neuropsychology: The Official Journal of the National Academy of Neuropsychologists, 7*(3), 193–211.

Griesbach, G. S. (2011). Exercise after traumatic brain injury: Is it a double-edged sword? *PM & R: The Journal of Injury, Function, and Rehabilitation, 3*(6 Suppl 1), S64–S72. doi:10.1016/j.pmrj.2011.02.008.

Griesbach, G. S., Hovda, D. A., & Gomez-Pinilla, F. (2009). Exercise-induced improvement in cognitive performance after traumatic brain injury in rats is dependent on BDNF activation. *Brain Research, 1288*, 105–115. doi:10.1016/j.brainres.2009.06.045.

Griesbach, G. S., Hovda, D. A., Molteni, R., Wu, A., & Gomez-Pinilla, F. (2004). Voluntary exercise following traumatic brain injury: Brain-derived neurotrophic factor upregulation and recovery of function. *Neuroscience, 125*(1), 129–139. doi:10.1016/j.neuroscience.2004.01.030.

Grool, A. M., Aglipay, M., Momoli, F., Meehan, W. P., Freedman, S. B., Yeates, K. O., ... Zemek, R. (2016). Association between early participation in physical activity following acute concussion and persistent postconcussive symptoms in children and adolescents. *JAMA, 316*(23), 2504. doi:10.1001/jama.2016.17396.

Gunstad, J., & Suhr, J. A. (2001). "Expectation as etiology" versus "the good old days": Postconcussion syndrome symptom reporting in athletes, headache sufferers, and depressed individuals, *Journal of the International Neuropsychological Society, 7*, 323–333.

Harmon, K. G., Drezner, J., Gammons, M., Guskiewicz, K., Halstead, M., Herring, S., ... Roberts, W. (2013). American Medical Society for Sports Medicine position statement: concussion in sport. *Clinical Journal of Sport Medicine: Official Journal of the Canadian Academy of Sport Medicine, 23*(1), 1–18. doi:10.1097/JSM.0b013e31827f5f93.

Hou, R., Moss-Morris, R., Peveler, R., Mogg, K., Bradley, B. P., & Belli, A. (2012). When a minor head injury results in enduring symptoms: A prospective investigation of risk factors for postconcussional syndrome after mild traumatic brain injury. *Journal of Neurology, Neurosurgery, and Psychiatry, 83*(2), 217–223. doi:10.1136/jnnp-2011-300767.

Howell, D., Osternig, L., Van Donkelaar, P., Mayr, U., & Chou, L.-S. (2013). Effects of concussion on attention and executive function in adolescents. *Medicine and Science in Sports and Exercise, 45*(6), 1030–1037. doi:10.1249/MSS.0b013e3182814595.

Iverson, G., & Gioia, G. (2016). Returning to school following sport-related concussion. *Physical Medicine Rehabilitation Clinics North America, 27*(2), 429–436.

Iverson, G. L., & Lange, R. T. (2003). Examination of "postconcussion-like" symptoms in a healthy sample. *Applied Neuropsychology, 10*(3), 137–144. doi:10.1207/S15324826AN1003_02.

Jefferson, G., Cairns, H., Brain, W., & Gutmann, L. (1942). Discussion on rehabilitation after injuries of the central nervous system. *Proceedings of the Royal Society of Medicine, 35*(4), 295–308.

Jurdana, M., Jenko-Pražnikar, Z., Mohorko, N., Petelin, A., Jakus, T., Šimunič, B., & Pišot, R. (2015). Impact of 14-day bed rest on serum adipokines and low-grade inflammation in younger and older adults. *Age, 37*(6), 116.

Kempe, C. B., Sullivan, K. A., & Edmed, S. L. (2014). A critical evaluation of written discharge advice for people with mild traumatic brain injury: What should we be looking for? *Brain Injury, 9052,* 1–8. doi:10.3109/02699052.2014.937360.

Kerr, J., Swann, I. J., & Pentland, B. (2007). A survey of information given to head-injured patients on direct discharge from emergency departments in Scotland. *Emergency Medicine Journal, 24,* 330–332. doi:10.1136/emj.2006.044230.

Kozlowski, K. F., Graham, J., Leddy, J. J., Devinney-Boymel, L., & Willer, B. S. (2013). Exercise intolerance in individuals with postconcussion syndrome. *Journal of Athletic Training, 48,* 627–635. doi:10.4085/1062-6050-48.5.02.

Laurer, H. L., Bareyre, F. M., Lee, V. M., Trojanowski, J. Q., Longhi, L., Hoover, R., … McIntosh, T. K. (2001). Mild head injury increasing the brain's vulnerability to a second concussive impact. *Journal of Neurosurgery, 95*(5), 859–870. doi:10.3171/jns.2001.95.5.0859.

Lebrun, C. M., Mrazik, M., Prasad, A. S., Tjarks, B. J., Dorman, J. C., Bergeron, M. F., … Valentine, V. D. (2013). Sport concussion knowledge base, clinical practises and needs for continuing medical education: A survey of family physicians and cross-border comparison. *British Journal of Sports Medicine, 47*(1), 54–59. doi:10.1136/bjsports-2012-091480.

Leddy, J. J., Cox, J. L., Baker, J. G., Wack, D. S., Pendergast, D. R., Zivadinov, R., & Willer, B. (2012). Exercise treatment for postconcussion syndrome: A pilot study of changes in functional magnetic resonance imaging activation, physiology, and symptoms. *The Journal of Head Trauma Rehabilitation, 28*(4), 241–249. doi:10.1097/HTR.0b013e31826da964.

Lewinsohn, E., Hoberman, H., Teri, L., & Hautzinger, M. (1985). An integrative theory of depression. In S. Reiss & R. Bootzin (Eds.), *Theoretical issues in behavior therapy* (pp. 331–359). Academic Press, Cambridge, MA.

Lindström, I., Ohlund, C., Eek, C., Wallin, L., Peterson, L. E., Fordyce, W. E., & Nachemson, A. L. (1992). The effect of graded activity on patients with subacute low back pain: A randomized prospective clinical study with an operant-conditioning behavioral approach. *Physical Therapy, 72*(4), 279–290. doi:10.1093/ptj/72.4.279.

Longhi, L., Saatman, K. E., Fujimoto, S., Raghupathi, R., Meaney, D. F., Davis, J., … McIntosh, T. K. (2005). Temporal window of vulnerability to repetitive experimental concussive brain injury. *Neurosurgery, 56*(2), 364–374. doi:10.1227/01.NEU.0000149008.73513.44.

Majerske, C., Mihalik, J. P., Ren, D., Collins, M. W., Reddy, C. C., Lovell, M. R., & Wagner, A. K. (2008). Concussion in sports: Postconcussive activity levels, symptoms, and neurocognitive performance. *Journal of Athletic Training, 43*(3), 265–274.

Makki, A. Y., Leddy, J., Hinds, A., Baker, J., Paluch, R., Shucard, J., & Willer, B. (2016). School attendance and symptoms in adolescents after sport-related concussion. *Global Pediatric Health, 3,* 1–3. doi:10.1177/2333794X16630493.

Marsden, K., Strachan, N., Monteleone, B., Ainslie, P., Iverson, G., & Don, V. (2015). The relationship between exercise-induced increases in cerebral perfusion and headache exacerbation following sport-related concussion: A preliminary study. *Current Research: Concussion, 2*(1), 17–21.

Matuseviciene, G., Borg, J., Stålnacke, B.-M., Ulfarsson, T., & de Boussard, C. (2013). Early intervention for patients at risk for persisting disability after mild traumatic brain injury: A randomized, controlled study. *Brain Injury*, 27(3), 318–324. doi:10.3109/02699052.2012.7 50740.

McCrea, M., Guskiewicz, K., Randolph, C., Barr, W. B., Hammeke, T. A., Marshall, S. W., & Kelly, J. P. (2009). Effects of a symptom-free waiting period on clinical outcome and risk of reinjury after sport-related concussion. *Neurosurgery*, 65, 876–882. doi:10.1227/01. NEU.0000350155.89800.00.

McCrory, P., Johnston, K., Meeuwisse, W., Aubry, M., Cantu, R., Dvorak, J., … Schamasch, P. (2005). Summary and agreement statement of the 2nd International Conference on Concussion in Sport, Prague 2004. *British Journal of Sports Medicine*, 39(4), 196–204. doi:10.1136/ bjsm.2005.018614.

McCrory, P., Meeuwisse, W., Dvorak, J., Aubry, M., Bailes, J., Broglio, S., … Vos, P. E. (2017). Consensus statement on concussion in sport—the 5th international conference on concussion in sport held in Berlin, October 2016. *British Journal of Sports Medicine*. doi:10.1136/ bjsports-2017-097699.

McCrory, P., Meeuwisse, W. H., Aubry, M., Cantu, B., Dvorák, J., Echemendia, R. J., … Turner, M. (2013). Consensus statement on concussion in sport: The 4th International Conference on Concussion in Sport held in Zurich, November 2012. *British Journal of Sports Medicine*, 47(5), 250–258. doi:10.1136/bjsports-2013-092313.

Mccrory, P., Meeuwisse, W., Johnston, K., Dvorak, J., Aubry, M., Molloy, M., & Cantu, R. (2009). Consensus statement on concussion in sport – The 3rd International Conference on Concussion in sport, held in Zurich, November 2008 q. *Journal of Clinical Neuroscience*, 16(6), 755–763. doi:10.1016/j.jocn.2009.02.002.

Meerloo, A. (1949). Cerebral concussion: A psychosomatic survey. *Journal of Nervous and Mental Disorders*, 110, 347–353.

Mittenberg, W., Tremont, G., Zielinski, R. E., Fichera, S., & Rayls, K. R. (1996). Cognitive-behavioral prevention of postconcussion syndrome. *Archives of Clinical Neuropsychology: The Official Journal of the National Academy of Neuropsychologists*, 11(2), 139–145.

Moor, H. M., Eisenhauer, R. C., Killian, K. D., Proudfoot, N., Henriques, A. A., & Congeni, J. A. (2015). The relationship between adherence behaviors and recovery time in adolescents after a sports-related concussion: An observational study. *The International Journal of Sports Physical Therapy*, 10(2), 225–233.

Moser, R. S., Glatts, C., & Schatz, P. (2012). Efficacy of immediate and delayed cognitive and physical rest for treatment of sports-related concussion. *The Journal of Pediatrics*, 161(5), 922–926. doi:10.1016/j.jpeds.2012.04.012.

Moser, R. S., Schatz, P., Glenn, M., Kollias, K. E., & Iverson, G. L. (2015). Examining prescribed rest as treatment for adolescents who are slow to recover from concussion. *Brain Injury*, 29(1), 58–63. doi:10.3109/02699052.2014.964771.

Mychasiuk, R., Hehar, H., Ma, I., Candy, S., & Esser, M. J. (2016). Reducing the time interval between concussion and voluntary exercise restores motor impairment, short-term memory, and alterations to gene expression. *European Journal of Neuroscience*, 44(7), 2407–2417. doi:10.1111/ejn.13360.

Pilkington, F. (1937). The treatment of the mental after-effects of head injury. *Irish Journal of Medical Science*, 12, 742–745.

Relander, M., Troupp, H., & af Björkesten, G. (1972). Controlled trial of treatment for cerebral concussion. *British Medical Journal*, 4(5843), 777–779.

Russell, W. R. (1942). Medical aspects of head injury. *British Medical Journal*, 521–523.

Schneider, K. J., Leddy, J. J., Guskiewicz, K. M., Seifert, T., McCrea, M., Silverberg, N. D., … Makdissi, M. (2017). Rest and treatment/rehabilitation following sport-related concussion: A systematic review. *British Journal of Sports Medicine*. doi:10.1136/bjsports-2016-097475.

Silverberg, N. D., Berkner, P. D., Atkins, J. E., Zafonte, R., & Iverson, G. L. (2016). Relationship between short sleep duration and preseason concussion testing. *Clinical Journal of Sport Medicine: Official Journal of the Canadian Academy of Sport Medicine*, 26(3), 226–231.

Silverberg, N. D., Hallam, B. J., Rose, A., Underwood, H., Whitfield, K., Thornton, A. E., & Whittal, M. L. (2013). Cognitive-behavioral prevention of postconcussion syndrome in at-risk patients: A pilot randomized controlled trial. *The Journal of Head Trauma Rehabilitation, 28*(4), 313–322. doi:10.1097/HTR.0b013e3182915cb5.

Silverberg, N. D., & Iverson, G. L. (2013). Is rest after concussion "the best medicine?": Recommendations for activity resumption following concussion in athletes, civilians, and military service members. *The Journal of Head Trauma Rehabilitation, 28,* 250–259. doi:10.1097/HTR.0b013e31825ad658.

Silverberg, N. D., Iverson, G. L., McCrea, M., Apps, J. N., Hammeke, T. A., & Thomas, D. G. (2016). Activity-Related Symptom Exacerbations After Pediatric Concussion. *JAMA Pediatrics, 170*(10), 946–953. doi:10.1001/jamapediatrics.2016.1187.

Smith-seemiller, L., Fow, N. R., Kant, R., & Franzen, M. D. (2003). Presence of post-concussion syndrome symptoms in patients with chronic pain vs mild traumatic brain injury, *17.* doi:10.1 080/0269905021000030823.

Smorawinski, J., Nazar, K., Kaminska, E., Cybulski, G., Bicz, B., Greenleaf, J. E., … Kamin, E. (2001). Effects of 3-day bed rest on physiological responses to graded exercise in athletes and sedentary men Effects of 3-day bed rest on physiological responses to graded exercise in athletes and sedentary men. *Journal of Applied Physiology, 91*(1), 249–257.

Snell, D. L., Hay-Smith, E. J. C., Surgenor, L. J., & Siegert, R. J. (2013). Examination of outcome after mild traumatic brain injury: The contribution of injury beliefs and Leventhal's common sense model. *Neuropsychological Rehabilitation, 23*(3), 333–362. doi:10.1080/09658211.2 012.758419.

Stoller, J., Carson, J. D., Snow, C. L., Law, M., & Frémont, P. (2014). Do family physicians, emergency department physicians, and pediatricians give consistent sport-related concussion management advice? *Canadian Family Physician Médecin de Famille Canadien, 60*(6), 548–552.

Symonds, C. (1928). The differential diagnosis and treatment of cerebral states consequent upon head injuries. *British Medical Journal,* 829–832.

Tee, L. H., & Chee, N. W. C. (2005). Vestibular rehabilitation therapy for the dizzy patient. *Annals of the Academy of Medicine Singapore, 34,* 289–294.

Thomas, D. G., Apps, J. N., Hoffmann, R. G., McCrea, M., & Hammeke, T. (2015). Benefits of strict rest after acute concussion: A randomized controlled trial. *Pediatrics, 135*(2). doi:10.1542/peds.2014-0966.

Trotter, W. (1924). On certain minor injuries of the brain. *British Medical Journal,* 816–819.

Ustün, T. B., Chatterji, S., Kostanjsek, N., Rehm, J., Kennedy, C., Epping-Jordan, J., … Pull, C. (2014). *Defense Centers of Excellence Progressive Return to Activity Following Acute Concussion/Mild Traumatic Brain Injury: Guidance for the Primary Care Manager in Deployed and Non-deployed Settings DCoE Clinical Recommendation.*

VA/DoD. (2009). *Clinical Practice Guideline Management of Concussion/mild Traumatic Brain Injury.*

VA/DoD. (2016). *Management of Concussion-mild Traumatic Brain Injury (mTBI) clinical practice guidelines.*

Vagnozzi, R., Tavazzi, B., Signoretti, S., Amorini, A., Belli, A., Cimatti, M., … Lazzarino, G. (2007). Temporal window of metabolic brain vulnerability to concussions: Mitochondrial-related impairment—part I. *Neurosurgery, 61*(2), 379–388.

Vanderploeg, R. D., Belanger, H. G., & Kaufmann, P. M. (2014). Nocebo effects and mild traumatic brain injury: Legal implications. *Psychological Injury and Law, 7*(3), 245–254. doi:10.1007/s12207-014-9201-3.

Voris, H. (1950). Mild head injury (concussion). *American Journal of Surgery, 80,* 707–713.

Walters, A. S., & Williamson, G. M. (1999). The role of activity restriction in the association between pain and depression: A study of pediatric patients with chronic pain. *Children's Health Care.* doi:10.1207/s15326888chc2801_3.

Watt, J. (1938). Head injuries: A treatise from the viewpoint of diagnosis, prognosis and treatment. *American Journal of Surgery, 41,* 272–274.

Whittaker, R., Kemp, S., & House, A. (2007). Illness perceptions and outcome in mild head injury: A longitudinal study. *Journal of Neurology, Neurosurgery, and Psychiatry, 78*(6), 644–646. doi:10.1136/jnnp.2006.101105.

Wiebe, D., Nance, M., Houseknecht, E., Grady, M., Otto, N., Sandsmark, D., & Master, C. (2016). Ecologic momentary assessment to accomplish real-time capture of symptom progression and the physical and cognitive activities of patients daily following concussion. *JAMA Pediatrics, 170*(11), 1108–1110.

Williamson, G. M. (2000). Extending the activity restriction model of depressed affect: Evidence from a sample of breast cancer patients. *Health Psychology: Official Journal of the Division of Health Psychology, American Psychological Association, 19*(4), 339–347. doi:10.1037/0278-6133.19.4.339.

Zemek, R., Eady, K., Moreau, K., Farion, K. J., Solomon, B., Weiser, M., & DeMatteo, C. (2015). Canadian pediatric emergency physician knowledge of concussion diagnosis and initial management. *CJEM, 17,* 115–122. doi:10.1017/cem.2014.38.

# chapter seven

# Early management recommendations
## What should be done now that we know it is a concussion?

*Roger Zemek and Josh Stanley*

## Contents

## Introduction

Once a minor head injury has been evaluated with an established concussion diagnosis, it is important to consider comorbidities that may influence recovery. Existing comorbid medical conditions, mental health disorders (e.g., depression, anxiety, learning deficits and attention deficit hyperactivity disorder [ADHD]), and additional associated injuries (Johnston et al., 2004; McCrory et al., 2017) may necessitate a multidisciplinary approach. This may require referral to other health-care practitioners including physiotherapists, occupational therapists, neuropsychologists, psychiatrists, or psychologists (see Chapters 8 through 11). If other, more severe head injuries, including hemorrhage and skull fractures, are suspected, CT imaging and neurosurgical intervention may be required (see Chapter 5) (Giza et al., 2013; Halstead et al., 2010; Hofman et al., 2000; Jagoda et al., 2008; McAllister et al., 2001; Ontario Neurotrauma Foundation, 2013; Sabini and Reddy, 2010). In addition, if a patient displays any *red flag* symptoms, physicians may consider prolonged observation or admission for further assessment and monitoring even in the presence of normal neuroimaging (see Chapter 5) (Gioia et al., 2008; Jagoda et al., 2008; Putukian et al., 2013).

After the initial assessment, the clinician should determine a treatment plan for the patient and provide both verbal information and written handouts. Providing information sheets has been shown to benefit patients and their caregivers; studies have found a greater improvement in parental understanding of treatment when provided instruction sheets (Waisman et al., 2005). Furthermore, lower symptoms levels, such as sleep disturbances, anxiety, and psychological distress are also associated with the provision of written information on symptoms, coping strategies, and expected recovery course (Ponsford et al., 2001). This chapter will focus on the various components of the treatment plan: (1) anticipatory guidance on the timeline of expected recovery, suggestions to permit optimal recovery (e.g., proper sleep hygiene), and recommendations for injury prevention; (2) cognitive and physical rest; and (3) nonpharmacological and, if necessary, pharmacological therapy for specific symptoms.

## Anticipatory guidance: The maintenance of healthy living and promotion of healthy habits to optimize recovery

### Expected recovery and return to activities

When educating patients and/or their families, it is important to normalize symptoms by explaining that they are common and expected. The anticipated outcomes and recovery should also be discussed (Riechers and Ruff, 2010). Specifically, physicians can provide reassurance to patients and their families that, despite differences amongst patients in the exact time course of recovery, majority of patients will make a full recovery and will have symptom resolution within a few days or weeks (Carroll et al., 2004; Ganesalingam et al., 2008; Halstead et al., 2010; McCrory et al., 2005; Motor Accidents Authority of NSW, 2008; NSW Ministry of Health, 2011; Ontario Neurotrauma Foundation, 2013; Rose et al., 2015). However, a minority of patients may experience symptoms for up to 3 months (Lundin et al., 2006; NSW Ministry of Health, 2011; Ontario Neurotrauma Foundation, 2013; Rose et al., 2015). Furthermore, recovery in children may be longer than in adults (Halstead et al., 2010; McCrory et al., 2005; McCrory et al., 2017), as approximately one-third of children presenting to the ED will have symptoms persisting at 1 month (Babcock et al., 2013; Barlow et al., 2011; Zemek et al., 2016). Physicians should also emphasize that careful observation and follow-up is necessary for patients with persistent symptoms beyond one month of injury (persistent post-concussive symptoms or PPCS). Certain risk factors, including severity of initial symptoms following injury, post-concussive migraine headaches and depression, and preexisting mental health disorders or migraines, may predict slower recovery and/or more persistent symptoms with sport-related concussions (McCrory et al., 2017). Clinical risk scores also exist that may facilitate prediction of PPCS. A recent clinical risk score based on nine clinical variables demonstrated superior ability to predict the likelihood of PPCS in children when combined with physician judgment compared with physician judgment alone (see Chapter 5, part 4) (Zemek et al., 2016). Physicians should discuss the burden and distress that parents and/or caregivers of children and adolescents with concussions may experience (Carroll et al., 2004; Ganesalingam et al., 2008). By doing all of the above, it may help to limit anxiety related to concussions, establish realistic expectations about recovery, prevent reinjury, enhance recovery, and limit symptom impact on daily functioning (Bell et al., 2008; Ferguson et al., 1999; Ganesalingam et al., 2008).

Many patients and their families may inquire about the timeline to return to various activities. Return to school, work, and sports will be discussed in greater detail in Chapters 12, 13, and 14, respectively. In brief, all guidelines emphasize a gradual, step-wise return to their life roles and activities, including sports, school, and work (Choe and Giza, 2015; Cifu et al., 2009; Halstead et al., 2010; McCrory et al., 2017; Scorza et al., 2012).

For example, the parachute *After a Concussion Guidelines for Return to Play* incorporates recommendations of the 2012 Zurich consensus statement on sport-related concussions by suggesting at least 24 hours before progressing to the next step (McCrory et al., 2013; Parachute Canada, 2013) (http://www.parachutecanada.org/downloads/resources/ return-to-play-guidelines.pdf). This has been further reaffirmed in the most recent 2016 Berlin consensus statement on sport-related concussions (McCrory et al., 2017). However, recommendations vary slightly in the amount of time required before a patient can progress to a step that is closer to normal functioning; this variation is most likely due to the paucity of definitive trials examining the comparative effectiveness of rest versus exertion (Schneider et al., 2013).

## Positive behaviors to promote recovery

After providing anticipatory guidance on expected recovery and return to activities to patients diagnosed with concussion, physicians should outline healthy behaviors and lifestyle modifications that may promote recovery and prevent long-term negative outcomes. Physicians should provide education about proper sleep hygiene. This includes maintaining a consistent bedtime and wakeup time schedule and establishing a fixed bedtime routine. Avoiding or minimizing caffeine, alcohol, or nicotine, limiting activities such as eating, reading, or television in the bedroom, and turning off electronic devices, such as cell phones and computers, a minimum of 30 minutes before bedtime may also facilitate better sleep habits (Cifu et al., 2009; Meehan, 2011; Motor Accidents Authority of NSW, 2008; Ontario Neurotrauma Foundation, 2013; Ouellet et al., 2012; Rao and Rollings, 2002; Riechers and Ruff, 2010; Sabini and Reddy, 2010). Maintaining proper sleep hygiene may be helpful in managing symptoms of concussion; specifically, it is recommended as first-line treatment for sleep disturbances including insomnia and hypersomnia (Arciniegas et al., 2005; Meehan, 2011; Rao and Rollings, 2002; Sabini and Reddy, 2010). Education surrounding sleep and fatigue symptoms and their triggers may be helpful in patient recovery; for example, physicians should explain to patients experiencing post-concussion fatigue that this symptom may be provoked spontaneously or with minimal exertion and should emphasize the importance of attempting to recognize triggers of fatigue (Harvey and Bryant, 1998; Ponsford et al., 2001).

Following traumatic brain injury (TBI) and concussion, patients may experience changes in their mental health, including irritability, changes in mood, and anxiety (Bailey et al., 2014; Ilie et al., 2014; Jagoda et al., 2008; Johnston et al., 2004; Meares et al., 2007; Motor Accidents Authority of NSW, 2008; Sabini and Reddy, 2010), all of which may impact their relationships with friends and family and their participation in leisure activities. For example, patients post-injury may be missing social interactions normally occurring through sports and recreational activities. Other social activities may be hampered due to symptom exacerbation; headaches and fatigue may be exacerbated by certain settings, such as going out to the movies or restaurants, due to bright lights and/or loud noises. To avoid social isolation, it is, therefore, important for physicians to encourage their patients to engage in social activities with modifications, such as interacting with a smaller group of individuals or avoiding situations that may trigger or worsen symptoms for that specific patient (Zemek et al., 2014). By providing this guidance, recovery may be promoted with a reduction in the risk of mental health issues and social isolation that has been associated with concussions and traumatic brain injury (Ilie et al., 2014; Jonsson and Andersson, 2012; Zemek et al., 2014).

## *Avoidance of reinjury, alcohol, recreational drugs, and driving*

Physicians should provide advice on the risk and complications of reinjury, which includes persistent symptoms and the rare but often lethal phenomenon of the second impact syndrome. This is especially important to discuss with pediatric patients and their parents or caregivers, as children and adolescents that return to sports prior to fully recovering may be at higher risk of sustaining another, potentially more severe, concussion, and may be more likely to be affected than adults (McCrea et al., 2004; McCrory, 2001). With the second impact syndrome, an additional impact to a brain that is in a vulnerable state of recovery can cause malignant cerebral edema and herniation, which has a mortality rate approaching 100% (Bey and Ostick, 2009; McCrea et al., 2004; McCrory, 2001; Wetjen et al., 2010). As well, children and adolescents that sustain multiple concussions have been found to report more somatic, cognitive, physical, and sleep disturbance-related symptoms, including headache, dizziness, problems with balance, nausea, and fatigue, compared with individuals with one or no concussions (Schatz et al., 2011). Therefore, it is recommended to avoid high speed and contact activities that may increase the risk of sustaining another concussion, particularly during this recovery period, until all symptoms have resolved (McCrory, 2001; McCrory et al., 2013). Furthermore, patients who have sustained numerous concussions should be referred to an expert in sport concussions to assist them with decisions regarding returning to play or retirement from contact sports (Choe and Giza, 2015; Giza et al., 2013; Sabini and Reddy, 2010; Schatz et al., 2011; Zemek et al., 2014).

As part of the early management of concussions, physicians should advise against the use of alcohol and other recreational drugs entirely for children and adolescents or until a patient is fully recovered in the case of adults. The goals of this recommendation are to avoid the use of alcohol as a means of self-medicating for their symptom relief, prevent the negative effects of drugs and alcohol, which may exacerbate or mimic certain symptoms of concussions such as nausea and difficulty concentrating, and preclude impaired judgment that may result in harmful risk-taking behavior (Motor Accidents Authority of NSW, 2008; Swaine et al., 2008; Zemek et al., 2014).

Physicians should provide guidance regarding driving for patients with concussions. Driving is complicated process that requires the coordination of various functions that may be affected by concussion, including reaction time, balance, visual perception, and higher order cognition such as attention and executive function (Canadian Medical Association, 2012; Preece et al., 2010, 2013). One study found that patients with mild TBI were significantly slower to respond to traffic hazards in a computerized hazard perception test compared with patients with minor orthopedic injuries (Preece et al., 2010). However, despite the dangers and risks of driving post-concussion, many individuals may not reduce their driving exposure accordingly (Preece et al., 2013). To ensure patient and public road safety, it is recommended that patients with concussions avoid driving for at least 24 hours and instead have physical and cognitive rest. Patients should not drive until their symptoms resolve, and they can fully concentrate (Canadian Medical Association, 2012; Motor Accidents Authority of NSW, 2008). If a patient experiences any concerning symptoms, such as severe or worsening headache, confusion, or multiple episodes of vomiting, after the initial assessment, patients should refrain from driving and seek immediate medical attention before returning to drive (Motor Accidents Authority of NSW, 2008).

## Physical and cognitive rest

A central component in the acute management of concussions is prescribing physical and cognitive rest (Choe and Giza, 2015; Halstead et al., 2010; McCrory et al., 2017; Moser et al., 2012; Rose et al., 2015; Sabini and Reddy, 2010). Cognitive and physical rest involves refraining from aerobic exercise or athletic activities, time off work and school, limiting activities that require concentration and attention, and refraining from usage of electronic devices such as cell phones and computers (Meehan, 2011; Moser et al., 2012; Sabini and Reddy, 2010). This will be discussed in greater detail in Chapter 6 titled "Rest in concussion recovery." In brief, in the acute symptomatic period following concussion, an initial 24–48 hour period of rest is recommended (McCrory et al., 2017). Some evidence advocates in favor of prescribing physical and cognitive rest post-concussion, as it may help avoid prolonged recovery, improve cognitive performance, and decrease symptom reporting (Brown et al., 2014; Grool et al., 2016; Moser et al., 2012; Schneider et al., 2017). A recent study found a reduced risk of PPCS at 28 days in participants aged 5–18 with acute concussion that participated in physical activity within 7 days post-concussion compared with no physical activity (Grool et al., 2016). Conversely, there is a growing body of evidence that prolonged rest and activity restriction may delay recovery through increased psychological conditions including anxiety and depression, and physical deconditioning (Choe and Giza, 2015; DiFazio et al., 2015). As a result, there is no clear consensus regarding the ideal duration of rest (McCrory et al., 2017). This is reflected in dissimilar conflicting recommendations regarding return to play, return to learn, and return to work (see Chapters 12 through 14 on return to school, work, and sports, respectively).

## Pharmacological and nonpharmacological treatments by symptoms

Although management of concussions typically involves anticipatory guidance, behavioral and activity modifications, and some degree of physical and cognitive rest, no single pharmacological or nonpharmacological therapy exists to treat concussions (Scorza et al., 2012). Rather, as concussion often presents as a constellation of signs and symptoms following injury, in addition to the aforementioned management, treatment can be targeted toward each patient's specific symptoms (McCrory et al., 2017; Motor Accidents Authority of NSW, 2008; Scorza et al., 2012). The following sections discuss management of some common symptoms of concussions. It is important to note that, although pharmacological agents may be used to treat various post-concussion signs and symptoms, there is limited evidence regarding their efficacy (Borg et al., 2004; Comper et al., 2005; McCrory, 2002; Rose et al., 2015; Scorza et al., 2012).

### Headaches

One of the most common symptoms that may require therapy following concussions is headache (Blinman et al., 2009; DiTommaso et al., 2014; Guskiewicz et al., 2000; King et al., 1995; Paniak et al., 2002; Sabini and Reddy, 2010). Written questionnaires, such as the PedMIDAS tool, can be utilized to assess for headache severity, frequency, and its impact on activities in their life (Hershey et al., 2001). Nonpharmacological management

*Table 7.1* Medication for acute headaches associated with pediatric concussion

|  | Ibuprofen | Naproxen | Acetaminophen |
|---|---|---|---|
| Dose | 5–10 mg/kg/dose PO q6-8h as needed | 5 mg/kg/dose PO q8-12h as needed PO q12h as needed | 10–15 mg/kg/dose PO/ rectal suppository q4h as needed |
| Maximum dosage | 600 mg/dose or 40 mg/kg/day | 500 mg/dose or 1000 mg/day | 75 mg/kg/day or 4000 mg/day |

*Source:* Dosages from: CHEO Pharmacy, *CHEO Pediatric Doses of Commonly Prescribed Medications*, 2011. http:// nperesource.casn.ca/wp-content/uploads/2017/03/CHEOPediatricDosesofCommonlyPrescribed MedicationsJune6.pdf; Lau, E., *The Hospital for Sick Children 2013/2014 Drug Handbook and Formulary* (*The Hospital for Sick Children*), Toronto, 2013; Taketomo, C.K. et al., *Pediatric & Neonatal Dosage Handbook*, Lexi-Comp, Hudson, OH, 2012.

for headaches is encouraged first and includes obtaining adequate rest, sleep, and ensuring sufficient breaks from activities that require concentration or effort. However, medication may be required acutely to manage headaches. Within the adult population, simple analgesics, such as nonsteroid anti-inflammatory drugs (NSAIDs), acetamino-phen, acetylsalicyclic (ASA), or combination analgesics with codeine or caffeine, may be indicated, with recommended use less than 15 days per month (Choe and Giza, 2015; Cifu et al., 2009; Ontario Neurotrauma Foundation, 2013). Similar medication can be used in the pediatric population; specifically, acetaminophen, ibuprofen, and, for adolescents, naproxen (DiTommaso et al., 2014; Pinchefsky et al., 2015; Rose et al., 2015; Sabini and Reddy, 2010). Appropriate pediatric dosages can be found in Table 7.1. Before prescribing NSAIDs, such as naproxen or ibuprofen, it is important to rule out intracranial hemorrhage as NSAIDs may exacerbate bleeding (Halstead et al., 2010; Scorza et al., 2012; Zemek et al., 2014). Another potential complication from frequent use of acute headache medication, including NSAIDs and simple analgesics, is medication-overuse headache (Cifu et al., 2009; Kuczynski et al., 2013; Meehan, 2011). In one study of adolescent patients with chronic post-traumatic headaches, 70.1% were characterized as likely suffering from medication-overuse headache (Heyer and Idris, 2014). Hence, it is important to avoid excessive, around-the-clock use of these acute headache medications in order to prevent medication-overuse headache and/or chronic post-traumatic headache (Heyer and Idris, 2014; Kuczynski et al., 2013; Meehan, 2011).

For persistent, nonresolving headaches, further follow up with a primary care physician or headache specialist may be required. A focused headache history may help more accurately classify the type of headache and alter subsequent treatment (e.g., tension or cluster type, migrainous, rebound, and fatigue related) (Choe and Giza, 2015; Kuczynski et al., 2013; Sabini and Reddy, 2010). Further management may involve both nonpharmacological therapy, such as good sleep hygiene, cognitive behavioral therapy (CBT), and stress reduction, and pharmacological treatment, including amitriptyline, topiramate, and melatonin (Choe and Giza, 2015; Cifu et al., 2009; Eccleston et al., 2012; Kuczynski et al., 2013; Meehan, 2011; Pinchefsky et al., 2015; Rose et al., 2015; Sabini and Reddy, 2010). Further details on how to manage persistent problems including headaches will be discussed in Chapter 15 (How to manage persistent problems).

## Fatigue and sleep disturbances

Sleep disturbances, including hypersomnia or insomnia, and fatigue are common symptoms of concussion (King et al., 1995; Paniak et al., 2002; Riechers and Ruff, 2010;

Stulemeijer et al., 2006). The former may have a negative impact on fatigue itself, as well as the concentration capabilities, sense of well-being, and behavior of patients who have sustained concussions (Sabini and Reddy, 2010). Therefore, management of these symptoms is critical to long-term outcomes and recovery. As previously discussed, education on proper sleep hygiene is recommended as first-line management (Arciniegas et al., 2005; Meehan, 2011; Rao and Rollings, 2002; Sabini and Reddy, 2010). The use of medication can be considered in situations where sleep hygiene measures fail to improve sleep duration; melatonin, trazodone, amitriptyline, nortriptyline, or ramelteon may be considered, whereas benzodiazepines are generally not recommended (Arciniegas et al., 2005; Lucke-Wold et al., 2015; Maldonado et al., 2007; Meehan, 2011; Sabini and Reddy, 2010). For persistent, nonresolving fatigue despite good sleep hygiene and management of other neuropsychiatric or somatic problems post-concussion, further investigations and referrals to other specialists, including neuropsychiatry, may be required before initiating medical therapy, such as psychostimulants or amantadine (Arciniegas et al., 2005). Further information regarding these topics will be discussed in Chapters 11 (The role of the psychologist and psychiatrist in concussion management) and 15 (How to manage persistent problems).

## References

Arciniegas DB, Anderson CA, Topkoff J, and McAllister TW (2005). Mild traumatic brain injury: A neuropsychiatric approach to diagnosis, evaluation, and treatment. *Neuropsychiatr. Dis. Treat. 1*, 311–327.

Babcock L, Byczkowski T, Wade SL, Ho M, Mookerjee S, and Bazarian JJ (2013). Predicting postconcussion syndrome after mild traumatic brain injury in children and adolescents who present to the emergency department. *JAMA Pediatr. 167*, 156–161.

Bailey NW, Hoy KE, Maller JJ, Segrave RA, Thomson R, Williams N, Daskalakis ZJ, and Fitzgerald PB (2014). An exploratory analysis of go/nogo event-related potentials in major depression and depression following traumatic brain injury. *Psychiatry Res.—Neuroimaging 224*, 324–334.

Barlow M, Schlabach D, Peiffer J, and Cook C (2011). Differences in change scores and the predictive validity of three commonly used measures following concussion in the middle school and high school aged population. *Int. J. Sports Phys. Ther. 6*, 150–157.

Bell KR, Hoffman JM, Temkin NR, Powell JM, Fraser RT, Esselman PC, Barber JK, and Dikmen S (2008). The effect of telephone counselling on reducing post-traumatic symptoms after mild traumatic brain injury: A randomised trial. *J. Neurol. Neurosurg. Psychiatry 79*, 1275–1281.

Bey T and Ostick B (2009). The second impact syndrome. *West. J. Emerg. Med. 10*, 6–10.

Blinman TA, Houseknecht E, Snyder C, Wiebe DJ, and Nance ML (2009). Postconcussive symptoms in hospitalized pediatric patients after mild traumatic brain injury. *J. Pediatr. Surg. 44*, 1223–1228.

Borg J, Holm L, Peloso P, Cassidy J, Carroll L, von Holst H, Paniak C, and Yates D (2004). Nonsurgical intervention and cost for mild traumatic brain injury: Results of the WHO collaborating centre task force on mild traumatic brain injury. *J. Rehabil. Med. 43 Suppl*, 76–83.

Brown NJ, Mannix RC, O'Brien MJ, Gostine D, Collins MW, and Meehan WP (2014). Effect of cognitive activity level on duration of post-concussion symptoms. *Pediatrics 133*, e299–e304.

Canadian Medical Association (2012). CMA driver's guide (electronic source): Determining medical fitness to operate motor vehicles. Ottawa, Canada: Canadian Medical Association.

Carroll L, Cassidy JD, Peloso P, Borg J, von Holst H, Holm L, Paniak C, and Pépin M (2004). Prognosis for mild traumatic brain injury: Results of the who collaborating centre task force on mild traumatic brain injury. *J. Rehabil. Med. 36*, 84–105.

CHEO Pharmacy (2011). CHEO Pediatric Doses of Commonly Prescribed Medications. http://nperesource.casn.ca/wp-content/uploads/2017/03/CHEOPediatricDosesofCommonlyPrescribedMedicationsJune6.pdf.

Choe MC and Giza CC (2015). Diagnosis and management of acute concussion. *Semin. Neurol. 35*, 29–41.

Cifu D, Hurley R, Peterson M, Cornis-Pop M, Rikli PA, Ruff RL, Scott SG et al. (2009). VA/DoD clinical practice guideline for management of concussion/mild traumatic brain injury. *J. Rehabil. Res. Dev. 46*, CP1–CP68.

Comper P, Bisschop S, Carnide N, and Tricco A (2005). A systematic review of treatments for mild traumatic brain injury. *Brain Inj. 19*, 863–880.

DiFazio M, Silverberg ND, Kirkwood MW, Bernier R, and Iverson GL (2015). Prolonged activity restriction after concussion: Are we worsening outcomes? *Clin. Pediatr. (Phila). 55*, 443–451.

DiTommaso C, Hoffman JM, Lucas S, Dikmen S, Temkin N, and Bell KR (2014). Medication usage patterns for headache treatment after mild traumatic brain injury. *Headache 54*, 511–519.

Eccleston C, Palermo TM, Williams AC de D, Lwandowski A, Morley S, Fisher E, and Law E (2012). Psychological therapies for the management of chronic and recurrent pain in children and adolescents. *Cochrane Database Syst Rev 12*, 1–84.

Ferguson RJ, Mittenberg W, Barone DF, and Schneider B (1999). Postconcussion syndrome following sport-related head injury: Expectation as etiology. *Neuropsychology 13*, 582–589.

Ganesalingam K, Yeates KO, Ginn MS, Taylor HG, Dietrich A, Nuss K, and Wright M (2008). Family burden and parental distress following mild traumatic brain injury in children and its relationship to post-concussive symptoms. *J. Pediatr. Psychol. 33*, 621–629.

Gioia GA, Collins M, and Isquith PK (2008). Improving identification and diagnosis of mild traumatic brain injury with evidence: Psychometric support for the acute concussion evaluation. *J. Head Trauma Rehabil. 23*, 230–242.

Giza CC, Kutcher JS, Ashwal S, Barth J, Getchius TSD, Gioia GA, Gronseth GS et al. (2013). Summary of evidence-based guideline update: Evaluation and management of concussion in sports: Report of the guideline development subcommittee of the American academy of neurology. *Neurology 80*, 2250–2257.

Grool AM, Aglipay M, Momoli F, Meehan WP III, Freedman SB, Yeates KO, Gravel J et al. (2016). Association between early participation in physical activity following acute concussion and persistent postconcussive symptoms in children and adolescents. *JAMA 23*, 2504–2514.

Guskiewicz KM, Weaver NL, Padua DA, and Garrett WE (2000). Epidemiology of concussion in collegiate and high school football players. *Am. J. Sports Med. 28*, 643–650.

Halstead ME, Walter KD, and Council on Sports Medicine and Fitness (2010). American academy of pediatrics. Clinical report- sport-related concussion in children and adolescents. *Pediatrics 126*, 597–615.

Harvey A and Bryant R (1998). Acute stress disorder after mild traumatic brain injury. *J. Nerv. Ment. Dis. 186*, 333–337.

Hershey AD, Powers SW, Vockell AL, LeCates S, Kabbouche MA, and Maynard MK (2001). PedMIDAS: Development of a questionnaire to assess disability of migraines in children. *Neurology 57*, 2034–2039.

Heyer GL and Idris SA (2014). Does analgesic overuse contribute to chronic post-traumatic headaches in adolescent concussion patients? *Pediatr. Neurol. 50*, 464–468.

Hofman P, Nelemans P, Kemerink GJ, and Wilmink JT (2000). Value of radiological diagnosis of skull fracture in the management of mild head injury: Meta-analysis. *J. Neurol. Neurosurg. Psychiatry 68*, 416–422.

Ilie G, Mann RE, Boak A, Adlaf EM, Hamilton H, Asbridge M, Rehm J, and Cusimano MD (2014). Suicidality, bullying and other conduct and mental health correlates of traumatic brain injury in adolescents. *PLoS One 9*, 10–15.

Jagoda AS, Bazarian JJ, Bruns JJ, Cantrill S V, Gean AD, Howard PK, Ghajar J et al. (2008). Clinical policy: Neuroimaging and decisionmaking in adult mild traumatic brain injury in the acute setting. *Ann. Emerg. Med. 52*, 714–748.

Johnston KM, Bloom GA, Ramsay J, Kissick J, Montgomery D, Foley D, Chen J, and Ptito A (2004). Current concepts in concussion rehabilitation. *Curr. Sports Med. Rep. 3*, 316–323.

Jonsson C and Andersson EE (2012). Mild traumatic brain injury: A description of how children and youths between 16 and 18 years of age perform leisure activities after 1 year. *Dev. Neurorehabil. 16*, 1–8.

King NS, Crawford S, Wenden FJ, Moss NEG, and Wade DT (1995). The rivermead post concussion symptoms questionnaire: A measure of symptoms commonly experienced after head injury and its reliability. *J. Neurol.* 242, 587–592.

Kuczynski A, Crawford S, Bodell L, Dewey D, and Barlow KM (2013). Characteristics of post-traumatic headaches in children following mild traumatic brain injury and their response to treatment: A prospective cohort. *Dev. Med. Child Neurol.* 55, 636–641.

Lau E (2013). The Hospital for Sick Children 2013/2014 Drug Handbook and Formulary (*The Hospital for Sick Children*), Toronto.

Lucke-Wold BP, Smith KE, Nguyen L, Turner RC, Logsdon AF, Jackson GJ, Huber JD, Rosen CL, and Miller DB (2015). Sleep disruption and the sequelae associated with traumatic brain injury. *Neurosci. Biobehav. Rev.* 55, 68–77.

Lundin A, de Boussard C, Edman G, and Borg J (2006). Symptoms and disability until 3 months after mild TBI. *Brain Inj.* 20, 799–806.

Maldonado MD, Murillo-Cabezas F, Terron MP, Flores LJ, Tan DX, Manchester LC, and Reiter RJ (2007). The potential of melatonin in reducing morbidity-mortality after craniocerebral trauma. *J. Pineal Res.* 42, 1–11.

McAllister TW, Sparling MB, Flashman LA, and Saykin AJ (2001). Neuroimaging findings in mild traumatic brain injury. *J. Clin. Exp. Neuropsychol.* 23, 775–791.

McCrea M, Hammeke T, Olsen G, Leo P, and Guskiewicz K (2004). Unreported concussion in high school football players: Implications for prevention. *Clin. J. Sport Med.* 14, 13–17.

McCrory P (2001). Does second impact syndrome exist? *Clin. J. Sport Med.* 11, 144–149.

McCrory P (2002). Should we treat concussion pharmacologically? The need for evidence based pharmacological treatment for the concussed athlete. *Br. J. Sports Med.* 36, 3–5.

McCrory P, Johnston K, Meeuwisse W, Aubry M, Cantu R, Dvorak J, Graf-Baumann T, Kelly J, Lovell M, and Schamasch P (2005). Summary and agreement statement of the second international conference on concussion in sport, prague 2004. *Phys. Sportsmed.* 33, 29–44.

McCrory P, Meeuwisse W, Dvorak J, Aubry M, Bailes J, Broglio S, Cantu RC et al. (2017). Consensus statement on concussion in sport-the 5th international conference on concussion in sport held in Berlin, October 2016. *Br. J. Sports Med.* Published Online First: April 26, 2017. doi:10.1136/bjsports-2017-097699.

McCrory P, Meeuwisse WH, Aubry M, Cantu B, Dvorák J, Echemendia RJ, Engebretsen L et al. (2013). Consensus statement on concussion in sport: The 4th international conference on concussion in sport held in Zurich, November 2012. *Br. J. Sports Med.* 14, e1–e13.

Meares S, Shores E, Taylor A, Batchelor J, Bryant R, Baguley I, Chapman J, Gurka J, Dawson K, Capon L et al. (2007). Mild traumatic brain injury does not predict acute postconcussion syndrome. *J. Neurol. Neurosurg. Psychiatry* 79, 300–306.

Meehan WP (2011). Medical therapies for concussion. *Clin. Sports Med.* 30, 1–10.

Moser RS, Glatts C, and Schatz P (2012). Efficacy of immediate and delayed cognitive and physical rest for treatment of sports-related concussion. *J. Pediatr.* 161, 922–926.

Motor Accidents Authority of NSW (2008). *Guidelines for Mild Traumatic Brain Injury Following Closed Head Injury.* Sydney, Australia: Motor Accidents Authority of New South Wales.

NSW Ministry of Health (2011). *Adult Trauma Clinical Practice Guidelines: Initial Management of Closed Head Injury in Adults.* New South Wales, Australia: NSW Ministry of Health.

Ontario Neurotrauma Foundation (2013). *Guidelines for Concussion/Mild Traumatic Brain Injury and Persistent Symptoms.* Toronto, Canada: Ontario Neurotrauma Foundation.

Ouellet M, Beaulieu-Bonneau C, and Morin S (2012). Sleep-wake disturbances. In *Brain Injury Medicine: Principles and Practice*, 2nd edition, N. Zasler, D. Katz, and R. Zafonte (Eds.), New York: Demos Medical Publishing LLC.

Paniak C, Reynolds S, Phillips K, Toller-Lobe G, Melnyk A, and Nagy J (2002). Patient complaints within 1 month of mild traumatic brain injury: A controlled study. *Arch. Clin. Neuropsychol.* 17, 319–334.

Parachute Canada (2013). After a Concussion Guidelines for Return to Play. http://www.parachute-canada.org/downloads/resources/return-to-play-guidelines.pdf.

Pinchefsky E, Dubrovsky AS, Friedman D, and Shevell M (2015). Part II—Management of pediatric post-traumatic headaches. *Pediatr. Neurol.* 52, 270–280.

Ponsford J, Willmott C, Rothwell A, Cameron P, Ayton G, Nelms R, Curran C, and Ng K (2001). Impact of early intervention on outcome after mild traumatic brain injury in children. *Pediatrics 108*, 1297–1303.

Preece MHW, Geffen GM, and Horswill MS (2013). Return-to-driving expectations following mild traumatic brain injury. *Brain Inj. 27*, 83–91.

Preece MHW, Horswill MS, and Geffen GM (2010). Driving after concussion: The acute effect of mild traumatic brain injury on drivers' hazard perception. *Neuropsychology 24*, 493–503.

Putukian M, Raftery M, Guskiewicz K, Herring S, Aubry M, Cantu RC, and Molloy M (2013). Onfield assessment of concussion in the adult athlete. *Br. J. Sports Med. 47*, 285–288.

Rao V and Rollings P (2002). Sleep disturbances following traumatic brain injury. *Curr Treat Options Neurol. 4*, 77–87.

Riechers RG and Ruff RL (2010). Rehabilitation in the patient with mild traumatic brain injury. *Continuum (Minneap. Minn). 16*, 128–149.

Rose SC, Weber KD, Collen JB, and Heyer GL (2015). The diagnosis and management of concussion in children and adolescents. *Pediatr. Neurol. 53*, 108–118.

Sabini RC and Reddy CC (2010). Concussion management and treatment considerations in the adolescent population. *Phys. Sportsmed. 38*, 139–146.

Schatz P, Moser RS, Covassin T, and Karpf R (2011). Early indicators of enduring symptoms in high school athletes with multiple previous concussions. *Neurosurgery 68*, 1562–1567.

Schneider KJ, Iverson GL, Emery CA, McCrory P, Herring SA, and Meeuwisse WH (2013). The effects of rest and treatment following sport-related concussion: A systematic review of the literature. *Br. J. Sports Med. 47*, 304–307.

Schneider KJ, Leddy JJ, Guskiewicz KM, Seifert T, McCrea M, Silverberg ND, Feddermann-Demont N, Iverson GL, Hayden A, and Makdissi M (2017). Rest and treatment/rehabilitation following sport-related concussion: A systematic review. *Br. J. Sports Med*. Published Online First: March 24, 2017. doi:10.1136/bjsports-2016-097475.

Scorza KA, Raleigh MF, and O'Connor FG (2012). Current concepts in concussion: Evaluation and management. *Am. Fam. Physician 85*, 123–132.

Stulemeijer M, Van Der Werf S, Bleijenberg G, Biert J, Brauer J, and Evos P (2006). Recovery from mild traumatic brain injury: A focus on fatigue. *J. Neurol. 253*, 1041–1047.

Swaine BR, Gagnon I, Champagne F, Lefebvre H, Friedman D, Atkinson J, and Feldman D (2008). Identifying the specific needs of adolescents after a mild traumatic brain injury: A service provider perspective. *Brain Inj. 22*, 581–588.

Taketomo CK, Hodding JH, and Kraus DM (2012). *Pediatric & Neonatal Dosage Handbook*. Hudson, OH: Lexi-Comp.

Waisman Y, Siegal N, Siegal G, Amir L, Cohen H, and Mimouni M (2005). Role of diagnosis-specific information sheets in parents' understanding of emergency department discharge instructions. *Eur. J. Emerg. Med. 12*, 159–162.

Wetjen NM, Pichelmann MA, and Atkinson JL (2010). Second impact syndrome: Concussion and second injury brain complications. *J. Am. Coll. Surg. 211*, 553–557.

Zemek R, Barrowman N, Freedman SB, Gravel J, Gagnon I, Mcgahern C, Aglipay M, Sangha G, Boutis K, Beer D et al. (2016). Clinical risk score for persistent postconcussion symptoms among children with acute concussion in the ED. *JAMA 315*, 1014–1025.

Zemek R, Duval S, DeMatteo C, Solomon B, Keightley M, and Osmond M (2014). *Guidelines for Diagnosing and Managing Pediatric Concussion*. Toronto, Canada: Ontario Neurotrauma Foundation.

## chapter eight

# Physiotherapy and concussion
## What can the physiotherapist do?

*Kathryn J. Schneider and Isabelle Gagnon*

### Contents

Physiotherapy is an allied health-care profession. Physiotherapists have training in the assessment, diagnosis, and treatment of a variety of health conditions that result in range of alterations in physical function (Canadian Physiotherapy Association 2017). Physiotherapists primarily deal with restoration of function through techniques aimed at retraining proper movement patterns, exercise, manual therapy, education, and awareness. They are often regarded as *movement specialists* and are part of a multidisciplinary care team. There are a variety of different subdomains in physiotherapy that practitioners may primarily work and develop expertise in. These areas include the assessment and treatment of neurological, orthopedic, sports, cardiorespiratory, burns, aging, pediatrics, and others. Thus, the physiotherapist has a skill set that can facilitate recovery following concussion due to expertise in a variety of rehabilitative techniques. The purpose of this chapter is to provide an overview of the role of the physiotherapy and the physiotherapist in the area of concussion.

A variety of different symptoms may be present following a concussion (McCrory et al. 2013, Kerr et al. 2016). In addition, a variety of different systems may be responsible for these symptoms, many of which may respond to rehabilitation techniques (Schneider 2016). Some of the most commonly occurring symptoms following concussion are headache, dizziness, neck pain, fatigue, difficulty with exertion, and blurred vision (Benson et al. 2011, Kerr et al. 2016). Many of these symptoms may be secondary to dysfunction in systems that respond well to physiotherapy intervention. It is important to recognize that in many cases, physiotherapy may be appropriate, but in other cases, there may be medical investigations or intervention that may be more appropriate. Thus, a thorough assessment by the physiotherapist and/or managing physician is important prior to initiating treatment. The following section summarizes some of the symptom patterns, assessment tests, and treatment techniques that may be appropriate for physiotherapy treatment.

## Dizziness

Dizziness is often the second most commonly reported symptom following concussion (Benson et al. 2011). A challenge is that the term *dizziness* tends to be a catch all term that can incorporate a variety of different symptoms (including vertigo, presyncope, and imbalance). In addition, dizziness may occur secondary to a variety of causes, some of which require urgent medical referral, and others that have been found to benefit from physiotherapy treatment (Hilton and Pinder 2004, Hoffer et al. 2004, Ernst et al. 2005, Schneider et al. 2009, Alsalaheen et al. 2010, Schneider et al. 2014b).

Balance is a complex process of orienting one's self in space and requires equal and accurate input from numerous systems (Guskiewicz 2001). The primary sources of afferent input for balance are the vestibular labyrinth, the eye, and the proprioceptors (Herdman 2007). Input from these three groups of peripheral sensory receptors relays afferent information to the central balance systems (primarily the vestibular nucleus and cerebellum), as well as higher centers, to be processed. Efferent output then ensues through a variety of efferent outputs including the vestibulo-spinal, vestibulo-ocular, oculomotor, and cervico-ocular reflexes (Armstrong et al. 2008). There is a complex interaction between systems that allows for maintenance of an upright position in space and the ability to see clearly while moving. Any alterations, in any of the afferent systems, can result in a sensation of dizziness or unsteadiness (Kristjansson and Treleaven 2009). Thus, a thorough assessment of all potential systems that may be involved in dizziness is appropriate in the case of a patient who presents with dizziness following a concussion.

A complete history regarding the nature, duration, aggravating, and easing factors related to dizziness can guide the clinician to best identify the primary source of symptoms and direct treatment accordingly. A history of cardiovascular or peripheral vascular disease or risk factors may alert the clinician of the need to refer for further medical evaluation. It is also important to recognize that there may be other concurrent neurological conditions, medications, medication interaction, and other conditions that may be a source of dizziness and require medical evaluation and treatment. In some cases, the vestibular system or cervical spine may be involved.

## Nature of dizziness

Vertigo is a sensation of one's self or the room spinning. Lightheadedness tends to describe a sense of presyncope and may occur following a rapid change of position to a more upright posture. Other individuals may report a sensation of imbalance when in environments with altered sensory stimulus. In the case of suspected cervicogenic dizziness, lightheadedness or a sensation of feeling *off* is commonly reported (Reneker and Cook 2015).

## Duration of dizziness

It is important to delve into the duration of dizziness. For example, reports of seconds of vertigo on changing position from sitting to lying, rolling in bed, getting into and out of bed, looking up and looking down are suggestive of benign paroxysmal positional vertigo (BPPV), a peripheral vestibular disorder that is effectively treated with canalith repositioning maneuvers by a physiotherapist trained in vestibular rehabilitation (Hilton and Pinder 2002, Hilton and Pinder 2014). Individuals with BPPV present with a characteristic pattern of concurrent nystagmus and vertigo with position changes that lasts for seconds after position changes (Hilton and Pinder 2004, Herdman 2007). However, an individual reporting vertigo (spinning) following a hit to the head that gradually improves and dissipates to lightheadedness with head motions may have suffered what is believed to be a labyrinthine concussion. The mechanism by which this occurs is not yet well understood.

A variety of different vestibular disorders may occur following head trauma and have been reported to include BPPV, labyrinthine concussion, otolith dysfunction, and vestibular migraines to name a few (Ernst et al. 2005). In many cases, gold standard evaluation has not been performed, and suspected diagnoses are made based on clinical findings. Other reports are based on impairments identified on testing such as vestibulo-ocular dysfunction and motion sensitivity (Schubert and Minot 2004). In some cases, assessment tests that evaluate for self-reported provocation of symptoms are used (Mucha et al. 2014, Ellis et al. 2015). Future research to better understand the nature of vestibular disorders following concussion is warranted.

Cervicogenic dizziness tends to be a diagnosis of exclusion and is believed to occur secondary to altered proprioceptive input from the upper cervical spine (Kristjansson and Treleaven 2009). In the case of cervicogenic dizziness, patients typically report a sensation of feeling fogginess, feeling off or lightheaded and do not report vertigo (Kristjansson and Treleaven 2009). Dizziness tends to be accompanied by neck pain and/or cervicogenic headaches, and the intensity of dizziness tends to fluctuate with the neck pain and/or headache (Kristjansson and Treleaven 2009). Typical treatment for cervicogenic dizziness includes multifaceted treatment for the cervical spine (as described below), including sensorimotor and neuromotor retraining (Treleaven 2008). Assessment of the patient's ability to relocate their head to neutral in space and head/neck coordination can guide the physiotherapist in determining an appropriate treatment plan (Treleaven 2008, Kristjansson and Treleaven 2009).

## Benign paroxysmal positional vertigo

BPPV has been reported to occur in approximately 5% of individuals with persistent dizziness following concussion (Alsalaheen et al. 2010, Schneider et al. 2014b). BPPV is believed to occur when debris from the otolith is dislodged into the semicircular canal (SCC). Normally, the SCC is not sensitive to gravity. However, in the case of BPPV, the debris in the canal induces a mismatch whereby there is an excitatory input from the affected ear resulting in a false sense of motion and vertigo then ensues (Hilton and Pinder 2014). Due to the intricate links between the semi-circular canals and extraocular musculature, a distinct pattern of nystagmus results and can inform the clinician as to the location and type of BPPV. This vertigo and nystagmus last for seconds following position changes that cause movement of the debris in the affected canal, with the nystagmus and vertigo abating once the debris has settled to the most dependent portion of the canal (Hilton and Pinder 2014). Typical provoking movements include getting into and out of bed, rolling in bed, looking up, looking down, and fast head movements. The standard assessment test for BPPV is the Hallpike–Dix test in which the patient is rapidly moved into a supine position of 45° rotation and subsequently 30° extension. In the case of BPPV, a characteristic pattern of nystagmus at the same time as vertiginous symptoms would ensue and typically lasts for seconds. It is important to ensure that prior to doing this test, a neurological screen and cervical spine screen have been performed. In the case of a concomitant cervical spine injury, the test can be done with the neck in a neutral position with the bed tilted and body rolled as a unit (rather than in a rotated position of the cervical spine). In some cases, a horizontal SCC BPPV may be present and can be assessed using a roll test where the patient is supine and the head is rotated to the right or to the left while the head is resting on a pillow (to allow the head to be flexed 20°–30° and allow to head to be in the plane of the horizontal SCC) (Balatsouras et al. 2017). Treatment for BPPV occurs through the use of canalith repositioning maneuvers, with the appropriate maneuver being selected based on the provoking position for vertigo and the nystagmus that is seen (Balatsouras et al. 2017). The majority of BPPV occurs in the posterior canal and typically responds well to treatment with an Epley maneuver in as few as 1–2 treatments (Hilton and Pinder 2014). In individuals with post-traumatic BPPV following mild traumatic brain injury, multiple canals may be involved, recurrences may occur, and a greater number of treatments may be required than in idiopathic BPPV (Balatsouras et al. 2017).

## Peripheral vestibular hypofunction

Peripheral vestibular hypofunction has been reported to occur in approximately 10% of cases with persistent dizziness following sport-related concussion (Alsalaheen et al. 2010, Hong et al. 2014). Normally, both peripheral vestibular labyrinths will relay consistent and equal information regarding the head position in space. In the case of a peripheral vestibular hypofunction, one labyrinth does not sense motion as well as it should, and thus, a mismatch of information between the right and left peripheral vestibular input ensues. Initially, individuals feel a sensation of vertigo due to this mismatch between the peripheral vestibular sensory receptors. However, it is believed that over time a tonic rebalancing of the central receptors occurs as well as sensorimotor reorganization. Thus, dizziness or lightheadedness with fast head motions tends to be a common complaint in individuals with this type of problem.

## Vestibulo-ocular reflex

The role of the vestibulo-ocular reflex (VOR) is to maintain a stable gaze during head motion. Thus, as one turns their head to the right, afferent input from the right peripheral vestibular system will trigger the oculomotor system to move the eyes equally and opposite to the head movement (in this case to the left) to maintain a stable eye position in space with head motion (Schubert and Minot 2004). Alterations with VOR function have been reported to occur following head trauma, and individuals may report difficulty with seeing clearly when moving their head (Hoffer et al. 2004, Gottshall 2011). Clinical tests including a *head thrust test* (or head impulse test) and *dynamic visual acuity* (a behavioral measure of the VOR) may be useful to assess the function of the VOR (Herdman et al. 1998, Schubert et al. 2004, Herdman 2007).

## Central vestibular disorders

Central vestibular disorders may also occur following concussion. In some cases, a collection of impairments in function are present but do not point to any one specific disorder. Provided that there are no clinical indications of more severe pathology that warrants medical attention, these individuals may benefit from an impairment-based approach to rehabilitation (Brown et al. 2006). On the other hand, if an individual has a history and clinical findings suggestive of a peripheral vestibular hypofunction, but the *head thrust* is negative, direction-changing nystagmus is noted in eccentric gaze or skew deviation (vertical misalignment of the eyes) is present, a potential vascular source of symptoms should be suspected, and further urgent medical follow-up is warranted (Kattah et al. 2009).

Vestibular rehabilitation is a combination of impairment-based treatment techniques that are employed by the physiotherapist based on the individual clinical presentation (Hillier and Hollohan 2007, Herdman 2007). These treatment techniques may include adaptation (gaze stabilization), habituation, substitution, standing balance, dynamic balance exercises, and canalith repositioning maneuvers (for BPPV) (Schneider et al. 2014b, Hall et al. 2016). Vestibular rehabilitation has been shown to be safe and effective for individuals with BPPV and unilateral peripheral vestibular disorders (Hilton and Pinder 2004, Hillier and Hollohan 2007). Emerging research has also demonstrated that the vestibular rehabilitation is likely beneficial for individuals with persisting dizziness and balance disorders following concussion (Alsalaheen et al. 2010, Schneider et al. 2014b).

## Visual impairments

The visual and vestibular systems interact synergistically to provide spatial orientation and position feedback, to maintain gaze and postural stability during movements. Both the visual and vestibular systems gather afferent sensory information (mechanical from the vestibular system and photo-optic from the visual system) and transfer it to higher order areas of the brain, where it is decoded and where efferent responses are generated as motor responses of the eye, head, or body (Bent et al. 2002). Although experiencing blurred vision can be a consequence of a lack of optimal integration of the VOR, visual complaints after concussion can also be the result of impairments to the oculomotor system itself, or to other central structures involved in the processing or interpretation of visual information (Barnett and Singman 2015).

The visual system registers both movements of the objects in the environment and the body's movements within the environment, thus contributing not only to the perception of the environment itself but also to postural control in a significant manner (Albright 1984, Braddick et al. 2003, Tohyama and Fukushima 2005, Slobounov et al. 2006). The system consists of mainly three components: central vision, ambient vision (peripheral), and retinal slip. The central vision specializes in object motion perception and object recognition; whereas peripheral vision is sensitive to movement scene and is thought to dominate both perception of self-motion and postural control. Peripheral vision is particularly sensitive to moving scenes, with movement influencing the extremes of a periphery. Retinal slip, or when rapidly moving objects are *slipping* across portions of the retina and trigger the optokinetic reflex to refocus objects, is used as a feedback for a compensatory sway.

A very large portion of the brain's networks is involved in processing visual information (Noguchi et al. 2005, Farivar et al. 2009). With the diffuse nature of the pathophysiology evidenced post-concussion, visual complaints are, not surprisingly, very common. The physiotherapist is not a specialist of vision impairments, and referrals to neuro-optometrists and neuro-ophthalmologists will be required for individuals with persisting visual difficulties. However, the physiotherapist is a first-line health professional who is uniquely positioned to provide care to acutely concussed individuals. Initial screening and early intervention for motor and perceptual problems of the visual system may be initiated by the physiotherapist to avoid delays in identification of these difficulties, recognizing the lack of evidence regarding the effectiveness of these interventions specifically for the concussed individual.

## Oculomotor system

Although the visual system is complex, perception of visual stimuli requires not only proper acuity and accommodation but also motor control of the eyes muscles. Coordinated eye movements will allow fixation, smooth pursuits, saccades, as well as vergence. Although instrumented tests are the gold standard in the assessment of oculomotor function (electro-oculography, infrared reflective devices, video-oculography), simple clinical procedures exist to screen for deficits in eye motility and can be administered by the trained physiotherapist as part of the initial assessment of the individual with a concussion (Vidal et al. 2012, Rine and Wiener-Vacher 2013). At present, the effects of visual rehabilitative techniques following concussion are not well established. However, in the case of oculomotor dysfunction, optometric vision rehabilitation strategies, and a referral to a vison rehabilitation specialist may be of benefit. The specialty-trained physiotherapist may play a role in initiating simple first-line rehabilitation strategies which will aim to improve eye movement control, eye focus, and coordination as well as eye teaming. Specifically, the physiotherapist may implement pursuit and saccadic exercises, as well as convergence exercises (e.g., pencil push-ups, Brock strings, and 3-Dot cards) (McGregor 2014, Horwood et al. 2014). Further vision therapy including lenses, prisms, and patching/occluding will typically be introduced by the second-line services.

## Visual perception

Beyond the coordination of eye movements, perception of visual stimuli is dependent on both the integrity of broad networks dedicated to the transmission of afferent input and processing of information. Recent work suggesting that deficits in higher order static and dynamic visual perception (Brosseau-Lachaine et al. 2006, 2008, Piponnier et al. 2016), as well as in dynamic visual attention (Kowalski et al. 2015) may be identified following concussion is triggering interest in developing intervention strategies targeting these functions. These remain largely experimental in nature, but interventions such as visual reaction time training (Clark et al. 2015) or multiple object tracking (Faubert and Sidebottom 2012) are showing promise and may emerge in the coming years as viable options with this population.

## Neck pain and headaches

There are a variety of structures in the cervical spine that may be affected by concussion and may produce neck pain and/or headaches following trauma, including the facet joints, musculature, and nerve roots (Bogduk 1982, Bogduk 2004, Bogduk and Govind 2009, Page 2011). The convergence of input from the upper cervical spine to the trigeminal nucleus is believed to be the pathway by which the cervical spine refers pain to the head (Bogduk 2001, Page 2011). An ongoing challenge is to identify if the cervical spine is a source of symptoms or if the originating cause of a headache and/or neck pain is from a concussive injury itself. Differentiation of cervical and concussion injuries is an area of much needed future research as there is no one test that will definitively *rule out* a concussive injury in the case of suspected cervical spine involvement. Thus, in individuals with persisting neck pain and headaches following concussion, the cervical spine should be evaluated as a potential source of symptoms that may be amenable to physiotherapy treatment, with the understanding that in many cases, a concomitant concussion may have occurred.

The upper three cervical spine joints can refer pain into the head and have been reported to be sources of pain following trauma (Treleaven et al. 1994). The lateral joint at the C1/C2 level has been reported to refer pain from the suboccipital to the occiput and vertex or into the neck, forehead, ear, and orbit (Cooper et al. 2007, Bovim and Sand 1992). The C2/C3 facet joints have been reported to refer pain to the lateral occiput, mastoid, and above but not encompassing the ear (Cooper et al. 2007). The C3/C4 facets often are affected in combination with other levels so may be more difficult to determine a pattern; however, pain typically may refer to the occipital and suboccipital region, vertex, or forehead and/or posterolateral neck (Cooper et al. 2007). At levels below C4, pain is referred into the neck, shoulders, and thoracic spine region but not to the head (Cooper et al. 2007). A combination of three positive tests on manual spinal examination (MSE), palpation for segmental tenderness (PST), and an active extension rotation test (ERT) have been shown to positively predict individuals with facet joint-mediated pain (Schneider et al. 2013, 2014a). Conversely, individuals who have a negative test on either the MSE or PST test most likely do not have facet joint-mediated pain (Schneider et al. 2014a). These tests have been shown to be highly reliable and have high degrees of positive and negative predictive ability in individuals with suspected facet joint mediated pain (Schneider et al. 2013). The C1-3 nerve roots may also be a source of referred pain to the head (Bogduk 2004). There is an intimate relationship with cervical spine fibers and the trigeminal nucleus (Bogduk 2001). Greater occipital nerve blocks have also been reported to alleviate headaches in individuals who have suffered a concussion (Dubrovsky et al. 2014).

The musculature of the cervical spine region may also be a source of neck pain and headaches (Fernandez-de-las Penas et al. 2010, Fernandez-de-las-Penas et al. 2011, Page 2011). Common locations of active trigger points that have been reported to produce headaches from the cervical spine musculature include the sternocleidomastoid, splenius capitis, masseter, upper trapezius, levator scapulae, superior oblique, and the suboccipital muscles (Fernandez-de-las Penas et al. 2010, Fernandez-de-las-Penas et al. 2011, Fernandez-de-las Penas et al. 2012, Florencio et al. 2016). Individuals with neck pain have also been found to have greater accessory muscle activation with arm movements when compared with controls without neck pain (Falla et al. 2004). Individuals with neck pain have also been found to perform more poorly than control subjects on a test of craniocervical flexion (Jull et al. 2004). Alterations in performance on the craniocervical flexion test have been reported to be associated with dysfunction of the deep cervical flexors (Falla et al. 2004). Craniocervical flexion retraining exercises have been shown to be effective in the treatment of cervicogenic headaches (Jull et al. 2002). There is also a body of literature that has demonstrated that multimodal care and a combination of manual therapy and exercise are more effective than other strategies for individuals that have neck pain (Gross et al. 2004, Hurwitz et al. 2008). In addition, functional exercise and specific training appear to be more effective than general training (Jull et al. 2002, Hurwitz et al. 2008). Thus, the cervical spine may be a source of ongoing symptoms following concussion and should be evaluated. A combination of treatment techniques including neuromotor retraining, soft tissue techniques, sensorimotor exercises, and manual therapy may be of benefit. The precise characteristics of cervical spine involvement following concussion are not yet well defined, and ongoing research is needed to better understand the link between the cervical spine and concussion symptoms. The physiotherapist is well positioned to play an active role in the treatment of the cervical spine following concussion.

A randomized controlled trial evaluated a combination of cervical and vestibular rehabilitation in individuals with persisting symptoms of dizziness, neck pain, and/or headaches for greater than 10 days following concussions (Schneider et al. 2014b). Individuals who were treated with physiotherapy were 3.91 (95% CI; 1.34-11.34) times more likely to be medically cleared by 8 weeks compared with a control group who rested and followed a protocol of graded exertion (Schneider et al. 2014b). Thus, a more active approach to treatment involving physiotherapy treatment in which the cervical spine and/or vestibular system may be a source of ongoing treatment may facilitate recovery (Schneider et al. 2017).

## Exercise

Physiotherapists are also actively involved in the prescription and monitoring of exercise for individuals with ongoing symptoms following a concussion. There is evidence that low-level aerobic exercise may be of benefit to facilitate recovery following concussion (Gagnon et al. 2009, Gagnon et al. 2016). This topic is covered in depth in Chapter 15.

## Putting it all together: A case study example

A 14-year-old female hockey player suffered a sport-related concussion during a game where she collided with another player and subsequently fell to the ice. She reported instant symptoms of dizziness (spinning) and a headache. She was observably unsteady on her feet as she was helped to the bench. She did not have a loss of consciousness and was oriented to person, place, and time. She followed up with a local sport-medicine physician and was diagnosed with a sport-related concussion. She rested for the initial 2-3 days after the injury (cognitively and physically) and gradually began to increase her activities of daily living but continued to report headaches in the suboccipital region that would refer to her forehead when they increased in intensity. She also reported dizziness with fast head movements. These symptoms persisted for 10 days, at which time she was seen by a physiotherapist.

At the time of the initial assessment she reported symptoms of sensitivity to visual stimulus, dizziness with fast head movements, ongoing suboccipital headaches that increased with prolonged positions (i.e., such as with any school/computer/phone activities for greater than 20 minutes) and when turning her head quickly. She had clinical findings suggesting a peripheral vestibular hypofunction and cervicogenic headaches. Initial treatment included postural education when sitting (i.e., avoidance of a forward head posture and maintaining a neutral cervical spine position), craniocervical flexion and extension neuromotor control exercises, gaze stabilization, and standing balance exercises. On follow-up one week later, she reported only 1–2 headaches in the previous week and was able to perform craniovertebral flexion and extension motions with minimal superficial muscle activity while maintaining a neutral lower cervical spine position. She also reported that she no longer had sensitivity to visual stimulus, and that dizziness only occurred when moving her head quickly. At this time, she was given habituation exercises for the directions of motion that she was sensitive to motion (in her case horizontal head turns and bending), and her neuromotor control exercises were also progressed. She was also given exercises to address difficulties with walking and turning her head as well as tandem gait. She was progressed to stick handling gaze stabilization exercises to allow training in a context-specific environment. In consultation with her physician, she also began some low-level aerobic exercise each day (starting with 15 minutes per day) that did not provoke symptoms. At her final appointment one week later, she reported being asymptomatic at rest and with all of her exercises. She had also been free of symptoms when walking for 30 minutes and had begun to increase the intensity of her exercise and had remained asymptomatic. Her physician then gave her clearance to progress through the remainder of the return to play protocol. At this time, further sport-specific motions were tested in clinic, to which she was not dizzy and was able to complete well. She progressed through the return to sport strategy and was subsequently medically cleared and returned to play the following week. Throughout the process, the physiotherapist was in continual contact with the sport-medicine physician regarding progress.

## Summary

The physiotherapist brings a unique multisystem skill set to the team with expertise in recovery of function through a variety of techniques. The physiotherapist also works regularly and closely with the patient and family throughout their recovery period. Thus, the physiotherapist is often in a unique position within the health-care team to gain an understanding of additional areas that the individuals may be struggling and can relay this information to the health-care team and facilitate further referral if indicated. On field management, assessment and treatment of the cervical spine, vestibular system, visual system, and exercise prescription are some of the areas that physiotherapists are frequently involved in. For individuals with ongoing symptoms, physiotherapy treatment may be of benefit.

## References

Albright, T. D. 1984. Direction and orientation selectivity of neurons in visual area MT of the macaque. *J Neurophysiol* 52 (6):1106–1130.

Alsalaheen, B. A., A. Mucha, L. O. Morris, S. L. Whitney, J. M. Furman, C. E. Camiolo-Reddy, M. W. Collins, M. R. Lovell, and P. J. Sparto. 2010. Vestibular rehabilitation for dizziness and balance disorders after concussion. *JNPT* 34 (2):87–93. doi: 10.1097/NPT.0b013e3181dde568.

Armstrong, B., P. McNair, and P. Taylor. 2008. Head and neck position sense. *Sports Med* 38 (2):101–117.

Canadian Physiotherapy Association. 2017. About physiotherapy. accessed January 29, 2017. https://physiotherapy.ca/about-physiotherapy.

Balatsouras, D. G., G. Koukoutsis, A. Aspris, A. Fassolis, A. Moukos, N. C. Economou, and M. Katotomichelakis. 2017. Benign paroxysmal positional vertigo secondary to mild head trauma. *Ann Otol, Rhinol Laryngol* 126 (1):54–60.

Barnett, B. P. and E. L. Singman. 2015. Vision concerns after mild traumatic brain injury. *Curr Treat Options Neurol* 17 (2):329. doi: 10.1007/s11940-014-0329-y.

Benson, B. W., W. H. Meeuwisse, J. Rizos, J. Kang, and C. J. Burke. 2011. A prospective study of concussions among national hockey league players during regular season games: The NHL-NHLPA concussion program. *CMAJ: = J de l'Asso Med Canadienne* 183 (8):905–911. doi: 10.1503/cmaj.092190.

Bent, L. R., B. J. McFadyen, and J. T. Inglis. 2002. Visual-vestibular interactions in postural control during the execution of a dynamic task. *Exp Brain Res* 146 (4):490–500. doi: 10.1007/s00221-002-1204-8.

Bogduk, N. 1982. The clinical anatomy of the cervical dorsal rami. *Spine* 7 (4):319–330.

Bogduk, N. 2001. Cervicogenic headache: Anatomic basis and pathophysiologic mechanisms. *Curr Pain Headache Rep* 5 (4):382–386.

Bogduk, N. 2004. The neck and headaches. *Neurol Clin N Am* 22:151–171.

Bogduk, N. and J. Govind. 2009. Cervicogenic headache: An assessment of the evidence on clinical diagnosis, invasive tests, and treatment. *Lancet Neurol* 8 (10):959–968. doi: 10.1016/S1474-4422(09)70209-1.

Bovim, G. and T. Sand. 1992. Cervicogenic headache, migraine without aura and tension-type headache. Diagnostic blockade of greater occipital and supra-orbital nerves. *Pain* 51 (1):43–48.

Braddick, O., J. Atkinson, and J. Wattam-Bell. 2003. Normal and anomalous development of visual motion processing: Motion coherence and "dorsal-stream vulnerability." *Neuropsychologia* 41 (13):1769–1784.

Brosseau-Lachaine, O., I. Gagnon, R. Forget, and J. Faubert. 2006. Complex visual information processing in children after mild traumatic brain injury. *J Vis* 6:638

Brosseau-Lachaine, O., I. Gagnon, R. Forget, and J. Faubert. 2008. Mild traumatic brain injury induces prolonged visual processing deficits in children. *Brain Inj* 22 (9):657–668. doi: 10.1080/02699050802203353.

Brown, K. E., S. L. Whitney, G. F. Mearchetti, D. M. Wrisley, and J. M. Furman. 2006. Physical therapy for central vestibular dysfunction. *Arch Phys Med Rehabil* 87:76–81.

Clark, J. F., A. Colosimo, J. K. Ellis, R. Mangine, B. Bixenmann, K. Hasselfeld, P. Graman, H. Elgendy, G. Myer, and J. Divine. 2015. Vision training methods for sports concussion mitigation and management. *J Vis Exp* (99):e52648. doi: 10.3791/52648.

Cooper, G., B. Bailey, and N. Bogduk. 2007. Cervical zygapophysial joint pain maps. *Pain Med* 8 (4):344–53. doi: 10.1111/j.1526-4637.2006.00201.x.

Dubrovsky, A. S., D. Friedman, and H. Kocilowicz. 2014. Pediatric post-traumatic headaches and peripheral nerve blocks of the scalp: A case series and patient satisfaction survey. *Headache* 54 (5):878–887.

Ellis, M. J., D. Cordingley, S. Vis, K. Reimer, J. Leiter, and K. Russell. 2015. Vestibulo-ocular dysfunction in pediatric sports-related concussion *J Neurosurg Pediatr*. doi: 10.3171/2015.1.PEDS14524.

Ernst, A., D. Basta, R. O. Seidl, I. Todt, H. Scherer, and A. Clarke. 2005. Management of posttraumatic vertigo. *Otolaryngol Head Neck Surg* 132 (4):554–558.

Falla, D. L., G. A. Jull, and P. W. Hodges. 2004. Patients with neck pain demonstrate reduced electromyographic activity of the deep cervical flexor muscles during performance of the craniocervical flexion test. *Spine* 29:2108–2114.

Farivar, R., O. Blanke, and A. Chaudhuri. 2009. Dorsal-ventral integration in the recognition of motion-defined unfamiliar faces. *J Neurosci* 29 (16):5336–5342. doi: 10.1523/JNEUROSCI.4978-08.2009.

Faubert, J. and L. Sidebottom. 2012. Perceptual-cognitive training of athletes. *J Clin Sport Psychol* 6:85–102.

Fernandez-de-las Penas, C., C. Grobli, R. Ortega-Santiago, C.S. Fischer, D. Boesch, P. Froidevaux, L. Stocker, R. Weissmann, and J. Gonzalez-Iglesias. 2012. Referred pain from myofascial trigger points in head, neck, shoulder and arm muscles reproduces pain symptoms in blue collar and white collar workers. *Clin J Pain* 28:511–518.

Fernandez-de-las Penas, C., H.-Y. Ge, C. Alonso-Blanco, J. Gonzalez-Iglesias, and L. Arendt-Nielsen. 2010. Referred pain areas of active myofascial trigger points in the head, neck and shoulder muscles, in chronic tension type headache. *J Bodyw Mov Ther* 14:391–396.

Fernandez-de-las-Penas, C., D. M. Fernandez-Mayoralas, R. Ortega-Santiago, S. Ambite-Quesada, D. Palacios-Cena, and J. A. Pareja. 2011. Referred pain from myofascial trigger points in head and neck-shoulder muscles reproduces head pain features in children with chronic tension type headache. *J Headache Pain* 12:35–43.

Florencio, L. L., G. N. Ferracini, T. C. Chaves, M. Palacios-Cena, C. Ordas-Bandera, J. G. Speciali, D. Falla, D. B. Grossi, and C. Fernandez-de-las Penas. 2016. Active trigger points in the cervical musculature determine altered activation of superficial neck and extensor muscles in women with migraine. *Clin J Pain*. doi: DOI:10.1097/AJP.0000000000000390.

Gagnon, I., L. Grilli, D. Friedman, and G. L. Iverson. 2016. A pilot study of active rehabilitation for adolescents who are slow to recover from sport-related concussion. *Scand J Med Sci Sports* 26:299–306. doi: 10.1111/sms.12441.

Gagnon, I., C. Galli, D. Friedman, L. Grilli, and G. L. Iverson. 2009. Active rehabilitation for children who are slow to recover following sport-related concussion. *Brain Inj* 23 (12):956–964. doi: doi:10.3109/02699050903373477.

Gottshall, K. 2011. Vestibular rehabilitation after mild traumatic brain injury with vestibular pathology. *NeuroRehabilitation* 29:167–171. doi: 10.3233/NRE-2011-0691.

Gross, A. R., J. L. Hoving, T. A. Haines, C. H. Goldsmith, T. Kay, P. Aker, and G. Bronfort. 2004. A cochrane review of manipulation and mobilization for mechanical neck disorders. *SPINE* 29 (14):1541–1548.

Guskiewicz, K. M. 2001. Postural stability assessment following concussion: One piece of the puzzle. *Clin J Sport Med* 11:182–189.

Hall, C. D., S. J. Herdman, S. L. Whitney, S. P. Cass, R. A. Clendaniel, T. D. Fife, J. M. Furman et al. 2016. Vestibular rehabilitation for peripheral vestibular hypofunction: An evidence-based clinical practice guideline. *JNPT* 40:124–154.

Herdman, S. J., R. J. Tusa, P. J. Blatt, A. Suzuki, P. J. Venuto, and D. Roberts. 1998. Computerized dynamic visual acuity test in the assessment of vestibular deficits. *Am J Otol* 19:790–796.

Herdman, S. J. 2007. *Vestibular Rehabilitation*. Edited by F. A. Davis Company. 3rd ed. Philadelphia, PA: F.A. Davis Company.

Hillier, S. L. and Hollohan, V. 2007. Vestibular rehabilitation for unilateral peripheral vestibular dysfunction. *Cochrane Database Syst Rev* 17 (4):CD005397.

Hilton, M. and Pinder, D. 2002. The epley manoeuvre for benign paroxysmal positional vertigo-a systematic review. *Clin Otolaryngol Allied Sci* 27 (6):440–445.

Hilton, M. and Pinder, D. 2004. The epley (canalith repositioning) manoeuvre for benign paroxysmal positional vertigo. *Cochrane Database Syst Rev* 2 (CD003162).

Hilton, M.P. and D.K. Pinder. 2014. The epley (canalith repositioning) manoeuvre for benign paroxysmal positional vertigo (Review). *Cochrane Database Syst Rev* (12). doi: 10.1002/14651858. CD003162.pub3.

Hoffer, M. F., K. R. Gottshall, R. Moore, B. J. Balough, and D. Wester. 2004. Characterizing and treating dizziness after mild head trauma. *Otol Neurotol: Off Publ Am Otol Soc, Am Neurotol Soc (and) Europ Acad Otol Neurotol* 25:135–138.

Hong, T. P., A. Scurfield, K. Schneider, M. Narous, M. Esser, and K. M. Barlow. 2014. Vestibular dysfunction following paediatric trainmatic brain injury—Prevalence and exploration of a novel diagnostic tool. *Brain Inj* 28:839.

Horwood, A. M., S. S. Toor, and P. M. Riddell. 2014. Change in convergence and accommodation after two weeks of eye exercises in typical young adults. *J AAPOS* 18 (2):162–168. doi: 10.1016/j.jaapos.2013.11.008.

Hurwitz, E. L., E. J. Carragee, G. van der Velde, L. J. Carroll, M. Nordin, J. Guzman, P. M. Peloso, L. W. Holm, P. Cote, S. Hogg-Johnson, J. D. Cassidy, S. Haldeman. 2008. Treatment of neck pain: Noninvasive interventions: Results of the bone and joint decade 2000–2010 task force on neck pain and its associated disorders. *Spine* 33:(4 Suppl)):S123–S152.

Jull, G., E. Kristjansson, and P. Dall'Alba. 2004. Impairment in the cervical flexors: A comparison of whiplash and insidious onset neck pain patients. *Man Ther* 9:89–94.

Jull, G., P. Trott, H. Potter, G. Zito, K. Niere, D. Shirley, J. Emberson, I. Marschner, and C. Richardson. 2002. A randomized controlled trial of exercise and manipulative therapy for cervicogenic headache. *Spine* 27 (17):1835–1843; discussion 1843.

Kattah, J. C., A. V. Talkad, D. Z. Wang, Y. H. Hsieh, and D. E. Newman-Toker. 2009. HINTS to diagnose stroke in the acute vestibular syndrome: Three-step bedside oculomotor examination more sensitive than early MRI diffusion-weighted imaging. *Stroke* 40 (11):3504–3510. doi: 10.1161/STROKEAHA.109.551234.

Kerr, Z. Y., S. L. Zuckerman, E. B. Wassermann, T. Covassin, A. Djoko, and T.P. Dompier. 2016. Concussion symptoms and return to play time in youth, high school and college American football athletes. *JAMA Pediatrics*. doi: 10.1001/jamapediatrics.2016.0073.

Kowalski, K., L. A. Corbin-Berrigan, J. Faubert, B. Christie, and I. Gagnon. 2015. Perceptual cognitive training in mild traumatic brain injury: Towards a sensitive marker of recovery. In *Proceedings of the 1st International Conference on Pediatric Acquired Brain Injury*, September 16-18, Liverpool, UK.

Kristjansson, E. and J. Treleaven. 2009. Sensorimotor function and dizziness in neck pain: Implications for assessment and management. *J Orthop Sports Phys Ther* 39 (5):364–377.

McCrory, P., W. H. Meeuwisse, M. Aubry, B. Cantu, J. Dvorák, R. J. Echemendia, L. Engebretsen et al. 2013. Consensus statement on concussion in sport: The 4th international conference on concussion in sport held in Zurich, November 2012. *Br J Sports Med* 47:250–258. doi: 10.1136/bjsports-2013-092313.

McGregor, M. L. 2014. Convergence insufficiency and vision therapy. *Pediatr Clin North Am* 61 (3):621–630. doi: 10.1016/j.pcl.2014.03.010.

Mucha, A., M. W. Collins, R. J. Elbin, J. M. Furman, C. Troutman-Enseki, R. M. DeWolf, G. Marchetti, and A. Kontos. 2014. A brief vestibular/ocular motor screening (VOMS) assessment to evaluate concussions. Preliminary findings. *Am J Sports Med*. doi: 10.1177/0363546514543775.

Noguchi, Y., Y. Kaneoke, R. Kakigi, H. C. Tanabe, and N. Sadato. 2005. Role of the superior temporal region in human visual motion perception. *Cereb Cortex* 15 (10):1592–1601. doi: 10.1093/cercor/bhi037.

Page, P. 2011. Cervicogenic headaches: An evidence-led approach to clinical management. *Int J Sports Phys Ther* 6 (3):254–266.

Piponnier, J. C., R. Forget, I. Gagnon, M. McKerral, J. F. Giguere, and J. Faubert. 2016. First- and second-order stimuli reaction time measures are highly sensitive to mild traumatic brain injuries. *J Neurotrauma* 33 (2):242–253. doi: 10.1089/neu.2014.3832.

Reneker, J. C. and C. E. Cook. 2015. Dizziness after sports-related concussion: Can physiotherapists offer better treatment than just "physical and cognitive rest?" *B J Sport Med* 49 (8):491–492.

Rine, R. M. and S. Wiener-Vacher. 2013. Evaluation and treatment of vestibular dysfunction in children. *NeuroRehabilitation* 32 (3):507–518. doi: 10.3233/NRE-130873.

Schneider, G. M., G. Jull, K. Thomas, A. Smith, C. Emery, P. Faris, C. Cook, B. Frizzell, and P. Salo. 2014a. Derivation of a clinical decision guide in the diagnosis of cervical facet joint pain. *Arch Phys Med Rehabil* 95 (9):1695–1701.

Schneider, G. M., G. Jull, K. Thomas, A. Smith, K. Schneider, and P. Salo. 2013. Intrarater and inter-rater reliability of select clinical test in patients referred for diagnostic facet joint blocks in the cervical spine. *Arch of Phys Med Rehabil* 94 (8):1628–1634.

Schneider, K. J. 2016. Sport-related concussion: Optimizing treatment through evidence-informed practice. *JOSPT* 46 (8):613–616. doi: 10.2519/jospt.2016.0607.

Schneider, K. J., J. Leddy, K. Guskiewicz, T. D. Seifert, M. McCrea, N. Silverberg, N. Feddermann-Demont, G. Iverson, K. A. Hayden, and M. Makdissi. 2017. Rest and specific treatments following sport-related concussion: A systematic review. *Br J Sports Med* 51(12):930–934.

Schneider, K. J., W. H. Meeuwisse, A. Nettel-Aguirre, L. Boyd, K. M. Barlow, and C. A. Emery. 2014b. Cervicovestibular physiotherapy in the treatment of individuals with persistent symptoms following sport related concussion: a randomised controlled trial. *Br J Sports Med* 48:1294–1298. doi: 10.1136/bjsports-2013-093267.

Schneider, K. J., W. H. Meeuwisse, and C. A. Emery. 2009. Symptom and functional improvements following a course of vestibular rehabilitation, manual therapy and spinal stabilization exercies in high performance athletes with complex concussions. *Clin J Sport Med* 19 (3):265–266.

Schubert, M. C. and L. B. Minot. 2004. Vestibulo-ocular physiology underlying vestibular hypofunction. *Phys Ther* 84 (4):373–385.

Schubert, M. C., R. J. Tusa, L. E. Grine, and S. J. Herdman. 2004. Optimizing the sensitivity of the head thrust test for identifying vestibular hypofunction. *Phys Ther* 84 (2):151–158.

Slobounov, S., T. Wu, M. Hallett, H. Shibasaki, E. Slobounov, and K. Newell. 2006. Neural underpinning of postural responses to visual field motion. *Biol Psychol* 72 (2):188–197.

Tohyama, K. and K. Fukushima. 2005. Neural network model for extracting optic flow. *Neural Netw* 18 (5–6):549–556.

Treleaven, J., G. Jull, and L. Atkinson. 1994. Cervical musculoskeletal dysfunction in post-concussional headache. *Cephalalgia* 14:273–279.

Treleaven, J. 2008. Sensorimotor disturbances in neck disorders affecting postural stability, head and eye movement control-Part 2: Case studies. *Man Ther* 13:266–275.

Vidal, P. G., A. M. Goodman, A. Colin, J. J. Leddy, and M. F. Grady. 2012. Rehabilitation strategies for prolonged recovery in pediatric and adolescent concussion. *Pediatr Ann* 41 (9):1–7. doi: 10.3928/00904481-20120827-10.

*chapter nine*

# Role of neuropsychology in sport concussion

## What can the neuropsychologist do?

*Vickie Plourde, Brian L. Brooks, Michael W. Kirkwood, and Keith O. Yeates*

## Contents

## Introduction

Neuropsychology is an essential discipline for evaluating, understanding, and managing the effects of sport-related concussion (SRC). Neuropsychologists are key personnel of any multidisciplinary team dealing with sport concussion, noting that no other discipline has established a similar repertoire of tools for understanding the neurobiopsychosocial impact of brain injury or disease. Neuropsychology has a rich history of studying concussion, with hundreds of studies aimed at understanding the effects of SRC. The purpose of this chapter is to provide an overview of neuropsychology and its role in SRC, addressing the field of neuropsychology broadly in understanding brain health and the role of neuropsychologists during acute, subacute, and chronic stages after concussion.

## Overview of neuropsychology

The National Academy of Neuropsychology (NAN) defines clinical neuropsychologists as independent health-care providers with expertise in the applied science of brain–behavior relationships and specialized training in assessing, treating, and rehabilitating patients with various neurological, medical, psychiatric, cognitive, and learning disorders. Neuropsychologists use psychological, neurological, cognitive, behavioral, and physiological principles, techniques, and methods to evaluate patients' functioning, establish, or confirm diagnoses, predict important functional outcomes, and propose interventions (refer to Barth et al., 2003 for the full definition).

Clinical neuropsychologists are trained to perform evidence-based neuropsychological assessment that consists of the integration of clinical expertise, outcome research, patient characteristics, and referral questions (Chelune, 2010; Schoenberg & Scott, 2011). A neuropsychological assessment typically includes an initial interview to collect data about developmental, medical, educational, and psychosocial history, as well as current functioning and symptoms and all other information that may be relevant to the referral question. This is followed by testing with standardized, population-referenced neuropsychological measures, assessing a range of cognitive skills according to patients' needs (Division 40, APA, 2010). This is followed by integration of all relevant information into a case formulation, together with recommendations for clinical management. Table 9.1 presents the different steps and range of domains that can be covered during a neuropsychological assessment.

*Table 9.1* Different steps and range of skills that can be covered during a neuropsychological assessment

| Assessment methods | Definition |
|---|---|
| Clinical interview | Interview with the patient (and sometimes relatives depending on circumstances) to collect information about the patient's demographics, history and preinjury functioning, details about the concussion, and current functioning. This interview is the first step of a neuropsychological assessment. When available, medical and school records are consulted prior to or after the interview. Neuropsychologists also note clinical observations during the initial interview and throughout the assessment. |
| Paper and pencil or computerized cognitive testing | Following the clinical interview, a formal neuropsychological assessment is performed using a variety of standardized and validated tests assessing multiple cognitive domains. |
| Intelligence | Intellectual functioning refers to a multidimensional construct of cognitive skills that help you adapt in your daily life (e.g., verbal and nonverbal reasoning skills). |
| Learning & Memory | Memory refers to encoding, retaining, and retrieving verbal and nonverbal information in a short (short-term memory) or a long (long-term memory) period of time. Learning corresponds to when the verbal or nonverbal information is encoded and consolidated in memory. Other types of memory can be assessed, such as declarative episodic (recall of autobiographical and context-specific events) or semantic memory (recall of general knowledge), and procedural memory (implicit memory about how to perform tasks). |
| Attention | Consists in the ability to focus to process verbal or visual information. Specific types of attention have been defined, such as selective (focus on a task while ignoring distractors), divided (focus to complete two simultaneous tasks), and sustained (maintain your interest on a task over time) attention skills. |
| Reaction time | Refers to time taken to *react* to a stimulus (e.g., time it takes to answer a simple task). |

*(Continued)*

*Table 9.1 (**Continued**)* Different steps and range of skills that can be covered during a neuropsychological assessment

| Assessment methods | Definition |
|---|---|
| Processing Speed | Time and efficiency in processing information and tasks, which can be chronologically divided in three steps: considering the information, making sense of it, and answering accordingly and in a timely manner. |
| Executive functions | Refers to higher order cognitive skills needed to adapt to environmental changes and deal with complex situations. These skills include but are not limited to, holding and manipulating information over brief periods of time (working memory), organizing, planning, inhibiting automatic responses (inhibition), shifting between task demands (cognitive flexibility), generating verbal or nonverbal responses (fluency), and analyzing and solving problems. They also comprise metacognitive skills, such as self-monitoring and self-awareness. |
| Visuospatial skills | Visuospatial skills include the ability to perceive visual information, to understand spatial relationships between visual items (e.g., visual discrimination, orientation in space), and to produce visual designs or constructions by coordinating visuospatial and motor skills. |
| Motor skills | Can include motor dexterity, strength, and speed. |
| Somatosensory skills | Somatosensory functioning corresponds to the senses of the body (e.g., tactile discrimination, pressure, vibration, olfactory sense, proprioception). |
| Language | Encompasses expressive (e.g., production of meaningful words, sentences, and nonverbal communicative cues) and receptive (e.g., understanding of words, sentences, nonverbal communicative cues) language skills can be assessed, as well as other language skills (e.g., pragmatics which refer to the use and comprehension of language in social contexts). |
| Academics | Can include the assessment of reading skills (e.g., phonological decoding, word reading, reading fluency, and reading comprehension), writing skills (e.g., spelling, grammar, syntax, text composition), and mathematical skills (e.g., calculating, geometry, applied problem resolution). |
| Questionnaires | Questionnaires are complementary to the neuropsychological tests and inform the neuropsychologist about multidimensional subjective symptoms the patient (and relatives) perceive and experience. |
| Concussion-related symptoms | Post-concussion symptoms can include physical/somatic, sleep, cognitive, and emotional symptoms, and some of these symptoms (e.g., headaches, pain, dizziness, sleep) can be addressed in greater detail. |
| Psychiatric, psychological, and behavioral functioning | This area of assessment covers a wide range of psychiatric and psychological symptoms and conditions, including, but not limited to, anxiety, post-traumatic stress, depression, somatization, substance abuse, resilience, adjustment, adaptability, and personality. |
| Social functioning | Includes social participation and support (e.g., participation to social activities, supportive environment), and social skills (e.g., how the person interacts with others). |
| Cognitive functioning | Corresponds to the assessment of subjective cognitive complaints, such as inattention symptoms, memory impairment, and executive functions deficits. |

*(Continued)*

*Table 9.1 (Continued)* Different steps and range of skills that can be covered during a neuropsychological assessment

| Assessment methods | Definition |
| --- | --- |
| Health-related quality of life | Refers to a multidimensional construct of how current functioning (e.g., physical, emotional, cognitive, academics, social) may impact on the patient's quality of life. |
| Validity testing | Different methods are integrated to test for effort, response bias, and malingering during the assessment, such as embedded validity tests, stand-alone performance validity tests, and validity scales in questionnaires. |
| Feedback session | After data collection, results' analysis, and interpretation are completed, the neuropsychologist meet the patient and relatives when appropriate, to provide a summary of the results, recommendations based on conclusions of the assessment, and to answer questions they may have. A detailed neuropsychological report usually follows the assessment and is sent to the patient or his parents (for children). |

*Source:* In part based on Iverson, G. L. et al., Cognitive impairment consequent to motor vehicle collisions: Foundations for clinical and forensic practice, in Duckworth, M. P., Iezzi, T., and O'Donohue, W. T. (Eds.), *Motor Vehicle Collisions: Medical, Psychosocial and Legal Consequences*, Academic Press, Cambridge, UK, pp. 243–309, 2008.

*Note:* Not all these areas are covered in every neuropsychological assessment. Learning and memory, attention, reaction time, processing speed, and executive functions are usually cognitive skills tested in any neuropsychological assessment (brief or comprehensive) whereas intelligence, visuospatial skills, motor skills, somatosensory skills, language, academic functioning can be included in comprehensive assessment.

# Consensus guidelines on sport concussion management: Role of neuropsychology

Neuropsychology has a longstanding history of studying brain disease and injury, with considerable foundational knowledge gained from World War II survivors who sustained brain injuries (see Lezak, Howieson, Bigler, & Tranel, 2012). Scientific interest in studying the behavioral repercussions of brain injuries in athletes has emerged over the past 4–5 decades, and studies reporting neuropsychological assessment and outcomes following SRC were published for the first time in the 1980s (Barth et al., 1989; see Webbe & Zimmer, 2015 for a detailed history of neuropsychology in SRC). Despite this relatively short history, sports neuropsychology has rapidly evolved and substantial work has already been conducted, which illustrates the value of neuropsychologists after SRC (e.g., textbooks on sports neuropsychology: Echemendia, 2006; Lovell, Barth, Collins, & Echemendia, 2004; Webbe, 2010). The growing interest in SRC has brought neuropsychologists to the forefront of providing assessment and intervention services, as well as conducting research and developing evidence-based care for athletes with SRC (Echemendia et al., 2012; Echemendia et al., 2013; Echemendia, Giza, & Kutcher, 2015; Kontos, Sufrinko, Womble, & Kegel, 2016). The involvement of neuropsychologists in SRC management paved the way toward the development of sport neuropsychology, "a sub-specialty of clinical neuropsychology that applies science and understanding of brain-behavior relationships to the assessment and treatment of sport-related brain injury" (Sports Neuropsychology Society, 2015).

In the context of SRC, neuropsychologists provide evidence-based assessment in order to evaluate symptoms, cognitive functioning, and psychological health, monitor recovery, and provide interventions or rehabilitation strategies (Iverson, 2007). When interpreting the results of their assessments, neuropsychologists carefully consider the athlete's background, preexisting functioning, other concurrent problems, and the psychometric properties of tests administered. According to the Sports Neuropsychology Society (2015), sports neuropsychologists require traditional training in clinical neuropsychology and additional training to learn how to apply their knowledge when providing assessment and intervention to athletes following concussion.

The central role of neuropsychologists in the management of SRC has been acknowledged in multiple consensus statements and clinical practice guidelines (Giza et al., 2013; Guskiewicz et al., 2004; Halstead & Walter, 2010; Harmon et al., 2013; McCrory et al., 2017). All these guidelines underscore that neuropsychological testing, including paper-and-pencil and computerized cognitive measures, can be useful to evaluate cognitive functioning following SRC and that results should be interpreted by a neuropsychologist for accurate understanding of their significance (West and Marion, 2014). Brief computerized cognitive testing can be part of a more comprehensive neuropsychological assessment, but should not be used as a replacement (McCrory et al., 2017). Neuropsychological assessment is also recognized as important when athletes present with complex symptoms or poor recovery after SRC (Harmon et al., 2013). The importance of neuropsychologists in the evaluation and management of SRC has been underscored by the American Academy of Clinical Neuropsychology, the American Board of Neuropsychology, the Society of Clinical Neuropsychology (Division 40 of the American Psychological Association), and the National Academy of Neuropsychology (Echemendia et al., 2012).

## Neuropsychological care after a sport-related concussion: Integration in a chronological and multidimensional model of recovery

Figure 9.1 presents a model illustrating the role of neuropsychologists during the various stages of recovery post-concussion. Each section of this chapter includes a summary of studies showing acute, subacute, and chronic effects of SRC and then discusses the role played by the neuropsychologist at each stage. The focus is mainly on athletes following SRC because of potential differences between athletes and the general population in terms of psychological and environmental factors affecting concussion recovery (see Rabinowitz, Li, & Levin, 2014 for a review of similarities and differences between sports or nonsport-related concussions). However, studies with individuals sustaining nonsports concussions are also reported when less empirical support is available specifically for SRC.

The model integrates individualized, patient-oriented, multidimensional, and evidence-based practices in neuropsychology, based on available published scientific evidence. However, given that additional studies are still required in many areas, this model should be considered an evolving framework about what neuropsychologists can add to multidisciplinary care.

### Acute period post-injury

*Acute symptoms and neuropsychological effects*: The acute period following SRC lasts about 3–5 days and is marked by sizable clinical effects and the beginning of clinical recovery on different levels, such as post-concussive symptoms, postural control, and cognitive functioning (McCrea et al., 2009; McCrea, Broshek, & Barth, 2015). There are multiple studies proposing, reviewing, and supporting the adoption of a multimodal approach when

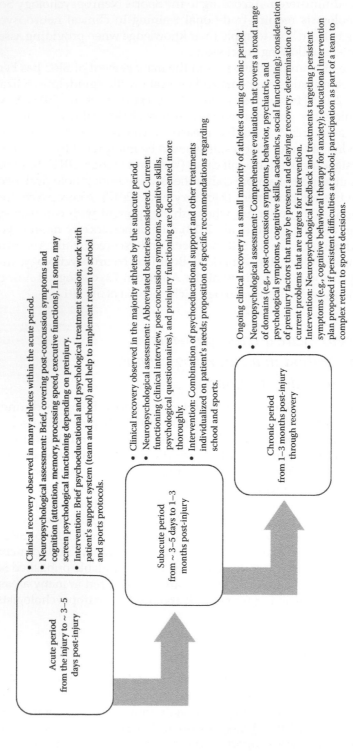

*Figure 9.1* Role of the neuropsychologist at different steps of recovery post-concussion.

doing on-field (sideline) assessment of concussions (Barr & McCrea, 2011; Echemendia et al., 2013; Kirkwood et al., 2008; McCrea, et al., 2009, 2015; McCrory et al., 2017; Okonkwo, Tempel, & Maroon, 2014). Moreover, 2 out of 11 meta-analyses published between 1997 and 2013 on the neuropsychological impact of concussion have been conducted on acute cognitive effects in adolescents or adults after sustaining SRC (Karr, Areshenkoff, & Garcia-Barrera, 2014a).

Broglio & Puetz (2008) conducted a meta-analysis of 39 articles among others to examine SRC outcomes with regard to self-reported symptoms, postural control, and cognition in the acute period (less than 24 hours to approximately 3 days post-injury). Results showed that all three domains (post-concussive symptoms—14 studies, postural control—6 studies, and cognitive testing—34 studies) are affected significantly during the acute period. The effect sizes for post-concussive symptoms immediately after the injury were significantly larger than the effect sizes for neurocognitive functioning, suggesting increased sensitivity of symptom reporting during this period. On the other hand, the fact that effect sizes for symptoms were larger than for other domains does not mean that objective evaluation of cognition or balance is not important. For example, acute cognitive testing in an emergency department with youth who sustained a concussion (about half of the sample sustained sports injuries) was predictive of poor outcome at one-month post-injury (Brooks et al., 2016a), suggesting that acute objective measurement of brain functioning can be advantageous not only for diagnosing concussion (Brooks, Khan, Daya, Mikrogianakis, & Barlow, 2014b) but also for prognosticating outcome (Brooks et al., 2016a).

Importantly, these three domains (symptoms, balance, cognition) may be differentially affected both between individuals and within the same person (Broglio & Puetz, 2008), reinforcing the importance of taking a multidimensional approach when making clinical decisions. Interestingly, Broglio & Puetz (2008) also compared effect sizes between the standardized assessment of concussion (SAC) cognitive screening, traditional paper-and-pencil neuropsychological measures, and computerized neuropsychological measures in the acute period following SRC. They found larger effect sizes using the SAC than more traditional paper-and-pencil or computerized neuropsychological measures. However, this result could be due to the time of assessment, which was often immediately after the injury when using the SAC while more often in the following days (but ≤ 3 days) with the other measures (Broglio & Puetz, 2008). The sensitivity of the SAC in the acute period has not always been replicated in other samples (Gorman, Hecht, Samborski, Lunos et al., 2016; Grubenhoff, Kirkwood, Gao, Deakyne, & Wathen, 2010; Putukian et al., 2015; Yengo-Kahn et al., 2016).

Belanger and Vanderploeg (2005) conducted a meta-analysis to identify potential deficits within neuropsychological domains during the acute period following SRC in adolescents and adults ($N = 21$ studies). They found acute cognitive effects (within 24 hours) on orientation (SAC) and attention, and more pronounced effects on memory skills (acquisition and retention) and global cognitive functioning, regardless of whether athletes with SRC were compared to a control group or to their preinjury scores (baseline). Importantly, the cognitive domain named as *attention* by Belanger and Vanderploeg (2005) included measures of reaction time and processing speed, which have been shown to be affected shortly after concussion in athletes and nonathletes (Babikian & Asarnow, 2009; Belanger, Curtiss, Demery, Lebowitz, & Vanderploeg, 2005; Brooks et al., 2014b; Peterson, Stull, Collins, & Wang, 2009). Surprisingly, SRC did not have a significant impact on executive functions, a result that differs from another meta-analysis in adolescents and adults sustaining concussion unrelated to sports that showed significant negative effects on executive functions (Belanger et al., 2005). The reasons for these divergent results remain unclear. Recent studies in the acute period post-concussion have shown that children and adolescents do not exhibit accuracy deficits in cognitive tasks, but they show slower reaction times on tasks of both attention (Crowe et al., 2015) and executive functions, such as inhibition and set-shifting (Brooks et al., 2014b). Moreover, slower shifting skills (ability to switch between cognitive tasks) have been identified in athletes who are 7 or more days post-injury (Karr, Garcia-Barrera, & Areshenkoff, 2014b), but these results have yet to be replicated during the acute period post-SRC. As executive functioning includes a broad set of skills (e.g., inhibition, planning, cognitive flexibility), future research will help clarify which of these skills are affected in the acute period following SRC.

*Role of the neuropsychologist in acute assessment and management*: The on-field presence of a well-trained professional in SRC is strongly recommended to establish the concussion mechanism, identify initial injury effects, rule out serious neck injury or other medical emergencies, and provide appropriate early management to athletes (Kirkwood et al., 2008; McCrea, Iverson, Echemendia, Makdissi, & Raftery, 2013b; Okonkwo et al., 2014). Neuropsychologists are rarely on field to assess acute functioning, but they can play a role as a consultant with sport teams and they also can conduct an acute brief assessment within the first days post-injury.

The use of validated and standardized instruments is recommended to accurately diagnose concussions, because informal questions following concussion may not be sensitive enough (Maddocks, Dicker, & Saling, 1995). Concerted efforts have been made to build a multidimensional screening measure to use on field with athletes after SRC. The sport concussion assessment test (SCAT) has been developed and revised, and is now in its fifth edition (SCAT5: Echemendia et al., 2017). This sideline assessment tool is available online and consists of the Glasgow Coma Scale (level of consciousness system), an orientation score using Maddocks questions (Maddocks et al., 1995), the post-concussion symptom scale (PCSS), a physical signs score, a coordination score, a balance examination using a modified version of the BESS (Guskiewicz, Riemann, Perrin, & Nashner, 1997), and a cognitive screening using the standardized assessment of concussion (SAC; McCrea, 2001). Interpretation of each score should be completed separately rather than using the total SCAT score (Echemendia et al., 2017; Guskiewicz et al., 2013). To adapt the SCAT5 to younger athletes, a child version (Child SCAT5; 5–12 years old) was developed (Davis et al., 2017), but additional studies on its validity and reliability are needed.

The evaluation of subjective post-concussive symptoms acutely after the injury is important to document symptoms that athletes may experience following the concussion and to help manage their recovery. There are many tools available to measure post-concussive symptoms (see Alla, Sullivan, Hale, & McCrory, 2009 for a review), including several that are supported by the National Institutes of Health Common Data Elements for TBI (McCauley et al., 2012; Wilde et al., 2010). Symptoms covered can be clustered into (1) physical/somatic (headache, nausea, balance, dizziness, sensitivity to light, and sensitivity to noise), (2) sleep (fatigue, difficulty sleeping, and drowsiness), (3) cognitive (feeling slowed down, feeling like in a fog, difficulty concentrating, and difficulty remembering), and (4) emotional/affective (irritability, sadness, nervousness, and more emotional) (see Merritt & Arnett, 2014; factor analysis of the post-concussion symptom scale). These rating scales have been shown good sensitivity after SRC in high school, university, and professional athletes (McCrea et al., 2015). Despite fewer studies overall with adolescents compared with adults (Davis & Purcell, 2014), good psychometric properties have been demonstrated for the post-concussion symptom inventory in children and adolescents (Sady, Vaughan, & Gioia, 2014). Administration of post-concussive symptoms rating scales to both children and their parents (Sady et al., 2014) is often recommended in cases of childhood SRC, to rate symptoms both pre- and a post-injury to better understand children's functioning prior to their concussion (Kirkwood et al., 2008).

As neuropsychologists are rarely on field, cognitive screening with the SAC or similar instruments may be conducted by team physicians or athletes' health-care providers, provided they have formal training in psychometrics and test administration and are, therefore, qualified to administer and interpret these acute assessments (Barr & McCrea, 2011). However, brief and limited objective cognitive screening measures should not be used to replace comprehensive neuropsychological assessment (Echemendia et al., 2013). Despite consensus about the importance of cognitive screening during the acute period (McCrea et al., 2013b), debate continues about whether a brief neuropsychological assessment should be part of acute SRC care (Iverson & Schatz, 2015). The main differences between a cognitive screening like the SAC and a brief neuropsychological assessment are the time involved (5 minutes compared to 20–30 minutes, respectively) and the range of skills covered (more limited in the cognitive screening model). For instance, the SAC covers orientation, immediate and delayed memory, and concentration skills (using only accuracy scores), whereas a brief neuropsychological assessment usually includes attention, reaction time, processing speed, working memory, short- and long-term verbal and visual memory skills, and executive functions such as fluency, inhibition, or cognitive flexibility (using both accuracy and speed scores). Moreover, although computerized versions of brief neuropsychological assessments can be administered by qualified health-care professionals, they should be interpreted by a neuropsychologist given their complexity and the need to consider the test's psychometric properties and patient's cognitive characteristics pre- and post-injury (Echemendia et al., 2012, 2013; Echemendia, Herring, & Bailes, 2009; Resch, McCrea, & Cullum, 2013). Unfortunately, neuropsychologists are still not always involved in the interpretation of brief neuropsychological assessments (see Covassin, Elbin, Stiller-Ostrowski, & Kontos, 2009; Meehan, D'Hemecourt, Collins, & Comstock, 2011; Moser, Schatz, & Lichtenstein, 2015 for examples).

One argument against the use of a brief neuropsychological assessment in the acute period is a study showing that paper-and-pencil neuropsychological testing in athletes within 2 days post-injury did not significantly increase sensitivity to detect cognitive impairment beyond the SAC cognitive screening (McCrea et al., 2005). However, other studies have suggested that computerized neuropsychological testing, more specifically ANAM (ANAM4 sports medicine battery automated neuropsychological assessment metrics), Axon sports/Cogstate sport (Cogstate Ltd.), and ImPACT (Lovell, 2013) can identify clinical impairment during the acute period after SRC (McCrea et al., 2013b; Nelson et al., 2016a) and can detect acute cognitive impact of the SRC in athletes hiding post-concussive symptoms (ImPACT; Schatz & Sandel, 2013). Iverson (2007) also has demonstrated the value of the ImPACT computerized cognitive test in athletes within 72 hours post-injury for predicting slower recovery from their concussion. They showed that athletes who took more than 10 days to recover were 18 times more likely to obtain three low scores on this computerized battery. Computerized cognitive testing has also been shown as safe, sensitive, and predictive of subsequent post-concussive symptoms in children seen in the emergency department acutely following their concussion (Brooks et al., 2014b, Brooks et al., 2016a; Brooks et al., 2016b). Computerized measures also have advantages, including their availability (and alternate forms) and their relatively simple administration (De Marco & Broshek, 2014; Rahman-Filipiak & Woodard, 2013). Finally, from a clinical perspective, Iverson and Schatz (2015) underline pros of using a brief neuropsychological assessment in the acute period, such as using results to provide early individualized management recommendations (e.g., driving, rest, return to school, work, sport).

In sum, based on available data, either a cognitive screening or a brief neuropsychological assessment can be used in the acute period to document potential acute cognitive impact following the injury, depending on resources, time, and team availability. In either case, environmental aspects such as the use of a quiet space, standardized testing material, and clear test instructions are important to reduce potential distractors during the cognitive screening or the brief neuropsychological assessment (Moser et al., 2015; Rahman-Filipiak & Woodard, 2013; Schatz, Neidzwski, Moser, & Karpf, 2010). Given divergent research results, however, additional studies are needed to examine the validity (does the test actually measure what it is intended to measure; Sherman, Brooks, Iverson, Slick, & Strauss, 2011) and predictive utility of both cognitive screening and brief neuropsychological assessment in the acute period following SRC. Future studies looking at test-retest reliabilities (are test scores consistent when administered twice over time; Sherman et al., 2011) are also warranted, as some studies have shown low test-retest reliabilities in both earlier editions of the SCAT screening tool (Chin, Nelson, Barr, McCrory, & McCrea, 2016; Hänninen et al., 2016) and computerized cognitive measures (McKay, Brooks, Mrazik, Jubinville, & Emery, 2014; Nelson et al., 2016a; Resch et al., 2013) when used in athletes. Moreover, test-retest reliabilities of these measures should be compared with traditional paper-and-pencil neuropsychological assessment, as a recent paper demonstrated that more *fluid* cognitive abilities, such as processing speed and executive functions, may be more difficult to assess in a reliable manner, regardless of the modality of neuropsychological testing, whether it be paper-and-pencil or computerized (Iverson & Schatz, 2015).

*Interventions during the acute recovery period.* Brief and early educational sessions provided to individuals with concussion can help to improve understanding of the typical clinical course and provide reassurance (Kirkwood et al., 2008; Leddy, Sandhu, Sodhi, Baker, & Willer, 2012). However, relatively little high-quality research has addressed the effectiveness of early educational interventions in improving post-concussive symptoms (Eliyahu, Kirkland, Campbell, & Rowe, 2016). Moreover, no known studies have examined the effectiveness of providing early educational interventions (or handouts) to athletes specifically after SRC (Conder & Conder, 2014).

Some evidence indicates that a brief psychological treatment session early after concussion could help prevent the development of persistent post-concussive symptoms (Mittenberg, Canyock, Condit, & Patton, 2001). These researchers identified key components of the session: education, cognitive restructuring, reassurance of a positive recovery, and a gradual return to activities. Neuropsychologists often include these components in their feedback following a brief neuropsychological assessment.

Regarding rest following the injury, data are still limited regarding its impact on post-concussion recovery (Schneider et al., 2013). Nevertheless, immediate removal from play following the concussion (Elbin et al., 2016b) and immediate physical and cognitive rest during the initial 1–2 days post-concussion (Taubman, Rosen, McHugh, Grady, & Elci, 2016) have been recommended (McCrory et al., 2017). An extended period of rest is not advised, however, as it can slow symptom recovery (Leddy, Baker, & Willer, 2016; Thomas, Apps, Hoffmann, McCrea, & Hammeke, 2015) and increase the risk of physical deconditioning, symptoms of anxiety and depression, and other psychological complications (DiFazio, Silverberg, Kirkwood, Bernier, & Iverson, 2016).

Neuropsychologists also have an important role to play in returning individuals to activities following the injury, including the provision of consultation to the athlete and school team involved in the acute management post-concussive. Studies have underlined the importance of informing school personnel (psychologist, teacher, nurse) about children and adolescents with acute concussion and educating them about concussion symptoms, clinical recovery, and management (Davies, Sandlund, & Lopez, 2016; Elbin et al., 2016b). Consultation to the school team can help identify students presenting with post-concussive symptoms, facilitate a graded and positive return to learn, and make accommodations available for the students when needed.

In addition to playing a consultative role, neuropsychologists are often members of interdisciplinary teams making decisions regarding return to school and other activities post-injury. Based on their assessment and available scientific evidence, neuropsychologists can propose recommendations for a return to school plan and accommodations best suited to the student's needs and current profile. Objectives of a gradual return to school and accommodations are to facilitate school functioning and recovery post-concussion. Despite not yet evidence based, detailed and graded returns to school protocols and accommodations for academics have been proposed (Gioia, 2014; Master, Gioia, Leddy, & Grady, 2012; McGrath, 2010; Rose, Weber, Collen, & Heyer, 2015b). For instance, academic accommodations during the acute period can include rest periods during the day, extended time for tests, or reduced homework load (Gioia, 2014). These return-to-learn protocols apply to primary and high schools and can be adapted to the college and university environments (Hall et al., 2015). Return to school is followed by return to sports. Again, a gradual protocol has been proposed (McCrory et al., 2017), with the use of a more conservative approach when returning children and adolescents back to high-risk activities (Kirkwood et al., 2008).

## Subacute period post-injury

*Subacute symptoms and neuropsychological effects*: The subacute period begins around 3–5 days after the concussion, at which point most athletes will continue to recover on neurological, symptomatic, and cognitive levels. For instance, in their meta-analysis, Broglio &Puetz (2008) showed that despite reduced effect sizes compared with the acute period, many athletes still experienced post-concussive symptoms as well as decreased postural control and neuropsychological functioning 3–14 days post-injury. These findings further underscore the utility of a multidimensional approach for addressing post-concussive symptoms, postural control, and neuropsychological functioning during the subacute period. The end of the subacute period has been set around 1 month, by which time the vast majority of athletes will have achieved full recovery (Belanger et al., 2005; Belanger & Vanderploeg, 2005; Broglio & Puetz, 2008; Crowe et al., 2015; McCrea et al., 2009; Zuckerman et al., 2012).

When assessing the presence of post-concussive symptoms subacutely in athletes, the number of previous assessments should be considered, given that it may moderate the extent to which post-concussive symptoms decrease within 14 days post-injury (Broglio & Puetz, 2008). Interestingly, studies have shown that the majority of athletes experience resolution of their post-concussive symptoms between a few weeks (Williams, Puetz, Giza, & Broglio, 2015) to within a month following the injury (Guskiewicz et al., 2003; Henry, Elbin, Collins, Marchetti, & Kontos, 2016; McCrea et al., 2003; Meehan et al., 2011). Nevertheless, a small proportion of athletes report persisting symptoms at one-month post-injury. In a clinical sample of 531 7–26-year-old athletes referred to a specialty clinic, Meehan, Mannix, Monuteaux, Stein, and Bachur (2014) used the post-concussion symptom scale to examine post-concussive symptoms at 12 ± 5 days after the injury and at 28 days post-injury. After controlling for different variables (age, sex, personal, and familial history of prior concussions, history of migraines and medical treatment for headaches, loss of consciousness and amnesia at the injury, performance on neurocognitive tests), they found that the number of post-concussive symptoms at the first assessment predicted prolonged symptoms at 28 days post-injury. Similar results in youth showed that worse post-concussive symptoms during the subacute period (mean of 10 days post-concussive) predicted longer duration of post-concussive symptoms (Heyer et al., 2016). Meehan et al. (2014) also showed that 14% of the athletes did not report elevated post-concussive symptoms at the first assessment but reported an elevated level of symptoms at 28 days post-injury, underlining the potential for nonconcussion factors to influence symptom reporting and the relevance of monitoring the evolution of symptoms during the subacute stage in athletes, even for those who report fewer symptoms during the acute period. Finally, the monitoring of potential comorbid psychological symptoms during the subacute period is also important, as a recent study in the emergency department showed that patients with higher post-concussive symptoms two weeks post-injury were also reporting higher levels of symptoms of depression, anxiety, and post-traumatic stress compared with those with few or no complaints (Scheenen et al., 2016).

Monitoring cognitive status during the subacute period following SRC is encouraged. Although functioning in most cognitive domains seems to return to normal after about one-week post-SRC (Belanger & Vanderploeg, 2005; Williams et al., 2015), Belanger and Vanderploeg (2005) have demonstrated some residual impact on delayed memory 10 days post-injury when athletes with SRC were compared with control participants. Moreover, they found no differences in cognitive effects following SRC between paper-and-pencil or computerized cognitive measures. However, because of statistical power issues, they only investigated differences between both types of measures on overall effect sizes and not between the acute and subacute periods of testing. Contrary to Belanger and Vanderploeg (2005), Broglio &Puetz (2008) have shown higher sensitivity of traditional paper-and-pencil neuropsychological than computerized cognitive testing or the SAC during the subacute period following SRC. These results converge with a recent study showing diminished utility of computerized cognitive tests to detect the cognitive effects of SRC after 8 days post-injury in high-school and collegiate athletes (Nelson et al., 2016a). These results suggest caution when interpreting computerized tests during the subacute period following SRC, and they reinforce the use of traditional neuropsychological tests as one component of a multidimensional clinical assessment (Nelson et al., 2016a).

Despite resolution of cognitive impairment within 10–14 days following concussion for the vast majority of athletes (e.g., Belanger & Vanderploeg, 2005; McCrea et al., 2003; Williams et al., 2015), a minority of athletes may experience cognitive deficits that persist longer. Indeed, studies have shown significant variability in the length of recovery between athletes post-SRC, with longer symptom recovery associated with more durable cognitive deficits (Iverson, Brooks, Collins, & Lovell, 2006; McCrea et al., 2013a). These results stress the need for analyses of individual trajectories to better delineate the temporal window of cognitive recovery following SRC.

*Role of the neuropsychologist in assessment and management subacutely*: Although no guidelines exist regarding assessment during the subacute period following SRC, McCrory et al. (2017) recommended a multidisciplinary approach by health professionals experienced in SRC for adult athletes who have not recovered after 10–14 days. At this stage, an abbreviated assessment provided by a neuropsychologist can be useful in guiding return to activities among athletes (McCrory et al., 2017), by providing an integrated overview of their current functioning, ensuring recovery and cognitive clearance before return to sports, and providing guidance about returning to school.

When athletes report persisting post-concussive symptoms and complaints one to two weeks following their concussion, the goal of the abbreviated neuropsychological assessment is to better understand their persistent symptoms. Importantly, post-concussive symptoms can be associated with injury-related factors (McCrea et al., 2013a; Merritt, Rabinowitz, & Arnett, 2015), but they are also not specific to concussion, as they can be present in healthy people (Iverson et al., 2015; Iverson & Lange, 2003; Jinguji et al., 2012) and often reflect preexisting or comorbid conditions, such as attention deficit hyperactivity disorder (ADHD) and learning disabilities (Elbin et al., 2013; Zuckerman, Lee, Odom, Solomon, & Sills, 2013), noncredible effort and symptom exaggeration (Araujo et al., 2014; Kirkwood, Grubenhoff, Peterson, Connery, & Baker, 2014), and migraines (Mannix et al., 2014). Symptoms that persist for weeks or longer are rarely explained entirely by the concussion per se (Iverson & Lange, 2011; Ruff, 2011). By identifying reasons that may help explain the persistent symptoms, neuropsychologists are able to suggest individualized and potentially effective intervention options for these athletes (Connery, Peterson, Baker, Randolph, & Kirkwood, 2016; Kirkwood et al., 2008). The implementation of interventions following the assessment can also help reduce risk for a further increase in symptoms and the development of other related problems, such as anxiety or depression.

The initial step of the neuropsychological assessment during the subacute period after SRC should involve gathering information related to the concussion during a clinical interview with the athlete (and family, partner, or parents, depending on age and current state of functioning). Neuropsychologists collect information about the mechanism of injury, severity of the injury (e.g., confusion, amnesia, loss of consciousness, immediate symptoms), and the athlete's functioning during the hours and first few days following the injury (e.g., post-concussive symptoms, orientation, coordination and balance, physical, cognitive, and psychological state) to better understand the severity of the injury and its potential influence on recovery. They also obtain information about sideline assessments if completed to better document acute functioning after SRC and to pair objective measures with subjective recall of the injury and related symptoms.

The clinical interview is also a time for the neuropsychologists to collect data with regard to medical (e.g., past or current diagnostics, previous concussions, or other conditions), familial, academic, psychosocial, and occupational history, as well as current functioning in these areas. In some cases, and when available, additional information is obtained by consulting medical charts, collateral sources, or school records. Preinjury and current functioning is also assessed with questionnaires, including post-concussive symptoms, as well as behavior and psychosocial functioning. To better understand the athlete's current functioning, detailed information about preinjury functioning and how different the athlete perceives her/himself since the injury is gathered. For example, preexisting or current conditions such as attention deficit/hyperactivity disorder, learning disabilities, sleep disorders, pain, and behavior (e.g., oppositional behavior) or mental health problems (e.g., depression, anxiety, personality) are documented and may affect interpretation of test results as they can affect performance. Standardized rating scales or questionnaires are also included to corroborate these results with the information collected during the clinical interview, as well as to document severity of long-term symptoms and identify which areas are more affected. For instance, psychological functioning can be assessed using rating scales related to depression, anxiety, and resilience. Rating scales can also be administered to the injured athletes and their relatives to obtain their perceptions about their cognitive functioning (e.g., questionnaires about attention, memory, or executive functions). Questionnaires related to health behaviors and current quality of life can also be administered to assess potential impact of the actual complaints of the athlete on daily life and activities.

The assessment typically includes rating scales assessing post-concussive symptoms, which can be compared with those in the acute period of the injury to see if they are perceived as less severe, similarly severe, or worse than immediately after the injury. In addition, post-concussive symptoms can be further documented using more detailed rating scales of headaches, pain, sleep, and fatigue. Norms are available for most post-concussive symptom scales (see, e.g., Lovell et al., 2006), allowing scores to be compared between athletes with or without SRC, whether or not post-concussive symptoms were assessed during the acute period.

Neuropsychologists should exercise caution when asking about preinjury functioning or post-concussive symptoms without corroborating records, especially considering the effect that possible biases can have on the accuracy of identifying levels of post-concussive problems. For instance, some studies have shown higher levels of symptoms when assessed with rating scales compared to when they are assessed in a clinical interview (Elbin et al., 2016a; Iverson, Brooks, Ashton, & Lange, 2010). Moreover, a tendency to perceive preinjury functioning as better than it actually was, referred as the *good old days* bias, can interfere with preinjury reporting and lead to a post-injury inflation of symptoms reported on questionnaires, especially as the amount of time since injury increases (Brooks et al., 2014a; Lange, Iverson, & Rose, 2010).

Finally, a thorough evaluation of cognitive functioning is included in the neuropsychological assessment at this stage. The battery should include validity tests to ensure athletes who are fully engaged and exerting adequate effort during the exam as well as tests that cover key domains that are most likely impacted by SRC, such as attention, memory, reaction time, processing speed, and executive functions. These areas are measured by traditional paper-and-pencil neuropsychological tests or computerized cognitive testing, and results are compared with appropriate norms to obtain a valid profile of the athlete's cognitive functioning. In clinical practice, a hybrid approach, combining paper-and-pencil with computerized measures, may be informative and useful given pros and cons of both test modalities. However, no published studies have empirically assessed this approach (Echemendia et al., 2013).

*Interventions during the subacute recovery*: At this stage, the provision of education to individuals and their family regarding concussion clinical recovery and symptoms remains relevant. For instance, the provision of educational (e.g., information about post-concussive symptoms) and supportive (e.g., coping strategies) interventions during the subacute period have been associated with a lower level of stress 3 months post-injury in adults and children (Ponsford et al., 2001, 2002) and with less post-concussive symptoms 6 months post-injury (Wade, King, Wenden, Crawford, & Caldwell, 1998). Despite these results, a recent systematic review of randomized controlled trials concluded that educational and reassurance interventions alone may not be as effective as previously stated in preventing persistent post-concussive symptoms (Al Sayegh, Sandford, & Carson, 2010).

Another treatment with evidence of effectiveness in reducing post-concussive symptoms during the subacute period is cognitive behavioral therapy (CBT), which attempts to modify symptom perceptions and cognitions, through cognitive restructuring and instruction in coping strategies (Potter & Brown, 2012). The number of studies in this regard is limited, but promising results suggest that CBT delivered during the subacute period could be effective to help treat post-concussive symptoms (Al Sayegh et al., 2010; Silverberg et al., 2013). Other treatments have been proposed, including a mindfulness-based stress reduction program (Azulay, Smart, Mott, & Cicerone, 2013) and subacute monitored exercises (Elbin, Schatz, Lowder, & Kontos, 2014), but additional studies of their effectiveness during the subacute stage are warranted.

Finally, the athlete's return to activities, school/work, and sports continues to be monitored during the subacute period. Neuropsychologists can work with athletic and school personnel to ensure that athletes are recovering and receiving appropriate accommodations. Moreover, results from the neuropsychological assessment can be used to modify or add academic accommodations or a specific plan with the school to support the student's recovery and academic, psychological, and social functioning. In cases where return to play is slower than expected due to complications or persistent symptoms, social participation with the team and a social support system should be available to make sure that the individual does not develop depression or anxiety associated with social isolation or retirement from the team (Kirkwood et al., 2008).

## Chronic period post-injury

*Are there long-term effects after SRC?* The chronic period following SRC starts around 1–3 months post-injury and continues until complete recovery. At this stage, the vast majority of athletes have fully recovered from their concussion, at least in terms of symptoms, balance, and cognition, and have returned to sport. Indeed, multiple studies presented above have shown complete recovery in most athletes by one month after concussion. However, a small proportion of athletes present with persistent post-concussive problems that can last for months or even years. To date, it remains difficult to accurately determine the prevalence of athletes displaying long-term effects after SRC, in part because most studies report group differences and do not include analyses to document individual variability in the length of recovery. For example, meta-analyses previously presented did not provide data regarding the prevalence and presentation of persistent post-concussive symptoms in athletes (Karr et al., 2014a). Iverson (2010) provided an example of a minority of patients having a concussion and residual cognitive impairment but who were not identified when using group statistics. Fortunately, newer statistical approaches are currently being used to better capture individual variability in athletes' recovery following SRC, such as multivariate base rate analyses, individual reliable changes, trajectory analyses, and clinical algorithms to identify impairment (Iverson & Schatz, 2015).

The assessment of long-term post-concussive symptoms is important, because elevated symptomatology negatively impacts health-related quality of life (Losoi et al., 2016; Novak et al., 2016). Factors related to current functioning can influence individual perceptions and reports of long-term post-concussive symptoms (Broshek, De Marco, & Freeman, 2015), including life stress (Gouvier, Cubic, Jones, Brantley, & Cutlip, 1992; McClure, Zuckerman, Kutscher, Gregory, & Solomon, 2014), insufficient sleep (Silverberg, Berkner, Atkins, Zafonte, & Iverson, 2016), and recent strenuous exercise (Balasundaram, Sullivan, Schneiders, & Athens, 2013). Psychological factors also can influence or predict post-concussive symptom reporting (Broshek et al., 2015). Indeed, preexisting mental health issues (e.g., anxiety, depression) have been identified as predictors of long-term post-concussive symptoms in adults 1–6 months post-injury (Lingsma et al., 2015; Silverberg et al., 2015). Similar results have been obtained in athletes with SRC (Morgan et al., 2015) and in children with concussion (Peterson, Connery, Baker, & Kirkwood, 2015; Yeates et al., 2012; Zemek, Farion, Sampson, & McGahern, 2013). In high school and college athletes, preinjury somatization tendencies have been found to contribute to post-concussive symptom recovery via their influence on acute post-concussive symptom reporting (Nelson et al., 2016b), a finding consistent with two recent studies examining somatization in concussed pediatric patients recruited from hospital emergency departments (Grubenhoff et al., 2016; Root et al., 2016). Early post-injury anxiety also has been shown to be a robust independent predictor of symptomatic outcome at least one month following concussion (see Silverberg et al., 2015 for a systematic review). In addition to preexisting or early post-injury psychological symptoms, concurrent anxiety and depression symptoms have shown to predict long-term post-concussive symptoms (3–12 months) in patients with concussion, but also in control groups of healthy or orthopedically injured participants (Clarke, Genat, & Anderson, 2012; Losoi et al., 2016; Ponsford et al., 2012). Therefore, the nonspecificity of symptoms, as well as preinjury and concurrent psychological functioning, should be considered when assessing post-concussive symptoms.

Early post-injury neuropsychological functioning is also a robust-independent predictor of long-term post-concussive symptoms (Silverberg et al., 2015) and cognitive complaints (Clarke et al., 2012) in adults with concussion. These results reinforce the importance of looking beyond injury-related factors and to consider acute and subacute neuropsychological assessment following concussion and its potential predictive value of long-term symptomatic outcomes.

Finally, some questions remain unanswered regarding long-term effects after concussion. First, can concussion lead to secondary cognitive deficits, psychological problems, and psychiatric conditions lasting months and years after the injury or even appearing years after retiring from sports? An increasing amount of research is investigating these long-term outcomes, but there is still little evidence to suggest that chronic problems result entirely from concussions. Additional prospective and longitudinal studies are warranted before drawing conclusions on this topic (Ellis et al., 2015; Emery et al., 2016; Finkbeiner, Max, Longman, & Debert, 2016; Riggio & Jagoda, 2016; Solomon, Kuhn, & Zuckerman, 2016). The same conclusion holds regarding chronic traumatic encephalopathy, defined as "a progressive tauopathy with distinctive clinical and pathological features that occurs after repetitive mild traumatic brain injury" (McKee et al., 2013), with cognitive, behavioral, mood, and motor repercussions (Montenigro, Corp, Stein, Cantu, & Stern, 2015). Despite the media attention and lay interest in this condition, and some highly-publicized cases of athletes purported to have CTE, CTE remains controversial as a distinct disease entity (Randolph, 2014), and insufficient high-quality research exists to conclude that late-life problems in retired athletes are caused by recurrent concussions (McCrory, Meeuwisse, Kutcher, Jordan, & Gardner, 2013). Future studies are needed to define the clinical and pathological criteria of CTE, investigate risk in a randomly selected high risk sample (e.g., NFL players) versus a matched control group, document incidence and prevalence, and understand potential modifiers other than concussions, including neurodevelopmental disorders, psychological or psychiatric conditions, and genetic and environmental factors (for detailed reviews, see Asken et al., 2016; Ban, Madden, Bailes, Hunt Batjer, & Lonser, 2016; Davis, Castellani, & McCrory, 2015; Gardner, Iverson, & McCrory, 2014; Maroon et al., 2015; Montenigro et al., 2015; Solomon & Zuckerman, 2015).

*Neuropsychological assessment in those with slow or poor recovery from concussion*: In clinical practice, neuropsychologists can be involved in the acute and subacute periods following the injury, but they are widely recognized as adding incremental value in the face of persistent symptoms after concussion. At this stage, the role of the neuropsychologist is to conduct comprehensive neuropsychological assessment with athletes who do not return to their preinjury functioning to better understand why they may be experiencing residual symptoms. The evaluation can help identify factors related to reported symptoms and ensure accurate diagnosis (Connery et al., 2016; Kirkwood et al., 2008) and can also detect the presence of comorbid conditions and help the neuropsychologist provide appropriate recommendations. Ultimately, the goal is to obtain an objective, multidimensional profile of the athlete's functioning, to help provide an updated management care plan and interventions adapted to current functioning. The implementation of interventions seeks to improve the athlete's functioning and achieve recovery. Depending on current functioning at the time of the evaluation, results can also help to guide return to activities (school, work, and sports).

A comprehensive neuropsychological assessment is typically longer (~5–6 hours for all components) than an abbreviated neuropsychological assessment and covers a broader range of skills with more depth. Similar to an abbreviated assessment, neuropsychologists first should conduct a clinical interview and consult available records to better understand how the patient's preinjury and current functioning can impact on recovery as well as to better understand functional impact of the concussion and long-term symptoms. A biopsychosocial conceptualization of poor outcomes from concussion (Iverson, 2012) can be a very helpful framework for neuropsychologists for organizing the data from the clinical interview and records. Questionnaires and cognitive testing covering a wide range of domains are then completed. Similar to the postacute stage, validity testing is again a necessary initial step to objectively rule out the possibility of feigning and exaggeration that are frequently in compensation-seeking concussion settings (Binder & Rohling, 1996) and also in adult and child patients seen clinically post-concussion (Araujo et al., 2014; Kirkwood et al., 2014; Mittenberg, Patton, Canyok, & Condit, 2002). At this stage postinjury, additional questionnaires can be added according to the athlete's complaints and clinical presentation. These data are helpful to assess the severity of symptoms reported by the athlete, to better understand their role in explaining long-term effects, and their impact on daily life functioning. Moreover, in addition to a broad cognitive assessment, questionnaires or tests assessing for instance, social cognition and skills, adaptive skills, problem-solving skills, familial and academic functioning (in children and adolescents), and intellectual abilities can be integrated to further document current potential impact of these skills on their daily life.

*Interventions to improve concussion recovery when symptoms persist*: An important benefit of conducting a comprehensive neuropsychological assessment in individuals presenting with persistent post-concussive symptoms is the identification of injury and noninjury factors explaining these symptoms and the consequent identification of individualized treatment targets. A recent study showed that a one-time neuropsychological consultation (3 hours in length, including interview, brief testing, and feedback) 2–12 months post-injury in children and adolescents may help decrease persistent post-concussive symptoms reported 1 week and 3 months postconsultation (Kirkwood, Peterson, Baker, & Connery, 2016). The feedback included general education about concussion, information related to injury and noninjury factors related to the patient's specific symptoms, and recommendations (Kirkwood, Peterson, Connery, Baker, & Forster, 2015).

In addition to neuropsychologically based feedback, other interventions can be offered at this stage, tailored according to the athlete's symptoms (Kirkwood et al., 2008). For instance, CBT can be considered to develop problem-solving and coping skills, and to work on post-concussive symptoms or other related issues, like mood and anxiety symptoms or sleep issues. Some promising results have been obtained. CBT treatment has been shown to improve long-term post-concussive symptoms (Potter, Brown, & Fleminger, 2016) while CBT for insomnia has been related to sleep improvement (Ouellet & Morin, 2007) in adults with mild to severe traumatic brain injuries. Moreover, interventions including CBT and motivational interviews adapted to cognitive impairment and focusing on anxiety and depression symptoms (Ponsford et al., 2016) and mindfulness-based cognitive therapy for depressive symptoms (Bédard et al., 2013) have shown significant alleviation of these symptoms.

Although the use of psychological therapy to treat persistent post-concussive symptoms is generally agreed upon, controversy continues regarding the use of cognitive remediation as an intervention during the chronic stage after concussion. Cicerone et al. (2011) systematically reviewed available studies and concluded that cognitive remediation of cognitive skills (attention, memory, and executive functions) could be useful with people presenting with persistent cognitive impairment following a mild to severe traumatic brain injury. However, others have discussed potential iatrogenic consequences of using cognitive remediation in patients with long-term post-concussive symptoms (e.g., increased sense of being cognitively impaired, increased somatization, shift from psychological work) (Kirkwood et al., 2008; Potter & Brown, 2012), highlighting the need for caution in the use of these interventions.

In some cases, athletes with persistent post-concussive symptoms can exhibit persistent school problems lasting for months to years. These students should have access to school supports, such as academic accommodations, individualized educational programs, and student support teams (Popoli, Burns, Meehan, & Reisner, 2014). In this context, neuropsychologists can work with school personnel to explain what factors play a role in the student's difficulties (e.g., ADHD, learning disorders, or psychological issues), as a concussion does not typically result in long-term academic problems (Kirkwood et al., 2008). Neuropsychologists can also help develop an individualized educational plan and propose accommodations tailored to each student needs and the neuropsychological evaluation's results. The student then can benefit from school assistance and more services than provided in the general school curriculum (Rose, Mcnally, & Heyer, 2015a).

Decisions regarding return to sports at this stage are particularly challenging. As discussed previously, symptoms that continue for months after the injury often reflect noninjury factors, and some authors have proposed that they should not necessarily exclude athletes from participation in exercise or sports (DiFazio et al., 2016). Indeed, active treatment approaches have shown promising positive effects on long-term post-concussive symptoms or return to sport participation in symptomatic participants. Such approaches include active rehabilitation, low-level and controlled exercise, and multimodal physiotherapy (Gagnon, Galli, Friedman, Grilli, & Iverson, 2009; Leddy et al., 2010; Schneider et al., 2013). This being said, decisions to return to sports should rest on an "individualized cost-benefit analysis weighing the potential risks of multiple insults to the brain and the psychosocial benefits of returning to play" (Kirkwood et al., 2008). Unfortunately, retirement needs to be considered in certain situations (e.g., multiple concussions, prolonged recovery, neurological sequelae, and secondary neuropsychological deficits); in such cases, an interdisciplinary workup is recommended, including a formal neuropsychological assessment (Laker, Meron, Greher, & Wilson, 2016). In the face of medical recommendations for retirement, low-level exercise and social support for the athlete can be important in preventing the development of secondary psychological problems (Laker et al., 2016).

## Conclusions and future directions

Neuropsychology is the study of brain and behavior, a focus that is clearly important in the evaluation and management of athletes after SRC. The neuropsychologist's level of involvement will vary depending on the presenting concerns and whether the athlete is at the acute, subacute, or chronic stage post-injury. Limited resources are a reality in most cases of SRC, and often neuropsychologists are primarily involved during the subacute and chronic time periods to help provide multidisciplinary care for those who have prolonged or unusual recovery. Clinical practices and evidence-based care in patients with SRC will evolve in coming years, guided by research discoveries and increased knowledge of SRC and its clinical presentations. Indeed, several questions remain about post-concussion outcomes and which factors can modify how athletes recover from a concussion. Interest continues to grow in better understanding the potential long-term impact of multiple concussions and subconcussive blows (Belanger, Spiegel, & Vanderploeg, 2010; Belanger, Vanderploeg, & McAllister, 2016). Future studies using a multidimensional framework and longitudinal design will help answer these questions and identify risk and protective factors at the neurobiological and psychosocial levels predicting outcomes post-injury (McCrea et al., 2015). Another important area of future research is the validation of existing measures and the development of new measures to accurately assess outcomes post-concussion. Additional studies regarding the relevance of baseline testing are also necessary before endorsing its clinical value. Ultimately, this work will help support positive clinical recovery trajectories following SRC in athletes.

## References

Al Sayegh, A. A., Sandford, D. D., & Carson, A. J. (2010). Psychological approaches to treatment of postconcussion syndrome: A systematic review. *Journal of Neurology, Neurosurgery, and Psychiatry, 81*(10), 1128–1134. http://doi.org/10.1136/jnnp.2008.170092

Alla, S., Sullivan, S. J., Hale, L., & McCrory, P. (2009). Self-report scales/checklists for the measurement of concussion symptoms: A systematic review. *British Journal of Sports Medicine, 43*(Suppl 1), i3–i12. http://doi.org/10.1136/bjsm.2009.058339

Araujo, G. C., Antonini, T. N., Monahan, K., Gelfius, C., Klamar, K., Potts, M., ... Bodin, D. (2014). The relationship between suboptimal effort and postconcussion symptoms in children and adolescents with mild traumatic brain injury. *The Clinical Neuropsychologist, 28*(5), 786–801. http://doi.org/10.1080/13854046.2014.896415

Asken, B. M., Sullan, M. J., Snyder, A. R., Houck, Z. M., Bryant, V. E., Hizel, L. P., ... Bauer, R. M. (2016). Factors influencing clinical correlates of chronic traumatic encephalopathy (CTE): A review. *Neuropsychology Review, 26*(4), 340–363. http://doi.org/10.1007/s11065-016-9327-z

Azulay, J., Smart, C., Mott, T., & Cicerone, K. (2013). A pilot study examining the effect of mindfulness-based stress reduction on symptoms of chronic mild traumatic brain injury/postconcussive syndrome. *Journal of Head Trauma Rehabilitation, 28*(4), 323–331. http://doi.org/10.1097/HTR.0b013e318250ebda

Babikian, T., & Asarnow, R. (2009). Neurocognitive outcomes and recovery after pediatric TBI: Meta-analytic review of the literature. *Neuropsychology, 23*(3), 283–296. http://doi.org/10.1037/a0015268

Balasundaram, A. P., Sullivan, J. S., Schneiders, A. G., & Athens, J. (2013). Symptom response following acute bouts of exercise in concussed and non-concussed individuals–A systematic narrative review. *Physical Therapy in Sport, 14*(4), 253–258. doi: 10.1016/j.ptsp.2013.06.002

Ban, V. S., Madden, C. J., Bailes, J. E., Hunt Batjer, H., & Lonser, R. R. (2016). The science and questions surrounding chronic traumatic encephalopathy. *Neurosurgical Focus, 40*(4), E15. http://doi.org/10.3171/2016.2.FOCUS15609

Barr, W. B., & McCrea, M. (2011). Diagnosis and assessment of concussion. In F. Webbe (Ed.), *The Handbook of Sport Neuropsychology* (pp. 91–112). New York, NY: Springer Publishing Company.

Barth J. T, Alves W. M., Ryan, T. V., Macciocchi, S. N., Rimel, R. W., Jane, J. A., & Nelson, W. E. (1989). Mild head injury in sports: Neuropsychological sequelae and recovery of function. In H. Levin, J. Eisenberg, & A. Benton, (Eds.), *Mild head injury* (pp. 257–275). New York, NY: Oxford University Press.

Barth, J. T., Pliskin, N., Axelrod, B., Faust, D., Fisher, J., Harley, J. P., ... Silver, C. (2003). Introduction to the NAN 2001 definition of a clinical neuropsychologist: NAN policy and planning committee. *Archives of Clinical Neuropsychology, 18*(5), 551–555. http://doi.org/10.1016/S0887-6177(02)00146-4

Bédard, M., Felteau, M., Marshall, S., Cullen, N., Gibbons, C., Dubois, S., ... Moustgaard, A. (2013). Mindfulness-based cognitive therapy reduces symptoms of depression in people with a traumatic brain injury: Results from a randomized controlled trial. *Journal of Head Trauma Rehabilitation, 29*(4), E13–E22. doi:10.1097/HTR.0b013e3182a615a0

Belanger, H. G., & Vanderploeg, R. D. (2005). The neuropsychological impact of sports-related concussion: A meta-analysis. *Journal of the International Neuropsychological Society, 11*, 345–357. doi:10.1017/S1355617705050411

Belanger, H. G., Curtiss, G., Demery, J. A., Lebowitz, B. K., & Vanderploeg, R. D. (2005). Factors moderating neuropsychological outcomes following mild traumatic brain injury: A meta-analysis. *Journal of the International Neuropsychological Society, 11*(3), 215–227. http://doi.org/10.1017/S1355617705050277

Belanger, H. G., Spiegel, E., & Vanderploeg, R. D. (2010). Neuropsychological performance following a history of multiple self-reported concussions: A meta-analysis. *Journal of the International Neuropsychological Society, 16*, 262–267. doi:10.1017/S1355617709991287

Belanger, H. G., Vanderploeg, R. D., & McAllister, T. (2016). Subconcussive blows to the head: A formative review of short-term clinical outcomes. *Journal of Head Trauma Rehabilitation, 31*(3), 159–166. doi:10.1097/HTR.0000000000000138

Binder, L., & Rohling, M. (1996). Money matters: A meta-analytic review of the effects of financial incentives on recovery after closed-head injury. *American Journal of Psychiatry, 153*(1), 7–10.

Broglio, S. P., & Puetz, T. W. (2008). The effect of sport concussion on neurocognitive function, self-report symptoms and postural control: A meta-analysis. *Sports Medicine, 38*, 53–67. doi:10.2165/00007256-200838010-00005

Brooks, B. L., Daya, H., Khan, S., Carlson, H. L., Mikrogianakis, A., & Barlow, K. M. (2016a). Cognition in the emergency department as a predictor of recovery after pediatric mild traumatic brain injury. *Journal of the International Neuropsychological Society, 22*, 379–387. doi:10.1017/S1355617715001368

Brooks, B. L., Kadoura, B., Turley, B., Crawford, S., Mikrogianakis, A., & Barlow, K. M. (2014a). Perception of recovery after pediatric mild traumatic brain injury is influenced by the "good old days" bias: Tangible implications for clinical practice and outcomes research. *Archives of Clinical Neuropsychology, 29*, 186–193. doi:10.1093/arclin/act083

Brooks, B. L., Khan, S., Daya, H., Mikrogianakis, A., & Barlow, K. M. (2014b). Neurocognition in the emergency department after a mild traumatic brain injury in youth. *Journal of Neurotrauma, 31*(20), 1744–1749. doi:10.1089/neu.2014.3356

Brooks, B. L., Low, T. A., Daya, H., Khan, S., Mikrogiankis, A., & Barlow, K. M. (2016b). Test or rest? Computerized cognitive testing in the emergency department after pediatric mild traumatic brain injury does not delay symptom recovery. *Journal of Neurotrauma, 33*, 1–6. doi:10.1089/neu.2015.4301

Broshek, D. K., De Marco, A. P., & Freeman, J. R. (2015). A review of post-concussion syndrome and psychological factors associated with concussion. *Brain Injury, 29*(2), 228–237. doi:10.3109/02699052.2014.974674

Chelune, G. J. (2010). Evidence-based research and practice in clinical neuropsychology. *The Clinical Neuropsychologist, 24*(3), 454–467. doi:10.1080/13854040802360574

Chin, E. Y., Nelson, L. D., Barr, W. B., McCrory, P., & McCrea, M. A. (2016). Reliability and validity of the sport concussion assessment tool-3 (SCAT3) in high school and collegiate athletes. *The American Journal of Sports Medicine, 44*(9), 2276–2285. doi:10.1177/0363546516648141

Cicerone, K. D., Langenbahn, D. M., Braden, C., Malec, J. F., Kalmar, K., Fraas, M., ... Ashman, T. (2011). Evidence-based cognitive rehabilitation: Updated review of the literature from 2003 through 2008. *Archives of Physical Medicine and Rehabilitation, 92*(4), 519–530. doi:10.1016/j.apmr.2010.11.015

Clarke, L. A., Genat, R. C., & Anderson, J. F. (2012). Long-term cognitive complaint and post-concussive symptoms following mild traumatic brain injury: The role of cognitive and affective factors. *Brain Injury, 26*(3), 298–307. doi:10.3109/02699052.2012.654588

Conder, R., & Conder, A. A. (2014). Neuropsychological and psychological rehabilitation interventions in refractory sport-related post-concussive syndrome. *Brain Injury, 29*(2), 249–262. doi:10.3109/02699052.2014.965209

Connery, A. K., Peterson, R. L., Baker, D. A., Randolph, C., & Kirkwood, M. W. (2016). The role of neuropsychological evaluation in the clinical management of concussion. *Physical Medicine and Rehabilitation Clinics of North America, 27*(2), 475–486. doi:10.1016/j.pmr.2015.12.001

Covassin, T., Elbin, R. J., Stiller-Ostrowski, J. L., & Kontos, A. P. (2009). Immediate post-concussion assessment and cognitive testing (ImPACT) practices of sports medicine professionals. *Journal of Athletic Training, 44*(6), 639–644. doi:10.4085/1062-6050-44.6.639

Crowe, L., Collie, A., Hearps, S., Dooley, J., Clausen, H., Maddocks, D., ... Anderson, V. (2015). Cognitive and physical symptoms of concussive injury in children: A detailed longitudinal recovery study. *British Journal of Sports Medicine*. Advance online publication. doi:10.1136/bjsports-2015-094663

Davies, S. C., Sandlund, J. M., & Lopez, L. B. (2016). School-based consultation to improve concussion recognition and response. *Journal of Educational & Psychological Consultation, 26*, 49–62. doi:http://dx.doi.org/10.1080/10474412.2014.963225

Davis, G. A., & Purcell, L. K. (2014). The evaluation and management of acute concussion differs in young children. *British Journal of Sports Medicine, 48*(2), 98–101. doi:10.1136/bjsports-2012-092132

Davis, G. A., Castellani, R. J., & McCrory, P. (2015). Neurodegeneration and sport. *Neurosurgery, 76*(6), 643–655. doi:10.1227/NEU.0000000000000722

Davis, G. A., Purcell, L., Schneider, K. J., Yeates, K. O., Gioia, G. A., Anderson, V., ... Kutcher, J. S. (2017). The child sport concussion assessment tool 5th ed. (Child SCAT5). *British Journal of Sports Medicine*, online publication. doi:10.1136/bjsports-2017-097492

De Marco, A. P., & Broshek, D. K. (2014). Computerized cognitive testing in the management of youth sports-related concussion. *Journal of Child Neurology, 31*(1), 68–75. doi:10.1177/0883073814559645

DiFazio, M., Silverberg, N. D., Kirkwood, M. W., Bernier, R., & Iverson, G. L. (2016). Prolonged activity restriction after concussion: Are we worsening outcomes? *Clinical Pediatrics, 55*(5), 443–451. doi:10.1177/0009922815589914

Division 40, American Psychological Association—APA, (2010). Clinical neuropsychology. Retrieved from: www.apa.org/ed/graduate/specialize/neuro.aspx)

Echemendia, R. J. (2006). *Sports neuropsychology: Assessment and management of traumatic brain injury.* New York, NY: Guilford Press.

Echemendia, R. J., Giza, C. C., & Kutcher, J. S. (2015). Developing guidelines for return to play: Consensus and evidence-based approaches. *Brain Injury, 29*(2), 185–194. doi:10.3109/02699052.2014.965212

Echemendia, R. J., Herring, S., & Bailes, J. (2009). Who should conduct and interpret the neuropsychological assessment in sports-related concussion? *British Journal of Sports Medicine, 43*(Suppl 1), i32-i35. doi:10.1136/bjsm.2009.058164

Echemendia, R. J., Iverson, G. L., McCrea, M., Broshek, D. K., Gioia, G. A., Sautter, S. W., ... Barr, W. B. (2012). Role of neuropsychologists in the evaluation and management of sport-related concussion: An inter-organization position statement. *Archives of Clinical Neuropsychology, 27*, 119–122. doi:10.1093/arclin/acr077

Echemendia, R. J., Iverson, G. L., McCrea, M., Macciocchi, S. N., Gioia, G. A., Putukian, M., & Comper, P. (2013). Advances in neuropsychological assessment of sport-related concussion. *British Journal of Sports Medicine, 47*(5), 294–298. doi:10.1136/bjsports-2013-092186

Echemendia, R. J., Meeuwisse, W., McCrory, P., Davis, G. A., Putukian, M., Leddy, J., ... Herring, S. (2017). The sport concussion assessment tool 5th ed. (SCAT5). *British Journal of Sports Medicine*, online publication. doi:10.1136/bjsports-2017-097506

Elbin, R. J., Knox, J., Kegel, N., Schatz, P., Lowder, H. B., French, J., ... Kontos, A. P. (2016a). Assessing symptoms in adolescents following sport-related concussion: A comparison of four different approaches. *Applied Neuropsychology: Child, 5*(4), 294–302. doi:10.1080/21622965.2015.1077334

Elbin, R. J., Kontos, A. P., Kegel, N., Johnson, E., Burkhart, S., & Schatz, P. (2013). Individual and combined effects of LD and ADHD on computerized neurocognitive concussion test performance: Evidence for separate norms. *Archives of Clinical Neuropsychology, 28*(5), 476–484. doi:10.1093/arclin/act024

Elbin, R. J., Schatz, P., Lowder, H. B., & Kontos, A. P. (2014). An empirical review of treatment and rehabilitation approaches used in the acute, sub-acute, and chronic phases of recovery following sports-related concussion. *Current Treatment Options in Neurology, 16*, 320. doi:10.1007/s11940-014-0320-7

Elbin, R. J., Sufrinko, A., Schatz, P., French, J., Henry, L., Burkhart, S., ... Kontos, A. P. (2016b). Removal from play after concussion and recovery time. *Pediatrics, 138*(3), e20160910. doi:10.1542/peds.2016-0910

Eliyahu, L., Kirkland, S., Campbell, S., & Rowe, B. H. (2016). The effectiveness of early educational interventions in the emergency department to reduce incidence or severity of postconcussion syndrome following a concussion: A systematic review. *Academic Emergency Medicine, 23*(5), 531–542. doi:10.1111/acem.12924

Ellis, M. J., Ritchie, L. J., Koltek, M., Hosain, S., Cordingley, D., Chu, S., ... Russell, K. (2015). Psychiatric outcomes after pediatric sports-related concussion. *Journal of Neurosurgery. Pediatrics, 16*, 709–718. doi:10.3171/2015.5.PEDS15220

Emery, C. A., Barlow, K. M., Brooks, B. L., Max, J. E., Villavicencio-Requis, A., Gnanakumar, V., ... Yeates, K. O. (2016). A systematic review of psychiatric, psychological, and behavioural outcomes following mild traumatic brain injury in children and adolescents. *Canadian Journal of Psychiatry, 61*(5), 259–269. doi:10.1177/0706743716643741

Finkbeiner, N. W. B., Max, J. E., Longman, S., & Debert, C. (2016). Knowing what we don't know: Long-term psychiatric outcomes following adult concussion in sports. *Canadian Journal of Psychiatry, 61*(5), 270–276. doi:10.1177/0706743716644953

Gagnon, I., Galli, C., Friedman, D., Grilli, L., & Iverson, G. L. (2009). Active rehabilitation for children who are slow to recover following sport-related concussion. *Brain Injury, 23*(12), 956–964. doi:10.3109/02699050903373477

Gardner, A., Iverson, G. L., & McCrory, P. (2014). Chronic traumatic encephalopathy in sport: A systematic review. *British Journal of Sports Medicine, 48*, 84–90. doi:10.1136/bjsports-2013-092646

Gioia, G. A. (2014). Medical-school partnership in guiding return to school following mild traumatic brain injury in youth. *Journal of Child Neurology, 31*(1), 93–108. doi:10.1177/0883073814555604

Giza, C. C., Kutcher, J. S., Ashwal, S., Barth, J., Getchius, T. S. D., Gioia, G. A., ... Zafonte, R. (2013). Summary of evidence-based guideline update: Evaluation and management of concussion in sports. Report of the guideline development subcommittee of the american academy of neurology. *Neurology, 80*(24), 2250–2257. doi:10.1212/WNL.0b013e31828d57dd

Gorman, M., Hecht, S., Samborski, A., Lunos, S., Elias, S., & Stovitz, S. D. (2016). SCAT3 assessment of non-head injured and head injured athletes competing in a large international youth soccer tournament. *Applied Neuropsychology: Child*. Advance online publication. doi:10.1080/21622965.2016.1210011

Gouvier, W. D., Cubic, B., Jones, G., Brantley, P., & Cutlip, Q. (1992). Postconcussion symptoms and daily stress in normal and head-injured college populations. *Archives of Clinical Neuropsychology, 7*(3), 193–211.

Grubenhoff, J. A, Kirkwood, M., Gao, D., Deakyne, S., & Wathen, J. (2010). Evaluation of the standardized assessment of concussion in a pediatric emergency department. *Pediatrics, 126*(4), 688–695. doi:10.1542/peds.2009-2804

Grubenhoff, J. A., Currie, D., Comstock, R. D., Juarez-Colunga, E., Bajaj, L., & Kirkwood, M. W. (2016). Psychological factors associated with delayed symptom resolution in children with concussion. *Journal of Pediatrics, 174*, 27–32.e1. doi:10.1016/j.jpeds.2016.03.027

Guskiewicz, K. M., Bruce, S. L., Cantu, R. C., Ferrara, M. S., Kelly, J. P., McCrea, M., ... Apuzzo, M. L. J. (2004). Recommendations on management of sport-related concussion: Summary of the national athletic trainers' association position statement. *Neurosurgery, 55*(4), 891–896. doi:10.1227/01.NEU.0000143800.49798.19

Guskiewicz, K., Mccrea, M., Marshall, S. W., Cantu, R. C., Randolph, C., Barr, W., ... Kelly, J. P. (2003). Cumulative effects associated with recurrent concussions in collegiate football players: The NCAA concussion study. *Journal of the American Medical Association, 290*(19), 2549–2555.

Guskiewicz, K. M., Register-Mihalik, J., McCrory, P., McCrea, M., Johnston, K., Makdissi, M., ... Meeuwisse, W. (2013). Evidence-based approach to revising the SCAT2: Introducing the SCAT3. *British Journal of Sports Medicine, 47*, 289–293. http://doi.org/10.1136/bjsports-2013-092225.

Guskiewicz, K., Riemann, B., Perrin, D., & Nashner, L. (1997). Alternative approaches to the assessment of mild head injury in athletes. *Medicine and Science in Sports and Exercise, 29,* S213–S221.

Hall, E. E., Ketcham, C. J., Crenshaw, C. R., Baker, M. H., McConnell, J. M., & Patel, K. (2015). Concussion management in collegiate student-athletes: Return-to-academics recommendations. *Clinical Journal of Sport Medicine, 25*(3), 291–296. doi:10.1097/jsm.0000000000000133

Halstead, M. E., & Walter, K. D. (2010). Sport-related concussion in children and adolescents. *Pediatrics, 126*(3), 597–615. doi:10.1542/peds.2010-2005

Hänninen, T., Parkkari, J., Tuominen, M., Iverson, G. L., Öhman, J., Vartiainen, M., & Luoto, T. M. (2016). Interpreting change on the SCAT3 in professional ice hockey players. *Journal of Science and Medicine in Sport.* doi:10.1016/j.jsams.2016.09.009

Harmon, K. G., Drezner, J. A., Gammons, M., Guskiewicz, K. M., Halstead, M., Herring, S. A., … Roberts, W. O. (2013). American medical society for sports medicine position statement: Concussion in sport. *British Journal of Sports Medicine, 47,* 15–26. doi:10.1136/bjsports-2012-091941

Henry, L. C., Elbin, R. J., Collins, M. W., Marchetti, G., & Kontos, A. P. (2016). Examining recovery trajectories after sport-related concussion with a multimodal clinical assessment approach. *Neurosurgery, 78*(2), 232–240. doi:10.1227/NEU.0000000000001041

Heyer, G. L., Schaffer, C. E., Rose, S. C., Young, J. A., McNally, K. A., & Fischer, A. N. (2016). Specific factors influence postconcussion symptom duration among youth referred to a sports concussion clinic. *Journal of Pediatrics, 174,* 33–38.e2. doi:10.1016/j.jpeds.2016.03.014

Iverson, G. (2007). Predicting slow recovery from sport-related concussion: The new simple-complex distinction. *Clinical Journal of Sport Medicine, 17*(1), 31–37. doi:10.1097/JSM.0b013e3180305e4d

Iverson, G. L. (2010). Mild traumatic brain injury meta-analyses can obscure individual differences. *Brain Injury, 24*(10), 1246–1255. doi:10.3109/02699052.2010.490513

Iverson, G. L. (2012). A biopsychosocial conceptualization of poor outcome from mild traumatic brain injury. In J. J. Vasterling, R. A. Bryant, & T. M. Keane (Eds.), *PTSD and mild traumatic brain injury* (pp. 37–60). New York, NY: The Guilford Press.

Iverson, G. L., & Lange, R. T. (2003). Examination of "postconcussion-like" symptoms in a healthy sample. *Applied Neuropsychology, 10*(3), 137–144. doi: 10.1207/S15324826AN1003_02

Iverson, G. L., & Schatz, P. (2015). Advanced topics in neuropsychological assessment following sport-related concussion. *Brain Injury, 29*(2), 263–275. doi:10.3109/02699052.2014.965214

Iverson, G. L., Brooks, B. L., & Ashton, V. L. (2008). Cognitive impairment consequent to motor vehicle collisions: Foundations for clinical and forensic practice. In M. P. Duckworth, T. Iezzi, & W. T. O'Donohue (Eds.), *Motor vehicle collisions: Medical, psychosocial and legal consequences* (pp. 243–309). Cambridge, UK: Academic Press.

Iverson, G. L., Brooks, B. L., Ashton, V. L., & Lange, R. T. (2010). Interview versus questionnaire symptom reporting in people with the postconcussion syndrome. *The Journal of Head Trauma Rehabilitation, 25*(1), 23–30. doi:10.1097/HTR.0b013e3181b4b6ab

Iverson, G. L., Brooks, B. L., Collins, M. W., & Lovell, M. R. (2006). Tracking neuropsychological recovery following concussion in sport. *Brain Injury, 20*(3), 245–252. doi:10.1080/02699050500487910

Iverson, G. L., Silverberg, N. D., Mannix, R., Maxwell, B. A., Atkins, J. E., Zafonte, R., & Berkner, P. D. (2015). Factors associated with concussion-like symptom reporting in high school athletes. *JAMA Pediatrics, 169*(12), 1132–1140. doi:10.1001/jamapediatrics.2015.2374

Iverson, G.L., & Lange, R. T. (2011). Post-concussion syndrome. In M. R., Schoenberg, & J. G. Scott (Eds.), *The little black book of neuropsychology: A syndrome based approach* (pp. 745–763). New York, NY: Springer.

Jinguji, T. M., Bompadre, V., Harmon, K. G., Satchell, E. K., Gilbert, K., Wild, J., & Eary, J. F. (2012). Sport concussion assessment tool–2: Baseline values for high school athletes. *British Journal of Sports Medicine, 46,* 365–370. doi:10.1136/bjsports-2011-090526

Karr, J. E., Areshenkoff, C. N., & Garcia-Barrera, M. A. (2014a). The neuropsychological outcomes of concussion: A systematic review of meta-analyses on the cognitive sequelae of mild traumatic brain injury. *Neuropsychology, 28*(3), 321–336. doi:10.1037/neu0000037

Karr, J. E., Garcia-Barrera, M. A., & Areshenkoff, C. N. (2014b). Executive functions and intraindividual variability following concussion. *Journal of Clinical and Experimental Neuropsychology, 36*(1), 15–31. doi:10.1080/13803395.2013.863833

Kirkwood, M. W., Grubenhoff, J. A., Peterson, R. L., Connery, A. K., & Baker, D. A. (2014). Injury postconcussive symptom exaggeration after pediatric mild traumatic brain postconcussive symptom exaggeration after pediatric mild traumatic brain injury. *Pediatrics, 133*(4), 643–650. doi:10.1542/peds.2013-3195

Kirkwood, M. W., Peterson, R. L., Baker, D. A., & Connery, A. K. (2016). Parent satisfaction with neuropsychological consultation after pediatric mild traumatic brain injury. *Child Neuropsychology,* Advanced online publication. doi:10.1080/09297049.2015.1130219

Kirkwood, M. W., Peterson, R. L., Connery, A. K., Baker, D. A., & Forster, J. (2015). A pilot study investigating neuropsychological consultation as an intervention for persistent postconcussive symptoms in a pediatric sample. *The Journal of Pediatrics, 169,* 244–249e1. doi:10.1016/j.jpeds.2015.10.014

Kirkwood, M. W., Yeates, K. O., Taylor, H. G., Randolph, C., Mccrea, M., & Anderson, V. A. (2008). Management of pediatric mild traumatic brain injury: A neuropsychological review from injury through recovery brain injury. *The Clinical Neuropsychologist, 22*(5), 769–800. doi:10.1080/13854040701543700

Kontos, A. P., Sufrinko, A., Womble, M., & Kegel, N. (2016). Neuropsychological assessment following concussion: An evidence-based review of the role of neuropsychological assessment pre- and post-concussion. *Current Pain and Headache Reports, 20,* 38. doi:10.1007/s11916-016-0571-y

Laker, S. R., Meron, A., Greher, M. R., & Wilson, J. (2016). Retirement and activity restrictions following concussion. *Physical Medicine and Rehabilitation Clinics of North America, 27*(2), 487–501. doi:10.1016/j.pmr.2016.01.001

Lange, R. T., Iverson, G. L., & Rose, A. (2010). Post-concussion symptom reporting and the "good-old-days" bias following mild traumatic brain injury. *Archives of Clinical Neuropsychology, 25*(5), 442–450. doi:10.1093/arclin/acq031

Leddy, J. J., Baker, J. G., & Willer, B. (2016). Active rehabilitation of concussion and post-concussion syndrome. *Physical Medicine and Rehabilitation Clinics of North America, 27*(2), 437–454. doi:10.1016/j.pmr.2015.12.003

Leddy, J. J., Kozlowski, K., Donnelly, J. P., Pendergast, D. R., Epstein, L. H., & Willer, B. (2010). A preliminary study of subsymptom threshold exercise training for refractory post-concussion syndrome. *Clinical Journal of Sport Medicine, 20,* 21–27. doi:10.1097/JSM.0b013e3181c6c22c

Leddy, J. J., Sandhu, H., Sodhi, V., Baker, J. G., & Willer, B. (2012). Active rehabilitation of concussion and post-concussion syndrome. *Sports Health: A Multidisciplinary Approach, 4*(2), 147–154. doi:10.1177/1941738111433673

Lezak, M. D., Howieson, D. B., Bigler, E. D., & Tranel, D. (2012). *Neuropsychological assessment* (5th ed.). New York, NY: Oxford University Press.

Lingsma, H. F., Yue, J. K., Maas, A. I., Steyerberg, E. W., Manley, G. T., Cooper, S. R., ... Yuh, E. L. (2015). Outcome prediction after mild and complicated mild traumatic brain injury: External validation of existing models and identification of new predictors using the TRACK-TBI pilot study. *Journal of Neurotrauma, 32,* 83–94. doi:10.1089/neu.2014.3384

Losoi, H., Silverberg, N., Wäljas, M., Turunen, S., Rosti-Otajärvi, E., Helminen, M., ... Iverson, G. L. (2016). Recovery from mild traumatic brain injury in previously healthy adults. *Journal of Neurotrauma, 33,* 766–776. doi:10.1089/neu.2015.4070

Lovell, M. R. (2013). *Immediate post-concussion assessment testing (ImPACT) test: clinical interpretive manual online ImPACT 2007–2012.* Pittsburgh, PA: ImPACT Applications Inc.

Lovell, M. R., Iverson, G. L., Collins, M. W., Podell, K., Johnston, K. M., Pardini, D., ... Maroon, J. C. (2006). Measurement of symptoms following sports-related concussion: Reliability and normative data for the post-concussion scale measurement of symptoms following sports-related concussion: Reliability and normative data for the post-concussion scale. *Applied Neuropsychology, 13*(3), 3166–174. doi:10.1207/s15324826an1303

Lovell, M., Barth, J., Collins, M., & Echemendia, R. (2004). *Traumatic brain injury in sports.* Boca Raton, FL: CRC Press.

Maddocks, D., Dicker, G. D., & Saling, M. M. (1995). The assessment of orientation following concussion in athletes. *Clinical Journal of Sport Medicine, 5,* 32–35.

Mannix, R., Iverson, G. L., Maxwell, B., Atkins, J. E., Zafonte, R., & Berkner, P. D. (2014). Multiple prior concussions are associated with symptoms in high school athletes. *Annals of Clinical and Translational Neurology, 1*(6), 433–438. doi:10.1002/acn3.70

Maroon, J. C., Winkelman, R., Bost, J., Amos, A., Mathyssek, C., & Miele, V. (2015). Chronic traumatic encephalopathy in contact sports: A systematic review of all reported pathological cases. *PLoS ONE, 10*(2), 1–16. doi:10.1371/journal.pone.0117338

Master, C. L., Gioia, G. A., Leddy, J. J., & Grady, M. F. (2012). Importance of "Return-to-Learn" in pediatric and adolescent concussion. *Pediatric Annals, 41*(9), e180–e185. doi:10.3928/00904481-20120827-09

McCauley, S. R., Wilde, E. A., Anderson, V. A., Bedell, G., Beers, S. R., Campbell, T. F., ... Yeates, K. O. (2012). Recommendations for the use of common outcome measures in pediatric traumatic brain injury research. *Journal of Neurotrauma, 29*(4), 678–705. doi:10.1089/neu.2011.1838

McClure, D. J., Zuckerman, S. L., Kutscher, S. J., Gregory, A. J., & Solomon, G. S. (2014). Baseline neurocognitive testing in sports-related concussions: The importance of a prior night's sleep. *The American Journal of Sports Medicine, 42*(2), 472–478. doi:10.1177/0363546513510389

McCrea, M. (2001). Standardized mental status testing on the sideline after sport-related concussion. *Journal of Athletic Training, 36*(3), 274–279.

McCrea, M., Barr, W. B., Guskiewicz, K. M., Randolph, C., Marshall, S. W., Cantu, R. C., ... Kelly, J. P. (2005). Standard regression-based methods for measuring recovery after sport-related concussion. *Journal of the International Neuropsychological Society, 11*, 58–69. doi:10.1017/S1355617705050083

McCrea, M., Broshek, D. K., & Barth, J. T. (2015). Sports concussion assessment and management: Future research directions. *Brain Injury, 29*(2), 276–282. doi:10.3109/02699052.2014.965216

McCrea, M., Guskiewicz, K. M., Marshall, S. W., Barr, W., Randolph, C., Cantu, R. C., ... Kelly, J. P. (2003). Acute effects and recovery time following concussion in collegiate football players: The NCCA concussion study. *Journal of the American Medical Association, 290*(19), 2556–2563. doi:10.1001/jama.290.19.2556

McCrea, M., Guskiewicz, K., Randolph, C., Barr, W. B., Hammeke, T. A, Marshall, S. W., ... Kelly, J. P. (2013a). Incidence, clinical course, and predictors of prolonged recovery time following sport-related concussion in high school and college athletes. *Journal of the International Neuropsychological Society, 19*(1), 22–33. doi:10.1017/S1355617712000872

McCrea, M., Iverson, G. L., Echemendia, R. J., Makdissi, M., & Raftery, M. (2013b). Day of injury assessment of sport-related concussion. *British Journal of Sports Medicine, 47*, 272–284. doi:10.1136/bjsports-2013-092145

McCrea, M., Iverson, G. L., McAllister, T. W., Hammeke, T. A., Powell, M. R., Barr, W. B., & Kelly, J. P. (2009). An integrated review of recovery after mild traumatic brain injury (MTBI): Implications for clinical management. *The Clinical Neuropsychologist, 23*(8), 1368–1390. doi:10.1080/13854040903074652

McCrory, P., Meeuwisse, W. H., Kutcher, J. S., Jordan, B. D., & Gardner, A. (2013). What is the evidence for chronic concussion-related changes in retired athletes: Behavioural, pathological and clinical outcomes? *British Journal of Sports Medicine, 47*(5), 327–330. doi:10.1136/bjsports-2013-092248

McCrory, P., Meeuwisse, W., Dvorak, J., Aubry, M., Bailes, J., Broglio, S., ... Vos, P. E. (2017). Consensus statement on concussion in sport—The 5th international conference on concussion in sport held in Berlin, October 2016. *British Journal of Sports Medicine*, online publication. doi:10.1136/bjsports-2017-097699

McGrath, N. (2010). Supporting the student-athlete's return to the classroom after a sport-related concussion. *Journal of Athletic Training, 45*(5), 492–498. doi:10.4085/1062-6050-45.5.492

McKay, C. D., Brooks, B. L., Mrazik, M., Jubinville, A. L., & Emery, C. A. (2014). Psychometric properties and reference values for the impact neurocognitive test battery in a sample of elite youth ice hockey players. *Archives of Clinical Neuropsychology, 29*(2), 141–151. doi:10.1093/arclin/act116

McKee, A. C., Stein, T. D., Nowinski, C. J., Stern, R. A., Daneshvar, D. H., Alvarez, V. E., ... Cantu, R. C. (2013). The spectrum of disease in chronic traumatic encephalopathy. *Brain, 136*(1), 43–64. doi:10.1093/brain/aws307

Meehan, W. P., D'Hemecourt, P., Collins, C. L., & Comstock, R. D. (2011). Assessment and management of sport-related concussions in United States high schools. *American Journal of Sports Medicine, 39*(11), 2304–2310. doi:10.1177/0363546511423503

Meehan, W. P., Mannix, R., Monuteaux, M. C., Stein, C. J., & Bachur, R. G. (2014). Early symptom burden predicts recovery after sport-related concussion. *Neurology, 83,* 2204–2210. doi:10.1212/WNL.0000000000001700

Merritt, V. C., & Arnett, P. A. (2014). Premorbid predictors of postconcussion symptoms in collegiate athletes. *Journal of Clinical and Experimental Neuropsychology, 36*(10), 1098–1111. doi:10.1080/13803395.2014.983463

Merritt, V. C., Rabinowitz, A. R., & Arnett, P. A. (2015). Injury-related predictors of symptom severity following sports-related concussion. *Journal of Clinical and Experimental Neuropsychology, 37*(3), 265–275. doi:10.1080/13803395.2015.1004303

Mittenberg, W., Canyock, E. M., Condit, D., & Patton, C. (2001). Treatment of post-concussion syndrome following mild head injury. *Journal of Clinical and Experimental Neuropsychology, 23*(6), 829–836. doi:10.1076/jcen.23.6.829.1022

Mittenberg, W., Patton, C., Canyok, E. M., & Condit, D. C. (2002). Base rates of malingering and symptom exaggeration. *Journal of Clinical and Experimental Neuropsychology, 24*(8), 1094–1102.

Montenigro, P. H., Corp, D. T., Stein, T. D., Cantu, R. C., & Stern, R. A. (2015). Chronic traumatic encephalopathy: Historical origins and current perspective. *Annual Review of Clinical Psychology, 11,* 309–330. doi:10.1146/annurev-clinpsy-032814-112814

Morgan, C. D., Zuckerman, S. L., Lee, Y. M., King, L., Beaird, S., Sills, A. K., & Solomon, G. S. (2015). Predictors of postconcussion syndrome after sports-related concussion in young athletes: A matched case-control study. *Journal of Neurosurgery. Pediatrics, 15*(6), 589–598. doi:10.3171/2014.10.PEDS14356.Disclosure

Moser, R. S., Schatz, P., & Lichtenstein, J. D. (2015). The importance of proper administration and interpretation of neuropsychological baseline and postconcussion computerized testing. *Applied Neuropsychology: Child, 4*(1), 41–48. doi:10.1080/21622965.2013.791825

Nelson, L. D., LaRoche, A. A., Pfaller, A. Y., Lerner, E. B., Hammeke, T. A., Randolph, C., … McCrea, M. A. (2016a). Prospective, head-to-head study of three computerized neurocognitive assessment tools (CNTs): Reliability and validity for the assessment of sport-related concussion. *Journal of the International Neuropsychological Society, 22*(1), 24–37. doi:10.1017/S1355617715001101

Nelson, L. D., Tarima, S., Laroche, A. A., Hammeke, T. A., Barr, W. B., Guskiewicz, K., … McCrea, M. A. (2016b). Preinjury somatization symptoms contribute to clinical recovery after sport-related concussion. *Neurology, 86,* 1856–1863. doi:10.1212/WNL.0000000000002679

Novak, Z., Aglipay, M., Barrowman, N., Yeates, K. O., Beauchamp, M. H., Gravel, J., … Zemek, R. L. (2016). Association of persistent postconcussion symptoms with pediatric quality of life. *JAMA Pediatrics,* E1–E8. doi:10.1001/jamapediatrics.2016.2900

Okonkwo, D. O., Tempel, Z. J., & Maroon, J. (2014). Sideline assessment tools for the evaluation of concussion in athletes: A review. *Neurosurgery, 75*(4), S82–S95. doi:10.1227/NEU.0000000000000493

Ouellet, M. C., & Morin, C. M. (2007). Efficacy of cognitive-behavioral therapy for insomnia associated with traumatic brain injury: A single-case experimental design. *Archives of Physical Medicine and Rehabilitation, 88*(12), 1581–1592. doi:10.1016/j.apmr.2007.09.006

Peterson, R. L., Connery, A. K., Baker, D. A., & Kirkwood, M. W. (2015). Preinjury emotional-behavioral functioning of children with lingering problems after mild traumatic brain injury. *The Journal of Neuropsychiatry and Clinical Neurosciences, 27,* 280–286. doi:10.1176/appi.neuropsych.14120373

Peterson, S. E., Stull, M. J., Collins, M. W., & Wang, H. E. (2009). Neurocognitive function of emergency department patients with mild traumatic brain injury. *Annals of Emergency Medicine, 53*(6), 796–803.e1. doi:10.1016/j.annemergmed.2008.10.015

Ponsford, J., Cameron, P., Fitzgerald, M., Grant, M., Mikocka-Walus, A., & Schönberger, M. (2012). Predictors of postconcussive symptoms 3 months after mild traumatic brain injury. *Neuropsychology, 26*(3), 304–313. doi:10.1037/a0027888

Ponsford, J., Lee, N. K., Wong, D., McKay, A., Haines, K., Alway, Y., … O'Donnell, M. L. (2016). Efficacy of motivational interviewing and cognitive behavioral therapy for anxiety and depression symptoms following traumatic brain injury. *Psychological Medicine, 46,* 1079–1090. doi:10.1017/S0033291715002640

Ponsford, J., Willmot, C., Rothwell, A., Cameron, P., Ayton, G., Nelms, R., … Ng, K. (2001). Impact of early intervention on outcome after mild traumatic brain injury in children. *Pediatrics, 108*(6), 1297–1303.

Ponsford, J., Willmott, C., Rothwell, A., Cameron, P., Kelly, A.-M., Nelms, R., & Curran, C. (2002). Impact of early intervention on outcome following mild head injury in adults. *Journal of Neurology, Neurosurgery, and Psychiatry, 73*(3), 330–332. doi:10.1136/jnnp.73.3.330

Popoli, D. M., Burns, T. G., Meehan, W. P., & Reisner, A. (2014). CHOA concussion consensus: Establishing a uniform policy for academic accommodations. *Clinical Pediatrics, 53*(3), 217–224. doi:10.1177/0009922813499070

Potter, S. D. S., Brown, R. G., & Fleminger, S. (2016). Randomised, waiting list controlled trial of cognitive–behavioural therapy for persistent postconcussional symptoms after predominantly mild–moderate traumatic brain injury. *Journal of Neurology, Neurosurgery & Psychiatry, 87*, 1075–1083. doi:10.1136/jnnp-2015-312838

Potter, S., & Brown, R. G. (2012). Cognitive behavioural therapy and persistent post-concussional symptoms: Integrating conceptual issues and practical aspects in treatment. *Neuropsychological Rehabilitation, 22*(1), 1–25. doi:10.1080/09602011.2011.630883

Putukian, M., Echemendia, R., Dettwiler-Danspeckgruber, A., Duliba, T., Bruce, J., Furtado, J. L., & Murugavel, M. (2015). Prospective clinical assessment using sideline concussion assessment tool-2 testing in the evaluation of sport-related concussion in college athletes. *Clinical Journal of Sport Medicine, 25*(1), 36–42. doi:10.1097/JSM.0000000000000102

Rabinowitz, A. R., Li, X., & Levin, H. S. (2014). Sport and nonsport etiologies of mild traumatic brain injury: Similarities and differences. *Annual Review of Psychology, 65*, 301–331. doi:10.1146/annurev-psych-010213-115103

Rahman-Filipiak, A. A. M., & Woodard, J. L. (2013). Administration and environment considerations in computer-based sports-concussion assessment. *Neuropsychology Review, 23*(4), 314–334. doi:10.1007/s11065-013-9241-6

Randolph, C. (2014). Is chronic traumatic encephalopathy a real disease? *Current Sports Medicine Reports, 13*(1), 33–37. doi:10.1249/JSR.0000000000000022

Resch, J. E., McCrea, M. A., & Cullum, C. M. (2013). Computerized neurocognitive testing in the management of sport-related concussion: An update. *Neuropsychology Review, 23*(4), 335–349. doi:10.1007/s11065-013-9242-5

Riggio, S., & Jagoda, A. (2016). Concussion and its neurobehavioural sequelae. *International Review of Psychiatry*, Advanced online publication. doi:10.1080/09540261.2016.1220927

Root, J. M., Zuckerbraun, N. S., Wang, L., Winger, D. G., Brent, D., Kontos, A., & Hickey, R. W. (2016). History of somatization is associated with prolonged recovery from concussion. *Journal of Pediatrics, 174*, 39–44.e1. doi:10.1016/j.jpeds.2016.03.020

Rose, S. C., Mcnally, A., & Heyer, L. (2015a). Returning the student to school after concussion: What do clinicians need to know? *Concussion, 1*, 37–47. doi:10.2217/cnc.15.4

Rose, S. C., Weber, K. D., Collen, J. B., & Heyer, G. L. (2015b). The diagnosis and management of concussion in children and adolescents. *Pediatric Neurology, 53*, 108–118. doi:10.1016/j.pediatrneurol.2015.04.003

Ruff, R. M. (2011). Mild traumatic brain injury and neural recovery: Rethinking the debate. *NeuroRehabilitation, 28*(3), 167–180. doi:10.3233/NRE-2011-0646

Sady, M. D., Vaughan, C. G., & Gioia, G. A. (2014). Psychometric characteristics of the postconcussion symptom inventory in children and adolescents. *Archives of Clinical Neuropsychology, 29*(4), 348–363. doi:10.1093/arclin/acu014

Schatz, P., & Sandel, N. (2013). Sensitivity and specificity of the online version of ImPACT in high school and collegiate athletes. *American Journal of Sports Medicine, 41*(2), 321–326. doi:10.1177/0363546512466038

Schatz, P., Neidzwski, K., Moser, R. S., & Karpf, R. (2010). Relationship between subjective test feedback provided by high-school athletes during computer-based assessment of baseline cognitive functioning and self-reported symptoms. *Archives of Clinical Neuropsychology, 25*(4), 285–292. doi:10.1093/arclin/acq022

Scheenen, M. E., Spikman, J. M., de Koning, M. E., van der Horn, H. J., Roks, G., Hageman, G., & van der Naalt, J. (2016). Patients "at risk" of suffering from persistent complaints after mild traumatic brain injury: The role of coping, mood disorders, and post-traumatic stress. *Journal of Neurotrauma, 33*, 1–7. doi:10.1089/neu.2015.4381

Schneider, K. J., Iverson, G. L., Emery, C. A., Mccrory, P., Herring, S. A., & Meeuwisse, W. H. (2013). The effects of rest and treatment following sport-related concussion: A systematic review of the literature. *British Journal of Sports Medicine, 47*, 304–307. doi:10.1136/bjsports-2013-092190

Schoenberg, M. R., & Scott, J. G. (2011). The neuropsychology referral and answering the referral question. In M. R. Schoenberg & J.G. Scott (Eds.), *The little black book of neuropsychology: A syndrome based approach* (pp. 1–37). New York, NY: Springer.

Sherman, E. M. S., Brooks, B. L., Iverson, G. L., Slick, D. J., & Strauss, E. (2011). Reliability and validity in neuropsychology. In M. R. Schoenberg & J. G. Scott (Eds.), *The little black book of neuropsychology: A syndrome based approach* (pp. 873–892). New York, NY: Springer.

Silverberg, N. D., Berkner, P. D., Atkins, J. E., Zafonte, R., & Iverson, G. L. (2016). Relationship between short sleep duration and preseason concussion testing. *Clinical Journal of Sport Medicine, 26*(3), 226–231. doi: 10.1097/JSM.0000000000000241.

Silverberg, N. D., Gardner, A. J., Brubacher, J. R., Panenka, W. J., Li, J. J., & Iverson, G. L. (2015). Systematic review of multivariable prognostic models for mild traumatic brain injury. *Journal of Neurotrauma, 32*(8), 517–526. doi:10.1089/neu.2014.3600

Silverberg, N., Hallam, B., Rose, A., Underwood, H., Whitfield, K., Thornton, A., & Whittal, M. (2013). Cognitive-behavioral prevention of postconcussion syndrome in at-risk patients: A pilot randomized controlled trial. *Journal of Head Trauma Rehabilitation, 28*(4), 313–322. doi:10.1097/HTR.0b013e3182915cb5

Solomon, G. S., & Zuckerman, S. L. (2015). Chronic traumatic encephalopathy in professional sports: Retrospective and prospective views. *Brain Injury, 29*(2), 164–170. doi:10.3109/02699052.2014.965205

Solomon, G. S., Kuhn, A. W., & Zuckerman, S. L. (2016). Depression as a modifying factor in sport-related concussion: A critical review of the literature. *The Physician and Sportsmedicine, 44*(1), 14–19. doi:10.1080/00913847.2016.1121091

Sports Neuropsychology Society. (2015). *Sports neuropsychology: Definition, qualifications, and training guidelines—An official position of the sports neuropsychology society.* Retrieved from http://sports-neuropsychologysociety.com/forms/SNS-Definition-Sports-Neuropsychologist.pdf

Taubman, B., Rosen, F., McHugh, J., Grady, M. F., & Elci, O. U. (2016). The timing of cognitive and physical rest and recovery in concussion. *Journal of Child Neurology, 31*(14), 1555–1560. doi:10.1177/0883073816664835

Thomas, D. G., Apps, J. N., Hoffmann, R. G., McCrea, M., & Hammeke, T. (2015). Benefits of strict rest after acute concussion: A randomized controlled trial. *Pediatrics, 135*(2), 213–223. doi:10.1542/peds.2014-0966.

Wade, D. T., King, N. S., Wenden, F. J., Crawford, S., & Caldwell, F. E. (1998). Routine follow up after head injury: A second randomised controlled trial. *Journal of Neurology, Neurosurgery, and Psychiatry, 65*(2), 177–183. doi:10.1136/jnnp.65.2.177

Webbe, F. (2010). *The handbook of sport neuropsychology.* New York, NY: Springer Publishing Company.

Webbe, F. M., & Zimmer, A. (2015). History of neuropsychological study of sport-related concussion. *Brain Injury, 29*(2), 129–138. doi:10.3109/02699052.2014.937746

West, T. A., & Marion, D. W. (2014). Current recommendations for the diagnosis and treatment of concussion in sport: A comparison of three new guidelines. *Journal of Neurotrauma, 31*(2), 159–168. doi:10.1089/neu.2013.3031

Wilde, E. A., Whiteneck, G. G., Bogner, J., Bushnik, T., Cifu, D. X., Dikmen, S., … Von Steinbuechel, N. (2010). Recommendations for the use of common outcome measures in traumatic brain injury research. *Archives of Physical Medicine and Rehabilitation, 91*(11), 1650–1660.e17. doi:10.1016/j.apmr.2010.06.033

Williams, R. M., Puetz, T. W., Giza, C. C., & Broglio, S. P. (2015). Concussion recovery time among high school and collegiate athletes: A systematic review and meta-analysis. *Sports Medicine, 45*, 893–903. doi:10.1007/s40279-015-0325-8

Yeates, K. O., Taylor, H. G., Rusin, J., Bangert, B., Dietrich, A., Nuss, K., & Wright, M. (2012). Premorbid child and family functioning as predictors of post-concussive symptoms in children with mild traumatic brain injuries. *International Journal of Developmental Neuroscience, 30*(3), 231–237. doi:10.1016/j.ijdevneu.2011.05.008

Yengo-Kahn, A. M., Hale, A. T., Zalneraitis, B. H., Zuckerman, S. L., Sills, A. K., & Solomon, G. S. (2016). The sport concussion assessment tool: A systematic review. *Neurological Focus, 40*(4), E6. doi:10.3171/2016.1.FOCUS15611.

Zemek, R. L., Farion, K. J., Sampson, M., & McGahern, C. (2013). Prognosticators of persistent symptoms following pediatric concussion: A systematic review. *JAMA Pediatrics, 167*(3), 259–265. doi:10.1001/2013.jamapediatrics.216

Zuckerman, S. L., Lee, Y. M., Odom, M. J., Solomon, G. S., & Sills, A. K. (2013). Baseline neurocognitive scores in athletes with attention deficit–spectrum disorders and/or learning disability: Clinical article. *Journal of Neurosurgery: Pediatrics, 12*(2), 103–109. doi: 10.3171/2013.5.PEDS12524

Zuckerman, S. L., Lee, Y. M., Odom, M. J., Solomon, G. S., Forbes, J. A., & Sills, A. K. (2012). Recovery from sports-related concussion: Days to return to neurocognitive baseline in adolescents versus young adults. *Surgical Neurology International, 3*, 130. doi:10.4103/2152-7806.102945

*chapter ten*

---

# The role of the occupational therapist in concussion management

## What can the occupational therapist do?

*Carol DeMatteo, Nick Reed, and Kathy Stazyk*

## Contents

It's all about activity!

## Introduction

This chapter presents a commentary on the inclusion of occupational therapy (OT) services during the management of concussion which includes sport concussion but also concussion from other causes. The profession of occupational therapy is not largely recognized or utilized within the world of sport concussion or when rehabilitating athletes following a concussion; yet the inclusion of OT in the rehabilitation of children youth and adults with acquired brain injury is paramount and not questioned. The importance of an interdisciplinary approach to sport-related concussion management has already been promoted internationally as the best practice (McCrory et al. 2005, 2009), but OT is often not a part of that team.

This chapter aims to address the need for improved management of concussion by considering the person, environment, and occupation during the delivery of an occupational therapy-based approach to rehabilitation. It is first important to understand the theory and approach of occupational therapy, which offers distinct and unique approaches to manage youth concussions. Occupational therapy in essence is the promotion of participation in productive and meaningful activities of daily life.

Occupational therapists are university-trained, regulated health professionals whose unique training enables them to understand not only the medical and physical limitations of a disability or injury but also the psychosocial factors that affect an individual's ability to function independently. Their approach is based on research that proves that an individual's ability to engage in occupation increases health and well-being (Law 2002; Law et al. 1998).

- Occupation gives meaning to life
- Occupation is an important determinant of health, well-being, and justice
- Occupation organizes behavior
- Occupation develops and changes over a lifetime
- Occupation shapes and is shaped by environments

Supporting individuals to engage in occupations differently than they have experienced previously can evoke new thoughts, feelings, and actions, and can result in positive changes in their lives (Kielhofner 2009). OT can, on a very practical level, help to solve the problems that interfere with one's ability to do the things that are important to them and that they need, want, and love to do. It can also help to prevent problems or minimize their effects; all very important realities after concussion.

Common practice in the management of concussive injury is the return to activity, school and sport, which speaks to the importance of getting individuals back to participating in all aspects of their lives, and this is congruent with OT's priority on participation. OTs can play a vital role in the successful attainment of these goals.

The combinations of symptoms associated with sport-related concussion can have a significant impact on occupational performance and participation, both on and off the playing field.

All types of concussive injuries, as well as a prolonged recovery from concussion or repeated concussions, can lead to long-term outcomes that include: (1) changes in neurocognitive functioning including processing speed, memory, and concentration (Lau et al. 2012), psychiatric illness such as mood disorders (Stazyk et al. 2017), post-traumatic stress disorder, anxiety, and obsessive compulsive disorder (Bryant et al. 2010); (2) behavioral changes that can include difficulties with attention, initiation, impulse control, and organizational skills (McKinlay et al. 2002; Daneshvar et al. 2011); and (3) post-concussive syndrome or protracted symptoms of at least 3 months (Daneshvar et al. 2011). These outcomes often result in functional difficulties that include decreased participation, school performance difficulties, and decreased quality of life (Parsons et al. 2013; DeMatteo et al. 2014). Although there are studies in the literature that highlight functional changes such as disruption to school performance and performance of instrumental activities of daily living, little attention has been paid to the evolution of participation over time. One study looking at the effects of concussion on leisure activities a year after injury has shown a

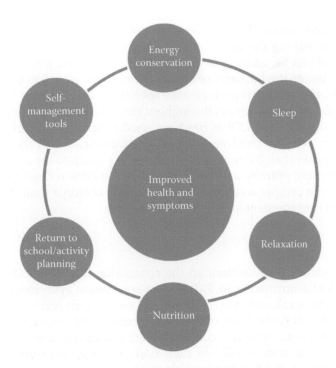

*Figure 10.1*   The OT approach to the individual with concussive injury.

statistically significant reduction in instrumental daily activities as well as social, physical, and cultural activities (Jonsson and Andersson 2012).

Occupational therapists can assume a variety of roles specific to the safe return of athletes to their meaningful daily occupations and full participation in their daily lives after concussive injury (Reed 2011). This chapter will outline sport-related concussion from an occupational perspective and aims to expand the scope of occupational therapy practice into the world of sport and concussion management, specifically how OT approaches the recovery and can enable return to full participation after concussive injury. Figure 10.1 illustrates the main areas incorporated into the OT approach to concussive injury.

## Evaluation

### Development of client-centered rehabilitation goals

A core competency across rehabilitation professions, including occupational therapy, is practicing in a client-centered manner. Client-centered practice emphasizes equality, sharing, and partnership between the therapist and the client (Fearing and Clark 2000). Using a client-centered approach, rehabilitation goals specific to the performance of functional activities that are meaningful and important (e.g., return to sport, return to school, and activities of daily living) can be identified collaboratively among the therapist, the client/patient, and their family. It has been reported that increased attention to client priorities during goal setting and treatment can lead to improved client motivation, satisfaction, and rehabilitation outcomes (Law et al. 1995; Law et al. 2005; Sumsion and Smyth 2000).

One measure that can be used to identify occupational performance issues following sport-related concussion in a client-centered manner is the Canadian Occupational Performance Measure (COPM) (Law et al. 2005). This measure allows the therapist and the client to collaboratively identify occupational performance issues (OPI—e.g., the activities in their life they are having the most difficulty doing) in the areas of self-care, productivity, and leisure that can be addressed within the rehabilitation process. In addition, the COPM allows one to rate the importance of the OPI for them as well as their related performance, and satisfaction with this performance specific to the identified OPIs. The rating is done prior to rehabilitation and again throughout the rehabilitation process as an outcome measure (Law et al. 1990). The COPM has been used effectively with clients over the age of 8 years; however, younger children often require modification of the interviewing and rating process (Poulsen et al. 2015). A client-centered approach to rehabilitation is inherent to occupational therapy practice and combined with the Person environment occupation (PEO) theory makes a unique and valuable contribution within a multidisciplinary sport-related concussion management and rehabilitation team.

## Symptoms

The OT shares with other professions in the concussion field the ability to do a physical and neurological examination including post-concussion symptoms (physical, cognitive, emotional/behavioral, and sleep symptoms); however, the focus or application of the information gained is different from other health professionals. Symptoms are viewed not simply as symptoms (e.g., difficulty concentrating), but rather how a symptom impacts one's ability to perform functionally in their daily life (e.g., impaired ability to absorb material at school and attend to a full lesson).

Symptoms are carefully explored with respect to how they are affecting daily routine, type of activity and level, school work, leisure, and mood. This includes the following:

- Evaluation of preferred activities
- Explore alternative activities
- Set the scene for balancing what can be done within symptomology

## Sensory challenges

OTs traditionally pay close attention in their evaluation to sensory performance and challenges. Adaptation of the environment can then be implemented to compensate for sensory disturbances and help improve functioning in specific settings. Sensory problems are frequently described after concussion. Visual and auditory hypersensitivity are common and debilitating for the youth wanting to return to school. The OT can determine the threshold of tolerance of various stimuli and help the youth, family, and school make the necessary adaptations. These changes may mean that the student wears sunglasses in school, earphones or avoids noisy classes for the present, such as music or even conversational language classes. Individualized recommendations are made based on the intensity of stimuli, type of stimuli, and environmental considerations of stimuli. Adaptations will be different for each individual depending on careful evaluation, collaboration, and consideration of the client/patient's abilities, goals, and preferences.

## Exertion challenge

As part of a good evaluation, an OT must know their client's tolerance for activity to help them and those involved in their life (family, friends, coach, teacher, and employer) know where to begin, how much is tolerated, and how much is too much. As recent international sport concussion management recommendations suggest a short period of rest (24–48 hours) followed by gradual resumption of activity that does not cause or exacerbate post-concussion symptoms (McCrory et al. 2017), this part of the evaluation is critical in understanding and educating others about the types of activities, the intensity and duration tolerated without exacerbating symptoms. Exertion challenges are becoming part of the standard practice post-concussive injury and should be part of the OTs assessment. There are a number of exertion protocols that have been shown to be helpful (Leddy et al. 2010; DeMatteo et al. 2015a).

## Cognitive function

Traditionally, in the field of brain injury rehabilitation, OTs are responsible for screening cognitive difficulties such as attention and concentration that are affecting functional activities such as schoolwork and daily routines. The neuropsychologist is responsible for the full neurocognitive intensive examination, but often the OT will be the one to help the injured individual implement the cognitive rehabilitation strategies in daily routines.

Many patients recovering from concussion do not have access to a full neuropsychological assessment, nor is it usually necessary unless the individual is experiencing sequelae from multiple concussions or prolonged cognitive symptoms post-concussive injury and academic failure.

However, having some indication of cognitive function is important. Today, many youth athletes have baseline testing as part of the requirement of their sport. The results of this baseline test can be most valuable to the OT evaluating the patient post-concussion. Even more valuable is to observe the patient as he or she completes a cognitive task which can provide very helpful observations of concentration, attention, and any exacerbation of symptoms resulting from functional activity that is meaningful to the client, such as reading, thinking, or screen stimuli. All observations during administration provide invaluable information for planning, particularly for return to school strategies.

## Mood, risk for depression/anxiety

Post-concussion symptoms related to mood and mental health are prevalent. As part of an interdisciplinary approach to care, it is paramount that the evaluation of mood-related deficits (depression and anxiety) be part of the concussion management process (Stazyk et al. 2017). In situations where a full interdisciplinary team is available to the client, it is likely that the team's physician or neuropsychologist will carry out an assessment for mood and mental health-related deficits. OTs can support the development and implementation of rehabilitation strategies with clients to help manage these symptoms (identifying triggers for negative thoughts and feelings and developing related coping strategies, and adapting environments to be more conducive to positive thoughts and feelings). In situations where OT is the sole provider, they are likely to engage in both the assessment and management of mood-related symptoms. The OT can explore mood in a number of ways although an increasing focus and reliance on evidence-based systematic evaluation has been strongly recommended and should include standardized measures (D'Angelo and Augenstein 2012). In children and youth, standardized self-report measures such as the child depression index (CDI; Kovacs 2012) or the screen for child anxiety-related disorders (SCARED; Birmaher et al. 1999) which are self-report measures designed with both parent and child versions for both children and adolescents up to

18 years, and are among some of the measures available to assess depression and anxiety for all ages. The clinical dilemma of overlapping symptoms between concussion and depression (sleep disturbances, emotional, and cognitive symptoms) is an ongoing issue. Using these standardized assessments may help determine whether the symptoms go beyond those caused by the head injury by examining responses to specific items where the overlap occurs. In addition, interviewing is a vital part of the systematic evaluation. Concerns noted through talking with the client can be confirmed with results from the standardized measures. Alternately, the completed questionnaires can be used to begin the dialog about how the individual is feeling and what can be done to give them hope that things will change so that they will be able to participate in activities they love to do once again.

The early detection of depression after concussive injury is vital to provide timely intervention and prevent the accompanying negative outcomes, recurrence, chronicity, and comorbid mental disorders (Frühe et al. 2012). Targeted screening in high-risk patients has been a highly recommended approach to identify patients with depression (Sharp and Lipsky 2002) but has rarely been implemented with those who have had a concussion. Concussion increases the risk for elevated depressive symptoms. If other known indicators which increase the risk of depression, such as a first-degree relative with history of depression, chronic pain, impoverished home environment, major life changes, fatigue, or sleep disturbance, are flagged during initial evaluation, then the post-concussion population at higher risk for depression could be identified (Macmillan et al. 2005).

The OT can assist in the rehabilitation and management of mood, including depression and anxiety, by supporting the client to develop coping strategies that can include identifying and engaging in alternative activities that promote positive thoughts and feelings, adapting the client's environment to be more conducive to promoting positive thoughts and feelings and helping the client recognize and respond to triggers for negative feelings before these feelings become exacerbated. Parental and family coping styles also have an impact on family dynamics and positive outcomes following concussion. These can also be evaluated and managed with support from an OT using a family-centered philosophy. For example, if this is an individual who is a high risk taker with low-impulse control and has only one interest such as hockey and he/she may see no hope and be resistant to following a graduated and cautious approach to recovery, the challenge will be greater for the family and the OT in finding alternative strategies that are appealing to the youth, to maintain participation, hope for recovery, and positive emotions.

## Special considerations: Child and adolescent development

Child and adolescent development is always considered with the OT evaluation, putting all performance problems in the context of age appropriate expectation and preinjury performance. This may include close examination of preinjury school records, any existing developmental or learning problems, or sensory motor problems. Preference is given to the use of standardized measures with developmental population norms for assessing balance, strength, endurance, agility, and coordination. Reaction time, visual motor skills, and fine motor skills are all best evaluated with a norm-referenced tool. Some of the more common measures used by OTs to evaluate these areas are The Movement ABC (Henderson and Sugden 1992) and the Bruininks Ozseretsky test of motor proficiency (Bruininks and Bruininks 2005). Even if there is no premorbid baseline data, this type of measure can illustrate where the youth is functioning compared with expectations for age and determine if this result is seemingly different from reported premorbid function of a high-level athlete and academic high achiever. Tests can then be repeated to show change over time and demonstrate recovery both for the youth and family but also the OT and clinical team.

## Intervention

### Education and support of the client and those involved in their lives (family and school)

The treatment of concussion should not occur in isolation from families. Parental and/or loved-one's uncertainty and distress affect the family after an injury such as concussion and particularly when symptoms do not abate. Specific to youth, parents can be overly cautious and protective or, conversely, question the need for concussion management strategies. Research has shown that after concussion, the number one need for adolescents and their parents is "clear information about the consequences of the injury and the course of recovery" (Swaine et al. 2008). Educational intervention directly after concussion has been shown to affect outcomes (Snell et al. 2009). Families often need ongoing support as they experience uncertainty and doubt in managing symptoms as well as navigating school and health-care systems. Parents of children with concussion experience psychological distress and are at increased risk for anxiety and depression themselves (Ganesalingam et al. 2008; Wade et al. 2006).

OTs can play a significant role in support and education of individuals who sustain a concussion, as well as their families. This role evolves from the client-centered goal setting established at the first meeting. This sets the stage for a proactive intensive relationship that allows in depth exploration of their daily lives. As OTs help their clients to discover alternative ways of doing things or alternative activities, they also give reassurance that recovery will occur. Communicating this reassurance provides hope and validation to those impacted by concussion along with the message that this injury needs to be taken seriously. The OT's unique perspective and focus on the importance of participation and activity and the contribution of these to health and well-being give the concussed individual an understanding that managing their symptoms is about getting them back to activity safely NOT keeping them out of activity. Individuals who sustain a concussion, and people close to them, can feel anxious about not participating in daily activities and related consequences (e.g., completion of school work and impact on grades). They may also struggle with isolation, boredom, and inactivity because of the perceived restrictiveness of common return to activity guidelines or recommendations made by their health professional team. The OT can solve the problem with the client and those involved in their lives on how to best interpret and implement these guidelines and advice, respectively. Using a youth returning to the classroom after a concussion as an example, the OT can work with the youth, family, and teachers to determine what activities are permissible at which stages of concussion management guidelines to promote optimal participation and well-being. The process of occupational therapy is based on task analyses, which provides the foundation for activity planning. Knowing what the physical, mental, and environmental demands of an activity are and balancing this information with the goals, abilities, and symptom level of the youth is a complex process that many families cannot undertake themselves without support.

OTs with their unique understanding of the role of occupation and meaningful activity to a person's life are aware of the emotional impact of implementing activity restrictions when introducing concussion management protocols to concussed youth. Discussion with clients and their families about finding ways to remain socially connected and maintain a sense of self through valued activities may help prevent some of the losses experienced by the concussed individuals who go through prolonged recoveries. This will also help to sooth some of the conflict within families as parents try to impose activity restrictions on their child with the injury.

## Return to activity planning

The decision regarding when and how to return to activity following concussion is one of the most difficult and controversial areas in concussion management. There is a growing body of evidence that demonstrates that, with education, comprehensive assessment, and rehabilitation, symptom resolution will occur sooner (for some) and secondary problems like depression and school failure may be prevented (Maugans et al. 2012; Hung et al. 2014).

Although post-concussion symptoms are thought to resolve quicker in adults (10%–20% of concussed adults continue to have symptoms after 10 days [McCrory et al. 2013]) than in children and youth (30% of concussed children and youth continue to have symptoms after 30 days [Zemek et al. 2016]), there remains a cohort of individuals with concussion that may be restricted from high-level activity for a significant period of time.

The recommended management of concussion is a balance of rest with gradual return to activities (Buzzini and Guskiewicz 2006; Daneshvar et al. 2011; Toledo et al. 2012); the proper balance, however, can be very difficult. For example, children are advised to rest when they are symptomatic; however, prolonged rest can lengthen the recovery time and contribute to depression (Leddy et al. 2010). Going back to activity too soon, on the other hand, can exacerbate current symptoms and may even elicit the return of symptoms and lengthen recovery. Preinjury stress has been shown to contribute to protracted symptoms (Smyth et al. 2014). Additional stressors associated with prolonged symptoms, including the loss of meaningful activity and disruption to everyday routines, are thought to contribute to the onset of depression (Silverberg and Iverson 2013). Managing concussion recovery when it is combined with the onset of depression is, therefore, complex.

Standard concussion management uses the 6-stage Zurich return to play recommendations (McCrory et al. 2013) now updated in the Berlin consensus statement, (McCrory et al. 2017). This statement and much of the literature now suggest a more conservative approach to the management of children/youth with concussion. However, it is still unclear as to what "more conservative" entails. When they are symptomatic, children and youth are advised to rest without any stimuli or normal activity for a period of time. As stated above, recent international sport concussion management recommendations suggest a short period of rest (24–48 hours) followed by gradual resumption activity that does not cause or exacerbate post-concussion symptoms (McCrory et al. 2017). Other literature suggests, however, that depression and anxiety may result, further interfering with the child's ability to function and participate (Alexander 1992; Berlin et al. 2006; Guskiewicz et al. 2007; Max et al. 2012). Prolonged rest can lengthen recovery time and contribute to depression and deconditioning (Leddy et al. 2007); therefore, guidelines for children must contain a balance of activity and rest to promote physical, emotional, and cognitive recovery. The CanChild guidelines for concussion management for children 5–18 years (DeMatteo et al. 2012a,b, 2015b,c,d), which will also be referred to below, were developed with reference to the original Zurich guidelines (McCrory et al. 2013), now updated by the Berlin consensus (McCrory et al. 2017), also have similar 6 stages of return to activity as the Zurich and Berlin return to play recommendations.

Management issues are different (DeMatteo et al. 2015c) depending on the pattern of recovery and until now were not differentiated in existing protocols. This new approach of providing different levels of rest and graduated recovery depending on the length of symptom presentation reflects the complicated course of healing that requires more than a *one size fits all* set of recommendations.

All children are advised that there can be no high-level physical activity or contact sport if symptoms are present. However, rest does not equal social isolation or sensory deprivation. There are many light daily activities that can be tolerated well by individuals without symptom exacerbation and are within symptom tolerance. OT task analysis and energy conservation approaches help determine which are the best activities for the individual child or youth.

The restricted normal activity period can be challenging for families to enforce. Finding activities that involve little movement and reduced multimodal sensory stimulation, which precludes much computer, cell phone use, and videogames, is difficult. New evidence is emerging that light physical activity sooner, even before all symptoms resolve, may be the best approach (Thomas et al. 2015). Also, cognitive activity may prove to be more taxing on brain recovery than physical exercise (Brown et al. 2014). There is also evidence suggesting that excessive physical or cognitive activity may not be the cause of symptom exacerbation in some youth (Iverson et al. 2016). All of this new evidence supports the individualized activity planning.

We suggest the formula:

Individual goals + Pre morbid persona

+ Symptom profile (time and intensity)

= Individualized return to activity profile

Additional education, reassurance, and supportive problem solving may be required so that families understand the short-term duration and type of this decreased activity and rest in stage 1 and the limits and gradual increase in activity in steps 2 and 3 (McCrory et al. 2013, 2017; DeMatteo et al. 2015b).

In the CanChild Return to Activity Guidelines developed for children and youth 5–18 years (DeMatteo et al. 2012a, 2015b), step 2 recommends 10 to 15 minutes of light exercise twice daily. It is recommended that children who experience symptoms beyond 2 weeks need to begin step 2 carefully and may need to modify time parameters and experiment with types of gentle activity. It is important to get these children moving and participating in activities that they enjoy to prevent any adverse effects such as deconditioning and symptoms of depression and anxiety yet balance this with continued brain healing and recovery (Leddy et al. 2007; Cotman et al. 2007; Majerske et al. 2008; Shrey et al. 2011). The client, and their family, may continue to require support and management through all stages of return to activity including contact sport to adapt each step to minimize symptom exacerbation while maximizing participation and quality of life.

## Return to school planning

One of the most stressful activities post-concussion for school-aged children and young adults is returning to school (Brown et al. 2014), and this will be discussed in more detail in another chapter. For youth specifically, their major role and occupation are that of student. As such, particularly in youth, supporting the return to school process for those who have experienced a concussion is a primary focus of OT. Participating in school is vital to social development, academic learning, and preparation for future roles; therefore, special attention must be given to returning to school (Buzzini and Guskiewicz 2006; Daneshvar et al. 2011; Baillargeon et al. 2012; Toledo et al. 2012; Arbogast et al. 2013; Gioia 2016). Both parents and children have been reported to have concerns and anxiety about academic performance after concussion. School absence and dropping grades have been reported in 30% of children post-injury (Arbogast et al. 2013; Parsons et al. 2013). Prolonged recovery from concussion exacerbates this problem, as reported by a tertiary care sports medicine clinic that found 61% of children reported a decline in grades, 69% needed school accommodations, and this increased to 87% when the youth were depressed (Corwin et al. 2014). Childhood concussion can significantly affect school attendance and achievement especially when recovery is longer than expected.

Given that being a student is the primary occupation from childhood through to young adulthood, an emphasis on returning to school should be a top priority for OTs working with these children and adolescents even more so than return to sport. However, research has highlighted that more emphasis is placed on return to sport by health-care providers. A medical chart review showed that primary care physicians were providing return to school instructions to only 27.5% of patients as compared with return to sport instructions to 51.6% of patients (Arbogast et al. 2013). This imbalance may reflect the absence of research about post-concussive school issues, and thus, empirical evidence for specific methods and timelines for returning children to school are not yet available. The best approach will always be individual and take into consideration the youth, the class environment, and the requirements of the task.

Little guidance, however, is available as to how much rest is needed, how much time off school is recommended, and what to do when students have difficulty with school routines.

Return-to-school decisions are characteristically based on the presence or absence of symptoms and an overarching dogma that missing school is not acceptable. It is not always understood that, emotional symptoms, fatigue, and difficulty concentrating are concussion related (Fedor and Gunstad 2014), and therefore, many children may be returned to school too soon or with too much expectation (DeMatteo et al. 2010). The consequences of returning to school and other activity too early can include exacerbation of symptoms, prolonged recovery, and the risk of sustaining another similar injury (Swaine et al. 2007; Brown et al. 2014). Alternatively, there have been instances in which the recommendation of rest post-concussion has been misinterpreted and has led to children being away from school for months. Prolonged absence from school may be equally as devastating to the young person due to loss of academic standing, social isolation, and may contribute to depression and/or anxiety (Karlin 2011).

Returning to school within the first 2–4 weeks post-concussion with modifications and accommodations to ensure successful reintegration can ameliorate poor outcomes, including decreased quality of life (Gibson et al. 2013; DeMatteo et al. 2014).

OTs regularly work in schools and with schools to facilitate students with disabilities and impairments to integrate smoothly and successfully in school. Adapting the school environment and curriculum for successful achievement of curriculum expectations by the individual student with injury or disability is a common role for the OT.

In the concussion field, the OT can assist in making decisions about successful return to school that will not exacerbate symptoms and will allow participation in social and academic activities as soon as possible.

Similar to the return to activity (RTA) protocol, pediatric concussion management for return to school should be conservative and individualized (Purcell 2006, 2012; Davis and Purcell 2013; DeMatteo et al. 2015d).

The CanChild return to school (RTS) protocol (DeMatteo et al. 2012b, 2015d) developed primarily by occupational therapists for ages 5–18 years specifically focuses on return to school, not just return to learning. The premise is that it is beneficial to have the child return to their school environment first and then to establish when readiness for learning can occur. Although the youth may not have the cognitive ability to participate in new learning at first, the school environment represents normality and a social environment that has routine and support from teachers and friends with a reassurance of recovery.

The OT focus is in getting the youth back to school by using four main techniques of adaptation:

*Timetable/attendance*: May start with 1 hour a day or 2 hours a week; whatever amount does not exacerbate symptoms. Which days are best? Mornings or afternoons? All must be carefully considered.

*Curriculum modifications*: It must be in consultation with the school. This can include choice and number of subjects to begin with and gradually progress to full load. Less stressful subjects for that particular child should be resumed first. This will vary greatly; for one child, it may be French another Math. Recommendations regarding no homework and when to resume tests and which tests are included in this area.

*Environment adaptation*: This may include recommendations such as no school bus travel, no cafeteria, no gym, no heavy backpacks, no noisy class assembly, or computer classes. It may also require change in placement in the classroom, wearing earphones or dark glasses to limit sensory stimuli.

*Activity modification*: May include recommendations like short periods of class time followed by rest in a quiet place, which gym activities are possible and limit screen time, and reading to 15 minute blocks initially up to 4 times per day.

The student with prolonged symptoms may require the above modifications which are stage 3 of regulatory technical standards guidelines for a significant period of time. It may also be required that the OT advocates for the youth to be given an Aegrotat standing to avoid the increased pressure of trying to redo and catch up all work that was missed in addition to learn new work and do all tests and assignments.

Aegrotat standing is the granting of credit for a course in which the required examination was not taken. The credit will be a mark/grade based on evaluation of achievement in the term work in the course. Aegrotat standing may be granted only for a student who has been unable to take the required final examination for medical or compassionate reasons.

This is a well known and accepted process in the education system at all levels even postsecondary. It also fits with the universal learning philosophy which emphasizes that not every student has to complete evaluations in the same way as long as course objectives are met. A recent study found that accommodations were provided for only 16% of high-school athletes with concussion (Parsons et al. 2013). Advocating for these accommodations with practical solutions as to how they could work in the learning environment is one of the most important roles of the OT with youth after concussion. The consequences of prolonged school absence and decreased academic performance result in a loss of a sense of competence and self-worth as well as increasing anxiety about homework and school success (Karlin 2011). These losses, compounded by anxiety and/or depression, are associated with school refusal and negative psychosocial outcomes (Casoli-Reardon et al. 2012; Kearney 2008).

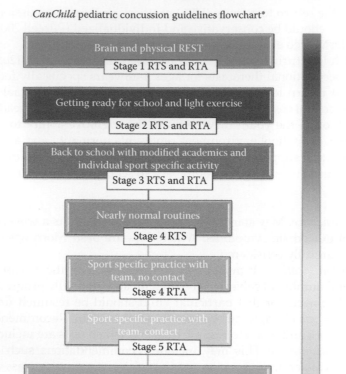

CanChild pediatric concussion guidelines flowchart*

Brain and physical REST
Stage 1 RTS and RTA

Getting ready for school and light exercise
Stage 2 RTS and RTA

Back to school with modified academics and individual sport specific activity
Stage 3 RTS and RTA

Nearly normal routines
Stage 4 RTS

Sport specific practice with team, no contact
Stage 4 RTA

Sport specific practice with team, contact
Stage 5 RTA

Full return to activity and school
Stage 5 RTS and 6 RTA

*To be used in supplement with the *CanChild* return to activity (RTA) and return to school (RTS) guidelines

*Figure 10.2* Integrating return to activity guidelines with return to school guidelines.

It is highly recommended that RTS stages should be followed in conjunction with the RTA protocol (DeMatteo et al. 2012a,b, 2015b) as suggested in Figure 10.2. A youth should never return to a full school program, if he or she is only allowed to be at step 3 moderate activity in the activity protocol. Likewise, if a youth cannot participate fully in his or her academic program, then he or she should not be playing full contact or step 6 full activity and contact sport.

## *"Rest" and the concept of energy conservation*

A concussion results in an *energy crisis* for the brain where a significant amount of energy is required to heal the injured brain (Giza and Hovda 2014). As a result, it is important to rest after a concussion to promote healing and feeling well. An analogy that can be used to convey this concept is that of a *gas tank*. One can view the brain and body as a gas tank in which everything that we do in our day (both physical and cognitive activities) is going to use some of the fuel (or energy) in that gas tank. After a concussion, due to this energy crisis, there is less fuel (or energy) in the tank available for use. To have the energy needed to promote recovery and feel well following a concussion, it is important that we keep this tank as full as possible. Although the recommendation of rest after a concussion may be clear to most (e.g., do not return to school or take part in sport-related activities), it is often less clear to most how rest can be incorporated into all aspects of daily life and be done in a way that promotes participation in activities that are not making post-concussion symptoms intolerable and are not putting individuals at risk for further concussion until medically cleared to do so. As a member of an interdisciplinary sport-related concussion team, occupational therapists can assume the role of educating the athlete and their family on the importance of rest during their recovery, and how rest can be incorporated into their daily activities. Furthermore, occupational therapists can provide the athlete and family with client-centered energy conservation strategies to reduce both physical and cognitive exertion and to promote opportunities to replenish lost energy. Providing clients from a wide range of clinical populations with energy conservation strategies is a common practice in occupational therapy, where general education on avoiding excessive exertion and individualized client-centered plans specific to particular daily activities can be delivered.

One approach to conserving energy can be referred to as the four P's (Canadian Association of Occupational Therapists 2012). OTs can help individuals who have experience concussion learn about and apply the concepts of prioritizing, planning, pacing, and positioning (physically and environmentally) to the completion of daily tasks, can assist in limiting unnecessary physical and cognitive demands of the athlete and can contribute to both achieving the goal of appropriate rest until post-concussive symptoms have resolved and promoting effective reintegration into daily activities. *Prioritizing* helps those with a concussion to determine what activities they will engage in a given day, week, or month and answer the question of if you only have so much fuel or energy to use, what will you decide to use it on? *Planning* helps those with a concussion to determine when they are going to engage in the activities they decide are of the most importance while considering times of day when one feels best (or worst) and what other activities (and how much fuel they may have used) will also be taking place during the same day, week, or month. *Pacing* helps those with a concussion determine how they are going to engage in the activities they decide are of the most importance while considering the need to not do too much for too long and take rest breaks from any physical or cognitive activity. *Positioning* helps those with a concussion determine where they are going to engage in the activities that are of most importance while considering the environment that the activity is taking place and if that environment can be changed or adapted to take place in a quiet or distraction-free area to help limit using unnecessary energy.

In addition to helping those with a concussion develop and apply strategies around what to do and when, how, and where to do it, OT can also contribute to the multidisciplinary care of athletes with concussion by helping them to identify and apply basic concepts of general wellness to ensure that the brain and body have optimal amounts of energy, and one can feel the best they possibly can at any given stage of their concussion recovery. General wellness strategies include: (1) sleep hygiene—this can include strategies like creating a sleep routine with regular bedtime and awakening times, using the bedroom for sleeping only (e.g., not for homework or studying), and avoiding stimulants before bed (food, caffeine, and technology); (2) relaxation training—this can include working with clients to identify situations or factors that trigger stress and developing strategies and skills such as deep breathing, visualization, avoidance to manage stress; (3) nutrition—this can include helping clients to identify their eating and hydration patterns and promote regular well-balanced meals and snacks and regular intake of water while avoiding sugary drinks, caffeine, or alcohol; (4) self-management tools—this can include helping individuals with concussion to develop planning calendars, methods to track their post-concussion symptoms, and what types of activity or rest makes them better or worse, and activity logs to record how much activity one is doing during their stages of recovery.

These self-management tools can help provide individuals with the support they need to engage in their rehabilitation in between health-care team appointments and also can act as a great resource for members of the health-care team to review activity levels and progress of the concussed individual to inform rehabilitation approaches and return to activity decision-making.

## Rehabilitation as needed

As mentioned earlier, OT is one of the multidisciplinary team members included in the best practice guidelines for acquired brain injury. The occupational therapy rehabilitation treatment repertoire is still available to children, youth, and adults with concussion, in addition to the areas listed above. Within the parameters of child development, it may be important to habilitate new skills not yet achieved or rehabilitate lost skills due to injury. The OT will determine with the child and family if a remediation approach or a compensatory approach is best suited to the stage of recovery and needs of the child. Usually with the concussed youth, one is hoping for recovery so skills are remediated. Yet in the early days of recovery, when symptoms may be severe, some compensatory and adapted activities may be needed temporarily such as those described in the previous return to school section. The use of activity, strategies, and activity/environmental modification is at the basis of occupational therapy to improve the individual's skill and function, with the ultimate goal of restoration of full participation in roles and occupations.

The areas of focus of the OT intervention through activity can include

- Neurocognitive function such as attention and memory
- Psycho emotional function such as anxiety and depression
- Physical function such as balance, coordination, and strength
- Visual motor skills

Facilitating the youth's high performance in multitasking activities that combine all of the above will prepare him or her well for safe return to the sports arena or whatever their chosen activity.

The OT will usually choose the environment or its replica, in which the skill needs to happen for the successful achievement of the youth's goal. So if it is the playing field or the classroom, it will be the place for therapy not in a clinic room working on skills in isolation from where the task needs to happen.

## Prevention

The OT intervention which helps to plan a new approach to activity and participation in a very practical way within symptom limitations and includes sport, school, and other activities goes a long way to preventing social isolation and depression and hopefully repeat injury and prolonged symptoms.

## Occupational therapy research

To date, OT research in the field of concussion has focused a great deal on balancing activity and symptoms and developing appropriate guidelines for school and activity post-concussion that are specific to children. The importance of education and peer education strategies and community engagement has also been an area of strength. Attention to the emotional impact and depression post-concussive injury has also been a focus. The future directions of OT research in concussion points to the importance of engagement in meaningful activities in the process of recovery.

## Summary

The OT will assist those with concussion, along with those involved in their lives (families, friends, teachers, and coaches), with returning to the activities that they need, want, and love to do. By evaluating what it is that their clients want to do most; considering the symptoms and deficits that are impeding performance; and, supporting the development of strategies that help concussed individuals determine what to do and when, how, and where to do it, OTs can provide a unique emphasis on participation. As part of an interdisciplinary health team, OTs can support in making the link between how one is feeling/what deficits they may have as a result of the concussion and what they can do functionally during their recovery as it relates to activities of meaning and importance. OTs can adapt return to activity (school and play) guidelines to his or her specific situation, symptoms, and occupational desires and demands—the fine tuning of activity and participation without exacerbating symptoms is the essence of the approach.

The OT can assist with incremental changes resulting in a positive outcome with a structured simple program. The OT will assist each child and youth in finding their equilibrium point of activity versus symptoms. Probably the biggest contribution to the multidisciplinary concussion team is the focus on the importance of engagement in meaningful activities in the process of recovery.

---

### Case study/Vignette

Sarah is a 16-year-old high-school student and an above average A student. While at cheerleading practice seven months ago, Sarah sustained a mild traumatic brain injury or concussion as it was called, when she was accidentally kicked in the head practicing their routine for Nationals. She was disoriented, confused, had amnesia, and experienced nausea and vomiting. Her coach called for an ambulance to take Sarah to the hospital, where a CT scan was performed. The CT scan was normal, showing no evidence of intracranial injury. Sarah was admitted for observation overnight and discharged the following morning. Because Nationals were only a month away, Sarah continued to practice, despite the fact that she was still experiencing difficulty concentrating, headaches, dizziness, and light sensitivity. Two weeks later she sustained another blow to the head during practice. Her neurological examination was normal, but her doctor recommended that she does not cheerlead for 3–6 months or until symptom free, to allow recovery. Sarah was devastated, worried that this will affect her future cheerleading scholarship in the USA. Her father who attends all clinic visits with her seems at a loss as to what to do to help Sarah, and he obviously feels much guilt related to the fact that Sarah sustained a second injury; so he allows her to make the decisions. She does not follow the doctor's advice as she is continuing to do 2 hour daily workouts with the team but does not compete. Seven months later she continues to experience headaches and dizziness, difficulty concentrating in class and trouble with fact retention, leading to a decline in her grades and she will need to repeat grade 12.

Some questions for the reader to consider:

- Do you think that the outcome could have been different?
- What changes would you suggest in management to get a more positive outcome for Sarah?
- When and what would you suggest at first diagnosis?
- How would you manage Sarah's refusal to follow recommendations?

Some possible strategies that could be applied from an OT perspective and in the context of a larger interdisciplinary rehab team:

## STAGE 1: FIRST INJURY

After diagnosis and in conjunction with the physician, the OT would carefully assist Sarah and her family in monitoring and self-managing her symptoms to determine how they respond to activity so that an activity profile of what she can tolerate even in the early stages of recovery could be implemented.

This activity profile will try to provide alternatives to cheerleading based on her personality, interests, and symptoms so that she does not experience grief and loss but can see hope of returning to her preferred active lifestyle safely and soon as possible. This is also where the strategies of rest and energy conservation are so important. These will help her to achieve the balance of activity with symptom exacerbation and progress she needs while still symptomatic.

As a very social competitive teenager, perhaps visits with one friend at a time and simple card, game competition could be tolerated while in stage 1 so that she is not totally bored, depressed, and feeling hopeless. Due to Sarah's symptom profile of headaches and dizziness, difficulty concentrating, and memory problems, full return to school is not indicated, but the OT can work with Sarah and her family and the school to determine which classes may be the least cognitively challenging to begin with and begin an early modified reentry into school with limited hours and limited expectations that can expand as symptoms lessen in intensity. The family will need some assistance in knowing how they can best help which may be in the area of nutrition, sleep hygiene, setting limits, and emotional support as well as practicalities of scheduling such as driving to school, while Sarah is not able to take the bus or walk. This is an emotionally stressful time for the family as well.

## STAGE 2: SECOND INJURY

As it was clear, Sarah did not follow advice and returned to full completion and in her vulnerable state received a second injury. Intervention becomes more of a challenge as symptoms are more intense, the pressure of failure and loss of scholarship are high. As Sarah is defiant and not thinking clearly both due to her age and her injury, it is very important to include the family in all planning, and although Sarah is of age to exclude her family, we know that her father has been very involved, and Sarah will most likely be open to this. It will be a big burden on them to support her through these challenging times. The family can be helped to problem solve how they can do this by examining the family roles and schedules and help them come up with strategies that might work for everyone coping with Sarah's symptoms and moods and future anxiety and in fact their own anxiety about what has happened to her, their guilt, and their fear that she may not recover fully now. Similar strategies to those in stage 1 should be used but with much more OT emphasis on Sarah participating in meaningful activities to her as she is at high risk for depression due to loss and pain. Both the physiotherapist and the neuropsychologist will be key collaborators with the OT in achieving this participation with Sarah. She will need cognitive help with school and physical help for balance and neck issues to be able to participate in more activities, social and academic and to keep her physically fit. It is also important to consider referring Sarah to a mental health clinician for counseling. Depending on the setting, this could be a social worker, counsellor, or sometimes the psychologist, or OT can take on this role.

### STAGE 3: SEVEN MONTHS LATER

Vocation and realistic future plans within existing abilities and graduation from high school become the highest priorities and the main focus of OT. Alternatives become even more important for Sarah as she lost her scholarship for cheerleading due to failing grade 12. Nor could she do cheerleading physically with chronic headaches and memory/concentration issues. Maintaining her sense of self, and hope that she can still achieve many successes without cheerleading is the ultimate goal.

## References

Alexander, MP. 1992. Neuropsychiatric correlates of persistent postconcussive syndrome. *Head Trauma Rehabilitation* 7 (2): 60–69.

Arbogast, K, A McGinley, C Master, M Grady, R Robinson, and M Zonfrillo. 2013. Cognitive rest and school-based recommendations following pediatric concussion: The need for primary care support tools. *Clinical Pediatrics* 52 (5): 397–402. doi:10.1177/0009922813478160.

Baillargeon, A, M Lassonde, S Leclerc, and D Ellemberg. 2012. Neuropsychological and neurophysiological assessment of sport concussion in children, adolescents and adults. *Brain Injury* 26 (3): 211–220. doi:10.3109/02699052.2012.654590.

Berlin, A, W Kop, and P Deuster. 2006. Depressive mood symptoms and fatigue after exercise withdrawal: The potential role of decreased fitness. *Psychosomatic Medicine* 68 (2): 224–230. doi:10.1097/01.psy.0000204628.73273.23.

Birmaher, B, S Khetarpal, M Cully, D Brent, and S Mckenzie. 1999. Screen for child anxiety related disorders (SCARED): Child version. *Journal of the American Academy of Child and Adolescent Psychiatry* 38 (10): 1230–1236. doi:10.1097/00004583-200310000-00009.

Brown, N, R Mannix, M O'Brien, D Gostine, M Collins, and WP Meehan Iii. 2014. Effect of cognitive activity level on duration of post-concussion symptoms. *Pediatrics* 133 (2): e299–e304. doi:10.1542/peds.2013-2125.

Bruininks, R and B Bruininks. 2005. *Bruininks-Oseretsky Test of Motor Proficiency*. 2nd ed. Minneapolis, MN: Pearson.

Bryant, R, M O'Donnell, M Creamer, A McFarlane, C Richard Clark, and D Silove. 2010. The psychiatric sequelaie of traumatic injury. *American Journal Psychiatry* 167 (3): 312–320.

Buzzini, SR and K Guskiewicz. 2006. Sport-related concussion in the young athlete. *Current Opinion in Pediatrics* 18 (4): 376–382. doi:10.1097/01.mop.0000236385.26284.ec.

Casoli-Reardon, M, N Rapport, D Kulick, and S Reinfeld. 2012. Ending school avoidance. *Educational Leadership* 70 (2): 50–55.

Corwin, DJ, MR Zonfrillo, CL Master, KB Arbogast, MF Grady, RL Robinson, AM Goodman, and DJ Wiebe. 2014. Characteristics of prolonged concussion recovery in a pediatric subspecialty referral population. *The Journal of Pediatrics*: 1–9. doi:10.1016/j.jpeds.2014.08.034.

Cotman, C, N Berchtold, and L Christie. 2007. Exercise builds brain health: Key roles of growth factor cascades and inflammation. *Trends in Neurosciences* 30 (9): 464–472. doi:10.1016/j.tins.2007.06.011.

D'Angelo, E and T Augenstein. 2012. Developmentally informed evaluation of depression: Evidence-based instruments. *American Journal Psychiatry* 21 (2): 279–298. doi:10.1016/j.chc.2011.12.003.

Daneshvar, D, D Riley, C Nowinski, A McKee, R Stern, and R Cantu. 2011. Long-term consequences: Effects on normal development profile after concussion. *Physical Medicine and Rehabilitation Clinics of North America* 22 (4): 683–700, ix. doi:10.1016/j.pmr.2011.08.009.

Davis, G and L Purcell. 2013. The evaluation and management of acute concussion differs in young children. *British Journal of Sports Medicine* 48 (April): 98–101. doi:10.1136/bjsports-2012-092132.

DeMatteo, C, K Stazyk, L Giglia, W Mahoney, SK Singh, R Hollenberg, JA Harper, et al. 2015d. A balanced protocol for return to school for children and youth following concussive injury. *Clinical Pediatrics* 54 (8): 783–792. doi:10.1177/0009922814567305.

DeMatteo, CA, SE Hanna, R Yousefi-Nooraie, C-YA Lin, WJ Mahoney, MC Law, and D McCauley. 2014. Quality-of-life after brain injury in childhood: Time, not severity, is the significant factor. *Brain Injury* 28 (1): 114–121. doi:10.3109/02699052.2013.848380.

DeMatteo, C, D Mccauley, K Stazyk, J Harper, J Adamich, S Randall, and C Missiuna. 2015c. Post-concussion return to play and return to school guidelines for children and youth: A scoping methodology. *Disability and Rehabilitation* 37 (12): 1107–1112. doi:10.3109/09638288.2014.952452.

DeMatteo, C, K Stazyk, S Singh, L Giglia, R Hollenberg, C Malcolmson, W Mahoney, et al. 2015b. Development of a conservative protocol to return children and youth to activity following concussive injury. *Clinical Pediatrics* 54 (2): 152–163.

DeMatteo, C, K Volterman, P Breithaupt, E Claridge, J Adamich, and B Timmons. 2015a. Exertion testing in youth with mild traumatic brain injury/concussion. *Medicine and Science in Sports and Exercise* 47 (11). doi:10.1249/MSS.0000000000000682.

DeMatteo, C, S Singh, L Giglia, WJ Mahoney, C Missiuna, R Hollenberg, J Harper, C Malcolmson, and K Stazyk. 2012b. Concussion management in children: Return to school guidelines. Hamilton. https://canchild.ca/system/tenon/assets/attachments/000/000/291/original/MTBI-return_to_school_brochure.pdf.

DeMatteo, C, S Singh, L Giglia, W Mahoney, R Hollenberg, C Malcolmson, K Stazyk, J Harper, and C Missiuna. 2012a. Concussion management in children: Return to activity guidelines. Hamilton. https://canchild.ca/system/tenon/assets/attachments/000/000/292/original/Return_To_Activity_Brochure.pdf.

DeMatteo, C, S Hanna, W Mahoney, R Hollenberg, L Scott, M Law, A Newman, C-Y Lin, and L Xu. 2010. My child doesn't have a brain injury, he only has a concussion. *Pediatrics* 125 (2): 327–334. doi:10.1542/peds.2008-2720.

Fearing, V, and J Clark, Eds. 2000. *Individuals in Context: A Practical Guide to Client-Centered Practice*. Thorofare, NJ: Slack.

Fedor, A and J Gunstad. 2014. Limited knowledge of concussion symptoms in college athletes. *Applied Neuropsychology: Adult* 22 (April 2015). 2015: 1–6. doi:10.1080/23279095.2013.860604.

Frühe, B, AK Allgaier, K Pietsch, B Saravo, M Baethmann, and G Schulte-Körne. 2012. Is the children's depression inventory short version a valid screening tool in pediatric care? A comparison to its full-length version. *Journal of Psychosomatic Research* 73 (5): 369–374. doi:10.1016/j.jpsychores.2012.08.016.

Ganesalingam, K, K Yeates, M Ginn, HG Taylor, A Dietrich, K Nuss, and M Wright. 2008. Family burden and parental distress following mild traumatic brain injury in children and its relationship to post-concussive symptoms. *Journal of Pediatric Psychology* 33 (6): 621–629. doi:10.1093/jpepsy/jsm133.

Gibson, S, L Nigrovic, M O'Brien, and W Meehan. 2013. The effect of recommending cognitive rest on recovery from sport-related concussion. *Brain Injury* 27 (7–8): 839–842. doi:10.3109/02699052.2013.775494.

Giza, CC and D Hovda. 2014. The new metabolic cascade of concussion. *Neurosurgery* 75 (0 4): S24–S33. doi:10.1227/NEU.0000000000000505.The.

Gioia, G. 2016. Medical-school partnership in guiding return to school following mild traumatic brain injury in youth. *Journal of Child Neurology* 2016, 31(1) 93–108.

Guskiewicz, K, S Marshall, J Bailes, M Mccrea, H Harding, A Matthews, J Mihalik, and R Cantu. 2007. Recurrent concussion and risk of depression in retired professional football players. *Medicine and Science in Sports and Exercise* 39 (6): 903–909. doi:10.1249/mss.0b013e3180383da5.

Henderson, S and D Sugden. 1992. *Movement Assessment Battery for Children (Movement ABC)*. Sidcup, KY: The Psychological Corporation, Ltd.

Hung, R, L Carroll, C Cancelliere, P Côté, P Rumney, M Keightley, J Donovan, BM Stålnacke, and J David Cassidy. 2014. Systematic review of the clinical course, natural history, and prognosis for pediatric mild traumatic brain injury: Results of the international collaboration on mild traumatic brain injury prognosis. *Archives of Physical Medicine and Rehabilitation* 95 (3 Suppl): S174–S191. doi:10.1016/j.apmr.2013.08.301.

Iverson, G, N Silverberg, M McCrea, J Apps, T Hammeke, and D Thomas. 2016. Activity-related symptom exacerbations after pediatric concussion. *JAMA Pediatric* 170 (10): 946–953.

Jonsson, C and E Andersson. 2012. Mild traumatic brain injury: A description of how children and youths between 16 and 18 Years of age perform leisure activities after 1 Year. *Developmental Neurorehabilitation* 16 (February): 1–8. doi:10.3109/17518423.2012.704955.

Karlin, AM. 2011. Concussion in the pediatric and adolescent population: "Different population, different concerns." *PM and R* 3 (10 Suppl. 2): S369–S379. doi:10.1016/j.pmrj.2011.07.015.

Kearney, C. 2008. School absenteeism and school refusal behavior in youth: A contemporary review. *Clinical Psychology Review* 28 (3): 451–471. doi:10.1016/j.cpr.2007.07.012.

Kielhofner, G. 2009. *Conceptual Foundation of Occupational Therapy Practice*. Philadelphia, PA: F.A. Davis Company.

Kovacs, M. 2012. *Children's Depression Inventory*, 2nd ed. North Tonawanda, NY: Multi-Health Systems.

Lau, B, M Collins, and M Lovell. 2012. Cutoff scores in neurocognitive testing and symptom clusters that predict protracted recovery from concussions in high school athletes. *Neurosurgery* 70 (2): 371–379.

Law, M. 2002. Participation in the occupations of everyday life. *American Journal of Occupational Therapy* 56 (6): 640–649.

Law, M, S Baptiste, M McColl, A Opzoomer, H Polatajko, and N Pollock. 1990. The canadian occupational performance measure: An outcome measure for occupational therapy. *Canadian Journal of Occupational Therapy* 57 (2): 82–87.

Law, M, S Steinwender, and L Leclair. 1998. Occupation, health and well-being. *Canadian Journal of Occupational Therapy* 65 (2): 81–91.

Law, M, S Baptiste, and J Mills. 1995. Client-centred practice: What does it mean and does it make a difference? *Canadian Journal of Occupational Therapy* 62 (5): 250–257.

Law, M, S Baptiste, A Carswell, M Ann McColl, H Polatajko, and N Pollock. 2005. Targeted application of the canadian occupational performance measure. *Canadian Journal of Occupational Therapy* 72 (5): 298–300.

Leddy, J, K Kozlowski, J Donnelly, D Pendergast, L Epstein, and B Willer. 2010. A preliminary study of subsymptom threshold exercise training for refractory post-concussion syndrome. *Clinical Journal of Sport Medicine* 20 (1): 21–27. doi:10.1097/JSM.0b013e3181c6c22c.

Leddy, JJ, K Kozlowski, M Fung, D Pendergast, and B Willer. 2007. Regulatory and autoregulatory physiological dysfunction as a primary characteristic of postconcussion syndrome: Implications for treatment. *NeuroRehabilitation* 22: 199–205.

MacMillan, H, C Patterson, and N Wathen. 2005. Screening for depression in primary care: Task force on preventive health care. *Canadian Medical Assocation Journal* 172 (1): 33–35. doi:10.1503/cmaj.1030823.

Majerske, C, J Mihalik, D Ren, M Collins, CC Reddy, M Lovell, and A Wagner. 2008. Concussion in sports: postconcussive activity levels, symptoms, and neurocognitive performance. *Journal of Athletic Training* 43 (3): 265–274.

Maugans, T, C Farley, M Altaye, J Leach, and K Cecil. 2012. Pediatric sports-related concussion produces cerebral blood flow alterations. *Pediatrics* 129 (1): 28–37. doi:10.1542/peds.2011-2083.

Max, J, E Wilde, E Bigler, M MacLeod, A Vasquez, A Schmidt, S Chapman, G Hotz, T Yang, and H Levin. 2012. Psychiatric disorders after pediatric traumatic brain injury: A prospective, longitudinal controlled study. *Neuropsychiatry Clin Neurosci* 24 (4): 427–436.

McCrory, P, K Johnston, W Meeuwisse, M Aubry, R Cantu, and J Dvorak. 2005. Summary and agreement statement of the 2nd international conference on concussion in sport, Prague 2004. *British Journal of Sports Medicine* 39 (4): 196–204.

McCrory, P, M, William, D, Jiří Aubry, M Bailes, J Broglio, S Cantu, RC Cassidy, D, Echemendia, R Castellani, RJ Davis et al. 2017. Consensus statement on concussion in sport—the 5th international conference on concussion in sport held in Berlin, October 2016. *Br J Sports Med*: 1–10. doi:10.1136/bjsports-2017-097699.

McCrory, P, W Meeuwisse, K Johnston., J Dvorak, M Aubry, M Molloy, and R Cantu. 2009. Consensus statement on concussion in sport: The 3rd international conference on concussion in sport held in Zurich, November 2008. *Journal of Athletic Training* 44 (4): 434–448.

McCrory, P, W Meeuwisse, M Aubry, B Cantu, J Dvorak, R Echemendia, L Engebretsen, et al. 2013. Consensus statement on concussion in sport: The 4th international conference on concussion in sport held in Zurich, November 2012. *British Journal of Sports Medicine* 47 (5): 250–258. doi:10.1136/bjsports-2013-092313.

McKinlay, A, J Dalrymple-Alford, J Horwood, and D Fergusson. 2002. Long term psychosocial outcomes after mild head injury in early childhood. *Journal of Neurology, Neurosurgery and Psychiatry* 73 (0022–3050 (Print): 281–288.

Parsons, J, RC Bay, and T Valovich-McLeod. 2013. School absence, academic accommodation and health-related quality of life in adolescents with sport-related concussion. *British Journal of Sports Medicine* 47 (5): e1.

Poulsen, A, J Ziviani, and M Cuskelly, Eds. 2015. *Goal Setting and Motivation in Therapy: Engaging Children and Parents.* London, UK and Philadelphia, PA: Jessica Kingsley Publishers.

Purcell, L. 2006. Identification and managment of children with sport-related concussions. *Paediatrics & Child Health* 11.

Purcell, L. 2012. Evaluation and management of children and adolescents with sports-related concussion. *Paediatrics & Child Health* 17 (1): 31–34.

Reed, N. 2011. Sport-related concussion and occupational therapy: Expanding the scope of practice. *Physical & Occupational Therapy in Pediatrics* 31 (3): 222–224. doi:10.3109/01942638.2011.589719.

Sharp, L and M Lipsky. 2002. Screening for depression across the lifespan: A review of measures for use in primary care settings. *American Family Physician* 66 (6): 1001–1008.

Shrey, D, G Griesbach, and C Giza. 2011. The pathophysiology of concussions in youth. *Physical Medicine and Rehabilitation Clinics of North America* 22 (4): 577–602. doi:10.1016/j.pmr.2011.08.002.

Silverberg, N and G Iverson. 2013. Is rest after concussion "The best medicine?": Recommendations for activity resumption following concussion in athletes, civilians, and military service members. *Journal of Head Trauma Rehabilitation* 28 (4): 250–259. doi:10.1097/HTR.0b013e31825ad658.

Smyth, K, S Sandhu, S Crawford, D Dewey, J Parboosingh, and KM Barlow. 2014. The role of serotonin receptor alleles and environmental stressors in the development of post-concussive symptoms after pediatric mild traumatic brain injury. *Developmental Medicine and Child Neurology* 56 (1): 73–77. doi:10.1111/dmcn.12263.

Snell, D, L Surgenor, E Jean Hay-Smith, and R Siegert. 2009. A systematic review of psychological treatments for mild traumatic brain injury: An update on the evidence. *Journal of Clinical and Experimental Neuropsychology* 31 (1): 20–38. doi:10.1080/13803390801978849.

Stazyk, K, C DeMatteo, S Moll and C Missiuna. 2017. Depression in youth recovering from concussion:Correlates and predictors *Brain Injury* 22:1–8. doi: 10.1080/02699052.2017.1283533. (Epub ahead of print)

Sumsion, T and G Smyth. 2000. Barriers to client-centredness and their resolution. *Canadian Journal of Occupational Therapy* 67 (1): 15–21.

Swaine B, I Gagnon, F Champagne, H Lefebvre, D Friedman, J Atkinson, D Feldman 2008. Identifying the specific needs of adolescents after a mild traumatic brain injury: A service provider perspective *Brain Injury* 22:581–588.

Swaine, B, C Tremblay, R Platt, G Grimard, X Zhang, and I Barry Pless. 2007. Previous head injury is a risk factor for subsequent head injury in children: A longitudinal cohort study. *Pediatrics* 119 (4): 749–758. doi:10.1542/peds.2006-1186.

Thomas, DG, J Apps, R Hoffmann, M McCrea, and T Hammeke. 2015. Benefits of strict rest after acute concussion: A randomized controlled trial. *Pediatrics* 135 (2): 213–223. doi:10.1542/peds.2014-0966.

Toledo, E, A Lebel, L Becerra, A Minster, C Linnman, N Maleki, D Dodick, and D Borsook. 2012. The young brain and concussion: Imaging as a biomarker for diagnosis and prognosis. *Neuroscience & Biobehavioral Reviews* 36 (6): 1510–1531. doi:10.1016/j.neubiorev.2012.03.007.The.

Wade, S, J Carey, and C Wolfe. 2006. An online family intervention to reduce parental distress following pediatric brain injury. *Journal of Consulting and Clinical Psychology* 74 (3): 445–454. doi:10.1037/0022-006X.74.3.445.

Zemek, R, N Barrowman, S Freedman, J Gravel, I Gagnon, C Mcgahern, M Aglipay, et al. 2016. Clinical risk score for persistent postconcussion symptoms among children with acute concussion in the ED. *JAMA* 315 (10): 1014–1025. doi:10.1001/jama.2016.1203.

*chapter eleven*

# The role of the psychologist and psychiatrist in pediatric concussion management
## What can they do for me?

*Michael Takagi, Emma Thompson, and Vicki Anderson*

## Contents

## Introduction

Concussion, a subset of the spectrum of mild traumatic brain injury (TBI), is a significant public health concern and comprises up to 90% of all child TBI. Indeed, in the United States, approximately 1 of every 220 pediatric patients seen in an emergency department (ED) is diagnosed with a concussion, representing 144,000 ED visits annually (Meehan and Mannix 2010). Similarly, in Australia, by the time children reach 10 years of age, 20% (approximately 51,000 children) will have had at least one head injury requiring medical treatment (Harmon et al. 2013). For adult populations, the majority of individuals who sustain a concussion will return to pre-injury levels of functioning within 2 weeks (McCrory et al. 2017). We know substantially less about recovery trajectories for children who sustain a concussion; however, it has been hypothesized that children take longer to recover relative to adults, and recent research indicates that approximately 40% of children remain symptomatic at 2-weeks post-injury (Hearps et al. 2017). Children who remain symptomatic long-term can develop significant cognitive, academic, emotional-behavioral, and occupational difficulties that are associated with reduced participation and overall quality of life. These persistent post-concussive symptoms (PPCS) include a broad spectrum of physical, cognitive, emotional, and behavioral difficulties. Most post-concussion symptoms are nonspecific (e.g., headache, fatigue, difficulty concentrating); thus it can be challenging to identify the etiology of prolonged symptoms. For example, a patient presenting with chronic headaches, fatigue, and difficulty concentrating may have suffered a vestibular injury, or they may be experiencing depression.

Treating and caring for children and adolescents who have sustained a concussion is a complex task that requires a multidimensional approach. Psychological and mental health factors are important areas of focus for clinicians when considering post-concussion management. This includes consideration of the circumstances surrounding the injury (e.g., a motor vehicle accident, sports injury, assault), preexisting mental health diagnoses (e.g., depression, anxiety, somatization), protective and predisposing personality features (e.g., resilience, perfectionism), as well as family and demographic variables (e.g., age, sex, family dynamics).

In this chapter, we review the contribution of psychological and mental health factors to the development and maintenance of PPCS in children and adolescents. Specifically, we will focus on: (1) common mental health difficulties post-concussion; (2) key personal and demographic factors to consider for concussion management; (3) the nature of the injury in relation to mental health challenges post-injury; and (4) an illustrative case study to highlight key clinical concepts.

## Definitions

The terms *concussion* and *mild traumatic brain injury* are often used synonymously (McCrory et al. 2017). Various diagnostic criteria overlap significantly (e.g., the Concussion in Sport Group consensus statement versus the American Congress of Rehabilitation Medicine criteria for mild traumatic brain injury), which leads to inconsistent terminology and methodological heterogeneity. With that in mind, for the purpose of this chapter, the terms *concussion* and *mild traumatic brain injury* will be used interchangeably and when discussing research evidence, the terminology of the original study will be used.

For the present chapter, several concepts will be illustrated through data and experience garnered from the Take CARe (Concussion Assessment and Recovery Research) pediatric concussion study. Take CARe is a single-center, prospective, longitudinal cohort study conducted in Melbourne, Australia at the Murdoch Children's Research Institute (MCRI) and the Royal Children's Hospital (RCH). For detailed information on the study protocol, see Bressan et al. (2016). In brief, children aged between 5 and 18 who present to the ED of RCH within 48 hours of sustaining a concussion are screened for eligibility. Recruited participants are assessed in the ED and demographic, clinical symptom, and injury-related data are collected. Participants are followed up in a dedicated concussion clinic at 1–4 days, 2-weeks, 1-month, and 3-months post-injury. Clinical, cognitive, symptom, psychological, and economic data are collected at each time point. Further, a clinician (e.g., clinical neuropsychologist, rehabilitation pediatrician) experienced in concussion management assesses each participant at each time point. Recruitment for Take CARe began in mid-2013 and 377 participants have been recruited to date.

## Common mental health difficulties post-concussion

A recent systematic review identified that, overall, relatively few rigorous prospective studies have examined psychological, behavioral, and psychiatric outcomes following mTBI (Emery et al. 2016). Specifically, (Emery et al. 2016) identified 30 articles investigating the topic mental health and behavioral difficulties in children and adolescents following mTBI. The authors concluded that there is little evidence to support the notion that psychological, behavioral, and/or psychiatric problems persist beyond the acute/subacute period for most young people; but children and adolescents with a history of multiple mTBIs and preexisting mental health difficulties (e.g., depression) were at risk for longer-term problems. The authors also acknowledge that additional research is necessary and future studies should focus on high-quality prospective longitudinal cohort studies to evaluate changes in mental health over time. The following section provides an overview of research into common mental health concerns observed following pediatric concussion.

### Mood disorders

Mood disorders are characterized by the presence of sad, empty, or irritable moods that are accompanied by somatic and cognitive changes and significantly impact an individual's capacity to function (American Psychiatric Association 2013). Mood disturbance is a relatively common feature following concussion (Ellis et al. 2015); however, it can be difficult to tease apart the origins and nature of depressive symptomatology in this population. For example, Kontos and colleagues (Kontos et al. 2012) examined depressive symptoms in a sample of high-school and collegiate athletes at several time points post-injury. Relative to baseline, they identified significant increases in depressive symptoms at 2, 7, and 14 days post-concussion (Kontos et al. 2012). This finding supports the notion of a causative link between concussion and mood disturbance in the acute and post-acute periods. Elevated mood symptoms have also been identified beyond the post-acute period. Luis and colleagues (Luis and Mittenberg 2002) identified a significantly higher incidence of mood disorders at 6 months for children experiencing mTBI compared to orthopedic controls. This study also found the incidence of post-injury mood disorders did not differ between children who had experienced a mild TBI versus moderate/severe TBI. Another study in adolescents found that, even after controlling for sex, age, parental mental health and socioeconomic status, a history of concussion was associated with a 3.3 times greater risk for having a diagnosis of depression (Chrisman and Richardson 2014). In a sample of children experiencing a sport-related concussion, 52.6% of participants with a novel psychiatric disorder post-injury met the criteria for a depressive disorder (Ellis et al. 2015).

These findings are not universal, however, with a retrospective study by Hawley et al. (2003) failing to identify any cases of clinically significant or subthreshold depression in individuals who had experienced mTBI between the ages of 5–15 years. This study had considerable heterogeneity in time since injury, which may account for their findings (mean 2.29 years, range 6 months to 5 years). In contrast, it has also been highlighted that the chronic symptoms of concussion can present as mood disturbance (Grady 2010). These chronic symptoms can include frequent headaches, fatigue, cognitive disturbance, labile mood, and irritability, which are also common symptoms of depression.

Interestingly, it has been hypothesized that common recommendations for concussion management (e.g., prolonged rest until symptoms return to baseline) may have iatrogenic effects (Thomas et al. 2015, DiFazio et al. 2016). In other words, prolonged absence from everyday activities (e.g., school, sport, socialization, screens) may contribute to the development of anxiety and/or depressive symptoms, which can be hard to distinguish from the primary consequences of the injury (Lewinsohn et al. 1997, Karlin 2011, DiFazio et al. 2016). Although prescribed rest is a widely used intervention for concussion management (McCrory et al. 2017), particularly in the acute period post-injury, a recent paper by DiFazio et al. (2016) proposed a model explaining how prolonged activity restriction after concussion may worsen outcomes post-concussion. They highlight three mechanisms by which this may occur: (1) via provoking anxiety in children/parents, (2) via depression and other psychological complications, and (3) via physical deconditioning following extended rest. They suggest the expectation of symptoms from serious injury may in fact create or exacerbate the experience of symptoms post-injury via provoking anxiety (i.e., the nocebo effect; 1). Additionally, by withdrawing from daily validating activities (e.g., sport, school, social interaction, and hobbies), whether prescribed or self-imposed, the individual is more likely to struggle coping with ongoing symptoms and more likely to experience psychological complications. After injury, the ability to participate in normal activity is a critical factor for psychological well-being; thus depressive and psychological complications may also worsen outcomes post-concussion (2). Finally, deconditioning and exercise intolerance can occur after a relatively brief period and some of the manifestations of deconditioning can mimic post-concussion symptoms (e.g., fatigue, dizziness; (3). These notions are supported by Thomas et al. (2015), who found that strict rest post-concussion was associated with more daily post-concussive symptoms and slower symptom resolution when compared to usual care (1–2 days' rest followed by a stepwise return to normal activity). Although preliminary, these findings suggest further research into the effectiveness of prolonged rest post-concussion is required.

## Anxiety disorders

Of the common mental health concerns following concussion in children, anxiety is perhaps the most thoroughly researched. This is not surprising given that in the general population anxiety is considered among the most common and debilitating of mental health disorders that occur in childhood and adolescence (Rockhill et al. 2010).

Anxiety disorders are characterized by excessive fear (an emotional response to real/ perceived imminent threat) and anxiety (anticipation of future threat), but differ from each other in terms of the stimulus that induces the fear, anxiety, or avoidance behavior (American Psychiatric Association 2013). In the context of pediatric concussion, it is hypothesized that the development of novel anxiety disorders post-injury may be the result of experiencing a life-threatening event or overwhelming stressor associated with the circumstances of the injury, which in turn impacts mental health, or alternatively, they may arise due to an organic cause resulting from the trauma to the brain (Moore et al. 2006). A recent systematic review of outcomes post TBI found that regardless of severity, children who had a TBI were at a greater risk for developing an anxiety disorder post-injury, even at one-year post-concussion (Albicini and McKinlay 2015). In terms of mTBI more specifically, this finding has been supported, with a number of studies identifying incidence of anxiety disorders for children who had experienced mTBI versus controls (Luis and Mittenberg 2002, Hawley 2003). A longitudinal study by Max and colleagues found that 11% of children with mTBI had novel diagnoses of anxiety, and 20% had subclinical anxiety disorders at 6 months follow-up (Max et al. 2011). It has thus been suggested that brain injuries, even at the milder end, increase a child's risk for subsequent internalizing symptoms and disorders (Luis and Mittenberg 2002).

Within the Take CARe study, anxiety symptoms are among the most commonly encountered mental health difficulties post-injury. Occasionally, the young person will have a preexisting anxiety diagnosis, but more often they or their parents will give qualitative descriptions that are consistent with anxiety symptoms (e.g., "he definitely worries enough for the whole family," "I've always been a perfectionist"). The following is a common clinical scenario: (1) A child/adolescent with subclinical anxiety symptoms sustains a concussion and experiences typical post-concussion symptoms (headache, fatigue, cognitive difficulties); (2) Most symptoms significantly improve/resolve within a 10–14 day period; (3) The young person experiences normal physical or cognitive phenomena (e.g., headache, word-finding difficulties, error of capture) and falsely ascribes the phenomena to lingering concussion symptoms; (4) This results in a state of hypervigilance, which has the effect of worsening perceived concussion symptoms (e.g., attention-related memory difficulties); (5) The individual experiences heightened anxiety about the perceived impact of the concussion, which creates a vicious cycle of worsening symptoms and increasing anxiety. This can have a profound impact upon the young person's quality of life, including withdrawing from school/social/sporting activities, often at the request of treating clinicians. There are a range of potential responses within this clinical scenario, with frank conversion disorder occurring in rare cases. This highlights the importance of considering anxiety symptoms when diagnosing and managing young people who have sustained a concussion.

## Post-traumatic stress disorder

Post-traumatic stress disorder (PTSD) is characterized by re-experiencing, dysphoric/anhedonic, hyperarousal, and/or dissociative symptoms following exposure to a traumatic event/s (American Psychiatric Association 2013). Given that mTBI can occur within the context of a distressing event, such as a car accident, it has been suggested that the most expected mental health outcome post-mTBI is PTSD (Moore et al. 2006). In a study of children aged 15 years and above 8.8% of individuals with mTBI met the criteria for PTSD compared to 2.2% of controls (Lagarde et al. 2014). Similarly, in a sample of adolescents aged 14–17 years, those who sustained an mTBI without intracranial hemorrhage reported greater PTSD symptoms over follow-up compared to those with injuries to their arm (O'Connor et al. 2012). These findings are not consistent, however, with other studies failing to find significantly higher incidence of PTSD symptoms for children with mTBI compared to orthopedic injuries (Hajek et al. 2010), nor children experiencing a road traffic accident with and without mTBI (Mather et al. 2003).

Within the Take CARe study, we examined post-traumatic stress symptoms (PTSS) in young people aged 5–18 who experienced a concussion. One hundred and twenty children aged 8–18 years reported PTSS for 3 months following concussion diagnosis using the Child PTSD Symptom Scale; age, sex, injury mechanism, loss of consciousness, previous concussions, prior hospitalization, prior diagnosis of depression or anxiety, and acute PCS were assessed as risk-factors. Results revealed that 16% of children had clinically significant PTSS 2 weeks post-concussion, declining to 10% at 1 month and 6% at 3 months post-injury. We concluded that the majority of children are resilient to PTSS post-concussion, but a substantial minority of children experience PTSS acutely and some continue to experience PTSS months after injury. Further, it is our experience that avoidance is a common PTSD characteristic among young people who have sustained a concussion. For example, children not returning to sport for fear of further injury or not playing 100% for fear of injury, which results in a loss of confidence. This notion is supported in the adult literature and Lagarde and colleagues (2014) found that the greatest contrast between mTBI and noninjured patients on PTSD dimensions was the avoidance dimension (20.4% vs. 6.0%). In contrast, Hajek et al. (2010) did not find a main effect of group for avoidance or re-experiencing dimensions when comparing children with mTBI and orthopedic controls. Despite the overlap between PTSD and PCS (Hajek et al. 2010), the nature of the relationship between mTBI and PTSD remains unclear.

## Adjustment disorder

Adjustment disorder refers to the development of emotional or behavioral symptoms in response to a specific and identifiable stressor, within three months of the onset of the stressor (American Psychiatric Association 2013). In order to reach the criteria for a diagnosis there must be either significant impairment to the individuals functioning or disproportionate distress in comparison to the severity/intensity of the stressor (American Psychiatric Association 2013). Very limited research exists on the development of adjustment disorder post-concussion in children. One study by Massagli and colleagues, however, found that 6% of children had an adjustment disorder diagnoses in the three year period post-concussion (Massagli et al. 2004).

## Malingering/symptom exaggeration/noncredible effort

Research in the adult mTBI population suggests that whilst most individuals who experience mTBI make a full recovery, a subset experience persistent symptoms that may seem inconsistent with the severity of their injury (Silver 2012). Cases of outright malingering are less likely to occur in pediatric populations, but it is unclear how often noncredible effort is given during assessment, particularly in pediatric concussion. Kirkwood and colleagues (2014) examined the relationship between credible effort test performance and symptom report. They hypothesized that children who failed credible effort testing would report significantly more post-concussive symptoms. Interestingly, 12% of their sample (191 children aged 8–17 years) failed credible effort testing post-mTBI, and these children endorsed significantly more post-concussive symptoms compared to those who passed the test, even after controlling for other factors (Kirkwood et al. 2014). Further, the authors found that those with a premorbid history of anxiety were significantly more likely to fail the validity test (Kirkwood et al. 2014). This finding supports results of an earlier study by the same group, which found that 15% of children post-mTBI behaved noncredibly on effort testing (Green et al. 2014). These findings suggest that for a subset of children post-concussion, enduring symptoms may reflect symptom exaggeration or feigning, and those with a premorbid history of anxiety may be particularly vulnerable.

## Chronic pain/chronic fatigue

Research in the adult concussion literature suggests that chronic pain is a common symptom post TBI (for all severities) (Nampiaparampil 2008). Among civilians with mTBI the prevalence of chronic pain has been estimated at 75.3%, with chronic headache particularly common (Nampiaparampil 2008). Chronic pain in children with mTBI, however, remains largely unexplored. It thus remains unclear the extent to which this symptomatology is seen in children who have experienced mTBI.

Fatigue is a frequent physical/somatic symptom in the early period post-concussion, and it is also a feature of several conditions common in PCS. In other words, fatigue in the initial stage post-concussion is best explained by temporary physiological changes in the brain (e.g., neurometabolic disruptions, alterations in cerebral blood flow) (Leddy et al. 2012), but after the typical recovery period (i.e., 14-days), fatigue symptoms are better explained by other factors (e.g., emerging mental health difficulties, physical deconditioning). From the individual's perspective, fatigue is continuous and uninterrupted, but the etiology of the fatigue changes. This can have a significant impact upon a child's quality of life and mental health and reduces their ability to participate in important activities (e.g., school, sport, and leisure activities) (Sady et al. 2011, Babcock et al. 2013, Crichton et al. 2015).

## Behavioral problems

Behavioral problems post-mTBI in children has been an area of great research interest and it has been suggested that mTBI can be associated with persistent behavioral problems post-injury (Hawley 2003). In one study, 20% of children with mTBI had reported behavioral problems and 60% temper problems (Hawley 2003). Another study found that 10% of children had issues with hyperactivity in the three years post concussion (Massagli et al. 2004). Children with mTBI have also been shown to experience elevated adverse psychological outcomes, in terms of hyperactivity, inattention and conduct, compared to controls, however only for children with more severe mTBI (requiring an inpatient stay) (McKinlay et al. 2002). Although there is evidence to suggest that behavioral problems post concussion are common, the extent to which these are directly precipitated by the mTBI remains largely unknown.

## Conversion disorder/somatization

Somatic symptom and related disorders are characterized by prominent somatic symptoms that are associated with significant distress and impairment (American Psychiatric Association 2013). Conversion disorder, which falls within this category of mental health problems, is characterized by symptoms and/or signs affecting voluntary motor or sensory function that cannot be explained by a neurological or other general medical condition (Kozlowska et al. 2007). In pediatric practice, although in low prevalence, conversion disorder is described as having a high impact on both the individual and the health system (Kozlowska et al. 2007). Emerging evidence suggests elevated somatizing symptoms may be associated with poorer recovery post-concussion (Root et al. 2016, Grubenhoff et al. 2016). In one study, children with delayed symptom recovery at one month reported significantly greater preinjury somatizing tendencies (Grubenhoff et al. 2016). It remains unclear, however, whether individuals with somatization experience delayed symptom recovery due to delayed recovery from the neuronal injury experienced in mTBI or whether delayed recovery reflects differences in symptom perception and reporting (Root et al. 2016). Nonetheless, these preliminary findings suggest somatization as potentially a confounding factor in symptom presentation and/or recovery following pediatric concussion (Root et al. 2016). Given the association between somatization and elevated and persistent health service use (e.g., numerous medical investigations, admissions, imaging) this is an important area of future research.

## Key personal factors to consider

### Age

Age is certainly an important factor to consider when assessing a young person who has sustained a concussion, but there is conflicting evidence as to how age may impact outcomes post-injury. Some studies indicate that younger age at injury appears to be most consistently associated with greater risk for mental health concerns, particularly anxiety, post-mTBI (Albicini and McKinlay 2015). It has been suggested that not only are younger children more susceptible to concussion, but that they also need more time to recover, and are more susceptible to experiencing long-term effects (Karlin 2011). This is not a universally accepted finding however; other studies have found that younger age and poorer outcomes are seen after more severe brain injuries, but this relationship is not found in milder injuries (Anderson et al. 2009, Anderson et al. 2011). Further, other studies have found that older age is associated with greater risk of delayed recovery (Zemek et al. 2016) and developing psychiatric illness post-mTBI (Massagli et al. 2004). It has been suggested that perhaps this may reflect increasing awareness and demands on cognitive functioning, and in turn frustration, with increased age (Li and Liu 2013). It is thus suggested that perhaps the impact of age on recovery depends in part on the broader environment of the child, and thus consideration should be given to the demands and expectations within the child's environment, as well as their sensitivity to them, when assessing children post-concussion.

### Sex

A search of the literature reveals mixed findings with relation to sex and mental health outcomes post-concussion have been identified. Massagli and colleagues (2004) found that males and females without a psychiatric history had a similar risk for developing a psychiatric illness post-mTBI. For those with a psychiatric history, however, males were at a 70% greater risk (Massagli et al. 2004). In contrast, Ellis et al. (2015) investigated sport-related concussion in children and found that those who went on to experience psychiatric symptoms post-injury were significantly more likely to be female (Ellis et al. 2015). Another study failed to find any association between sex and PCS (Olsson et al. 2013). The extent to which sex influences psychological outcomes following mTBI thus remains unclear.

### Personality traits

To our knowledge, only a handful of studies have investigated the relationship between personality traits and outcome post-concussion in young people. Woodrome et al. (2011) found that the coping strategies utilized by children post-mTBI accounted for 10%–15% of the variance in children's symptoms over time. Wood and colleagues (2011, 2014) examined personality factors in the development and maintenance of symptoms following mTBI and fount that higher anxiety sensitivity and alexithymia (difficulty in experiencing, expressing, and describing emotional responses) were associated with greater number of post-concussion symptoms and greater psychological distress. Similarly, Hou et al. (2012) identified individuals with anxiety proneness and/or a history of somatic complaints as being more vulnerable to experiencing delayed recovery post-mTBI.

The relationship between personality factors and delayed recovery following concussion is an area we are currently investigating within the Take CARe study. Specifically, we are interested in examining perfectionism and resiliency and how these traits interact and influence outcomes post-injury. Based on our experience, a considerable number of young people who experience delayed recovery describe themselves as perfectionists (e.g., high achieving athletically, academically, and socially) and also appear to have a reduced capacity to recover quickly from the normal pattern of difficulties associated with concussion (e.g., symptoms for 10–14 days). We believe that these data will be of considerable clinical utility and assist in better characterizing young people who are at high risk of experiencing PPCS.

## Family dynamics

Limited research has investigated the impact of family functioning and adjustment on psychological outcomes of the child post-mTBI. It has been suggested that elevated family burden and stress after mTBI is limited (Ganesalingam et al. 2008); however, this finding is not universal. Parents of children with complicated mTBI have been shown to report significantly elevated overall family and child related burden compared to parents of children with orthopedic injuries, despite the majority of families adapting well (Stancin et al. 2008). Despite mixed findings regarding the impact of mTBI on family functioning, it appears that a family's level of functioning is important to the child's outcomes post-mTBI (Yeates et al. 2012). Interestingly, a recent study found that group differences between mTBI and orthopedic injuries in terms of somatic symptoms were more pronounced in families with more resources and better functioning (Yeates et al. 2012). It was proposed that perhaps children from higher functioning families with more resources may be more vulnerable to the impact of mTBI, perhaps due to higher demands, expectations, or levels of monitoring present in their immediate environment (Yeates et al. 2012). Whilst family functioning appears important to psychological and recovery outcomes post pediatric TBI (Ellis et al. 2015), the direction of this relationship remains unclear.

## Parental mental health

Unsurprisingly, family history of internalizing disorders has been found to be associated with greater risk of developing an anxiety disorder following childhood mTBI (Albicini and McKinlay 2015). In a recent study into psychiatric disorders post pediatric sport-related concussion, 40% of individuals who had post-injury psychiatric diagnoses reported a family history of psychiatric illness (Ellis et al. 2015). Similarly, a recent systematic review identified that elevated psychosocial adversity was associated with greater risk of developing an anxiety disorder post-mTBI (Albicini and McKinlay 2015). Parents' psychological status and adjustment following their child's injury also appears important. A study by Olsson and colleagues found that parent anxiety predicted the trajectory of change of their child's PCS from 6 to 18 months post-mTBI (Olsson et al. 2013). Additionally, the authors found that child PPCS at 6 months was predicted by parent preinjury distress levels, and child PPCS at 18 months was predicted by higher levels of parent distress at 6 months (Olsson et al. 2013). Current research evidence supports the notion that both family history of mental health concerns as well as parents' current mental health impact the psychological adjustment of the child post-concussion.

## Preexisting subclinical mental health symptoms

As highlighted in earlier sections, preexisting mental health concerns are consistently associated with prolonged symptoms and recovery following concussion in children (Karlin 2011, Kirkwood et al. 2014, Albicini and McKinlay 2015). Corwin and colleagues (2014) found that preexisting depression was associated with 2.2 times longer recovery from concussion compared to those without (Corwin et al. 2014). Similarly, children with preexisting anxiety took twice as long to be fully cleared compared to those without (Corwin et al. 2014). Interestingly, it has also been shown that greater somatizing tendencies (preinjury) were associated with threefold greater symptoms of recovery (Grubenhoff et al. 2016). While the bulk of studies support the notion that young people with preexisting mental health difficulties are more likely to experience delayed recovery post-concussion, other studies did not identify an association (Max et al. 2012, Eisenberg et al. 2013).

## Case study

This case study was selected to further clarify and illustrate several of the concepts and examples discussed earlier. The individual presented here was a participant in the Take CARe study and her personal details have been changed.

### Injury circumstances

Julie, a female high-school-aged student, sustained a concussion participating in field hockey; she was hit in the head with a hockey stick while going after the ball. She briefly lost consciousness and was taken to the side-lines. She had a headache, she was dizzy, disoriented, had trouble balancing, and her vision was blurred. After a few minutes of rest, she attempted to return to the game, but was unable to participate because of symptom exacerbation. She rested for the remainder of the day and attempted school the following day, but her symptoms worsened and her parents took her to RCH in the early afternoon. On presentation to the hospital, she had a Glasgow Coma Scale score of 15 and was experiencing the following symptoms: photophobia, fatigue, headache, nausea, balance difficulties, trouble concentrating, and labile mood. She was enrolled in the Take CARe study, assessed in the ED, and seen in the concussion clinic 3 days later (4 days post-injury).

### Initial assessment, 4 days post-injury

Julie attended the appointment with her mother, Kelly. On interview, both described Julie as an excellent student who was consistently at the top of her class. She was also an avid hockey player and participated in sport 5 days/week. She lived at home with her mother, father, and younger brother and had a good relationship with her family. She also had a good social network, with her closest friends being her fellow hockey players. Kelly also described Julie as, *perfectionistic* and that she had an *anxious temperament*. Kelly was concerned about Julie's recovery; she was surprised at how symptomatic Julie was and how long it was taking for her to recover. Julie echoed Kelly's concerns about the severity and duration of her symptoms. Julie had attempted to attend school the previous three days, but returned home early each day because of symptom exacerbation. Her primary symptoms were headache, fatigue, concentration difficulties, labile mood, irritability, and sleeping more than usual. Kelly and Julie were provided with psychoeducation about concussion and symptom management and advised that Julie should take 2–3 days' rest at home and then attempt school again. If her symptoms worsened at school, it was suggested that Julie find a quiet area of the school (e.g., the nurses office) and rest. If the symptoms did not abate after rest, return home. She was also advised not to return to sport, but to maintain light physical activity (e.g., walking) if her symptoms allowed.

## Second assessment, 2 weeks post-injury

At the second assessment, Julie and Kelly reported ongoing and worsening symptoms. Both were noticeably upset and Julie became teary at multiple points. She reported ongoing headaches, fatigue, concentration difficulties, unusual sleep patterns, and labile mood. Julie's parents were concerned about her symptoms and had begun strictly enforcing physical and cognitive rest shortly after the previous assessment. Julie could attend school, but no homework, sport, physical activity, screen time (e.g., TV, social media), or social interactions was permitted. On further questioning, Julie described feeling *flat* and feeling like she was *losing control*. Julie also said she was anxious about missing school and sport. Kelly said Julie was noticeably less vibrant, she slept frequently, and cried often.

The clinician consensus was that Julie's symptoms were best explained by psychological distress (e.g., anxiety symptoms surrounding missing school and sport, depressive symptoms due to activity restriction). Julie and Kelly were provided with psychoeducation about mental health and how her symptoms could be explained by psychological distress. Both were receptive and they were provided with the following advice:

1. Continue to attend school, gradually re-introduce homework.
2. Do not participate in sport, but re-introduce socialization. This included attending hockey practice to watch and socialize with friends and helping during games (e.g., keeping score).
3. Re-introduce physical activity. This should be done gradually, begin with light exercise. For example, begin by walking around the block. If symptoms are not present, increase the distance/pace of the walk the following day. Monitor symptoms and gradually and carefully work toward a light jog.
4. Once jogging could be tolerated without symptoms, a graded return to sport could begin (e.g., participating in warm-up activities).

Julie and her parents were satisfied with the advice and worked with her teachers and coaches to implement the recommendations. She was also referred to a clinical psychologist to address her mood and anxiety symptoms.

## Third assessment, 1 month post-injury

Julie and Kelly reported incremental improvement in symptoms in the first week following the previous assessment, but a substantial improvement in the second week. This improvement coincided with Julie's return to sport training. She attended practice approximately 3 weeks post-injury having gradually re-introduced physical activity. She participated in warm-up activities (e.g., jogging) with no symptoms. For the rest of the week, she continued to attend nightly practice, only participating in warm-up activities. She had also been attending full days at school with improving symptoms; her sleep had normalized, her mood had improved substantially, she was able to introduce homework, and her headaches had reduced in frequency and severity. Following the advice of concussion clinic staff and the supervision of Julie's parents and coaches, Julie gradually began increasing her participation at practice. This gradual return began with warm-up followed by sport-specific drills. There were no reported symptoms and the intensity and duration of Julie's practice participation was increased slightly. This process continued for 2 weeks, after which Julie was cleared and returned to sport full time.

## Fourth assessment, 3 months post-injury

At 3 months post-injury, both Julie and Kelly reported a return to normal functioning. Julie was performing well at school and sport and her symptoms had returned to pre-injury levels (e.g., occasional headaches). She had also been seeing a clinical psychologist, who worked with her on strategies to manage anxiety and stress.

## Conclusion

As highlighted in this chapter, mental health difficulties can significantly contribute to the development and maintenance of PPCS in children and adolescents. This includes pre-existing conditions, injury-related factors, personality traits, family dynamics, and social relationships. As such, it is critical for clinicians involved in pediatric concussion management to assess for mental health complications at all stages post-injury.

## References

Albicini, M. and A. McKinlay. 2015. A systematic review of anxiety disorders following mild, moderate and severe TBI in children and adolescents. In *A Fresh Look at Anxiety Disorders*, Federico Durbano (ed.). Intech Open, pp. 199–224.

Anderson, V., M. Spencer-Smith, and A. Wood. 2011. Do children really recover better? Neurobehavioural plasticity after early brain insult. *Brain* 134 (Pt 8):2197–2221. doi: 10.1093/brain/awr103.

Anderson, V., M. Spencer-Smith, R. Leventer, L. Coleman, P. Anderson, J. Williams, M. Greenham, and R. Jacobs. 2009. Childhood brain insult: Can age at insult help us predict outcome? *Brain* 132 (Pt 1):45–56. doi: 10.1093/brain/awn293.

American Psychiatric Association. 2013. *Diagnostic and Statistical Manual of Mental Disorders (DSM-5®)*: American Psychiatric Pub, Washington, D.C.

Babcock, L., T. Byczkowski, S. L. Wade, M. Ho, S. Mookerjee, and J. J. Bazarian. 2013. Predicting postconcussion syndrome after mild traumatic brain injury in children and adolescents who present to the emergency department. *JAMA Pediatrics* 167 (2):156–161. doi: 10.1001/jamapediatrics.2013.434.

Bressan, S., M. Takagi, V. Anderson, G. A. Davis, E. Oakley, K. Dunne, C. Clarke, M. Doyle, S. Hearps, V. Ignjatovic et al. 2016. Protocol for a prospective, longitudinal, cohort study of postconcussive symptoms in children: The Take C.A.R.e (Concussion Assessment and Recovery Research) study. *BMJ Open* 6 (1):e009427.

Chrisman, S. P. D. and L. P. Richardson. 2014. Prevalence of diagnosed depression in adolescents with history of concussion. *Journal of Adolescent Health* 54 (5):582–586.

Corwin, D. J., M. R. Zonfrillo, C. L. Master, K. B. Arbogast, M. F. Grady, R. L. Robinson, A. M. Goodman, and D. J. Wiebe. 2014. Characteristics of prolonged concussion recovery in a pediatric subspecialty referral population. *The Journal of Pediatrics* 165 (6):1207–1215.

Crichton, A., S. Knight, E. Oakley, F. E. Babl, and V. Anderson. 2015. Fatigue in child chronic health conditions: A systematic review of assessment instruments. *Pediatrics* 135 (4):e1015–e1031. doi: 10.1542/peds.2014-2440.

DiFazio, M., N. D. Silverberg, M. W. Kirkwood, R. Bernier, and G. L. Iverson. 2016. Prolonged activity restriction after concussion: Are we worsening outcomes? *Clinical Pediatrics* 55 (5):443–451.

Eisenberg, M. A., J. Andrea, W. Meehan, and R. Mannix. 2013. Time interval between concussions and symptom duration. *Pediatrics* 132 (1):8–17.

Ellis, M. J., L. J. Ritchie, M. Koltek, S. Hosain, D. Cordingley, S. Chu, E. Selci, J. Leiter, and K. Russell. 2015. Psychiatric outcomes after pediatric sports-related concussion. *Journal of Neurosurgery: Pediatrics* 16 (6):709–718.

Emery, C. A., K. M. Barlow, B. L. Brooks, J. E. Max, A. Villavicencio-Requis, V. Gnanakumar, H. L. Robertson, K. Schneider, and K. O. Yeates. 2016. A systematic review of psychiatric, psychological, and behavioural outcomes following mild traumatic brain injury in children and adolescents. *Can Journal of Psychiatry* 61 (5):259–269. doi: 10.1177/0706743716643741.

Ganesalingam, K., K. O. Yeates, M. S. Ginn, H. G. Taylor, A. Dietrich, K. Nuss, and M. Wright. 2008. Family burden and parental distress following mild traumatic brain injury in children and its relationship to post-concussive symptoms. *Journal of Pediatric Psychology* 33 (6):621–629.

Grady, M. F. 2010. Concussion in the adolescent athlete. *Current Problems in Pediatric and Adolescent Health Care* 40 (7):154–169.

Green, C. M., J. W. Kirk, A. K. Connery, D. A. Baker, and M. W. Kirkwood. 2014. The use of the rey 15-item test and recognition trial to evaluate noncredible effort after pediatric mild traumatic brain injury. *Journal of Clinical and Experimental Neuropsychology* 36 (3):261–267.

Grubenhoff, J. A., D. Currie, R. D. Comstock, E. Juarez-Colunga, L. Bajaj, and M. W. Kirkwood. 2016. Psychological factors associated with delayed resolution in children with concussion. *The Journal of Paediatrics* 174:27–32.

Hajek, C. A., K. O. Yeates, H. G. Taylor, B. Bangert, A. Dietrich, K. E. Nuss, J. Rusin, and M. Wright. 2010. Relationships among post-concussive symptoms and symptoms of PTSD in children following mild traumatic brain injury. *Brain Injury* 24 (2):100–109.

Harmon, K. G., J. Drezner, M. Gammons, K. Guskiewicz, M. Halstead, S. Herring, J. Kutcher, A. Pana, M. Putukian, and W. Roberts. 2013. American medical society for sports medicine position statement: Concussion in sport. *Clinical Journal of Sport Medicine* 23 (1):1–18. doi: 10.1097/JSM.0b013e31827f5f93.

Hawley, C. A. 2003. Reported problems and their resolution following mild, moderate and severe traumatic brain injury amongst children and adolescents in the UK. *Brain Injury* 17 (2):105–129.

Hearps, S., M. Takagi, F. E. Babl, S. Bressan, K. Truss, G. A. Davis, C. Godfrey, C. Clarke, M. Doyle, V. Rausa, K. Dunne, and V. Anderson. 2017. Validation of a score to determine time to postconcussive recovery. *Pediatrics* 139.

Hou, R., R. Moss-Morris, R. Peveler, K. Mogg, B. P. Bradley, and A. Belli. 2012. When a minor head injury results in enduring symptoms: A prospective investigation of risk factors for postconcussional syndrome after mild traumatic brain injury. *Journal of Neurol Neurosurg Psychiatry* 83 (2):217–223. doi: 10.1136/jnnp-2011-300767.

Karlin, A. M. 2011. Concussion in the pediatric and adolescent population: "Different population, different concerns". *Physical Medicine and Rehabilitation* 3 (10):S369–S379.

Kirkwood, M. W., R. L. Peterson, A. K. Connery, D. A. Baker, and J. A. Grubenhoff. 2014. Postconcussive symptom exaggeration after pediatric mild traumatic brain injury. *Pediatrics* 133 (4):643–650.

Kontos, A. P., T. Covassin, R. J. Elbin, and T. Parker. 2012. Depression and neurocognitive performance after concussion among male and female high school and collegiate athletes. *Archives of Physical Medicine and Rehabilitation* 93 (10):1751–1756.

Kozlowska, K., K. P. Nunn, D. Rose, A. Morris, R. A. Ouvrier, and J. Varghese. 2007. Conversion disorder in Australian pediatric practice. *Journal of the American Academy of Child & Adolescent Psychiatry* 46 (1):68–75.

Lagarde, E., L. R. Salmi, L. W. Holm, B. Contrand, F. Masson, R. Ribereau-Gayon, M. Laborey, and J. D. Cassidy. 2014. Association of symptoms following mild traumatic brain injury with posttraumatic stress disorder versus postconcussion syndrome. *The Journal of the American Medical Association Psychiatry* 71 (9):1032–1040.

Leddy, J. J., H. Sandhu, V. Sodhi, J. G. Baker, and B. Willer. 2012. Rehabilitation of concussion and post-concussion syndrome. *Sports Health* 4 (2):147–154. doi: 10.1177/1941738111433673.

Lewinsohn, P. M., J. R. Seeley, and I. H. Gotlib. 1997. Depression-related psychosocial variables: Are they specific to depression in adolescents? *Journal of Abnormal Psychology* 106 (3):365.

Li, L. and J. Liu. 2013. The effect of pediatric traumatic brain injury on behavioral outcomes: A systematic review. *Developmental Medicine & Child Neurology* 55 (1):37–45.

Luis, C. A. and W. Mittenberg. 2002. Mood and anxiety disorders following pediatric traumatic brain injury: A prospective study. *Journal of Clinical and Experimental Neuropsychology* 24 (3):270–279.

Massagli, T. L., J. R. Fann, B. E. Burington, K. M. Jaffe, W. J. Katon, and R. S. Thompson. 2004. Psychiatric illness after mild traumatic brain injury in children. *Archives of Physical Medicine and Rehabilitation* 85 (9):1428–1434.

Mather, F. J., R. L. Tate, and T. J. Hannan. 2003. Post-traumatic stress disorder in children following road traffic accidents: A comparison of those with and without mild traumatic brain injury. *Brain Injury* 17 (12):1077–1087.

Max, J. E., E. A. Wilde, E. D. Bigler, M. MacLeod, A. C. Vasquez, A. T. Schmidt, S. B. Chapman, G. Hotz, T. T. Yang, and H. S. Levin. 2012. Psychiatric disorders after pediatric traumatic brain injury: A prospective, longitudinal, controlled study. *The Journal of Neuropsychiatry and Clinical Neurosciences* 24 (4):427–436.

Max, J. E., E. Keatley, E. A. Wilde, E. D. Bigler, H. S. Levin, R. J. Schachar, A. Saunders, L. Ewing-Cobbs, S. B. Chapman, and M. Dennis. 2011. Anxiety disorders in children and adolescents in the first six months after traumatic brain injury. *The Journal of Neuropsychiatry and Clinical Neurosciences* 23 (1):29–39.

McCrory, P., W. Meeuwisse, J. Dvorak, M. Aubry, J. Bailes, S. Broglio, R. C. Cantu, D. Cassidy, R. J. Echemendia, R. J. Castellani et al. 2017. Consensus statement on concussion in sport-the 5th international conference on concussion in sport held in Berlin, October 2016. *British Journal of Sports Medicine*. doi: 10.1136/bjsports-2017-097699.

McKinlay, A., J. C. Dalrymple-Alford, L. J. Horwood, and D. M. Fergusson. 2002. Long term psychosocial outcomes after mild head injury in early childhood. *Journal of Neurology, Neurosurgery & Psychiatry* 73 (3):281–288.

Meehan, W. P. and R. Mannix. 2010. Pediatric concussions in United States emergency departments in the years 2002 to 2006. *The Journal of Pediatrics* 157 (6):889–893.

Moore, E. L., L. Terryberry-Spohr, and D. A. Hope. 2006. Mild traumatic brain injury and anxiety sequelae: A review of the literature. *Brain Injury* 20 (2):117–132.

Nampiaparampil, D. E. 2008. Prevalence of chronic pain after traumatic brain injury: A systematic review. *The Journal of the American Medical Association* 300 (6):711–719.

O'Connor, S. S., D. F. Zatzick, J. Wang, N. Temkin, T. D. Koepsell, K. M. Jaffe, D. Durbin, M. S. Vavilala, A. Dorsch, and F. P. Rivara. 2012. Association between posttraumatic stress, depression, and functional impairments in adolescents 24 months after traumatic brain injury. *Journal of Traumatic Stress* 25 (3):264–271.

Olsson, K. A., O. T. Lloyd, R. M. LeBrocque, L. McKinlay, V. A. Anderson, and J. A. Kenardy. 2013. Predictors of child post-concussion symptoms at 6 and 18 months following mild traumatic brain injury. *Brain Injury* 27 (2):145–157.

Rockhill, C., I. Kodish, C. DiBattisto, M. Macias, C. Varley, and S. Ryan. 2010. Anxiety disorders in children and adolescents. *Current Problems in Pediatric and Adolescent Health Care* 40 (4):66–99.

Root, J. M., N. S. Zuckerbraun, L. Wang, D. G. Winger, D. Brent, A. Kontos, and R. W. Hickey. 2016. History of somatization is associated with prolonged recovery from concussion. *The Journal of Pediatrics* 174:39–44.

Sady, M. D., C. G. Vaughan, and G. A. Gioia. 2011. School and the concussed youth: Recommendations for concussion education and management. *Physical Medicine and Rehabilitation Clinics of North America* 22 (4):701–719, ix. doi: 10.1016/j.pmr.2011.08.008.

Silver, J. M. 2012. Effort, exaggeration and malingering after concussion. *Journal of Neurology, Neurosurgery & Psychiatry* 83 (8):836–841.

Stancin, T., S. L. Wade, N. C. Walz, K. O. Yeates, and H. G. Taylor. 2008. Traumatic brain injuries in early childhood: Initial impact on the family. *Journal of Developmental & Behavioral Pediatrics* 29 (4):253–261.

Thomas, D. G., J. N. Apps, R. G. Hoffmann, M. McCrea, and T. Hammeke. 2015. Benefits of strict rest after acute concussion: A randomized controlled trial. *Pediatrics* 135 (2):213–23. doi: 10.1542/peds.2014-0966.

Wood, R. L., G. O'Hagan, C. Williams, M. McCabe, and N. Chadwick. 2014. Anxiety sensitivity and alexithymia as mediators of postconcussion syndrome following mild traumatic brain injury. *Journal of Head Trauma Rehabilitation* 29 (1):E9–E17. doi: 10.1097/HTR.0b013e31827eabba.

Wood, R. L., M. McCabe, and J. Dawkins. 2011. The role of anxiety sensitivity in symptom perception after minor head injury: An exploratory study. *Brain Injury* 25 (13–14):1296–1299. doi: 10.3109/02699052.2011.624569.

Woodrome, S. E., K. O. Yeates, H. G. Taylor, J. Rusin, B. Bangert, A. Dietrich, K. Nuss, and M. Wright. 2011. Coping strategies as a predictor of post-concussive symptoms in children with mild traumatic brain injury versus mild orthopedic injury. *Journal of International Neuropsychology Society* 17 (2):317–326. doi: 10.1017/S1355617710001700.

Yeates, K. O., H. G. Taylor, J. Rusin, B. Bangert, A. Dietrich, K. Nuss, and M. Wright. 2012. Premorbid child and family functioning as predictors of post-concussive symptoms in children with mild traumatic brain injuries. *International Journal of Developmental Neuroscience* 30 (3):231–237.

Zemek, R., N. Barrowman, S. B. Freedman, J. Gravel, I. Gagnon, C. McGahern, M. Aglipay, G. Sangha, K. Boutis, D. Beer et al., and Team Pediatric Emergency Research Canada Concussion. 2016. Clinical risk score for persistent postconcussion symptoms among children with acute concussion in the ED. *The Journal of the American Medical Association* 315 (10):1014–1025. doi: 10.1001/jama.2016.1203.

*section three*

---

*Recovery and beyond*

## chapter twelve

# Return to school
## When and how should return to school be organized after a concussion?

*Gerard A. Gioia*

### Contents

### Introduction

Traumatic brain injury (TBI) is recognized as a significant public health concern with *mild* TBI (mTBI) as the most common presentation. There is also a growing understanding of the necessity of the student's successful return to school and provision of appropriate supports (Davis et al., 2017; Halstead et al., 2013). Beyond the statements of need, the empirical literature is growing in efforts to define the type of needs and associated supports (e.g., Ransom et al., 2016; Glang et al., 2014). Despite the recovery of most children and adolescents with mTBI within four weeks (Zemek et al., 2016), the process of returning to school is not a simple issue. As with any other medical or neurological disorder, it requires a collaborative relationship between the health-care provider, school personnel, family, and student. To accomplish the goal of a successful and productive return, the need exists to operationalize the process for all involved (Gioia, 2016).

This chapter proposes a pathway for health-care providers and schools to standardize the practical management of the student with mTBI. School return must also be contextualized within the full continuum of mTBI care from its initial diagnosis to its final recovery. This pathway spans the point of initial communication with the school of the student's injury through to its full recovery and resumption of the student's preinjury school program. To ensure proper school reentry, the family and student must receive active and coordinated guidance across the care continuum by the informed health-care provider and the prepared school team.

Regarding terminology, we use the term mTBI in this chapter, to include the term *concussion*, defined as a TBI induced by traumatic biomechanical forces secondary to direct or indirect forces to the head. It produces a disturbance of brain function that is related to dysfunction of neurometabolism (Giza and Hovda, 2014) and neurotransmission (Smith et al., 2003) rather than macrostructural injury and is typically associated with normal structural neuroimaging findings (i.e., CT scan, MRI). The mTBI typically does not involve a loss of consciousness with only 12.9% reported in the large Canadian 5P pediatric emergency department (ED) study (Zemek et al., 2016). The injury results in a constellation of symptoms manifested in physical, cognitive, emotional, and sleep-related domains. Duration of symptoms is variable and may last for as short as several minutes and last for as long as several days, weeks, or months in some cases. The most recent estimate of time to recovery in the pediatric 5P study indicates that 30% of children and adolescents remain symptomatic past four weeks (Zemek et al., 2016).

## Partnering in the neighborhood of mild traumatic brain injury care

The care of children and adolescents with mTBI occurs across a number of settings, from its initial presentation and diagnosis to its final recovery. In returning the student to school, the mTBI care continuum must be understood, including the unique and complementary roles each partner plays. Active role definition and performance will not only optimize the student's positive movement toward clinical recovery but also their successful reintegration into school.

The mTBI *neighborhood* can potentially include a variety of health-care providers such as emergency and urgent care practitioners, sports medicine clinicians, as well as primary care and specialty care providers. Fundamentally, mTBI is a medical/neurological diagnosis requiring the active role of the health-care provider in defining its clinical symptom manifestation and guiding its active treatment (Gioia, 2015, 2016). This brain injury should never be viewed as simply *a concussion* with passive nonmedical management as this will increase risk of reinjury and a more complicated recovery (Terwilliger et al., 2016). In the early stage of an mTBI, important medical decisions must be made about the timing of the student's return to school, the types of tolerable daily activities that the student may engage in, and the degree of participation or restriction in physical (sport and recreation) and social activities. To ensure coordinated guidance across recovery, direct and explicit communication across the care system is critically important.

The school setting though not a health-care setting per se, nevertheless, plays a particularly important role in the mTBI care continuum as the *job* of the student places physical, cognitive, and social demands on the recovering brain. For a variety of reasons, students should be reintegrated back into their school environment as soon as possible. This process must, however, be done with careful and strategic preparation. School personnel, as the experts in the educational process, is charged with the important task of facilitating this reentry, making the individualized symptom-targeted adjustments and accommodations to the student's academic, social, and physical program. At the same time, the school should not be making these programmatic adaptations in isolation. The health-care provider must provide an accurate and timely diagnosis with appropriate management guidance based on the student's unique injury presentation, providing for a smooth handoff to the school. Each of the mTBI *neighbors* must carry out their unique yet complementary roles and tasks with collaborative communication.

## Mild TBI and school learning and performance

Special education programming for students with severe TBI in the United States has existed since the 1990 amendment to P.L. 94-142 (Education for All Handicapped Children) to address their academic needs (http://idea.ed.gov/explore/view/p/,root,regs,300,A,300%252E8,c,12). In contrast, only recently have the educational needs of students with mTBI been recognized. In 2010, the CDC published its initial *Heads Up* toolkit for schools (https://www.cdc.gov/headsup/schools), providing an overview of the issues that schools might face and the types of problems and associated supports that they might be provided to the returning student. That same year McGrath (2010) began the discussion, specifically within the sport mTBI arena, providing a framework for athletic trainers to support the academic needs of student athletes who were returning to school. Sady et al. (2011) followed up with a further description of the likely effects of an mTBI on the student's academic learning and performance and also discussed the effects of excessive, unsupported cognitive activity on the student's recovery. Furthermore, system-level requirements to provide school-based supports were also discussed in this paper. At a broader organizational level, the American Academy of Pediatrics (AAP) (Halstead et al., 2013) and the Canadian Pediatric Society (CPS) (Purcell, 2014) communicated the importance of the return to school process in their statements to the North American pediatric community. Since that time, the momentum has continued with a host of authors writing about the importance of supporting the student's return (e.g., Popoli et al., 2014; DeMatteo, McCauley et al., 2015).

Most recently, the pediatric subgroup reviewed the available empirical literature on sport-related concussion (SRC) in children and adolescents for the 2016 International Concussion in Sport Group meeting in Berlin, Germany including the question "What factors must be considered in 'return to school' following concussion and what strategy or accommodations should be followed?" (Davis et al., 2017). Eleven articles were reviewed revealing five factors that influence the return to school process: (1) Age: adolescents tend to take longer to recover, longer to return to school and are more concerned about possible adverse academic effects than younger children; (2) Symptom load/severity: students with a greater number of and more severe symptoms tend to take longer to return to school and require more academic accommodations; (3) School resources: schools with concussion policies that focus on student/parent education demonstrate best-practice management, provide more academic supports, and are more likely to form school-based concussion management teams; (4) Medical follow-up after injury: students who receive medical follow-up are more likely to receive academic supports in their school return; and (5) Effects on certain subjects: certain subjects are more challenging during concussion recovery (i.e., math, reading/language arts). Stemming from this literature, five recommendations were generated:

1. "All schools are encouraged to have a concussion policy that includes education on SRC prevention and management for teachers, staff, students, and parents and should offer appropriate academic accommodations and support to students recovering from SRC.
2. Students should have regular medical follow-up following an SRC to monitor recovery and help with return to school.
3. Students may require temporary absence from school after injury.
4. Clinicians should assess risk factors/modifiers that may prolong recovery and require more/prolonged/formal academic accommodations. In particular, adolescents may require more academic support during concussion recovery.
5. Further research is required to determine the appropriate return to school accommodations for children and adolescents with prolonged SRC symptoms." (p. 8)

Effects of mTBI on Learning and Performance. To set the scene for the operational pathway that follows, a brief description is provided of the potential effects of mTBI on the student's learning and performance in school as well as critical system issues that should be considered. The effects of mTBI on the student can take a variety of forms and are related to their particular symptom manifestation, which can be described within four basic symptom categories—physical, cognitive, emotional, and sleep. McGrath (2010), Sady et al. (2011), and the aforementioned CDC school toolkit all describe these possible academic effects. Several studies provide empirical evidence of adverse academic effects. Ransom et al. (2015) described the types of self- and parent-reported effects on academic learning and performance in elementary, middle, and high-school students diagnosed with mTBI. In comparison with students with recent mTBI who had recovered, actively symptomatic students and their parents reported significantly higher levels of concern for the impact of mTBI on school performance and significantly more school-related problems than recovered peers and their parents. 88% of students in the symptomatic group reported at least one school problem related to symptoms interfering with school performance (e.g., headaches, fatigue, problems concentrating), and 77% reported diminished academic skills (e.g., difficulty taking notes, spending more time on homework, problems studying) in comparison with a minority of students in the just recovered group. High school reported significantly more adverse academic effects than middle and elementary school students. Greater severity of post-mTBI symptoms was associated with more school-related problems and worse academic effects, regardless of time since injury. A recent paper by Ransom et al. (2016) found that higher levels of post-concussion executive dysfunction and symptom burden were significant predictors of greater academic problems. Wasserman et al. (2016) describe greater overall academic dysfunction (e.g., attention, memory problems, and increased exertion-related symptoms), using a self-report measure, at one week but not at one-month post-injury in student–athletes who sustained mTBI compared with an orthopedic injury control group. Baker et al. (2015) performed a retrospective telephone survey (14.9 months post-injury) of 13–19-year-old students and found that symptom severity was most predictive of problems in school, including the number of days missed. Certain symptoms had a greater relationship to school problems including headache, reduced concentration and memory, and fatigue. None of these studies report whether a systematic mTBI-support structure was in place at the schools, leaving unanswered the possible contribution of the school program and environment to the student's academic challenges.

Academic Supports. In addition to describing the effects of the mTBI on academic learning and performance and the Berlin summary recommendations, a number of papers provide logical guidance regarding adjustments and accommodations to support the student. As part of the support process to start, a gradual reintroduction into the school environment and academic program is recommended by a number of authors (McGrath, 2010; Gioia, 2015, 2016; Gioia et al., 2016; Sady et al., 2011; Master et al., 2012; Purcell et al., 2016; DeMatteo, Stazyk et al., 2015) although, to date, no research has provided specific evidence-informed guidelines for this gradual return. Interestingly, in the spirit of the active rehabilitation movement (Leddy et al., 2016; Collins et al., 2016; Gagnon et al., 2009), none of these more recent papers recommend that the student be withheld from school until fully asymptomatic. Most recommend an orderly progression based on the student's symptom status and the student's tolerance for engaging in academic activity. We provide an example of a 6-stage gradual return process (Gioia, 2016) with the proposed levels of acceptable school-related activity at each stage and criteria to consider in advancing the student to the next stage. Further research is needed to validate appropriate recommendations for academic support (Carson et al., 2014).

While there are as of yet no hard and fast evidence-based guidelines as to when a student would return to school following an mTBI, the health-care provider and the parents of the injured student must nevertheless address this issue. It is generally recommended that most students remain out of school only one or two days to facilitate the acute recovery process. In a randomized controlled trial of children and adolescents with mTBI, students who were restricted from school and other activities for only 1–2 days exhibited better recovery indicators than those who were restricted for five days (Thomas et al., 2015). Thus, most students will likely do well with restriction from school for only a brief period, whereas a small percent may require a longer period due to more significant symptom severity. This decision must be an individualized decision based on the child/adolescent's symptom burden. Corwin et al. (2014) reported that higher symptom burden was related to a greater number of days out of school prior to return, but this sample was a higher acuity, specialty clinic sample and does not provide guidance on a general rule. It may be that certain symptom patterns have a particular relationship to the timing of school return. For example, Corwin et al. (2015) found that students with vestibular symptoms—either abnormal gaze stability (VOR) or abnormal tandem gait—took a significantly longer time to return to school (median 59 days vs 6 days, $P = .001$). Without an evidence-based guide to the optimal time to return to school, the severity of the symptom burden should be considered. Gioia (2016) and Halstead et al. (2013) recommend a test trial of cognitive activity prior to school return to determine if 30 minutes of school activity can be tolerated. If so, return to school—at least a partial day—is recommended. This decision on the timing of the student's return to school highlights the critical importance of a medical examination soon after the injury.

Communication. A developing literature exists to reinforce the need for active communication between the health-care provider, family, and school. Zuckerbraun and colleagues (2014) demonstrated that educating parents in the ED with explicit information about mTBI symptoms, and their management helped parents to advocate for their children in returning to school and other activities. In this study, a return to school letter provided from the ED facilitated greater academic assistance given to the student upon return to school. In addition, Grubenhoff and colleagues (2015) reported that families who pursued outpatient clinic services following a visit to the ED received greater academic accommodations than those who did not receive follow-up outpatient services, suggesting that communication between the health-care provider and school benefited the student.

## Improving the systems of mild traumatic brain injury care

Policies and Procedures. To promote the systematic delivery of individual student supports, preparation and readiness are needed by the school and health-care systems. Written policies and procedures are critical guiding organizational documents to direct the school and health-care providers in providing systematic care to students across recovery (Davis et al., 2017; Gioia et al., 2016). Implementation of active policies to provide academic supports has been advocated for students with mTBI (Sady et al., 2011; Popoli et al., 2014; DeMatteo, Stazyk et al., 2015; Baker et al., 2014). The benefits of active policies for mTBI service in the schools were demonstrated in the Brain 101 program (http://brain101.orcasinc.com/) in Oregon (Glang et al., 2014) where school administrators were directed to create mTBI management policy and procedures, resulting in student athletes and parents demonstrating significantly greater mTBI knowledge, knowledge application, and behavioral intention to implement effective mTBI management practices. Recent examples of statewide mTBI policies for supporting school return can be found in North Carolina (Newlin & Hooper, 2015; http://www.nchealthyschools. org/legislation/stateboard/) and Ontario, Canada (http://www.edu.gov.on.ca/extra/ eng/ppm/158.pdf). Ideally, school-based policies should address (1) a brief description of mTBI, (2) definition of the school *receiving team* to guide reentry, (3) the gradual process to assist the student's return into school life (learning, social activity, and so on), (4) a process for communicating with the health-care provider(s) and family, and (5) criteria for when students can safely return to physical activity and full cognitive activity (Gioia et al., 2016).

In the health-care field, no state or national professional body has developed formal policies or procedures to prepare their respective members to develop competencies in the return to school process. The athletic training community has been the most active in researching its members' knowledge and preparation to support the student's academic return (Kasamatsu et al., 2016; Williams et al., 2015). As previously noted, the AAP (Halstead et al., 2013) and CPS (Purcell, 2014) have written on the importance of addressing return to school needs of students with mTBI, but as of yet neither national body has been active in developing a practical training program for pediatricians.

Defining Roles. As a key element of the policy and procedure process, mTBI-specific roles should be defined within the schools to efficiently and effectively manage the return and support processes (CDC, 2012; Sady et al., 2011; Glang et al., 2014; Gioia, 2016; Gioia et al., 2016). A writing group of the National Collaborative on Childhood Brain Injury (NCCBI) proposed guidance to state and local boards of education on the essential components of a statewide educational infrastructure to support the management of students with mTBI (Gioia et al., 2016). State and local policy considerations are emphasized to promote implementation of a consistent process, including five key components: (1) definition and training of the interdisciplinary school team; (2) professional development of the school and medical communities; (3) identification, assessment, and progress monitoring protocols; (4) a flexible set of intervention strategies to accommodate students' recovery needs; and (5) systematized protocols for active communication among medical, school, and family team members. These consensus-based elements are practical guides for effective program implementation.

A very practical example of specific school-based roles is presented by the BrainSTEPS program (www.brainsteps.net) in Pennsylvania where two primary roles are defined: (1) medical/symptom monitor and (2) an academic program monitor. The medical/symptom monitor liaisons with the community health-care provider and monitors the symptom status of the student in school, using a standardized symptom scale, and reporting this status to the academic program monitor. The academic program monitor oversees and guides the academic support process, linking the student symptom status with specific accommodations and adjustments, and liaisoning with the student, teachers, and medical/symptom monitor. These two roles do not necessarily have defined personnel as each school's resources can vary but ideally the medical/symptom monitor role would be handled by a school health person (e.g., nurse), psychologist, or athletic trainer. The academic program monitor should have knowledge and experience with academic programming, ideally defined as a guidance counselor, administrator, or teacher.

Education and Training. Education and training of school personnel are also a critical component of an mTBI-supportive school environment. Needless to say, the knowledge of school personnel is a necessary step in providing the appropriate support services. As previously noted, the Brain 101 Concussion Playbook program (Glang et al., 2014; Oregon Center for Applied Science, 2007) demonstrated the facilitating effect of training school staff and students in mTBI knowledge and process. The knowledge and support of school administrators are also a key component in providing top-down support of returning students. Heyer et al. (2015) surveyed principals' knowledge and practices related to mTBI management, reporting that only 37% of principals had mTBI training in the past year. Those with training were more likely to promote training of other school faculty although most principals indicated a willingness to provide students with short-term academic accommodations. Only a minority, however, communicated with families using a written academic plan. Kasamatsu et al. (2016) and Williams et al. (2015) surveyed athletic trainers' practices in supporting the academic supports of student–athletes, identifying their important role in the return to school process. Importantly, the athletic trainers are employed directly by their schools and with more school-related experience were more familiar with academic supports. Finally, Davies et al. (2016) describe the importance of system-level training in mTBI management, including school psychologists, to the positive supports of students with mTBI.

## Components of the school mild traumatic brain injury management pathway

In the previous sections, we have lobbied hard for the need for a well-prepared collaborative partnership between the health-care provider(s) and the school to implement proper school management following an mTBI, each possessing unique and complementary areas of expertise. In the following, we specify the roles for the health-care provider(s) and the school personnel. For the school roles, we borrow heavily from the excellent BrainSTEPS program and add definition to the health-care provider role to provide a complementary, coordinated system.

Health-care Provider Role. The primary role of the health-care provider—whether primary care provider or emergency/urgent care—is to conduct the initial medical evaluation, define the student's symptom profile, and communicate this information to the school for their use in developing a plan of supports. There are a number of potential ways to communicate with the school—we recommend the use of a return to school letter (sample provided in Appendix A), as its use produced a demonstrable increase in student supports (Zuckerbraun et al., 2014). The information in this letter provides the basis for the school experts to develop a feasible educational plan to support the student's return. Key elements of the return to school letter should include (a) the proposed date of return to school (if it can be determined), (b) the student's current symptoms, and (c) necessary safety restrictions. Receipt of the return to school letter provides the school with the necessary information to translate the identified symptoms into symptom-targeted academic accommodations, providing individualized support to the recovering student.[13] As previously noted, the use of this return to school letter resulted in a significant positive effect in facilitating school management as with a significantly greater number of children receiving academic supports compared with the control group that did not use the letter. In addition to the earlier components in the letter, some health-care providers may be comfortable in providing specific recommendations for school adjustments and accommodations. In the spirit of collaboration, these recommendations should be given consideration by the school though not obligatory until the educational experts examine their relevance and capacity for implementation.

School Personnel Role. In the handoff from the mTBI-informed health-care provider—defining the student's symptom profile—the school must be prepared to receive the injured student and translate the symptom pattern into appropriate individualized supports. Although the same goal and general process of supporting the student's successful return applies to all, each school is unique in their environment and resources (e.g., personnel, skillsets, assigned duties). In addition, the clinical manifestations of an mTBI vary from student to student. As a result, we do not advocate a *one size fits all* plan of mTBI management. The gradual return to school progression should be individually adapted (see Appendix B, ACE Gradual Return to School Guide). Each school management plan starts with a definition of the individualized medical/neurological needs of the injured student as specified by the health-care provider(s), proceeding to translate these needs into a workable educational support plan, to be implemented by a coordinated team of school personnel.

Borrowing from the excellent BrainSTEPS program, one school-based person should serve in a medical/symptom liaison role (e.g., nurse, school psychologist, or athletic trainer) who tracks symptoms periodically, monitors for improvement (or worsening), and communicates with the school team, health-care provider, and family. In addition, an academic liaison role (e.g., guidance counselor, school psychologist) should be defined to coordinate the cognitive/academic adjustments and accommodations, using an academic log to track and guide adjustments. Additional school members include the classroom teachers who must be observant of the cognitive and emotional effects of injuries detected in the classroom such as increased problems paying attention or concentrating, greater challenges remembering or learning new information, needing more time to complete tasks or assignments, greater irritability and less tolerance for stressors, and the possibility of increased headache or fatigue symptoms when doing schoolwork. Throughout the course of recovery, it is essential that students receive a consistent, positive, and supportive message from all school staff about performance expectations during recovery.

## Implementing the school mild traumatic brain injury management pathway

Returning students with mTBI to school is a multistep process that can be operational-ized in a systematic manner, utilizing the key personnel and roles previously described. Implementing a systematic process of school supports serves the combined clinical recov-ery and educational goals of the student. The pathway is intended to respect the practical workflow of the school setting, implementing the proper supports standardly and effec-tively. Such a pathway recognizes the likely need to adapt the process to the resources of a given school setting. Figure 12.1 presents the seven-step school mTBI management

### mTBI School Management Pathway Worksheet

| Step | Event | Action | Completion Date |
|---|---|---|---|
| | **Prior to School Return** | | |
| 1 | School notification of mTBI<br><br>Injury Date:_____ | MTBI Management Team alerted | |
| 2 | Healthcare Provider Communication/ Return to School Letter<br><br>Date of Return:_____ | a. Symptom Monitor: Reviews symptom status & contacts family<br><br>b. Academic Monitor: Coordinates with Symptom Monitor to construct academic management plan (e.g., STAMP) | a._____<br><br>b._____ |
| 3 | Academic Management Plan Created | Academic Monitor: Reviews Academic Management Plan with teachers to prepare for student's return | |
| | **Return to School** | | |
| 4 | First Day of Return to School | a. Symptom Monitor: Meets with student to re-assess symptom status, notes any changes<br><br>b. Academic Monitor: Makes final academic management plan changes; counsels student on plan | a._____<br><br>b._____ |
| 5 | Academic Management Plan implemented | a. Symptom Monitor: Arrange symptom monitoring schedule<br><br>b. Academic Monitor: Update teaching team if needed | a._____<br><br>b._____ |
| 6a | Progress Monitoring | a. Symptom Monitor: Periodic symptom updates with student, from family/ healthcare providers<br><br>b. Academic Monitor: Collects weekly updates from teachers | a._____<br><br>b._____ |
| 6b | Academic Management Plan Adjusted | Symptom Monitor & Academic Monitor discuss changes to academic management plan<br>Academic Monitor informs student/ teacher of changes | Adj 1_____<br>Adj 2_____<br>Adj 3_____ |
| 7a | Recovery/ Return to Full Academic Participation | Supports no longer required | a._____ |
| 7b | Complicated Recovery/ Additional Supports Assessed | Referral to HCP for further assessment of complicating factors, additional programming supports | b._____ |

*Figure 12.1* mTBI school management pathway.

pathway beginning with the school's initial notification of the injury and concluding when recovery has been achieved or a more complicated, protracted recovery has been identified, necessitating referral for specialized services.

This pathway serves to build a routine support process identifying the events, actions, and tools prior to school return and then when the student returns, developing, implementing, and modifying an individualized symptom—targeted academic support plan. We recommend adopting a school mTBI management pathway worksheet such as Figure 12.1 to guide and document the actions taken.

To illustrate the use of the pathway, we describe the case of JT, a 14-year-old ninth-grade male.

*JT is an active athlete who plays soccer, basketball, and lacrosse although his injury was sustained while skateboarding on a Monday afternoon. He has a history of one prior mTBI at age of 8 as a result of a fall that took 1 week to recover. He has no history of learning disabilities, attention-deficit/hyperactivity disorder (ADHD), anxiety, or depression. He also has no history of chronic headache. His recent injury resulted from falling from his skateboard and striking the back of his head on the ground. He was wearing a helmet at the time. There was no loss of consciousness, but JT does not recall 10 minutes after the injury (post-traumatic amnesia) and presented with an initial period of confusion. He was evaluated by his pediatrician that day using the acute concussion evaluation (ACE) and diagnosed with an mTBI. He recommended no school for two days. The symptom evaluation indicated physical symptoms of headaches, dizziness, fatigue, sensitivity to light, blurry vision; cognitive symptoms of fogginess, problems concentrating, and slow thinking; emotional symptoms of irritability; and sleeping more than usual. He was instructed by his pediatrician to stay home for two days with a relatively low level of activity and a likely return to school on the third day post-injury.*

## Step 1. School notification of mild traumatic brain injury

The school mTBI management pathway begins at the moment that the school is notified of a student that has sustained an mTBI. This will typically be the student's parent although it is possible that another member of the school provides the notification if the injury occurs on school grounds or in a school-sponsored activity (e.g., athletic trainer following a sport-related injury). The school must be prepared with a planned response regardless of whether it is an elementary, middle, or high-school student. The assigned mTBI medical and academic liasons are alerted and stand ready to prepare for the next steps in the development of a support plan. The injury date is noted as is the return date if known.

*In JT's case, the school was notified of the injury by his mother on Tuesday with the recommendation of no return until Thursday, with a likely half-day attendance the first two days. The mTBI liasons, consisting of the symptom monitor and academic monitor were alerted. A school mTBI management pathway worksheet (Figure 12.1) is initiated.*

## Step 2. Health-care provider communication/return to school letter

The school should receive a communication from the health-care provider, typically via the family, in the form of a return to school letter, detailing the student's injury, symptom profile, and likely date of return. Upon receipt of this communication from the health-care provider, the symptom monitor reviews the symptom status and the proposed date of return to school. The symptom monitor contacts the family and student to review the student's status and progress, and reviews the process of return (Steps 4–7) with a focus on the near-term events and actions. The academic monitor is alerted about the injury details and symptom status to be used in the development of an initial academic management plan.

*The symptom monitor, upon receipt of the return to school letter calls JT's family to check in on his status and informs them that an academic management plan will be developed based on the pediatricians initial symptom evaluation. She also requests a meeting with the student and parent on the first day of his return to review the initial academic management plan. The return to school letter indicates physical restrictions including no physical education class, no contact sports, and no physical activity during recess. The academic monitor notifies JT's teaching team of the injury and alerts them to the upcoming receipt of the academic management plan.*

## Step 3. Academic management plan created by academic monitor

The academic management plan is the tool that translates the student's symptom profile into specific accommodations to support their academic program. See the symptom-targeted academic management plan (STAMP) as an example in Appendix C. This tool is set up to directly translate the specific symptoms into related accommodations and adjustments to the student's academic program so as to not exacerbate the symptoms yet allow the student optimal participation in their school program. The accommodations and adjustments are only necessary to the extent that the symptoms have an adverse effect upon the student's academic learning and performance. It is possible that a student may present with certain symptoms that do not affect their academic learning and performance (e.g., dizziness when standing from a laying down position) or are very mild (e.g., resolving headache) and do not require an active accommodation or adjustment of the student's school program.

*Examination of the return to school letter for JT indicates five physical symptoms, three cognitive symptoms, and one emotional symptom to be addressed in his STAMP. The pediatrician also indicated that the symptoms worsen with cognitive activity although it is not yet known whether they worsen with physical activity. Translating the attention/ concentration problems into accommodations results in the recommendation for shorter assignments, breaking down the tasks/tests into chunks, and a lighter workload with less than 30 minutes of homework at night. His difficulties with processing speed were accommodated through allowances for extended time to complete his work. The fatigue and fogginess issue were addressed by allowing 10–15-minute rest breaks during classes. For the physical symptoms, interspersed rest breaks were recommended in addition to an allowance for a short nap in a quiet location, if necessary. His light sensitivity could be managed by allowing him to wear sunglasses and/or sitting away from bright lights. In addition, limiting exposure to the SmartBoard as well as other light emitting devices was recommended. His dizziness/balance problems were addressed by allowing him to transition to the next class before the bell rings to reduce walking through crowded hallways. His fatigue and lack of energy were managed by periodic rest breaks and passive participation if he could not keep up the work. Finally, irritability was addressed by attempting to reduce overall stimulation and stressors whenever possible. The STAMP was shared with JT's classroom teachers and adapted to the specific type of class and workload demands.*

## Step 4. First day of return to school

On the day that the student returns, the symptom monitor and academic monitor meet with the student and parent with several tasks to accomplish. The symptom monitor reassesses the student's symptom status for any changes in the intervening days to allow an up-to-date academic management plan. A sample symptom monitor form is presented in Appendix D. The symptom information is communicated to the academic monitor who makes the final changes to the plan, communicates the plan with the teachers, and counsels the student on the use of the STAMP to support their academic return. The student is informed that each teacher has been made aware of the adjustment/accommodation plan.

*Upon JT's return on Thursday, the symptom monitor meets with he and his parent to assess his symptom status. Over the three days since the injury, several of the symptoms have reduced in their intensity including the balance/dizziness and irritability. In addition, JT reports that on the prior day, he was able to read some light text in his history book for approximately 30 minutes without worsening his headaches, fatiguing him significantly, or having troubles concentrating on the material. The academic monitor reviews the adjusted STAMP with JT and his parent and gives them each a copy of the document. They discuss how these accommodations will be implemented and that his teachers have been made aware of the plan. The symptom monitor and academic monitor sets a follow-up schedule with JT to monitor his progress. On this first day of his return, which is only a half day, they ask JT to meet with them just prior to leaving so that they can assess the success of the initial day of his program and address any questions or concerns.*

## Step 5. Implementation of the academic management plan

In this stage of the school support pathway, the academic management plan is now implemented, which involves the symptom monitor meeting with the student to monitor his symptoms and the academic monitor meeting with the student and teachers periodically to review academic progress and/or problems. These meetings can be scheduled, based on the number and severity of symptoms, as either a daily process or every several days, depending on the need. During the initial days of the students return, it is probably worthwhile to check in with the student on a daily basis to ensure effective program implementation. Students with relatively milder symptoms may require less frequent meetings to monitor their progress, whereas students with more significant symptoms will likely require a tighter schedule of monitoring to ensure that the supports are appropriate.

*Given JT's relatively significant symptom profile, the decision was made to monitor his symptom status on a daily basis for the first week and then decide on the frequency after that time period. The monitoring of his academic progress was scheduled to occur on a weekly basis with JT and his teachers although the option was made available for JT to check in with the academic monitor at any point if any questions arose about the implementation of the academic management plan.*

## Step 6. Progress monitoring

Given the established schedule of progress monitoring, the student's symptom status and academic progress are monitored. The symptom monitor uses a formal symptom assessment scale (Appendix D) as gathered from the student and, in some cases, the parents and teachers. To keep the care team fully informed, this information is communicated periodically with the parents and the health-care provider(s). In the more typical recovery scenarios, new symptoms do not emerge and instead the number and severity of symptoms decrease. At times, however, particularly with complex recoveries, new symptoms may appear (e.g., anxiety, depressed mood), which require some additional accommodations to be made. In concert with the symptom monitor, the academic monitor collects weekly progress updates (see Appendix E for a sample academic monitor form) from the teachers and student regarding their participation and success as outlined in the STAMP and the gradual return to school plan. During these periodic monitoring meetings with the student and teachers, changes to the STAMP are made (e.g, reduction or removal of accommodations).

*JT's recovery over the first week was steady with a reduction in his headaches, sensitivity to light, fatigue, mental fogginess, and irritability. He began attending school full days as of the 3rd day of his return. The accommodations associated with these symptom targets were reduced and in some cases removed (e.g., no longer needing sunglasses for light sensitivity). JT's workload was gradually increased with 1 hour of homework now possible. The work that he missed was logged on the academic monitor form, with a decision by several of his teachers to excuse the less essential work assignments and quizzes.*

## Step 7. Recovery/Return to full academic participation

*Typical Recovery*: In the vast majority of cases, the student will demonstrate a gradual symptom resolution and recovery with positive movement toward full academic participation, including a full return to the school day as well as a gradual lessening of the symptom—targeted adjustments and accommodations. Given the variability in time to recovery, full return to the student's academic program may occur within a matter of several days or several weeks in the typical cases. As per the more recent epidemiological data, it is expected that up to 30% of students will not have reached full recovery by four weeks and will require some degree of continued academic supports.

*In the case of JT, he made a relatively typical recovery over the course of 3 weeks with gradual resolution of his symptoms and the associated adjustment of the necessary accommodations on the STAMP until none were needed, and he could participate fully in his academic program with no symptoms provoked by cognitive or physical activity. The symptom monitoring forms demonstrated this pattern of resolution of all symptoms to his preinjury baseline level, whereas the academic monitoring forms indicated JT's positive capacity to increase his amount of classwork and homework as well as his ability to now take quizzes and tests for which he was prepared.*

*Complicated Recovery/Additional Supports*: In the case of students whose symptoms have not resolved within 3–4 weeks' time, continued academic supports will be necessary. However, with active and regular communication between the school, parents, and the health-care providers, referrals to mTBI specialists and/or rehabilitation services for these students should be an expected matter of course. Depending on the student's pattern of persistent symptoms, the follow-up services will be specific to the persisting issues such as the need for headache management, vestibular rehabilitation, aerobic therapy; cognitive treatments for poor concentration or memory problems; or behavior medicine services for emotional symptoms such as increased anxiety or mood problems. With these active rehabilitation services in place, it is rare that students will require any additional accommodations after a period of several months. If, however, the need exists, a more formal process of initiating a 504 plan may be needed.

## Summary

Returning the student with mTBI to school is a central task in the care continuum, involving active communication and collaboration among the health-care, family, school, and student. To provide a smooth and effective return to school following mTBI, this neighborhood of partners must follow a shared process that is based on the needs of the student as they proceed toward recovery. To accomplish this goal, a seven-step operational pathway is described from the time of the school's first notification of the injury through to complete recovery, working with mTBI-prepared school liaisons (medical/symptom, academic) and employing a standardized process that works collaboratively with the health-care providers, family, and student to facilitate the systematic management of the student. Operationalizing and standardizing these processes by applying individualized symptom-targeted adjustments and accommodations, progress monitoring, and referral/ communication using the clinical pathway and tools will better serve the needs of students with mTBI returning to school. To ensure effective school reentry, the family and student must receive active and coordinated guidance across the care continuum by the informed health-care provider and the prepared school team. Each collaborative partner has a unique and complementary role that will not only optimize the student's successful reintegration into school but also contribute to a positive movement toward clinical recovery. Recommended actions and tools are provided to guide the school return process systematically.

Although this mTBI school management pathway provides a logical and systematic process for the health care, school, family, and student to follow, the field is still in need of further evidence to provide more precise guidance as recommended in the recent Berlin pediatric concussion statement (Davis et al., 2017). Issues requiring further study include the need to better predict the optimal timing to return the student to school incorporating as predictors the host of injury-related, personal, and environmental factors that produce the most effective recovery outcomes. The process would also benefit from further research of specific targeted interventions—specifying which adjustments and accommodations are critical for optimal school performance, at what time in the return process, delivered for how long, and tied to the student's specific clinical profile (subtype). In addition to student-centered research, the return to school process would benefit from further study of system-level interventions including demonstrating the effectiveness of team/role definition, training methods, and applications of the management pathway to different levels of schooling (elementary, middle, and high school).

# *Appendices*

## *Appendix A: ACE return to school letter*

### ACE POST-CONCUSSION
### RETURN TO SCHOOL LETTER

Dear School Staff:

_____ sustained a concussion on _____. Every concussion is different and recovery typically can take between several days to several weeks. While it is important for the student to return to school as soon as they can tolerate, the key to assisting recovery is to manage their physical and cognitive activity. Too much cognitive or physical activity can make symptoms worse and possibly prolong recovery, while too little activity can unnecessarily create anxiety and cause him/her to fall behind in their school work. As symptoms resolve and the student's learning/cognitive functioning returns to normal, they can gradually progress to their normal school day.

The student is currently reporting the following symptoms. They should be viewed as the targets for classroom accommodations and adjustments.

| PHYSICAL | | COGNITIVE | SOCIAL/EMOTIONAL |
|---|---|---|---|
| Headaches | Visual problems | Feeling foggy | Irritability / Easily Angered |
| Sensitivity to Light | Sensitivity to Noise | Memory loss | Nervousness |
| Vomiting | Nausea | Feeling slowed down | Sadness |
| Fatigue | Dizziness | Difficulty concentrating | Feeling more emotional |
| Balance Problems | Tingling | | |

Based on the current symptoms, he/she is ___ permitted to return to school. OR ___ is excused for ___ days. As general guidance, the student can return to school when:

(1) They can concentrate on school work for 30 minutes before symptoms worsen significantly, AND
(2) Symptoms reduce or disappear with cognitive rest breaks, allowing return to activity.

The student requires the following physical restrictions until cleared by a health professional:

* No physical activity during recess
* No PE class
* No Sports
   Other _____

Health Care Provider Signature _____     Date _____

Contact information: _____

---

### SCHOOL SUPPORTS

Students with post-concussion symptoms and/or neuropsychological dysfunction often need support to perform school related activities. The following accommodations and adjustments to the student's school program may be helpful to support the specific targeted symptoms.

| | |
|---|---|
| • Shortened day | • Support for prioritizing, organization and planning coursework |
| • Shortened classes | • No significant classroom or standardized testing |
| • Rest breaks during the day as needed | • Extended time to complete coursework, assignments, tests |
| • Reduced/modified homework | • Alternative/modified grading or reduced make up work |

*Appendix B: ACE gradual return to school guide*

## ACE Post-Concussion
### Gradual Return to School (GrRTS) Guide

***Use of the Gradual Return to School Guide:*** Every student's recovery from concussion is different. The five progressive stages were designed to give the medical provider and school team <u>general guidance</u> to assist the student's gradual return to school. The stages should not be viewed as absolute for every student if their symptoms do not warrant it. What is important is to strike a balance between providing the student with the necessary supports for symptom relief while progressing to their normal school schedule. Students with faster recoveries may skip a stage or two. Use of the ***Symptom Targeted Academic Management Plan*** should accompany this guide.

| Stage | Description | Level of Activity | Move to stage 2 when: |
|---|---|---|---|
| 1 | Return to School, Partial Day (1–3 hours) | • Attend 1–3 classes. Intersperse rest breaks.<br>• Scheduled rest breaks: ____ Rest breaks/ day in quiet area. ___ AM ___ PM ____ When symptoms worsen ("flash pass") ____ min.<br>• Expectations for productivity: Minimal.<br>• No classroom/ standardized tests. No homework.<br>• Attendance is primary goal<br>• Excused from Physical Education (PE) class. No recess. | ▪ Symptom status improving<br>▪ Tolerates 4–5 hours of activity-rest cycles<br>▪ 2–3 cognitive rest breaks built into school day |

| Stage | Description | Level of Activity | Move to stage 3 when: |
|---|---|---|---|
| 2 | Full Day, Maximal Supports (required throughout day) | • Attend most classes with 2–3 rest breaks (20–30 min).<br>• Scheduled rest breaks: ____ Rest breaks/ day in quiet area. ___ AM ___ PM ____ When symptoms worsen ("flash pass") ____ min.<br>• Expectations for productivity: Minimal – moderate.<br>• No classroom/ standardized tests.<br>• Homework < 60 minutes.<br>• Excused from Physical Education (PE) class. No recess. | ▪ Symptom number & severity improving<br>▪ Needs 1–2 cognitive rest breaks built into school day. |

| Stage | Description | Level of Activity | Move to stage 4 when: |
|---|---|---|---|
| 3 | Return to Full Day, Moderate Supports (provide in response to symptoms) | • Attend all classes with 1–2 rest breaks (20–30 min).<br>• Scheduled rest breaks: ____ Rest breaks/ day in quiet area. ___ AM ___ PM ____ When symptoms worsen ("flash pass") ____ min.<br>• Expectations for productivity: Moderate.<br>• No classroom/ standardized tests. Begin quizzes.<br>• Moderate homework 60–90 minutes .<br>• Design schedule for make-up work. Consider reducing or waiving missing/ outstanding work. Assign essential learning tasks.<br>• Excused from Physical Education (PE) class. No recess. | ▪ Continued symptom improvement<br>▪ Needs no more than 1 cognitive rest break per day |

| Stage | Description | Level of Activity | Move to stage 5 when: |
|---|---|---|---|
| 4 | Return to Full Day, Minimal Supports (Monitor final recovery) | • Attend all classes with 0–1 rest breaks (20–30 min) OR when symptoms worsen ("flash pass")<br>• Expectations for productivity: Moderate – maximum.<br>• Begin modified classroom tests (allow breaks, extra time, alternate formats). Number of classroom tests per day ____.<br>• Homework 90+ minutes.<br>• Begin to address make-up work.<br>• Excused from Physical Education (PE) class. No recess. | ▪ No active symptoms<br>▪ No exertional effects across the full school day. |

| Stage | Description | Level of Activity | Date of full return: |
|---|---|---|---|
| 5 | Full Return, No Supports Needed | • Full class schedule, no rest breaks.<br>• Maximum expectations for productivity.<br>• Address make-up work. | |

## *Appendix C: Symptom-targeted academic management plan (STAMP)*

To be completed by the Academic Monitor

**Student Name:** _____   **Date:** _____

Children's National.

### Symptom Targeted Academic Management Plan (STAMP)

Below, please see the symptoms they are currently experiencing. To promote recovery, the student will be provided with the following classroom accommodations that support their academic learning and performance:

| Symptom (check) | Functional school problem | Accommodation/ management strategy (select) |
|---|---|---|
| **Cognitive Symptoms** | | |
| Attention & concentration difficulties | Short focus on lecture, classwork, homework | Shorter assignments (odd/even problems, requiring outline or bullet points instead of full written responses)<br>Break down tasks and tests into chunks/segments<br>Lighter work load: Max. nightly homework (including studying): ___ min |
| Working memory (short-term memory) | Trouble holding instructions, lecture, reading material, thoughts in mind during tasks | Repetition<br>Written instructions<br>Provide student with teacher generated class notes |
| Memory consolidation/ retrieval | Retaining new information | Smaller chunks/segments to learn, repetition |
| | Accessing learned information | Recognition cues |
| Processing speed | Unable to keep pace with work load<br>Slower reading/writing/calculation<br>Difficulty processing verbal information effectively | Allowances for extended time to complete coursework, assignments, tests<br>Reduce/slowdown verbal information and check for comprehension |
| Cognitive Fatigue/ Fogginess | Decreased arousal, mental energy; trouble thinking clearly, formulating thoughts | Rest breaks during classes<br>Homework, and examinations in quiet location |
| **Physical Symptoms** | | |
| Headaches | Interferes with concentration | Intersperse rest breaks, shortened day if symptom does not subside |
| | Increased irritability | Allow for short naps in quiet location (e.g., nurse's office) |
| Light/ noise sensitivity | Symptoms worsen in bright or loud environments | Wear sunglasses/hat, seating away from bright sunlight<br>Limit exposure to SMART board, computers, provide class notes<br>Avoid noisy/crowded environments such as lunchroom, assemblies, chorus/music class, and hallways. Leave class early.<br>Allow student to wear earplugs as needed |
| Dizziness/ balance/ nausea | Unsteadiness when walking | Elevator pass |
| | Nausea or vomiting | Class transition before bell |
| Sleep disturbance | Decreased arousal, shifted sleep schedule, trouble falling asleep | Later start time<br>Shortened day or rest breaks |
| Fatigue | Lack of energy | Periodic rest breaks, short naps in quiet location<br>Passive participation |
| **Emotional Symptoms** | | |
| Irritability | Poor tolerance for stress | Reduce stimulation and stressors (e.g., overwhelmed with missing work) |
| Anxiety/ nervousness | Worried about falling behind, pushing through symptoms | Reassurance from teachers and team about accommodations, workload reduction, alternate forms of testing<br>Time built in for socialization |
| Depression/ withdrawal | Withdrawal from school or friends because of stigma or activity restrictions | Allow student to be engaged with peers during selected low stress/ extracurricular activities as tolerated<br>Lunch in a quiet room with friends |
| **Specific Academic Recommendations** | | |
| Subject specific difficulties | Writing | Provide alternatives to written output (word bank, oral response, etc.) |
| | Mathematics calculation | Use of calculator, reduced number of problems |
| | Reading comprehension | Shorter reading passages<br>Provide tools to assist with visual tracking or comprehension of information (e.g., use of audio books) |
| Make-up/Missing work | Trouble managing current load of make-up work | Waive previously missed work<br>Reduce amount of outstanding work (assign essential learning tasks) |
| Tests/quizzes | Unprepared for tests/quizzes | No/ Modified classroom testing (e.g., breaks, extra time, quiet location)<br>Limit number of classroom tests per day. _____ per day. |
| Other: | | |

## *Appendix D: Symptom monitoring log*

To be completed by the Symptom Monitor

**Concussion Symptom Monitoring Log**

Have the student rate each symptom that he/she is currently experiencing on a scale of 0 through 6.

**Student Name:**

| Rate Symptom | Date: | Date: | Date: | Date: | Date: |
|---|---|---|---|---|---|
| Physical | 0 = Not a problem | 3 = Moderate Problem | | 6 = Severe problem | |
| 1. Headaches | | | | | |
| 2. Fatigue | | | | | |
| 3. Visual problems | | | | | |
| 4. Dizziness | | | | | |
| 5. Balance problems | | | | | |
| 6. Sensitivity to light | | | | | |
| 7. Sensitivity to noise | | | | | |
| 8. Nausea | | | | | |
| 9. Vomiting | | | | | |
| 10. Numbness / tingling | | | | | |
| Cognitive | 0 = Not a problem | 3 = Moderate Problem | | 6 = Severe problem | |
| 11. Feeling mentally foggy | | | | | |
| 12. Problems concentrating | | | | | |
| 13. Problems remembering | | | | | |
| 14. Slow to respond/ complete work | | | | | |
| 15. Disorganized | | | | | |
| Emotional | 0 = Not a problem | 3 = Moderate Problem | | 6 = Severe problem | |
| 16. Irritability/ easily angered | | | | | |
| 17. Sadness | | | | | |
| 18. Nervousness | | | | | |
| 19. Feeling socially isolated | | | | | |
| 20. Feeling more emotional | | | | | |
| 21. Less able to cope with stress | | | | | |
| Other | | | | | |
| *Exertion | | | | | |
| *Overall Rating (0, 1, 2) | | | | | |
| *Activity (0,1) | | | | | |

**\* Please read the following questions and use the corresponding rating scales to complete the three items above\***

Exertion: Which symptoms worsen with Physical or Cognitive Activity? (place # of symptom inside corresponding box)

Overall Rating: To what degree do you feel "differently" than before the injury (not feeling like yourself)?
    0 = No difference/normal   1= A little different   2= Very different

Activity Level: Compared to what your typical activity (before the injury), your current level of activity has been:
    0= Less than usual   1= Same as usual

**Communication to Healthcare Provider/ Family:** The above table indicates monitoring of the student's symptoms.
Additional Information:

Concerns/ Questions:

- This material was adapted from the BrainSTEPS Program in Pennsylvania which is jointly funded by the Department of Health and the PA Department of Education, and implemented by the Brain Injury Association of PA.
- Any use or revision of this material should cite the Safe Concussion Outcome Recovery & Education (SCORE) program and receive permission from the authors (G. Gioia).

## *Appendix E: Academic monitoring tool*

To be completed by classroom teachers

**Academic Monitoring Tool**

Student Name:_____   Date:_____
Teacher:_____   Course/Class:_____

**Instructions:** Please fill out this form on a weekly basis to monitor the student's academic progress and concussion symptoms observed in the classroom. Discuss with the student the assignments that are essential to complete, what assignments can be modified, and what assignments will be excused. Discuss a reasonable timeline to complete the work. While the student is recovering, the focus should be on mastery and essential learning concepts.

*Please return to the Academic Monitor by this date: _____*

Please list the *essential* assignments (or attach electronic grade book) the student will need to complete the following week and any accommodations you think the student may need to complete the assignment. Once an assignment has been completed, please fill in the grade the student received.

| Due date | Assignments, classwork, homework, tests, or quizzes | Accommodations needed/ Additional comments | Grade/ score |
|---|---|---|---|
|  |  |  |  |
|  |  |  |  |
|  |  |  |  |
|  |  |  |  |
|  |  |  |  |
|  |  |  |  |
|  |  |  |  |
|  |  |  |  |

**This week the following post-concussive symptoms were observed that (more than usual prior to his/her concussion) (check).**

| Physical | | Thinking/Cognitive | Social/Emotional | |
|---|---|---|---|---|
| Headaches | Sensitivity to light | Feeling mentally foggy | Irritability/easily angered | Social isolation |
| Fatigue | Sensitivity to noise | Problems concentrating | Sadness | Less able to cope with stress |
| Visual problems | Nausea | Problems remembering | Nervousness | Feeling more emotional |
| Dizziness | Vomiting | Slow to respond / complete work | **Exertional Effects:** Do symptoms worsen with activities? | |
| Balance Problems | Numbness/ tingling | Disorganized | Physical Activity: Yes___ No___        Cognitive Activity: Yes___ No___ | |

Additional comments about this student:

What has improved (symptoms or performance)?

Has anything worsened (symptoms or performance)?

- This material was adapted from the BrainSTEPS Program in Pennsylvania which is jointly funded by the Department of Health and the PA Department of Education, and implemented by the Brain Injury Association of PA.
- Any use or revision of this material should cite the Safe Concussion Outcome Recovery & Education (SCORE) program and receive permission from the authors (G. Gioia).

# References

Baker JG, Rieger BP, McAvoy K, Leddy JJ, Master CL, Lana SJ, and Willer BS. (2014) Principles for return to learn after concussion. *International Journal of Clinical Practice, 68*(11), 1286–1288.

Baker JG, Leddy JJ, Darling SR, et al. (2015) Factors associated with problems for adolescents returning to the classroom after sport-related concussion. *Clinical Pediatrics, 54*(10), 961–968.

Centers for Disease Control and Prevention. Heads up to schools: Know your concussion ABCs [updated March 23, 2012]. Available at: http://www.cdc.gov/concussion/HeadsUp/schools.html. Accessed January 15, 2017.

Carson JD, Lawrence DW, Kraft SA, et al. (2014) Premature return to play and return to learn after a sport-related concussion: Physician's chart review. *Canadian Family Physician, 60*(6), e310–e315.

Collins MW, Kontos AP, Okonkwo DO, et al. (2016) Statements of agreement from the targeted evaluation and active management (TEAM) approaches to treating concussion meeting held in Pittsburgh, October 15–16, 2015. *Neurosurgery, 79*(6), 912–929. doi:10.1227/NEU.0000000000001447.

Corwin DJ, Zonfrillo MR, Master CL, et al. (2014) Characteristics of prolonged concussion recovery in a pediatric subspecialty referral population. *Journal of Pediatrics, 165*(6), 1207–1215.

Corwin DJ, Wiebe DJ, Zonfrillo MR, et al. (2015) Vestibular deficits following youth concussion. *Journal of Pediatrics, 166*(5), 1221–1225.

Davies S, Sandlund JN, and Lopez LB (2016) School-based consultation to improve concussion recognition and response. *Journal of Educational and Psychological Consultation, 26,* 49–62.

Davis GA, Anderson V, Babl FE, et al. (2017) What is the difference in concussion management in children as compared with adults? A systematic review. *British Journal of Sports Medicine,* published online April 28, 2017. doi:10.1136/bjsports-2016-097415.

DeMatteo C, McCauley D, Stazyk K, Harper J, Adamich J, Randall S, and Mussiuna C. (2015) Post-Concussion return to play and return to school guidelines for children and youth: A scoping methodology. *Disability and Rehabilitation, 37*(12), 1107–1112. doi:10.3109/09638288.2014.952452.

DeMatteo C, Stazyk K, Giglia L, et al. (2015) A balanced protocol for return to school for children and youth following concussive injury. *Clinical Pediatrics, 54*(8), 783–792.

Gagnon I, Galli C, Friedman D, Grilli L, and Iverson GL. (2009) Active rehabilitation for children who are slow to recover following sport-related concussion. *Brain Injury, 23,* 956–964.

Gioia GA. (2015) Multimodal evaluation and management of children with concussion: Using our heads and available evidence. *Brain Injury, 29*(2), 195–206. doi:10.3109/02699052.2014.965210.

Gioia GA. (2016) Medical-school partnership in guiding return to school following mild traumatic brain injury in youth. *Journal of Child Neurology, 31*(10), 93–108.

Gioia GA, Glang AE, Hooper SR, and Eagan-Brown B. (2016) Building statewide infrastructure for the academic support of students with mild traumatic brain injury. *Journal of Head Trauma Rehabilitation, 31*(6), 397–406. doi:10.1097/HTR.0000000000000205.

Giza CC and Hovda DA. (2014) The new neurometabolic cascade of concussion. *Neurosurgery,* 75(Suppl 4), S24–S33. doi:10.1227/NEU.0000000000000505.

Glang AE, Koester MC, Chesnutt JC, Gioia GA, McAvoy K, Marshall S, and Gau JM. (2014) The effectiveness of a web-based resource in improving postconcussion management in high schools. *Journal of Adolescent Health, 56*(1), 91–97. doi:10.1016/j.jadohealth.2014.08.011.

Grubenhoff JA, Deakyne SJ, Comstock RD, et al. (2015) Outpatient follow-up and return to school after emergency department evaluation among children with persistent post-concussion symptoms. *Brain Injury, 29*(10), 1186–1191.

Halstead ME, McAvoy K, Devore CD, et al. (2013) Returning to learning following a concussion. *Pediatrics, 132,* 948–957.

Heyer GL, Weber KD, Rose SC, Perkins SQ, and Schmittauer CE. (2015) High school principals' resources, knowledge, and practices regarding the returning student with concussion. *Journal of Pediatrics, 166*(3), 594–599.

Kasamatsu T, Cleary M, Bennett J, Howard K, and Valovich McLeod T. (2016) Examining academic support after concussion for the adolescent student-sahlete: Perspectives of the athletic trainer. *Journal of Athletic Training, 51*(2), 153–161.

Leddy JJ, Baker JG, and Willer B. (2016) Active rehabilitation of concussion and post-concussion Syndrome. *Physical Medicine & Rehabilitation Clinics of North America, 27*(2), 437–454. doi:10.1016/j.pmr.2015.12.003.

Master TL, Gioia GA, Leddy JJ, and Grady MF. (2012) The importance of a "return to learn" plan in pediatric and adolescent concussion. *Pediatric Annals, 41*(9), 1–6.

McGrath N. (2010) Supporting the student-athlete's return to the classroom after a sport-related concussion. *Journal of Athletic Training, 45,* 492–498.

Newlin E and Hooper S. (2015) Return to school protocols following concussion. *North Carolina Medical Journal, 76*(2), 107–108. doi:10.18043/ncm.76.2.107.

Oregon Center for Applied Science. Brain 101: The Concussion Playbook. (2007). http://brain101.orcasinc.com/

Popoli DM, Burns TG, Meehan WP, and Reisner A. (2014) CHOA concussion consensus: Establishing a uniform policy for academic accommodations. *Clinical Pediatrics, 53*(3), 217–224.

Purcell L. (2014) Sport-related concussion: Evaluation and management. *Paediatric Child Health, 19*(3), 153–158.

Purcell L, Harvey J, and Seabrook JA. (2016) Patterns of recovery following sport-related concussion in children and adolescents. *Clinical Pediatrics, 55*(5), 452–458.

Ransom DM, Vaughan CG, Pratson L, Sady MD, McGill CA, and Gioia GA. (2015) Academic effects of concussion in children and adolescents. *Pediatrics, 135*(6), 1043–1050. doi:10.1542/peds.2014-3434.

Ransom DM, Burns A, Youngstrom EA, Sady MD, Vaughan CG, and Gioia GA. (2016) Applying an Evidence-Based Assessment Model to Identify Students at Risk for Perceived Academic Problems following Concussion. *Journal of the International Neuropsychological Society*, 22(10), 1038–1049.

Sady MD, Vaughan CG, and Gioia GA. (2011) School and the concussed youth: Recommendations for concussion education and management. *Physical Medicine and Rehabilitation Clinics of North America*, 22, 701–719.

Smith DH, Meaney DF, and Shull WH. (2003) Diffuse axonal injury in head trauma. *Journal of Head Trauma Rehabilitation*, 18(4), 307–316.

Terwilliger VK, Pratson L, Vaughan CG, and Gioia GA (2016) Additional post-concussion impact exposure may affect recovery in adolescent athletes. *Journal of Neurotrauma*, 33, 761–765.

Thomas DG, Apps JN, Hoffmann RG, McCrea M, and Hammeke T. (2015) Benefits of strict rest after acute concussion: A randomized controlled trial. *Pediatrics*, 135(2), 213–223. doi:10.1542/peds.2014-0966.

Wasserman EB, Bazarian JJ, Mapstone M, Block R, and van Wijngaarden E. (2016) Academic dysfunction after a concussion among US high school and college students. *American Journal of Public Health*, 106(7), 1247–1253.

Williams RM, Welch CE, Parsons JT, and Valovich McLeod TC. (2015) Athletic trainers' familiarity with and perceptions of academic accommodations in secondary school athletes after sport-related concussion. *Journal of Athletic Training*, 50(3), 262–269.

Zemek R, Barrowman N, Freedman SB, et al. (2016) Clinical risk score for persistent postconcussion symptoms among children with acute concussion in the ED. *JAMA*, 315(10), 1014–1025. doi:10.1001/jama.2016.1203.

Zuckerbraun NS, Atabaki S, Collins MW, Thomas D, and Gioia GA. (2014) Use of modified acute concussion evaluation tools in the emergency department. *Pediatrics*, 133(4), 635–642.

## chapter thirteen

# Return to work

## When and how should I return to work after a concussion?

*Michelle McKerral and Geneviève Léveillé*

### Contents

### Introduction

As other chapters in this book have demonstrated, there is a growing literature and strength of evidence as to the best practices for prevention and early management of a sports or recreation related concussion, or mild traumatic brain injury (mTBI), with respect to cognitive and physical activities for youth, as well as for elite or professional adult athletes for whom their sport is their main occupational activity. However, many adults sustain a concussion during nonelite or recreational sports activities. For this group, a prompt return to work is their primary concern. It is well known that after a concussion, a subgroup of individuals will experience persistence of symptoms, and an atypical evolution. As explained in other chapters of this book, several interacting neuropathological and psychosocial factors are behind the initial post-concussion symptoms and their persistence over time, which can have a negative impact on an individual's daily activities and social roles, cause emotional distress and affect their quality of life. It is important to recognize the outward signs and to treat them through specific interventions at the right moment so as to reduce the risk of the long-term consequences associated with a concussion. These consequences can have an impact on returning to work and maintaining employment.

This chapter will first present an overview of published findings on concussion in adults, sustained during nonprofessional sports, as well as on recovery from mTBI as it relates to employment and other associated outcomes. Then, the best practice guidelines for early management of return to work after a concussion and of persisting symptoms (early and late referrals) will be described and summarized in an algorithm to help guide interventions. Finally, a detailed case study of specialized interdisciplinary rehabilitation interventions, with emphasis on the resumption of work-related activities following a concussion sustained during a recreational hockey match, will be presented with specific references to best practice guidelines and suggested tools.

## Sport-related head injury in adults and return to work outcomes

### Epidemiology of sports mTBI in working-age adults

There are no specific, readily available, epidemiological data on the subpopulation of working adults who sustain a concussion during sports activities. Nevertheless, it is known that in high-income countries the overall mTBI incidence rate is approximately 600 per 100,000 population, with about one third presenting to the emergency room. There is a high prevalence in teenagers and young adults, and the median age of individuals with a TBI is below 50 years (Cassidy et al., 2004; Public Health Agency of Canada, 2014; Roozenbeek et al., 2013; Ryu et al., 2009). Furthermore, there is information suggesting that, in North America, 90% of sports related TBIs are mild in severity. This represents approximately 5%–10% of all hospital-treated mTBIs and up to 20% of all head injuries. Males are affected two to three times more frequently than females and appear to show an increasing incidence (Fu et al., 2016; McKeever and Schatz, 2003; Selassie et al., 2013).

There is also strong evidence that a nonnegligible proportion of adults with a concussion, including one related to sports, may remain symptomatic beyond the expected recovery period. For these people, resumption of work-related activities could be potentially problematic if their concussion-related issues are not addressed readily or correctly. In fact, although the majority of people will recover from a concussion and will return to work within 3–6 months after their injury (Cancelliere et al., 2014), it is estimated that, if left untreated, anywhere between 5% and 15% of cases are at risk of developing chronic symptoms which will impact many areas of their lives (Ahman et al., 2013; Belanger et al., 2005; Carroll et al., 2004; Drake et al., 2000; Emanuelson et al., 2003; Guérin et al., 2005, 2006; Iverson, 2005; Kashluba et al., 2004; Stulemeijer et al., 2008). When post-concussion symptoms persist, often, by the time the person receives specific treatment or interventions for the problems associated with their concussion, they may have experienced numerous failed attempts to reintegrate their job at the same level of performance as before, and may be experiencing emotional distress in addition to the initial symptoms associated with their mTBI.

## Symptom and cognitive recovery beyond the first few weeks and implications for work

Although most individuals will fully recover and return to their usual occupational activities within three months after a concussion, studies on the *natural* evolution of mTBI (i.e., untreated other than medical treatment for physical injuries) show that 30% of adults report, three months after having been diagnosed in the emergency room with a *simple* mTBI (i.e., Glasgow Coma Scale 13–15, post-traumatic amnesia ≤ 24 hours, a negative CT scan), concentration and memory problems that impact their daily activities (Ponsford et al., 2011). In addition, individuals with mTBI are different from those seen in general trauma (i.e., without a head injury) since they show signs of various cognitive problems. Moreover, research shows that, 1 year after a *simple* mTBI, the most frequently reported symptoms are: concentration and memory problems, fatigue, anxiety, irritability, sleeping difficulties, and headaches (Dikmen et al., 2010). Adults who have sustained a *complex* mTBI (i.e., Glasgow Coma Score 13–15, post-traumatic amnesia ≤ 24 hours, positive CT scan) show additional symptoms, such as dizziness and anger. This symptomatology, along with the fact that these individuals report three or more symptoms, has been identified at least 50% more often in all types of mTBIs compared to adults having sustained a general trauma. These data from well controlled studies which describe the effects that can persist after a concussion are convincing. These effects manifest themselves not only as a particular symptomatology, as described above, but there can also be quantifiable cognitive deficits that must be followed for the first few weeks and be formally evaluated from neurological and neuropsychological perspectives when symptoms persist so as to propose a clear framework and the necessary interventions to ensure a successful return to work.

In the acute phase after a concussion, there are generally impairments in attention, learning, and memory, as well as speed of information processing, while in the medium and long term, it is the more subtle aspects of cognitive performance that remain the most often affected, such as speed of processing in cognitively demanding situations, complex attention, and working memory (i.e., executive components of attention and memory), together with fatigue (Vanderploeg et al., 2005). A complete neuropsychological evaluation is still, to date, the most valid and reliable method for measuring the cognitive impact of a concussion as well as for evaluating its potential effects on cognitive activities related to work tasks and demands. However, its ability to detect the effects of a concussion may decline over time, especially if sensitive neuropsychological tests that can most accurately identify these impairments in more complex cognitive processes are not used (Bigler et al., 2013). It should be noted that computer-based tests are being used more and more, particularly in the sports field, to identify the cognitive effects of concussion, and inform return-to-play decisions, usually by comparing test results to a baseline level. However, these tests can only provide a basic screening. They have shown validity in high level athletes with pre-established baselines, but they should not be used in place of a detailed neuropsychological evaluation when indicated (Maerlender et al., 2010). For adults having sustained mTBI, a comprehensive neuropsychological evaluation is recommended especially when cognitive symptoms persist for more than three months (Ontario Neurotrauma Foundation-ONF, 2013).

## Prognostic models, return to work, and related outcomes

In terms of outcome following a concussion, a systematic review of multivariate prognostic models provides evidence that close to 50% of individuals who have sustained an mTBI will eventually receive a mental health diagnosis, especially for depression (Silverberg et al., 2015). Moreover, depression has been linked with short-term (1 month) as well as longer term (1 year)

*Table 13.1* Factors associated with poor functional outcomes following
mTBI—return to work

---

Dizziness

Number of reported symptoms (approximately five or more)

Post-traumatic stress

Cognitive impairments on tests of memory and executive functioning

Reduced social interaction (compared to pre-injury)

Financial compensation-seeking

Loss of consciousness

Preexisting mental health difficulties (i.e., anxiety, depression, mania, psychotic symptoms)

Lower premorbid intelligence/cognitive ability

Pre-injury work history (i.e., prior work instability, lower earnings)

---

*Source:*   Ontario Neurotrauma Foundation, *Guidelines for Concussion/Mild Traumatic Brain Injury and Persistent Symptoms*, 2nd ed., (For adults, 18+ years of age), http://onf.org/documents/ guidelines-for-concussion-mtbi-persistent-symptoms-second-edition, 2013.

post-concussion symptom presentation (Wäljas et al., 2015). A recent study has shown that individuals with mTBI who reported persistent symptoms one year after their injury tend to have early signs of psychological distress (e.g., depression, traumatic stress) (Losoi et al., 2016). Also, it would appear that cognitive deficits can explain for the most part difficulties in social participation, especially return to work and other life activities and roles (Silverberg et al., 2015; Drake et al., 2000). Thus, even if a single specific multivariate prognostic model has not yet been able to adequately predict post-mTBI outcomes, there appears to be strong factors that could suggest a poorer prognosis, such as preexisting mental health issues and early post-mTBI neuropsychological functioning. Table 13.1 provides a list of the factors that have been frequently associated with poor functional outcomes, in particular return to employment, after mTBI. These risk factors must be taken into consideration when following up on an individual who has sustained a concussion as well as in the return to work process.

In addition, other factors have been found to be associated with poorer recovery from mTBI, for example, the early onset of pain, and in particular headache, within the first 24 hours following injury, the presence of nausea, reduced balance or dizziness after injury, older age, presence of life stressors at time of mTBI, and delay in returning to work (ONF, 2013). Differences according to sex should also be considered for return to work prognosis. Women tend to show greater persistence of post-concussion symptomatology, especially during child-bearing years, and although hormonal issues could play a role in recovery, women do not miss more work days than males do (Bazarian et al., 2010). However, it has been suggested that adults, especially women, who have high levels of anxiety initially following concussion have poorer outcomes following mTBI (Silverberg, 2015). Age has yielded more variable results in terms of its relationship with return to work following mTBI (Guérin et al., 2006; Stulemeijer et al., 2008), probably since it is likely to be associated with other social factors which have not been concomitantly studied. The level of social interaction and relationships at work, a supportive workplace and a job with greater decision-making latitude have been shown to be related to better employment outcomes post- mTBI (Ruffalo et al., 1999; Stergiou-Kita et al., 2016; Wehman et al., 2005).

It should also be pointed out that brain imaging tools, such as magnetic resonance imaging (MRI) and diffusion tensor imaging (DTI), have not been shown to systematically correlate with post-concussion symptomatology (Wäljas et al., 2015). However, it has been documented that mTBI individuals with positive brain MRI do take longer to return to work than individuals with negative imaging (Iverson et al., 2012). Still, since computed tomography is recommended only for people with certain risk factors and post-mTBI characteristics (Stiell et al., 2001) and since MRIs are rarely performed following a concussion, the majority of concussed individuals do not undergo any brain imaging procedure. Consequently, this variable cannot presently be used systematically at the individual patient level for prognosticating, or intervention decision-making with regard to outcomes such as return to work.

The previous paragraphs have emphasized factors which, when studied during the natural evolution of a concussion, can have an impact on recovery. It is clear that interacting neuropathological, physical, and psychosocial factors are at the bases of post-concussion symptoms and, in particular, their persistence in time. As such, early detection and treatment of modifiable health issues related to the concussion and to associated injuries (e.g., soft tissue, orthopedic) are thus particularly important in order to ensure optimal and unhindered recovery and return to work. This is highlighted by a study that showed that variables such as post-mTBI anxiety, depression, or pain, when present at the onset of specialized interdisciplinary intervention and treated within the first few months, do not represent a risk factor for poor return to work outcomes after mTBI (Guérin et al., 2006). Thus, interventions for mTBI, which are individualized, specific and well planned in relation to an individual's recovery curve, should facilitate a return to regular life activities (Guérin et al., 2006; Ponsford, 2005).

## Best practices for management of return to work after a concussion

### Intervention approaches for concussion and implications for resumption of work-related activities

Providing education and information on mTBI for the concussed adult, as well as for all health professionals, are of the utmost importance in order to prevent and overcome obstacles during recovery and to allow for an optimal return to activities within a reasonable time frame. A comprehensive definition of mTBI (e.g., that proposed by the WHO task force on mTBI; Carroll et al., 2004) is not always used and may result in missed diagnoses (Ryu et al., 2009). A health risk management approach should be applied to concussions, by promoting educational material that encourage early medical consultation when needed, management of early symptoms and of return to physical activities/sports and work. It should also propose a more complete curriculum related to concussion and TBI within medical training and all health-related academic programs. By identifying and following up more closely those at risk of slower recovery through an individualized approach to concussion management, while also taking the individuals' early recovery pattern and known risk factors into consideration, problems can be prevented when they return to work, thus considerably reducing the risk of long term effects related to concussion (Fayol et al., 2009; Guérin et al., 2005; Guérin and McKerral, 2008; ONF, 2013; Ouellet et al., 2016).

Evidence from sports medicine and exercise clinics that treat concussed adults suggests that longer recovery and restriction from contact/collision sports are seen in adults with more complex initial clinical presentation (e.g., higher post-concussion symptoms and neck scores) (Ouellet et al., 2016). It has also been advanced that a slower recovery from a sport-related concussion in some adults could potentially be due to a lack of uniformity in, and knowledge of, the management criteria for concussions in the emergency room and in the physician's office, resulting in a variation in the quality and coherence of advice given to concussed adults (Carson et al., 2016).

In the mTBI literature, positive effects of early intervention (e.g., intervention booklet, telephone counseling) have been reported, especially on stress levels, symptom reporting and their impacts on daily functioning, such as work (Bell et al., 2008; Kashluba et al., 2004; Ponsford et al., 2002). However, in those mTBI cases who received interventions, some individuals continued to show persistent symptoms in the year following their injury, indicating that in some cases further investigation of, and intervention for, specific symptom management and return to work-related activities were needed. There is also evidence from publicly funded specialized interdisciplinary rehabilitation contexts within a trauma continuum of care, which treat all referred mTBIs that show atypical recovery including those sustained in nonprofessional sports contexts, that a personalized intervention approach even with later referrals (e.g., 6 months post-mTBI) can have a positive impact on return to work outcomes and social participation (Desormeau and McKerral, 2010; Guérin et al., 2005, 2006; McKerral and Desormeau, 2009; Vincent et al., 2015). However, even in such an intervention context, reduced speed and efficacy in processing complex visual information, as well as longer referral delays, were related to less favorable return to work outcomes (Guérin et al., 2006; Lachapelle et al., 2008). This would appear to reinforce the importance of timely referral for specific cognitive behavioral or environmental interventions to reduce the impact of cognitive difficulties in the work environment.

It is interesting to note that approaches to studying and treating concussions in elite versus nonelite sport contexts, as well as sports versus nonsports contexts, are now merging in terms of the recommended management of persisting symptoms and return to daily activities. In fact, many clinicians and researchers believe that all individuals with a sport-related concussion, regardless of their level of participation, should be managed using a similar treatment paradigm and that both the exchange of ideas and cooperation between all professionals and scientists interested in mTBIs can enrich knowledge in the field and contribute to their best management (McCrory et al., 2013; Sojka, 2011). Particularly worthy of mention is the addition, in the most recent Concussion in Sport Group consensus statement, of recommendations for rehabilitation and referral when post-concussion symptoms persist beyond two weeks in adults, which include using *closely monitored active rehabilitation programmes* and a *collaborative approach to treatment* (McCrory et al., 2017).

## Best practice guidelines for return to work

A multifactorial conception of concussion is the basis for the most recent Guidelines for Concussion/Mild Traumatic Brain Injury and Persistent Symptoms published by the Ontario Neurotrauma Foundation (ONF, 2013). They were developed from the most recent and most conclusive data available as well as previously published guidelines for health professionals in applying the best practices with those showing persistent post-concussion symptoms. Return to work and the ability to maintain employment should be a central objective of the clinical follow-up of all concussed adults, and it is essential to quickly establish a framework for resumption of work-activities and a structure/timeframe for the various interventions required (McKerral and Léveillé, 2016). A progressive management of and return to the various activities and responsibilities involved in the workplace is suggested.

Firstly, as a form of early intervention it is recommended that, after a concussion, all adults receive, in the emergency room or physician's office, a written document containing recommendations for the initial rest period, progressive return to cognitive and physical activities, return to work, as well as information on the steps to take if symptoms persist (Ponsford, 2005) (e.g., Institut national d'excellence en santé et en services sociaux-INESSS, 2014). Ideally, there should be a follow-up visit with the physician within the next few weeks to monitor symptom recovery. A session on information and reassurance related to the symptomology and the generally favorable general prognosis is also recommended for those who present one or more

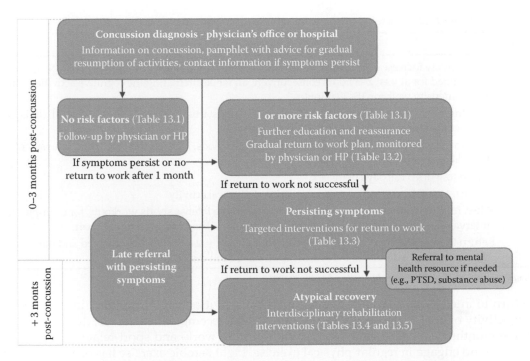

*Figure 13.1* Algorithm for guiding interventions for return to work following concussion.

risk factors (Table 13.1), and these individuals should receive follow-up care from a physician during the first few months after the concussion so as to structure the steps for return to work. Moreover, it is recommended that people whose recovery is progressing slower than expected during the first three months post-concussion receive additional interventions to guide return to work. Beyond three months post-injury, if impacts on daily activities and social roles persist, referral for specialized interdisciplinary rehabilitation interventions for atypically recovering mTBI is recommended (McKerral and Léveillé, 2016; ONF, 2013; Ponsford, 2005). A suggested algorithm to guide interventions for return to work following concussion in adults is presented in Figure 13.1, which refers to the specific intervention frameworks and modalities that are presented in the following paragraphs and tables.

Up to now, several recommendations for the return to intellectual and sports activities after a concussion have advocated rest until the symptoms dissipate. Despite the multitude of studies on concussion, none has yet established a validated specific rest period. Some studies tend to show that a progressive return to intellectual activities several days post-concussion, despite the persistence of certain symptoms, would offer more long term benefits than maintaining a complete and prolonged stoppage of activities, such as work. In that respect, the 2017 Concussion in Sport Group consensus statement recommends, after 24–48 hours post-concussion, gradual and progressive reactivation at a level that should not bring on or increase symptoms (McCrory et al., 2017). The complete exclusion of a person who has sustained a concussion from all regular activities could, in fact, have a negative impact symptoms recovery by increasing stress and anxiety related to the withdrawal from activities that are important for the individual (Brown et al., 2014; Ponsford et al., 2012; Wells et al., 2015).

General recommendations for progressive return to intellectual activities include returning to work for half-days, then part-time and finally full-time, with progressive adjustment in the work tasks according to the cognitive demands required to accomplish them (INESSS, 2014; Leclerc, 2016). There is general agreement in recommending the

*Table 13.2* General steps for guiding return to work in physically active adults

| Step | Description |
|---|---|
| 1 | Progressively increase cognitive activities (reading and computer work) until they can be maintained for at least 2–3 hours consecutively, all while alternating the cognitive activities with a low intensity walk for 15–20 minutes. |
| 2 | Once this first stage has been achieved, return to work starting with half days, at first 2 half days per week and then increasing to 5 half days per week. |
| 3 | In a similar way, but alternating with work days or periods, increase the length and intensity of the walks. |
| 4 | Return to work 3 full days per week. |
| 5 | If return to work goes well, increase intensity of physical activity. |
| 6 | When full-time return to work is possible, resume more intense sports workouts, for example, in intervals, and then undertake more specific activities related to the preferred sport. |
| 7 | Return to intensive sport should not be attempted until full-time work is achieved and the different stages of return to the specific sport have been completed. |

*Source:* Leclerc, S., *Le Médecin du Québec*, 51, 49–53, 2016.

return to intellectual as well as regular physical activities before resuming intense physical activity or contact sports. Table 13.2 outlines the recommended course, during the first three months post-concussion, for gradual return to work- and sport-related activities in adults who engage in regular physical exercise. Light aerobic exercise has been suggested as being a potentially powerful facilitator of symptom recovery and should be included in post-concussion management plans (Gagnon et al., 2009; Leddy et al., 2010). Evolution of symptoms should be measured using a validated tool, such as the Rivermead Post-Concussion Symptoms Questionnaire (King et al., 1995; ONF, 2013; Tinawi and Brière, 2016). These recommended steps should be monitored by a health professional (HP) specialized in concussion management, and a physician in cases where symptoms are particularly elevated and there are associated physical injuries and pain for example (e.g., see ONF Guidelines for recommendations for evaluation of all possible factors contributing to symptom presentation and for specific symptom management).

When symptoms persist beyond 4–6 weeks post-injury, in parallel to follow-up visits with the physician in order to adequately manage symptoms, additional targeted interventions by professionals with expertise in concussion management are recommended to support return to employment and to other activities. For example, the person may be referred to a physiotherapist to treat positional vertigo or to a neuropsychologist for neurocognitive screening if cognitive symptoms remain problematic. In addition, an occupational therapist can support return to work and activities by introducing specific symptom and work management strategies in relation to the nature and requirements of the person's job; suggested intervention modalities and stages are presented in Table 13.3.

## Specialized intervention for concussion with atypical evolution

In cases where an attempt to return to work within the first three months after the accident was inefficient, unproductive, or unsuccessful, specialized interventions for adults with atypically recovering concussions targeting increased support and treatment for symptom management and resumption of work related activities are recommended (McKerral and Léveillé, 2016; ONF, 2013; Ponsford, 2005).

As discussed earlier and in the previous chapters of this book, slow-to-recover mTBI is a multifactorial issue that can be associated with various types of impairments (e.g.,

*Table 13.3* Framework for structured interventions for return to work in the context of persisting symptoms

| Step | Description |
| --- | --- |
| 1 | Regular contact with the workplace and work related activities should be encouraged as soon as possible (e.g., e-mail, reading). |
| 2 | In parallel to the gradual resumption of cognitive and physical activities (including light aerobic exercise in adults who are not particularly physically active), incite the adoption of a lifestyle schedule similar to the usual work schedule incorporating, if possible, tasks similar to those done at work. |
| 3 | An evaluation of the work related tasks, demands and responsibilities should be performed to determine an appropriate return to employment plan, and to identify possible facilitators and barriers (ONF, 2013). |
| 4 | Compensatory tools and strategies should be proposed to promote optimal planning and organization abilities, and to reduce stress and anxiety related to returning to work (e.g., personal organizer, self-assessment grid for progressive return to work; see Appendix A). |
| 5 | A plan for return to work, detailing progression in terms of number of work hours and the required temporary adaptations (e.g., in terms of task complexity and quantity) should be presented to the employer (Appendix A). |

physical, cognitive, emotional) which impact on different areas of daily functioning. In this light, specialized post-concussion interventions are ideally applied within an interdisciplinary approach which is the same for adults who are actively involved in sports and those who are not. The core clinical team usually includes a physician or physiatrist (for those who do not have a treating doctor in the community, or for complex cases), a psychologist-neuropsychologist and an occupational therapist, to which can be added, if need be, a kinesiologist, a physiotherapist, or a social worker (Guérin et al., 2005; Guérin and McKerral, 2008). A clinical coordinator or case manager ensures, with the physician, the initial screening of the individual's mTBI related problems, quickly directs them to the appropriate professionals within the team, and supports them in applying the recommended intervention framework and guidelines. The coordinator also maintains a link with the individuals' treating doctor in the community during the rehabilitation period in cases where the team physician is not actively involved in the case.

Rehabilitation interventions consist firstly of evaluating the person to assess the level at which they were functioning before the concussion and establish the differences with their current state, and to get them psychologically and cognitively ready for the interventions to follow. For example, job requirements and responsibilities will be evaluated, and a neuropsychological evaluation will usually be performed in order to identify cognitive strengths and problems that could have an impact on the return to work process. A concise intervention plan is developed with the concussed individuals, with specific measurable and realistic objectives centered on their daily activities and social roles (e.g., life domains; Noreau et al., 2002) that are affected. Among the most commonly affected life domains of adults with atypically recovering mTBI are sleep, physical and psychological condition, household responsibilities, social contacts, leisure activities, and work. After 6–8 weeks, progress is assessed in terms of attainment of the predetermined goals, and so on until resumption of the targeted activities, for example, work. Interdisciplinary interventions rely on the person's strengths and promote experiences of success in achievement of their goals in order to increase self-efficacy with respect to resumption of employment and other daily activities and social roles. The principles and specificities of specialized intervention for adults who show atypical recovery from mTBI are presented, respectively, in Tables 13.4 and 13.5.

**Table 13.4** Principles of specialized intervention for atypically recovering mTBI

**Evaluate**

Post-injury functioning according to clinical team members, the individual seeking care and significant other.

Differences in abilities before the accident, as described by the individual, significant other, employer, and the patient's current state.

Factors linked to a poor outcome (Table 13.1).

**Prepare the patient for rehabilitation (when necessary)**

Medically: for example, pharmacological treatment for headaches, sleeping, anxiety/depression.

Psychologically: for example, reconnecting appropriately with emotions and identification of related needs.

Education and reassurance (even if this was already done during previous follow-ups) on the effects of mTBI, to reduce anxiety levels.

**General principles for intervention**

Dose correctly the objectives, expectations, level of activation, interventions.

Focus the objectives on the life domains judged most important by the individual.

Encourage adaptation to the temporary changes.

Act on the negative spiral (symptoms and loss of personal reference points → lack of comprehension of the situation → stress → fatigue → reduced activity → feeling of dissatisfaction and loss of control → increase in stress and fatigue) and dysfunctional cognitions.

Explore and use strategies to deal with the symptomology (e.g., physical activity, energy management, management of attention and memory resources, daily organization, control of emotional reactions, management of attitudes and behavior that contribute to symptom persistence).

Prioritize interdisciplinary intervention on a common factor (foster a domino effect, e.g., increase in energy → improvement in attention, better mood, less irritability).

Identify satisfactory functional reference points (previous ones or new ones).

In parallel and at appropriate moments in time, undertake the steps presented in Table 13.3.

*Source:*   McKerral, M. and Léveillé, G., *Le Médecin du Québec*, 51, 57–61, 2016.

**Table 13.5** Specific intervention according to the clinical complexity of the mTBI

*Simple* **intervention (e.g., referral around 3 months post-mTBI, few risk factors–Table 13.1)**

Education about mTBI, reassurance, validation of symptoms.

Temporary adaptation to difficulties, management of physical and mental resources and energy, physical reactivation

Promoting a gradual return to daily activities and social roles with an emphasis on return to work with specific support where needed.

Targeted medication (e.g., sleep, pain, anxiety), short term.

Short term and low intensity rehabilitation.

*Complex* **intervention (e.g., later referral, several risk factors–Table 13.1)**

Progressive increase in activation in terms of physical and mental condition and life domains.

Significant assistance with the return to work process.

Target self-management of symptoms.

Foster self-responsibility and self-determination.

Possible longer term polypharmacy (e.g., depression, sleep).

Longer and more intensive rehabilitation.

*Source:*   McKerral, M. and Léveillé, G., *Le Médecin du Québec*, 51, 57–61, 2016.

In rarer cases, where disabilities persist, the rehabilitation process should be more oriented toward the resumption of social roles by aiming for a professional reorientation or job tasks that better correspond to the individuals' abilities. Consulting partners within the health care and social services network is also recommended at any time during the intervention process if there are very complex co-morbid problems (e.g., post-traumatic stress disorder or PTSD, substance abuse).

Although there are very few published studies conducted within a specialized interdisciplinary rehabilitation context for atypically recovering adults with mTBI (e.g., Guérin et al., 2006), there is growing evidence that multidimensional approaches such as that described above has positive effects on return to work and social participation in general. For example, as shown in Figure 13.2, the social participation outcomes of mTBI individuals with persisting symptoms, measured at start and at end of interdisciplinary interventions with the Participation scale of the Mayo-Portland Adaptability Inventory–MPAI-4 (Malec, 2004), showed a significant improvement in overall participation, with significant reductions in difficulties with initiation, social contacts, leisure and recreational activities, responsibilities of independent living, transportation, and return to work (Vincent et al., 2015; Guerrette et al., 2017).

Such an approach to systematic outcome measurement with common data elements during the concussion/mTBI intervention process should be pursued in order to build, in a pragmatic but methodologically sound manner (e.g., by comparing outcomes between rehabilitation program completers and noncompleters; Altman et al., 2010; Wilde et al., 2010) and in parallel to conducting controlled trials where possible, a solid evidence base for treatment efficacy in this clinical population. Continued support and advocacy for early preventative treatment of concussion remains, of course, a necessity.

In order to conclude on this chapter, the next section will outline a case study of the interdisciplinary rehabilitation path of a woman having sustained a concussion during

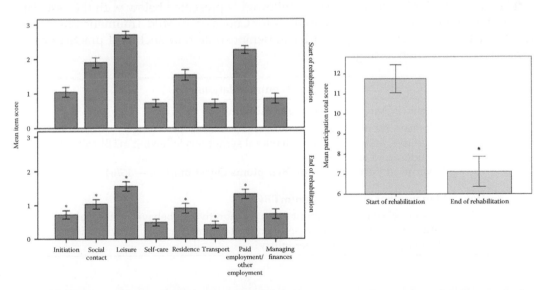

*Figure 13.2* Pre- and post-intervention social participation outcomes in 38 atypically recovering adults referred between 3 and 9 months post-mTBI (22F, 16M; mean age: 44.7 ± 15.5 years; mean duration of intervention: 6.8 ± 4.5 months). Individual items: 0-normal to 4-severe problem; Participation maximum total score: 30; higher scores indicate more impairment. Significant improvement indicated with an asterisk (p<.05, paired t-tests; large or moderate-to-large effect sizes).

sports and who showed an atypical recovery. Appropriate recommendations of published guidelines will be put forward while presenting the various intervention steps in order to appreciate their integration within the overall return to work process.

## Case study of specialized interdisciplinary interventions for concussion with focus on return to work

### Clinical history and general assessment/management considerations

Marie is a 32 year-old woman who was referred to an interdisciplinary rehabilitation program for individuals with mTBI which is focused on socio-professional integration, six months after sustaining a concussion caused by a hit to the head during a hockey game. She did not seek medical advice on the day of the injury. She completed a half-marathon the following day despite experiencing mild symptoms (headaches, nausea). Those symptoms grew significantly worse during the course of the day, pushing her to consult a doctor at a medical clinic the next day. The doctor prescribed a week-long medical leave from work, a brain scan and a neck X-ray (both negative), and pain medication. Her medical leave from work lasted more than four months and, while still experiencing symptoms and without any professional support, she attempted to resume her work, but her symptoms quickly worsened. She was then referred for intervention.

Before her mTBI, Marie was a full-time research professional. She regularly took part in sports activities, was in a serious relationship, and had a strong social network. At the moment of her referral for rehabilitation six months post-injury, she was trying to progressively return to work (15 hours per week). She had also reduced to the bare minimum all sports activities and was receiving help at home for household chores. She felt limited by her headaches and fatigue, which made it difficult to concentrate and caused nonrestorative sleep and sensitivity to noise.

The intervention process that Marie followed is presented below with the associated recommendations from the ONF Guidelines for Concussion/Mild Traumatic Brain Injury and Persistent Symptoms (2013) in order to demonstrate how such best practices can be applied in intervention settings.

---

Guideline recommendations

---

**Section 1  Diagnosis/Assessment of Concussion/mTBI**

☑   1.8   Clinicians should assess, monitor, and document persisting somatic, cognitive, and emotional/behavioral symptoms following mTBI using a standardized assessment scale.
**Rivermead Post Concussion Symptoms Questionnaire → 15/64**

**Section 2  Management of Concussion/mTBI**

☑   2.2   Persons who complain about somatic, cognitive, or behavioral difficulties after mTBI should be assessed and treated symptomatically even if it has been a prolonged time after injury

---

| Few persisting symptoms and risk factors |
| --- |
| Persisting headaches and neck pain |
| Fatigue (physical and mental, difficulty sleeping) |
| Difficulty concentrating |
| High-level job requirements (possible barrier) |

## *Professionals involved and targeted evaluations/interventions*

- Kinesiology: Coaching, guidance and neuromotor interventions during the progressive resumption of sports activities.
- Occupational therapy: Energy management and sleep schedule, reactivation, assessment of job requirements, guidance in the increase of daily tasks and work schedule, education and reassurance.
- Neuropsychology: Assessment of cognitive functions, mental health screening and support for adaptation, education, and reassurance.
- Physician: Complete medical evaluation and treatment of persisting headaches and sleeping problems.

| Guideline recommendations |
| --- |

### Section 4  General Recommendations Regarding Diagnosis/Assessment of Persistent Symptoms

☑ 4.3 The assessment should include a review of currently prescribed medications, over-the-counter medications/supplements, and substance use, including alcohol.

### Section 6  Post-Traumatic Headache

☑ 6.1 Take a focused headache history in order to identify the headache subtype(s) that most closely resembles the patient's symptoms. To aid in determining the specific phenotype of headache disorder present, refer to the International Classification of Headache Disorders (ICHD-II) classification criteria. Unfortunately, some post-traumatic headaches are unclassifiable.

☑ 6.2 Establish the degree of headache-related disability (i.e., missed work/school, decreased productivity, missed social/recreational activities, bedridden) to assist in stratifying a treatment approach (Headache Impact Test 6).

☑ 6.3 Perform a neurologic exam and musculoskeletal exam including cervical spine examination.

### Section 7  Persistent Sleep/Wake Disturbances

☑ 7.1 Every person with concussion/mTBI who has identified sleep problems should be screened for sleep/wake disturbances (e.g., insomnia, excessive daytime sleepiness).

☑ 7.4 Evaluate and treat sleep/wake problems eve in the presence of other problems (anxiety, depression, pain) since it can have positive effects on them.

**Section 8  Persistent Disorders**

☑     8.1     Given their prevalence and potential impact, all patients with persistent
               symptoms following concussion/mTBI should be screened for mental
               health symptoms and disorders, including:
               – Depressive disorders (PHQ-9)
               – Anxiety disorders (GAD-7), including post-traumatic stress disorder
                 (PTSD) (PC-PTSD, PCL-CV)
               – Irritability and other personality changes
               – Substance use disorders (CAGE Questionnaire)
               – Somatoform disorders

## Intervention process

The clinical team did not follow a linear *Evaluation → Intervention* model, but instead pursued simultaneous actions: *Evaluations—Interventions—Education*. For example, at the start, in parallel to evaluations were offered psychoeducation and reassurance interventions for temporary adjustments to difficulties, and education with regard to the expected evolution and the impact of stress on recovery. Many interventions to reassure Marie of her abilities were provided for the purpose of progressive activation, as was education for the recognition of signs foretelling symptoms and on how to manage them.

### Guideline recommendations

**Section 2  Management of Concussion/mTBI**

☑     2.3     The patient should be advised that a full recovery of symptoms is seen in
               the majority of cases.

☑     2.8     On presentation to health care providers, education about symptoms,
               including an advice card provided in writing and explained verbally,
               and reassurance should be provided to all patients and family members.
               Education should ideally be delivered at the time of initial assessment
               or minimally within one week of injury/first assessment.

☑     2.10    Education should be provided in printed material combined with verbal
               review and consist of:
               – Symptoms and expected outcomes
               – Normalizing symptoms (education that current symptoms are
                 expected and common after injury event)
               – Reassurance about expected positive recovery
               – Gradual return to activities and life roles
               – Techniques to manage stress

**Section 5  General Recommendations Regarding Management of Persistent
Symptoms**

☑     5.1     Patients should be advised that they are likely to experience one or more
               symptoms as a consequence of the concussion/mTBI that may persist
               for a short period of time and that this is usually expected (normal
               course)

**Section 11  Persistent Fatigue**

☑    11.1    Determine whether fatigue is a significant symptom by taking a focused history and reviewing the relevant items from administered questionnaires

---

*First intervention plan (established with the concussed individual 2 weeks post-referral; 8 weeks duration)*

Two objectives:

1. Jogging → **Achieved**
   How? Neuromotor stimulation, oculovestibular and spinal exercises, energy management and planning, medication for the headaches, and sleep-aid medication.
2. Increase work hours while maintaining a balanced lifestyle → **Achieved**

*Second intervention plan (8 weeks duration).* Two new objectives:

1. Maintain a full-time work schedule while keeping a balanced lifestyle → **Achieved**
   How? Energy management, restorative sleep, progressive work schedule and work load, weekly grid for self-observation, regular follow-ups with immediate supervisor, follow-up by the occupational therapist on the progressive return to work.
   **Rivermead Post Concussion Symptoms Questionnaire → 8/64**
2. Take part in sports activities, including hockey (possible contact sport) to Marie's satisfaction, while following the clinical team's advice → **Achieved**

---

Guideline recommendations

---

**Section 3  Sport-Related Concussion/mTBI**

☑    3.3    The cornerstone of concussion management is physical and cognitive rest until the acute symptoms resolve and then a graded program of exertion prior to medical clearance and return to play.
   – An initial period of rest in the acute symptomatic period following injury (24–48 hours) may be of benefit.
   – A sensible approach involves the gradual return to school and social activities (prior to contact sports) in a manner that does not result in a significant exacerbation of symptoms.

**Section 6  Post-Traumatic Headache**

☑    6.10    Prophylactic therapy should be considered if headaches are occurring too frequently or are too disabling, or if acute headache medications are contraindicated, poorly tolerated, or being used too frequently
   **→Pregabalin prescribed by physician**

### Section 7  Persistent Sleep/Wake Disturbances

☑    7.5    All patients with persistent sleep/wake complaints should be placed on a program of sleep hygiene in addition to other interventions (or as part of a program of cognitive-behavioral therapy).
→**For example, http://www.msktc.org/tbi/factsheets**

☑    7.7    If medications are to be used, then the aim should be to use medications that will not produce dependency and have minimal adverse effects for mTBI patients. The aim is to establish a more routine sleep pattern. Medications should be used on a short-term basis only.
→**Zopiclone prescribed by physician**

### Section 9  Persistent Cognitive Difficulties

☑    9.6    For cognitive sequelae following mTBI, the cognitive rehabilitation strategies that should be considered include compensatory strategies and remediation approaches. → **Weekly planner, personalized with support from occupational therapist (color-codes, energy levels, post-its, etc.)**

### Section 11  Persistent Fatigue

☑    11.3    If identified as a significant symptom, some key considerations that may aid in the management of persistent fatigue can include:
– Aiming for a gradual increase in activity levels that will parallel improvement in energy levels.
– Reinforce that pacing activities across the day will help patients to achieve more and to avoid exceeding tolerance levels.
– Encouraging good sleep hygiene (especially regularity of sleep/wake schedules, and avoidance of stimulants and alcohol), and proper relaxation times.
– Using a notebook or a diary to plan meaningful goals, record activity achievement, and identify patterns of fatigue.
– Acknowledging that fatigue can be exacerbated by a low mood or stress.
Provide patients with a pamphlet containing advice on coping strategies for fatigue
→**For example, http://www.msktc.org/tbi/factsheets**

### Section 12  Return-to-Activity/Work/School Considerations

☑    12.8    Individuals who continue to experience persistent impairments following mTBI, or those who have not successfully resumed pre-injury work duties following injury, should be referred for a fuller in-depth vocational evaluation by clinical specialists and teams (e.g., occupational therapist, vocational rehabilitation counselor, occupational medicine physician, neuropsychologist, speech language pathologist) with expertise in assessing and treating concussion/mTBI. This evaluation should include an assessment of the person, occupational and job demands, work environment, environmental supports, and facilitators and barriers to successful work/return to work.
→**For example, Position Analysis Questionnaire, Worker Role Interview**

*Overview of interventions and recovery*

With Marie, who was referred 6-months post-mTBI, a small clinical team (physician, occupational therapist, kinesiologist, neuropsychologist) was involved in her intervention plan over a four month period. The frequency of the interventions started at four to five hours per week and decreased progressively to about an hour per week. The team established, with Marie's collaboration and insight, two intervention plans and conducted a final assessment at the time of discharge. Total intervention duration was approximately 18 weeks, including a two-week evaluation period before the first intervention plan was developed.

Professionally, Marie adjusted her work schedule in order to follow the gradual planned progression in terms of schedule and work load. The clinical team noticed that some freedom in the planning and variation of tasks, her possibility to work from home (fewer distractions) as well as some flexibility in her work schedule were facilitating factors for the return to work. Moreover, she adjusted her at-home work station in a way to maintain her neck in a neutral position, which significantly reduces the onset of pain.

However, even with the positive effects of the interventions and the excellent involvement on Marie's part, her energy and resistance to fatigue remained fragile at end of interventions. The clinical team recommended that, if possible for her financially to do so, she adopt for a few months a 4-day (28 hours) per week work schedule. This would reduce the risk of relapse since the overall balanced management of work and other life activities had yet to be fully consolidated.

By doing so, Marie was able to resume her sports activities with confidence. Functionally, she attained a well-balanced schedule. She is now able to manage her energy well (prioritizes, plans and integrates break and rest periods as well as micro pauses, varies tasks and activities, maintains stability in the wake/sleep schedule, plans all activities in a personal organizer). She learned how to adopt a lifestyle that she describes as *wiser*. She also balances out the frequency and intensity of her sports activities so that they remain enjoyable.

## Appendix A

*Tools for planning and self-assessment of a gradual return to work*

A) Example of gradual return to work plan

| IDENTIFICATION OF THE PARTIES | |
|---|---|
| Employer: | Employee: |
| Workplace: | |
| **JOB TITLE** | |
| | |
| **DESCRIPTION OF JOB DUTIES** | |
| | |

| GOAL |
|---|
| Resumption of the role of employee, with a gradual increase in terms of work load and work schedule, in order to foster positive adaptation and build up endurance. |

| OBJECTIVES |
|---|
| 1. At work, the person applies energy management strategies by taking breaks and micro pauses and adjusts their work schedule and work load. |
| 2. The person completes the progressive return to work schedule, all while maintaining a balanced lifestyle. |
| 3. ... |

| TIME PERIOD | |
|---|---|
| From: | To: |
| Number of weeks: | |

| PROGRESSIVE RETURN TO WORK SCHEDULE | |
|---|---|
| **Week** | **Work schedule** |
| Weeks 1, 2 | 2 half-days per week |
| Weeks 3, 4 | 4 half-daysper week |
| Weeks 5, 6 | 1 full day and 3 half-days |
| Weeks 7, 8 | 2 full days and 2 half-days |
| Weeks 9, 10, 11 | 3 full days and 1 half-day |
| Weeks 12 | 4 full days |
| Week 13, 14 | Full time |

*This schedule can be modified at any time according to the employee's evolution, in agreement with all the parties involved.*

| FOLLOW-UP AND PARTICULAR CONDITIONS |
|---|

The progressive return to work will be supervised by _____,
occupational therapist. Phone number: _____ Extension: _____
Through:

– On-site (service provider) meetings, meetings at the work place or telephone follow-ups with the employee (frequency of meetings to be determined according to the employee's evolution).
– Occasional telephone follow-up with the immediate superior.
– Weekly self-assessment grid to be filled out by the employee and to be sent by email.

| SIGNATURES OF THE PARTIES INVOLVED |
|---|

| _____ | _____ |
|---|---|
| *Employer*      *Date* | *Employee*      *Date* |

B)  Example of self-assessment grid

Week worked: _____    Name: _____Date: _____

How many hours did I work this week: _____ and how was my energy level (energy scale 1 to 10, where 10 = full energy):
Morning: _____  Afternoon: _____  Evening:_____

Did I face any difficulties at work?                                                                          Yes ☐ No ☐
If so, what were the difficulties and what strategies did I use to compensate?
_____
_____

At work, did I keep my stress levels at an acceptable level?If so, how?                Yes ☐ No ☐
_____
_____

At work, was I able to manage my pain adequately?If so, how?                            Yes ☐ No ☐
_____
_____

Overall, I maintained healthy life habits (for example, getting enough sleep,
eating meals at regular hours).                                                                              Yes ☐ No ☐
_____
_____

Did I take on my regular tasks at home (for example, house cleaning),
my responsibilities, and maintain contact with family members?                       Yes ☐ No ☐
_____
_____

Did I take part in personal activities that I enjoy and that contribute to
my physical and mental well-being?                                                                      Yes ☐ No ☐
_____
_____

Am I satisfied with my energy management? Did I respect my limits?               Yes ☐ No ☐
_____
_____

Am I satisfied with my productivity level at work?                                               Yes ☐ No ☐
_____
_____

Does my performance meet the expected requirements at my recovery stage?    Yes ☐ No ☐
_____
_____

# References

Ahman S, Saveman BI, Styrke J, Björnstig U, Stålnacke BM (2013). Long-term follow-up of patients with mild traumatic brain injury: A mixed-method study. *J Rehabil Med* 45(8):758–764.

Altman IM, Swick S, Parrot D, Malec JF (2010). Effectiveness of community-based rehabilitation after traumatic brain injury for 489 program completers compared with those precipitously discharged. *Arch Phys Med Rehabil* 91(11): 1697–1704.

Bazarian JJ, Blyth B, Mookerjee S, He H, McDermott MP (2010). Sex differences in outcome after mild traumatic brain injury. *J Neurotrauma* 27(3): 527–539.

Belanger HG, Curtiss G, Demery JA, Lebowitz BK, Vanderploeg RD (2005). Factors moderating neuropsychological outcomes following mild traumatic brain injury: A meta-analysis. *J Int Neuropsychol Soc* 11(3): 215–227.

Bell KR, Hoffman JM, Temkin NR, Powell JM, Fraser RT, Esselman PC, Barber JK, Dikmen S (2008). The effect of telephone counselling on reducing post-traumatic symptoms after mild traumatic brain injury: A randomised trial. *J Neurol Neurosurg Psychiatr* 79(11): 1275–1281.

Bigler ED, Farrer TJ, Pertab JL, James K, Petrie JA, Hedges DW (2013). Reaffirmed limitations of meta-analytic methods in the study of mild traumatic brain injury: A response to Rohling et al. *Clin Neuropsychol* 27(2): 176–214.

Brown NJ, Mannix RC, O'Brien MJ, Gostine D, Collins MW, Meehan WP (2014). Effect of cognitive activity level on duration of post-concussion symptoms. *Pediatrics* 133(2): e299–e304.

Cancelliere C, Kristman VL, Cassidy JD, Hincapié CA, Côté P, Boyle E, Carroll LJ, Stålnacke BM, Nygren-de Boussard C, Borg J (2014). Systematic review of return to work after mild traumatic brain injury: Results of the International Collaboration on Mild Traumatic Brain Injury Prognosis. *Arch Phys Med Rehabil* 95(3 Suppl): S201–S209.

Carroll LJ, Cassidy JD, Holm L, Kraus J, Coronado VG (2004). Methodological issues and research recommendations for mild traumatic brain injury: The WHO Collaborating Centre Task Force on mild traumatic brain injury. *J Rehabil Med* 43: 113–125.

Carson JD, Rendely A, Garel A, Meaney M, Stoller J, Kaicker J, Hayden L, Moineddin R, Frémont P (2016). Are Canadian clinicians providing consistent sport-related concussion management advice? *Can Fam Physic* 62(6): e346–e353.

Cassidy JD, Carroll L, Peloso P, Borg J, Von Holst H, Holm L, Kraus J, Coronado V (2004). Incidence, risk factors and prevention of mild traumatic brain injury: Results of the WHO Collaborating Centre Task Force on Mild Traumatic Brain Injury. *J Rehabil Med* 36(43 Suppl): 28–60.

Desormeau J, McKerral M (2010). Quality of life 1 to 7 years after rehabilitation in people with a traumatic brain injury (TBI)—A pilot study. *J Int Neuropsychol Soc* 16 (Suppl 1): 67.

Dikmen S, Machamer J, Fann JR, Temkin NR (2010). Rates of symptom reporting following traumatic brain injury. *J Int Neuropsychol Soc* 16(3): 401–411.

Drake AI, Gray N, Yoder S, Pramuka M, Llewellyn M (2000). Factors predicting return to work following mild traumatic brain injury: A discriminant analysis. *J Head Trauma Rehabil* 15(5): 1103–1112.

Emanuelson I, Andersson E, Holmkvist R, Björklund R, Stalhammar D (2003). Quality of life and post-concussion symptoms in adults after mild traumatic brain injury: A population-based study in western Sweden. *Acta Neurol Scand* 108(5): 332–338.

Fayol P, Carrière H, Habonimana D, Dumond J-J (2009). Preliminary questions before studying mild traumatic brain injury outcome. *Ann Phys Rehabil Med* 52(6): 497–509.

Fu TS, Jing R, Fu WW, Cusimano MD (2016). Epidemiological trends of traumatic brain injury identified in the emergency department in a publicly-insured population, 2002–2010. *PLoS One* 11(1): e0145469.

Gagnon I, Galli C, Friedman D, Grilli L, Iverson GL (2009). Active rehabilitation for children who are slow to recover following sport-related concussion. *Brain Inj* 23(12): 956–964.

Guérin F, Dominique A, Léveillé G, Kennepohl S, Honoré W, Brière N, McKerral M (2005). Intervention based on the multifactorial nature of mild TBI. In Michallet, B. (Eds.) Interdisciplinary rehabilitation research and traumatic brain injury: New theoretical and clinical perspectives, Montréal: Carte Blanche Editions, pp. 145–157.

Guérin F, Kennepohl S, Léveillé G, Dominique A, Honore W, Brière N, McKerral M (2006). Vocational outcome indicators in atypically recovering mild TBI: A post-intervention study. *NeuroRehabil* 21(4): 295–303.

Guérin F, McKerral M (2008). Le traumatisme craniocérébral léger à évolution atypique: État de la question concernant l'intervention et le retour au travail. In: Banville, F. and Nolin, P. (Eds.) *Épidémie Silencieuse. Le Traumatisme Craniocérébral Léger: Symptômes et Traitement*, Montréal: Presses de l'Université du Québec, pp. 205–212. [Book in French]

Guerrette M-C, McKerral M, LaGarde G, Vincent P, Winter S, Miniciello R et al. (2017). Implantation multicentrique du Mayo-Portland Adaptability Inventory (MPAI-4) en réadaptation: Résultats d'évolution fonctionnelle de la clientèle traumatisée craniocérébrale (TCC). *2e Congrès Québécois de Recherche en Adaptation-Réadaptation*, Montreal, Canada, May 2017.

Institut national d'excellence en santé et en service sociaux (INESSS) (2014). Advice following a mild TBI, adults 16 years of age or older, for the gradual resumption of intellectual activities and physical or sports training. http://fecst.inesss.qc.ca/fileadmin/documents/Publications/DEPLIANT_ANGLAIS_ TCC_ADULTE_11042014.pdf. Accessed 10 October 2016.

Iverson G (2005). Outcome from mild traumatic brain injury. *Curr Opin Psychiatr* 18(3): 301–317.

Iverson GL, Lange RT, Wäljas M, Liimatainen S, Dastidar P, Hartikainen KM, Soimakallio S, Ohman J (2012). Outcome from complicated versus uncomplicated mild traumatic brain injury. *Rehabil Res Pract* 2012: 415740.

Kashluba S, Paniak C, Blake T, Reynolds S, Toller-Lobe G, Nagy J (2004). A longitudinal, controlled study of patient complaints following treated mild traumatic brain injury. *Arch Clin Neuropsychol* 19(6):805–816.

King NS, Crawford S, Wenden FJ, Moss NE, Wadw DT (1995). The Rivermead Post-Concussion Symptoms Questionnaire: A measure of symptoms commonly experienced after head injury and its reliability. *J Neurol* 242(9): 587–592.

Lachapelle J, Bolduc-Teasdale J, Ptito A, McKerral M (2008). Deficits in complex visual information processing after mild TBI: Electrophysiological markers and vocational outcome prognosis. *Brain Inj* 22(3): 265–274.

Leclerc S (2016). La reprise des activités après un TCC léger chez le sportif adulte. *Le Médecin du Québec* 51(1): 49–53. [Article in French]

Leddy JJ, Kozlowski K, Donnelly JP, Pendergast DR, Epstein LH, Willer B (2010). A preliminary study of subsymptom threshold exercise training for refractory postconcussion syndrome. *Clin J Sport Med* 20(1): 21–27.

Losoi H, Silverberg ND, Wäljas M, Turunen S, Rosti-Otajärvi E, Helminen M, Luoto TM, Julkunen J, Öhman J, Iverson GL (2016). Recovery from mild traumatic brain injury in previously healthy adults. *J Neurotrauma* 33(8): 766–776.

Maerlender L, Flashman A, Kessler S, Kumbhani R, Greenwald T, Tosteson, McAllister T (2010). Examination of the construct validity of ImPACT™ computerized test, traditional, and experimental neuropsychological measures. *Clin Neuropsychol* 24(8): 1309–1325.

Malec JF (2004). The Mayo-Portland participation index: A brief and psychometrically sound measure of brain injury outcome. *Arch Phys Med Rehabil* 85(12): 1989–1996.

McCrory P, Meeuwisse WH, Aubry M, Cantu B, Dvořák J, Echemendia RJ, Engebretsen L et al. (2013). Consensus statement on concussion in sport: The 4th International Conference on Concussion in Sport held in Zurich. *Br J Sports Med* 47: 250–258.

McCrory P, Meeuwisse WH, Dvořák J, Aubry M, Bailes J, Broglio S, Cantu RC et al. (2017). Consensus statement on concussion in sport–the 5th international conference on concussion in sport held in Berlin, October 2016. *Br J Sports Med* 51: 838–847.

McKeever CA, Schatz P (2003). Current issues in the identification, assessment, and management of concussions in sports-related injuries. *Appl Neuropsychol* 10(1): 4–11.

McKerral M, Desormeau J (2009). Impact of neuropsychological rehabilitation on return to work after TBI rehabilitation. *J Int Neuropsychol Soc* 15 (Suppl 2): 14.

McKerral M, Léveillé G (2016). Le traumatisme craniocérébral léger à évolution atypique: Intervention spécialisée et perspectives d'avenir. *Le Médecin du Québec* 51(1): 57–61. [Article in French]

Noreau L, Fougeyrollas P, Vincent C (2002). The LIFE-H: Assessment of the quality of social participation. *Technol Disabil* 14(3): 113–118.

Ontario Neurotrauma Foundation-ONF (2013). *Guidelines for Concussion/Mild Traumatic Brain Injury and Persistent Symptoms*(2nd ed) (For adults, 18+ years of age). http://onf.org/documents/guidelines-for-concussion-mtbi-persistent-symptoms-second-edition.

Ouellet J, Boisvert L, Fischer L (2016). Patients presenting to an outpatient sport medicine clinic with concussion. Retrospective observational analysis. *Can Famil Physic* 62(6): e340–e345.

Ponsford J (2005). Rehabilitation interventions after mild head injury. *Curr Opin Neurol* 18(6): 692–697.

Ponsford J, Cameron O, Fitzgerald M, Grant M, Mikocka-Walus A, Schönberger M (2012). Predictors of postconcussive symptoms 3 months after mild traumatic brain injury. *Neuropsychology* 26(3): 304–313.

Ponsford J, Cameron P, Fitzgerald M, Grant M, Mikocka-Walus A (2011). Long-term outcomes after uncomplicated mild traumatic brain injury: A comparison with trauma controls. *J Neurotrauma* 28(6): 937–946.

Ponsford J, Willmott C, Rothwell A, Cameron P, Kelly AM, Nelms R, Curran C (2002). Impact of early intervention on outcome following mild head injury in adults. *J Neurol Neurosurg Psychiatr* 73(3): 330–332.

Public Health Agency of Canada (2014). Mapping Connections: An understanding of neurological conditions in Canada. http://www.phac-aspc.gc.ca/publicat/cd-mc/mc-ec/index-eng.php.

Roozenbeek B, Maas AIR, Menon DK (2013). Changing patterns in the epidemiology of traumatic brain injury. *Nat Rev Neurol* 9(4): 231–236.

Ruffalo CF, Friedland JF, Dawson DR, Colantonio A, Lindsay PH (1999). Mild traumatic brain injury from motor vehicle accidents: Factors associated with return to work. *Arch Phys Med Rehabil* 80(4): 392–398.

Ryu WHA, Feinstein A, Colantonio A, Streiner DL, Dawson DR (2009). Early identification and incidence of mild TBI in Ontario. *Can J Neurol Sci* 36(4): 429–435.

Selassie AW, Wilson DA Pickelsimer EE, Voronca DC, Williams NR, Edwards JC (2013). Incidence of sport-related traumatic brain injury and risk factors of severity: A population-based epidemiologic study. *Ann Epidemiol* 23(12): 750–756.

Silverberg ND, Gardner AJ, Brubacher JR, Panenka WJ, Li JJ, Iverson GL (2015). Systematic review of multivariable prognostic models for mild traumatic brain injury. *J Neurotrauma* 32(8): 517–526.

Sojka P (2011). Sport and non-sport concussions. *Can Med Assoc J* 183(8): 887–888.

Stergiou-Kita M, Mansfield E, Sokoloff S, Colantonio A (2016). Gender influences on return to work after mild traumatic brain injury. *Arch Phys Med Rehabil* 97(2 Suppl): S40–S45.

Stiell IG, Wells GA, Vandemheen K, Clement C, Lesiuk H, Laupacis A, McKnight RD et al. (2001). The Canadian CT Head Rule for patients with minor head injury. *Lancet* 357(9266): 1391–1396.

Stulemeijer M, Van der Werf S, Borm GF, Vos PE (2008). Early prediction of favourable recovery 6 months after mild traumatic brain injury. *J Neurol Neurosurg Psychiatr* 79(8): 936–942.

Tinawi S, Brière N (2016). Le casse-tête du traumatisme craniocérébral léger. Pour voir clair dès le début. *Le Médecin du Québec* 51(1): 31–36. [Article in French]

Vanderploeg RD, Curtiss G, Belanger HG (2005). Long-term neuropsychological outcomes following mild traumatic brain injury. *J Int Neuropsychol Soc* 11(3): 228–236.

Vincent P, Chayer S, Léveillé G, Goulet P, Préville K, Mckerral M (2015). Implantation de l'Inventaire d'Adaptabilité Mayo-Portland-4 comme mesure des résultats en réadaptation: Collaboration et expérience de deux établissements. 10e Congrès québécois de réadaptation, October, Laval, Canada.

Wäljas M, Iverson GL, Lange RT, Hakulinen U, Dastidar P, Huhtala H, Liimatainen S, Hartikainen K, Öhman J (2015). A prospective biopsychosocial study of the persistent post-concussion symptoms following mild traumatic brain injury. *J Neurotrauma* 32(8): 534–547.

Wehman P, Targett P, West M, Kregel J (2005). Productive work and employment for persons with traumatic brain injury what have we learned after 20 years? *J Head Trauma Rehabil* 20(2): 115–127.

Wells EM, Goodkin HP, Griesbach GS (2015). Challenges in determining the role of rest and exercises in the management of mild traumatic brain injury. *J Child Neurol* 31: 86–92.

Wilde EA, Whiteneck GG, Bogner J, Bushnik T, Cifu DX, Dikmen S, French L et al. (2010). Recommendations for the use of common outcome measures in traumatic brain injury research. *Arch Phys Med Rehabil* 91(11): 1650–1660.

## chapter fourteen

# Return to sports
## When and how should I return to sports after a concussion?

*Ruben J. Echemendia*

### Contents

## Introduction

The return to play (RTP) decision following sport-related concussion (SRC) is arguably one of the most complicated decisions made by the sports medicine team. Although seemingly a simple exercise that involves identifying the injury, making a diagnosis, tracking recovery until the concussion has healed, and returning the athlete to sport, we now know that the decision process if far from simple. The RTP decision following SRC is made complex by (a) the nature of the injury itself, (b) the imprecise and varied definitions of concussion, (c) difficulty detecting the injury, (d) the variability in symptom expression that exists between and within athletes who sustain SRC, (e) the broad age range of athletes who sustain SRC, (f) and the risks of reinjury or possible long-term consequences associated with RTP. The injury itself is generally thought to be caused by the transmission of biomechanical forces to the brain either directly through contact with the head or indirectly through blows sustained by the torso (McCrory et al. 2013). Although the definition set forth by the concussion in sport group is widely used in sports medicine, there is no consensus definition that has been accepted broadly in the medical community. Similarly, despite many years of study, there is no clear threshold of force that has been identified to cause an SRC, making it difficult to determine what type and intensity of a blow are necessary to cause SRC (Guskiewicz and Mihalik 2011). Injury identification is also complicated by the lack of visible/behavioral indicators of concussion. For example, Echemendia and colleagues have reported that even with well-defined observable signs of concussions, approximately 53% of concussions in the National Hockey League (NHL) occur without the presence of an observable sign (Echemendia et al. 2017b). Unlike most other sports injuries, an SRC is invisible (there are no bandages, casts, and crutches) or cannot be identified through conventional imaging. The injury cannot conclusively be recognized by any objective bio-marker, and extensive work on the pathophysiology of the injury has uncovered a complex metabolic cascade that leads to dynamic fluctuations in symptoms (Giza and Hovda 2014). The emergence of psychological symptoms, resulting from both direct and indirect injury factors, along with possible iatrogenic effects of treatment complicates the picture even further. All of these factors are involved in managing athletes who are diagnosed with SRC and by extension making the decision to RTP, which then places the competitor at greater risk for additional injury and raises the possibility of long-term neurocognitive dysfunction. The purpose of this chapter is to untangle some of the elements of the RTP decision and discuss these elements in the context of the athlete's life. I will begin by out-lining the historical approaches to RTP, discuss the contemporary key elements or factors included in the RTP decision, and ultimately discuss the differences between RTP deci-sions and the decision to permanently retire an athlete from sport.

## Historical approaches to RTP

The existence of sport-related brain injury has been documented in early history (BC). Modern reports of concussion emerged in the sixteenth century (DeMarco and Barth 2014). Prior to the 1980s, sports concussions were largely believed to be a nuisance that was *part of the game*—a *ding*. These dings were to be shaken off and the player typically continued to play even though he or she may have been suffering from fairly significant symptoms. The tide began to turn as sports medicine professionals recognized that SRC may not be as benign an injury as once thought. Early attempts at standardizing RTP guidelines were an outgrowth of approaches designed to *grade* the injury or to provide a standardized index of injury severity. Grading scales such as those published by Cantu (1992, 1998), the Colorado Medical Society (CMS) (Committee 1990 (revised May 1991)), and the American Academy of Neurology (AAN, 1997) characterized concussion severity into three categories—mild (I), moderate (II), and severe (III), based on symptom dura-tion, amnesia, and loss of consciousness (LOC). Typically, any SRC with associated LOC was considered to be the most severe. For example, the CMS guidelines assigned concus-sion severity as follows: Grade I (Mild), Confusion without amnesia, No LOC; Grade II (Moderate), Confusion with amnesia, No LOC, and grade III (Severe), any LOC. Cantu (1986) was more specific: Grade I, PTA < 30 minutes, no LOC; Grade II, PTA less than 30 minutes but not to exceed 24 hours, LOC less than 5 minutes; and grade III, PTA greater than 24 hours and/or LOC greater than 5 minutes. By today's standards, these levels of LOC or PTA would be considered quite extreme.

The emphasis on LOC was largely a result of studies that associated moderate and severe traumatic brain injury (TBI) outcomes with duration of coma (Benson et al. 1976). However, the importance of LOC to outcome in SRC is not as clear as in moderate to severe TBI (Aubry et al. 2002; Erlanger et al. 2001; Guskiewicz et al. 2000, 2003; Maroon et al. 2000; Lovell et al. 1999; McCrea et al. 2002, 2003; McCrory et al. 2000). The identification of amnesia, either post-traumatic or retrograde, was also considered to be key indicator of concussion severity. As above, although the relationship between amnesia and outcome following moderate and severe TBI was well established (Levin et al. 1979, 1990; Levin and

Eisenberg 1979; Richardson 1990; Russell and Nathan 1946; Russell and Smith 1961; Sciarra 1984), the link between amnesia and outcome in SRC is far less clear (Fisher 1966; Leininger et al. 1990; McCrea et al. 2003; Maddocks et al. 1995) with some suggesting that amnesia is not a good predictor of severity in SRC (McCrory et al. 2009).

The concussion grading scales were associated with management and RTP guidelines for more severe injuries leading to more conservative management. For example, according to CMS, an athlete with a grade I concussion had to be symptom free with no amnesia for 20 minutes before returning to play; at grade II, the athlete had to be symptom free for 1 week prior to RTP; and those with grade III had to be symptom free for 2 weeks prior to RTP. Unfortunately, there was little agreement among the grading systems. For example, under the Cantu (1986) guidelines, grade I and II athletes had to be symptom free for one week, but those with grade III concussions were held out a minimum of one month following being symptom free for one week.

The guidelines also made an attempt at dealing with those athletes who had more than one concussion in a season. Under Cantu, a player with two grade II concussions in the same season was not allowed to RTP for one month after being symptom free. Under the AAN guidelines that same player could RTP after being asymptomatic for two weeks. Although these guidelines were very useful in drawing attention to the issues associated with SRC, there was significant criticism of the guidelines because they were not based on empirical data, they emphasized a *one size fits all* approach to concussion management irrespective of age or athlete history, and they created confusion given the number of different systems and inconsistences among systems.

## RTP contemporary approaches

In light of the criticisms leveled at existing guidelines, the sports medicine community sought to create RTP approaches that were individually tailored and either supported by, or at least informed by, the scientific literature. In November 2001, an international concussion consensus conference was held in Vienna by the Concussion In Sport Group (CISG) with a resulting consensus statement being published in 2002 (Aubry et al. 2002). The CISG convened expert international consensus panels in Prague (McCrory et al. 2005a), Zurich (McCrory et al. 2009, 2013), and more recently in Berlin (McCrory et al. 2017). The CISG has followed an evolving approach to its consensus conferences based on comprehensive reviews of the scientific literature (more recently formal systematic reviews), discussion of the findings by an expert panel with increased public input as the meetings evolved, and ultimately the dissemination of a consensus statement based on the conference proceedings.

The initial Vienna statement was seminal in that it set forth a new definition of sport concussion conceptualized as a complex pathophysiological process caused by biomechanical forces transmitted to the head, leading to functional rather than structural changes to the brain, which resulted in transient symptoms that resolved spontaneously following a sequential course (Aubry et al. 2002). The statement made note of the limitations of the existing concussion grading systems along with their RTP guidelines and made a significant departure from those approaches by emphasizing that SRC management must be individualized. Grading of the concussion was de-emphasized with grading only (if at all) occurring once concussion symptoms had resolved. A second significant departure from the existing models was the recommendation that athletes diagnosed with a concussion should not be returned to the same game or practice (unless under specific circumstances).

The most recent CISG consensus statement (McCrory et al. 2017) maintains continuity with prior documents regarding the management of athletes who sustain SRC. Key components include baseline testing, acute evaluation of athletes suspected of having sustained an SRC and removal of athletes. Significant changes have been made to the SCAT with the revision labeled as the SCAT5 (to be consistent with the 5th meeting of the CISG) (Echemendia et al. 2017d). The SCAT5 was designed to be used by health-care professionals in the evaluation of individuals 13 years old or older during the acute stage of the injury. The SCAT systematic review concluded that the diagnostic utility of the SCAT decays significantly after 3–5 days post-injury, which has implications for how and when the tool should be used (Echemendia et al. 2017a). It appears that the SCAT is useful in helping to diagnose concussion and for tracking recovery (particularly symptom recovery), but it is less useful as an instrument to assist in the RTP decision (Echemendia et al. 2017a). The Child SCAT5 is to be used in the acute phase of injury to evaluate children 5–12 years old who are suspected of having an SRC (Davis et al. 2017). The Concussion Recognition Tool 5 (Echemendia et al. 2017c) is a derivative of the Pocket SCAT, which was developed for use by nonmedically trained individuals to assist in the identification and provide basic management information for *suspected* SRC.

The SCAT5 differs from the SCAT3 in several important ways. The section on immediate/acute assessment was expanded to include additional information on emergency management and observable signs of possible concussion. The SAC immediate and delayed word recall lists provide the option of using a 10-word list to minimize ceiling effects. A rapid neurological screen has been added, which includes a cervical exam, rudimentary assessment of speech, postural stability, gait, oculomotor functioning, and a coordination test (finger to nose). Because the SCAT5 also covers adolescents who are 13 years and older, a return to school progression has been added, which includes suggestions for academic accommodations.

## Assessment

In light of the complexities associated with SRC, it should not be surprising that assessment and evaluation of the injury are multifaceted, differing with the question being asked as well as with the phase of the injury (e.g., acute and postacute). Below is a brief overview of current approaches to assessing SRC.

## Baseline evaluation

Baseline assessment has become a unique feature of most SRC assessment programs. Given the extent of *normal* variability in functioning that exists across players in multiple domains of functioning, the primary purpose of the baseline testing is to provide an estimate of a player's preinjury status. Although typically discussed only with respect to cognitive testing, it is important to note that comprehensive baseline assessments involve domains of functioning in addition to cognitive abilities (e.g., balance/postural stability, oculomotor functioning, health status, and psychological functioning). Specifically, with respect to cognitive assessment, recent research has called into question the utility of the baseline/retest approach over comparisons with normative approaches (Echemendia et al. 2012; Louey et al. 2014; McCrory et al. 2005b; Schatz and Robertshaw 2014). Despite the popularity of baseline testing, the success of within patient baseline/post-injury approach is largely dependent on the temporal stability (test-retest reliability) of the measures being used. If scores on tests remain stable from baseline to some point in the future, then the test is considered reliable and a good candidate for this approach. However, if the test varies significant and unsystematically from time 1 to time 2 without any intervening injury, then its utility in detecting clinically reliable change is diminished. Many neuropsychological measures have test-retest reliability estimates based on convenient time frames such as one week, one month, or even 6 months. In the sports domain, the time interval between baseline and post-injury assessment can be measured in months and years. Long-term test-retest reliability of commonly used neuropsychological measures has recently been assessed by several investigators. For example, Bruce and colleagues found low one-year test-retest reliability for multiple language versions of the immediate post-concussion assessment and cognitive test (ImPACT), the most commonly used computerized battery in professional sports (Bruce et al. 2014). Echemendia and colleagues also found low 2, 3, and 4 year test-retest reliability of ImPACT among samples of English speaking professional hockey players (Echemendia et al. 2016). Poor reliability reduces the sensitivity of a measure, increasing the likelihood that an athlete may RTP before full cognitive recovery.

Evidence has been published that the reliability of ImPACT can be improved by using alternate approaches to generating test composite scores. Using the Schatz and Maerlander (2013) two-factor approach in a sample of professional ice hockey players, Echemendia, Bruce, and colleagues demonstrated that ImPACT reliability could be improved significantly using a 2-factor approach (memory and processing speed) to interpret the test data (Bruce et al. 2016; Echemendia et al. 2016; Schatz and Maerlender 2013). Unfortunately, even though there is converging evidence that the two-factor solution of ImPACT improves reliability, it is yet been made available for commercial use. Bruce and colleagues also demonstrated improved reliability of ImPACT using an aggregate baseline approach; the average of two baseline tests and the two-factor solution provided adequate or better long-term reliability in professional hockey players (2016).

## Acute evaluation

There are three primary questions associated with the acute evaluation. First, is the athlete's injury life threatening? Second, are there indications that a player should be evaluated because of a suspected SRC? Third, does the player meet diagnostic criteria for SRC? Typically, an athletic trainer and/or team physician will conduct an acute evaluation in the game setting. The primary goal acutely is to identify whether the athlete is medically stable (e.g., airway, breathing, and cardiac functioning) and to assess for the possibility of spinal cord injury. If an athlete's symptoms are deteriorating, especially if there is deterioration to a comatose state of consciousness, the situation becomes a medical emergency where immediate transport by ambulance is required (Guskiewicz et al. 2009). The nature and extent of the evaluation may also be sports specific. For example, Fédération Internationale de Football Association (FIFA) has a limitation of three substitutions per team per game and pitch-side assessments typically cannot exceed 3 minutes. If additional time is needed for the evaluation, the team must either continue playing with one less player (a competitive disadvantage) or use a substitution, which is a clear disincentive to an adequate evaluation. The rules for most other professional sports allow for game stoppage and evaluation of players without a substitution penalty. The most widely used tool to assist in the diagnostic process acutely is the SCAT3, now the SCAT5.

Despite admonitions to the contrary, it is not unusual for athletes to continue to play while exhibiting symptoms of concussion, which risks additional injury and prolonged recovery (Elbin et al. 2016; Fraas et al. 2014; McCrea et al. 2004; Meehan et al. 2013). The identification of athletes with possible concussion has evolved to include the use of visible signs of concussion (e.g., loss of consciousness, vacant look, motor incoordination, or balance problems) to minimize reliance on self-reported symptoms. The identification of visible signs has progressed from observation of players by medical staff live during game play to more elaborate models that include spotter programs and video review (Bruce et al. 2017; Echemendia et al. 2017b; Fuller et al. 2016; Gardner 2015a, 2015b; Kemp et al. 2016; Makdissi and Davis 2016a, 2016b).

## Post-injury evaluation

Post-injury assessment of athletes involves either tracking recovery over time or making the RTP decision. As per the CISG guidelines, injured players are gradually introduced to activity as tolerated following a period of cognitive and physical rest. Neuropsychological (and other testing) is introduced either serially post-injury to assess the extent to which a player is recovering or after symptoms resolve to assist in making the RTP decision. Typically, players must be symptom free at rest and at levels of exertion consistent with competitive play and have returned to their estimated neurocognitive level of functioning.

# Culture/Language factors

The effects of increasing cultural and ethnic diversity present interesting challenges to the evaluation of players with SRC. Linguistic differences present formidable challenges since many of the most sensitive neuropsychological tests (Daugherty et al. 2016) used in the sports domain are language dependent (Jones 2014; Shuttleworth-Edwards et al. 2009), most notably with tests of verbal learning and memory. As is typical across most of neuropsychology, there is limited access to large-scale normative neuropsychological data for use with concussed athletes from varying language, ethnic, and educational backgrounds. As such, language-specific normative data are best obtained via local sport-specific data collection using a standardized battery of instruments that have appropriate translations and/or minimal language demands.

A well-developed body of the literature indicates that cultural factors influence performance on standardized and neuropsychological tests, despite the erroneous belief that some tests are free of *cultural bias* (Glymour et al. 2008; Lim et al. 2009; Pedraza and Mungas 2008). Consequently, neuropsychologists who work with athletes from diverse backgrounds are encouraged to adapt testing as needed and interpret findings with an awareness of the limitations that exist when working with individuals whose backgrounds and history are different from the majority culture.

# Physical versus physiological recovery

As noted above, the current approach to management of athletes with SRC is to allow gradual return to activity and competition once the athlete is neurocognitively back to baseline and free of concussion-related symptoms at rest and with exertion. However, recent research suggests that physiological recovery may persist beyond physical or symptomatic recovery. This is particularly important in light of data that the brain may be in a heightened state of vulnerability acutely after a concussive injury (Giza and Hovda 2014; Vagnozzi et al. 2010), and additional trauma during this period of vulnerability may lead to greater disruption in functioning (DeMarco and Barth 2014; Echemendia et al. 2017b; Giza and Hovda 2014). The precise identification of this period of vulnerability is difficult. As developing technology allows for more fine-grained detection of physiological changes, the likelihood of identifying atypical changes that are not clinically meaningful increases.

In other words, we are progressively moving into an arena where we can detect change but the interpretation of that change (i.e., normal vs. abnormal) is unclear. These advances pertain to neuroimaging, biomarkers, electrophysiology, blood flow, and so on, with each of these possibilities identifying different time courses for resolution (McCrory et al. 2017). As such, although some data suggest a prolonged course for physiological recovery that extends beyond the period of vulnerability to additional injury, there are no clear patterns or indicators that allow the clinician to identify when *true* or complete recovery has occurred. It is imperative that research continues in this area because finding greater clarity in the interpretation of data obtained by these measures has the potential of answering some of the most fundamental questions involved in the detection and management of SRC.

## Role of exercise/Active rehabilitation

The cornerstone of concussion management has been physical and cognitive rest until all concussion-related symptoms have abated (McCrory et al. 2009). Although intuitively appealing, the recommendation for rest has often been operationalized by some clinicians to include weeks and months of inactivity with ensuing increases in anxiety and depression. It should not be a surprise that if active athletes are *shut down*, the likelihood of creating additional unintended psychological symptoms increases significantly, particularly as the time of inactivity increases. For school-age children, this is critical because often the inactivity includes not being in school, which at times leads to extended homebound instruction. This isolation from their peers may lead to difficulties in social development.

There is a growing body of the literature which suggests that the judicious application of physical activity/exercise may enhance recovery from SRC. At a physiological level, exercise has been found to facilitate neuroplasticity and neurogenesis and to increase brain-derived neurotrophic factor (BDNF) (Griesbach et al. 2004, 2009), which in turn upsurges neuronal survival and long-term potentiation (increases neuronal signal transmission). Exercise increases vascular endothelial growth factor (VEGF) and insulin-like growth factor (IGF)—both of which increase vascularization and neuronal proliferation. At a psychological level, exercise decreases anxiety (Wipfli et al. 2008), improves self-esteem (Ekeland et al. 2004), sleep quality (Youngstedt 2005), and decreases headaches (Koseoglu et al. 2003). Also, fitness has been associated with increases in bilateral hippocampal volume in children (Chaddock et al. 2010a, 2010b).

In rodents, Griesbech and her colleagues executed a series of elegant studies to assess when and how to introduce exercise post-injury. Their initial study (Griesbach et al. 2009) demonstrated that exercise is useful in promoting recovery post-injury when introduced after a period of relative rest. In a subsequent study, they compared active exercise within one week of fluid percussion injury versus no exercise. Griesbach et al. (2007) found that rodents who were acutely exercised had decreased molecular markers of plasticity, which led to the conclusion that premature exercise compromises compensatory response to injury. In a third study, they found that the amount of the delay in exercise is related to injury severity with more severe injuries requiring greater delay (Griesbach et al. 2007). In sum, exercise following mTBI appears to facilitate recovery in animals. However, there appears to be a window of vulnerability during which the introduction of physical exercise may compromise recovery.

The evidence underlying the beneficial effects of active models of rehabilitation following SRC has been growing. I will briefly touch on two seminal studies. Leddy and colleagues (Willer et al. 2009) emphasized the physiological underpinning of exercise. They explained that post-concussion syndrome is due to physiological dysfunction of autonomic functions (including sympathetic activity) and impaired cerebral autoregulation. They noted that exercise increases parasympathetic activity, decreases sympathetic activation, and increases cerebral blood flow. Willer and colleagues recruited 12 slow to recover individuals, 6 of whom were athletes who continued to have symptoms at rest for more than 6 weeks but for less than 52 weeks. They asked these athletes to undergo a treadmill test until their symptoms increased. The goal of the intervention was to exercise these individuals to the point of exhaustion without an increase in symptoms being observed or reported. Participants were placed on a treadmill daily for 5–6 days per week at 80% of their symptom exacerbation threshold with gradual increases in intensity. Their findings led to the conclusion that the use of controlled exercise as a treatment modality was safe and effective in improving symptoms when compared with a nontreatment control group.

Isabelle Gagnon and her collaborators (Gagnon et al. 2009) created a comprehensive program with 16 slow-to-recover children and adolescents whose symptoms persisted 4 weeks beyond injury. Their program consisted of submaximal aerobic training, light sport-specific coordination exercise, visualization/imagery, and a home program for 20 minutes daily that combined the three prior treatment components. The results revealed that all children and adolescents exhibited a relatively rapid recovery and *returned to their normal lifestyles and sport participation*.

## Retirement

The decision of when to retire from sport or to terminate contact sport activity due to SRC is difficult and often lifealtering at most levels of play (Cantu 2009, 2013; Cantu and Register-Mihalik 2011; Echemendia and Cantu 2003). Although perhaps most prominent at the professional level, athletes in high school, college, and other levels of elite play also wrestle with this decision. Like most factors associated with SRC, the decision of when to retire from sport due to brain injury is complex. The scientific literature is scarce and filled with contradictory findings. We do not have an answer to the frequently asked question: how many is too many? At the very least, it is clear that no uniform standard can be applied to everyone. Consequently clinicians and athletes alike must struggle with which standard(s) to choose. Is it absolute number of concussions? Number of concussions in a season or a lifetime? Severity of concussions? Temporal spacing of concussions? Age of the athlete? Burden and duration of symptoms? Results of diagnostic testing (neuroimaging, neuropsychology, postural stability, blood serum markers)? Interference/deterioration of life functions? Psychosocial functioning? Or, some combination of all of the above?

When choosing one or more criteria for retirement, how do you balance economic/financial concerns, dramatic change in life goals, restructuring of family dynamics, loss of identity/purpose in life, lack of training/preparation for other activities, removal from peer group and/or negative views regarding being weak, soft, unmotivated. Importantly, whose choice is it? Is it the health-care provider, athlete, league/organization or parents? Do states have the right to legislate choice? Does choice vary by age or level of play?

These are clearly complicated questions, which I will not presume to answer here. My goal is to raise the questions and perhaps provide a framework that encourages and promotes open discussion of these difficult issues.

First, and foremost, retirement decisions should be a process, not an event.

It is rare that a single event will disqualify an athlete from play. I view the decision-making process as a series of cost/benefit analyses that should begin when

- Playing is no longer fun
- The thought of returning to play is scary
- When lesser and lesser provocation (impact) produces injury
- When injuries become more closely spaced
- When symptom duration is greater, and symptom duration persists longer
- When neurocognitive deficits persist

In addition to complex clinical questions, Echemendia and Bauer (2015) point out that RTP and retirement decisions often pose ethical dilemmas for clinicians. The decision process is fraught with tensions between preventing harm (e.g., *long term or permanent dysfunction*), doing no harm (e.g., preventing the athlete from playing a sport), and respecting [athlete] autonomy. For example, counseling or dictating that a player should/must retire requires weighing scientific evidence (or lack thereof) for the possibility of long-term neurocognitive dysfunction if the athlete continues playing versus the important role that playing a sport serves to the athlete's identity, self-esteem, career aspirations, social development, as well as academic and economic trajectory.

## Conclusion

The management and ultimate decision to RTP is complex and multifactorial. Although many in the sports medicine world would like simple, even singular tests to identify when a concussion has occurred and when it has ended, it is clear from the research thus far that a simple or singular answer will be elusive and perhaps even impossible given the complexities of brain function and its response to injury. It is incumbent on all clinicians who work with athletes diagnosed with SRC to avail themselves of the knowledge and resources of an interdisciplinary team when treating this injury. It is also clear that the RTP decision is often difficult and fraught with contradictory information and competing ethical considerations. Again the use of an interdisciplinary team to help inform the decision-making process can be useful. In the end, it is up to the clinician to stay abreast of the rapidly growing literature in this area and to accurately communicate what we know and do not know to the athletes we treat.

## References

American Academy of Neurology. 1997. Practice Parameter: The management of concussion in sports (summary statement). Report of the quality standards Subcommittee of the American Academy of Neurology. *Neurology* 48:581–585.

Aubry, M., R. Cantu, J. Dvorak, T. Graf-Baumann, K. Johnston, J. Kelly, M. Lovell, P. McCrory, W. Meeuwisse, and P. Schamasch. 2002. Summary and agreement statement of the first International Conference on Concussion in Sport, Vienna 2001. Recommendations for the improvement of safety and health of athletes who may suffer concussive injuries. *British Journal of Sports Medicine* 36 (1):6–10.

Benson, D. F., H. Gardner, and J. C. Meadows. 1976. Reduplicative paramnesia. *Neurology* 26 (2):147–151.

Bruce, J., R. Echemendia, W. Meeuwisse, P. Comper, and A. Sisco. 2014. 1 year test-retest reliability of ImPACT in professional ice hockey players. *Clinical Neuropsychology* 28 (1):14–25. doi:10.1080/13854046.2013.866272.

Bruce, J., R. Echemendia, L. Tangeman, W. Meeuwisse, P. Comper, M. Hutchison, and M. Aubry. 2016. Two baselines are better than one: Improving the reliability of computerized testing in sports neuropsychology. *Applied Neuropsychology Adult* 23 (5):336–342. doi:10.1080/23279095. 2015.1064002.

Bruce, J. M., R. Echemendia, W. Meeuwisse, M. Hutchison, P. Comper, and M. Aubry. 2017. Development of a risk prediction model among professional hockey players using visible signs of concussion. *British Journal of Sport Medicine*.

Cantu, R. C. 1986. Guidelines for return to contact sports after a cerebral concussion. *The Physician and Sportsmedicine* 14 (10):75–83. doi:10.1080/00913847.1986.11709197.

Cantu, R. C. 1992. Cerebral concussion in sport. Management and prevention. *Sports Medicine* 14 (1):64–74.

Cantu, R. C. 1998. Return to play guidelines after a head injury. *Clinics in Sports Medicine* 17 (1):45–60.

Cantu, R. C. 2009. When to disqualify an athlete after a concussion. *Current Sports Medicine Reports* 8 (1):6–7. doi:10.1249/JSR.0b013e31819677db.

Cantu, R. C. 2013. The role of the neurologist in concussions: When to tell your patient to stop. *JAMA Neurology* 70 (12):1481–1482. doi:10.1001/jamaneurol.2013.3231.

Cantu, R. C., and J. K. Register-Mihalik. 2011. Considerations for return-to-play and retirement decisions after concussion. *PM R* 3 (10 Suppl 2):S440–S444. doi:10.1016/j.pmrj.2011.07.013.

Chaddock, L., K. I. Erickson, R. S. Prakash, J. S. Kim, M. W. Voss, M. Vanpatter, M. B. Pontifex et al. 2010a. A neuroimaging investigation of the association between aerobic fitness, hippocampal volume, and memory performance in preadolescent children. *Brain Research* 1358:172–183. doi:10.1016/j.brainres.2010.08.049.

Chaddock, L., K. I. Erickson, R. S. Prakash, M. VanPatter, M. W. Voss, M. B. Pontifex, L. B. Raine, C. H. Hillman, and A. F. Kramer. 2010b. Basal ganglia volume is associated with aerobic fitness in preadolescent children. *Developmental Neuroscience* 32 (3):249–256. doi:10.1159/000316648.

Committee, Report of the Sports Medicine. 1990 (revised May 1991). *Guidelines for the Management of Concussion in Sports*. Denver, CO: Colorado Medical Society.

Daugherty, J. C., A. E. Puente, A. F. Fasfous, N. Hidalgo-Ruzzante, and M. Perez-Garcia. 2016. Diagnostic mistakes of culturally diverse individuals when using North American neuropsychological tests. *Applied Neuropsychology Adult* 1–7. doi:10.1080/23279095.2015.1036992.

Davis, G. A., L. Purcell, K. Schneider, K. O. Yeates, G. Gioia, V. Anderson, R. Ellenbogen et al. 2017. The child sport concussion assessment tool 5th edition (Child-SCAT5). *British Journal of Sports Medicine*.

DeMarco, A. P. and J. Barth. 2014. Historical perspectives of sport-related concussion: Definition, evaluation, and management. In R. J. Echemendia and G. L. Iverson (Eds.) *The Oxford Handbook or Sport-Related Concussion*. London, UK: Oxford University Press.

Echemendia, R., S. P. Broglio, G. A. Davis, K. Guskiewicz, K. A. Hayden, J. Leddy, W. P. Meehan et al. 2017a. What tests and measures should be added to the SCAT3 and related tests to improve their reliability, sensitivity and/or specificity in sideline concussion diagnosis? A systematic Review *British Journal of Sport Medicine* 51:895–901.

Echemendia, R., J. M. Bruce, W. Meeuwisse, M. Hutchinson, P. Comper, and M. Aubry. 2017b. Visible signs of concussion in the National Hockey League: A preliminary examination using observable signs to predict concussion diagnosis. *British Journal of Sports Medicine*.

Echemendia, R. J., J. M. Bruce, C. M. Bailey, J. F. Sanders, P. Arnett, and G. Vargas. 2012. The utility of post-concussion neuropsychological data in identifying cognitive change following sports-related MTBI in the absence of baseline data. *The Clinical Neuropsychologist* 26 (7):1077–1091. doi:10.1080/13854046.2012.721006.

Echemendia, R. J., J. M. Bruce, W. Meeuwisse, P. Comper, M. Aubry, and M. Hutchison. 2016. Long-term reliability of ImPACT in professional ice hockey. *The Clinical Neuropsychologist* 30 (2):328–337. doi:10.1080/13854046.2016.1158320.

Echemendia, R. J. and R. C. Cantu. 2003. Return to play following sports-related mild traumatic brain injury: The role for neuropsychology. *Applied Neuropsychology* 10 (1):48–55.

Echemendia, R., W. Meeuwisse, P. McCrory, G. A. Davis, M. Putukian, J. Leddy, M. Makdissi et al. 2017c. The concussion recognition tool 5th edition (CRT5). *British Journal of Sport Medicine*.

Echemendia, R., W. Meeuwisse, P. McCrory, G. A. Davis, M. Putukian, J. Leddy, M. Makdissi et al. 2017d. The sport concussion assessment tool 5th edition (SCAT5). *British Journal of Sport Medicine*.

Echemendia, R. J. and R. M. Bauer. 2015. Professional ethics in sports neuropsychology. *Psychological Injury and Law* 8 (4):289–299.

Ekeland, E., F. Heian, K. B. Hagen, J. Abbott, and L. Nordheim. 2004. Exercise to improve self-esteem in children and young people: A systematic Review. *Cochrane Database of Systematic Reviews*: CD003683. doi:10.1002/14651858.CD003683.pub2.

Elbin, R. J., A. Sufrinko, P. Schatz, J. French, L. Henry, S. Burkhart, M. W. Collins, and A. P. Kontos. 2016. Removal from play after concussion and recovery time. *Pediatrics* 138 (3). doi:10.1542/peds.2016-0910.

Erlanger, D., E. Saliba, J. Barth, J. Almquist, W. Webright, and J. Freeman. 2001. Monitoring resolution of postconcussion symptoms in athletes: Preliminary results of a web-based neuropsychological test protocol. *Journal of Athletic Training* 36 (3):280–287.

Fisher, CM. 1966. Concussion amnesia. *Diseases of the Nervous System* 16:826–830.

Fraas, M. R., G. F. Coughlan, E. C. Hart, and C. McCarthy. 2014. Concussion history and reporting rates in elite Irish rugby union players. *Physical Therapy in Sport* 15 (3):136–142. doi:10.1016/j.ptsp.2013.08.002.

Fuller, G. W., S. P. Kemp, and M. Raftery. 2016. The accuracy and reproducibility of video assessment in the pitch-side management of concussion in elite rugby. *Journal of Science & Medicine in Sport* 5:5. doi:10.1016/j.jsams.2016.07.008.

Gagnon, I., C. Galli, D. Friedman, L. Grilli, and G. L. Iverson. 2009. Active rehabilitation for children who are slow to recover following sport-related concussion. *Brain Injury* 23 (12):956–964.

Gardner, A., G. Iverson, M. Wojtowicz, C. Levi, M. Makdissi, T. Quinn, S. Shultz, D. Wright, P. Stanwell. 2015a. A systematic video analysis of concussion in the national rugby league. *Neurology* 84:no pagination.

Gardner, A. J., G. L. Iverson, T. N. Quinn, M. Makdissi, C. R. Levi, S. R. Shultz, D. K. Wright, P. Stanwell. 2015b. A preliminary video analysis of concussion in the National Rugby League. *Brain Injury*:1–4.

Giza, C. C. and D. A. Hovda. 2014. The new neurometabolic cascade of concussion. *Neurosurgery* 75 (Suppl 4):S24–S33. doi:10.1227/NEU.0000000000000505.

Glymour, M. M., J. Weuve, and J. T. Chen. 2008. Methodological challenges in causal research on racial and ethnic patterns of cognitive trajectories: Measurement, selection, and bias. *Neuropsychology Review* 18 (3):194–213. doi:10.1007/s11065-008-9066-x.

Griesbach, G. S., F. Gomez-Pinilla, and D. A. Hovda. 2004. The upregulation of plasticity-related proteins following TBI is disrupted with acute voluntary exercise. *Brain Research* 1016 (2):154–162. doi:10.1016/j.brainres.2004.04.079.

Griesbach, G. S., F. Gomez-Pinilla, and D. A. Hovda. 2007. Time window for voluntary exercise-induced increases in hippocampal neuroplasticity molecules after traumatic brain injury is severity dependent. *Journal of Neurotrauma* 24 (7):1161–1171. doi:10.1089/neu.2006.0255.

Griesbach, G. S., D. A. Hovda, and F. Gomez-Pinilla. 2009. Exercise-induced improvement in cognitive performance after traumatic brain injury in rats is dependent on BDNF activation. *Brain Research* 1288:105–115. doi:10.1016/j.brainres.2009.06.045.

Guskiewicz, K., R. Echemendia, and R. Cantu. 2009. Assessment and return to play following sports-related concussion. In *Orthopaedic Knowledge Update: Sports Medicine.*, edited by WB Kibler. Rosemont, IL: American Academy of Orthopaedic Surgeons.

Guskiewicz, K. M., M. McCrea, S. W. Marshall, R. C. Cantu, C. Randolph, W. Barr, J. A. Onate, and J. P. Kelly. 2003. Cumulative effects associated with recurrent concussion in collegiate football players: The NCAA Concussion Study. *JAMA: The Journal of the American Medical Association* 290 (19):2549–2555. doi:10.1001/jama.290.19.2549.

Guskiewicz, K. M., and J. P. Mihalik. 2011. Biomechanics of sport concussion: Quest for the elusive injury threshold. *Exercise and Sport Sciences Reviews* 39 (1):4–11. doi:10.1097/JES.0b013e318201f53e.

Guskiewicz, K. M., N. L. Weaver, D. A. Padua, and W. E. Garrett, Jr. 2000. Epidemiology of concussion in collegiate and high school football players. *The American Journal of Sports Medicine* 28 (5):643–650.

Jones, N. S., K. D. Walter, R. Caplinger, D. Wright, W. G. Raasch, C. Young. 2014. Effect of education and language on baseline concussion screening tests in professional baseball players. *Clinical Journal of Sport Medicine* 24 (4):284–288. doi:10.1097/JSM.0000000000000031.

Kemp, J. L., J. D. Newton, P. E. White, C. F. Finch. 2016. Implementation of concussion guidelines in community Australian Football and Rugby League-The experiences and challenges faced by coaches and sports trainers. *Journal of Science and Medicine in Sport/Sports Medicine Australia* 19 (4):305–310.

Koseoglu, E., A. Akboyraz, A. Soyuer, and A. O. WErsoy. 2003. Aerobic exercise and plasma beta endorphin levels in patients with migrainous headache without aura. *Cephalgia* 23 (10):972–976.

Leininger, B. E., S. E. Gramling, A. D. Farrell, J. S. Kreutzer, and E. A. Pech. 1990. Neuropsychological deficits in symptomatic minor head injury patients after concussion and mild concussion. *Journal of Neurology, Neurosurgery & Psychiatry* 53:293–296.

Levin, H. S. and H. M. Eisenberg. 1979. Neuropsychological outcome of closed head injury in children and adolescents. *Childs Brain* 5 (3):281–292.

Levin, H. S., H. E. Gary, Jr., H. M. Eisenberg, R. M. Ruff, J. T. Barth, J. Kreutzer, W. M. High Jr et al. 1990. Neurobehavioral outcome 1 year after severe head injury. Experience of the Traumatic Coma Data Bank. *Journal of Neurosurgery* 73 (5):699–709. doi:10.3171/jns.1990.73.5.0699.

Levin, H. S., V. M. O'Donnell, and R. G. Grossman. 1979. The Galveston Orientation and Amnesia Test. A practical scale to assess cognition after head injury. *The Journal of Nervous and Mental Disease* 167 (11):675–684.

Lim, Y. Y., K. H. Prang, L. Cysique, R. H. Pietrzak, P. J. Snyder, and P. Maruff. 2009. A method for cross-cultural adaptation of a verbal memory assessment. *Behavior Research Methods* 41 (4):1190–1200. doi:10.3758/brm.41.4.1190.

Louey, A. G., J. A. Cromer, A. J. Schembri, D. G. Darby, P. Maruff, M. Makdissi, and P. McCrory. 2014. Detecting cognitive impairment after concussion: Sensitivity of change from baseline and normative data methods using the CogSport/Axon cognitive test battery. *Archives Clinical Neuropsychology* 29 (5):432–441. doi:10.1093/arclin/acu020.

Lovell, M. R., G. L. Iverson, M. W. Collins, D. McKeag, and J. C. Maroon. 1999. Does loss of consciousness predict neuropsychological decrements after concussion? *Clinical Journal of Sport Medicine: Official Journal of the Canadian Academy of Sport Medicine* 9 (4):193–198.

Maddocks, D. L., G. D. Dicker, and M. M. Saling. 1995. The assessment of orientation following concussion in athletes. *Clinical Journal of Sport Medicine* 5:32–35.

Makdissi, M. and G. Davis. 2016a. The reliability and validity of video analysis for the assessment of the clinical signs of concussion in Australian football. *Journal of Science & Medicine in Sport* 11:11. doi:10.1016/j.jsams.2016.02.015.

Makdissi, M. and G. Davis. 2016b. Using video analysis for concussion surveillance in Australian football. *Journal of Science & Medicine in Sport* 11:11. doi:10.1016/j.jsams.2016.02.014.

Maroon, J. C., M. R. Lovell, J. Norwig, K. Podell, J. W. Powell, and R. Hartl. 2000. Cerebral concussion in athletes: Evaluation and neuropsychological testing. *Neurosurgery* 47 (3):659–669.

McCrea, M., K. M. Guskiewicz, S. W. Marshall, W. Barr, C. Randolph, R. C. Cantu, J. A. Onate, J. Yang, and J. P. Kelly. 2003. Acute effects and recovery time following concussion in collegiate football players: The NCAA Concussion Study. *JAMA: The Journal of the American Medical Association* 290 (19):2556–2563. doi:10.1001/jama.290.19.2556.

McCrea, M., T. Hammeke, G. Olsen, P. Leo, and K. Guskiewicz. 2004. Unreported concussion in high school football players: Implications for prevention. *Clinical Journal of Sport Medicine* 14 (1):13–17.

McCrea, M., J. P. Kelly, C. Randolph, R. Cisler, and L. Berger. 2002. Immediate neurocognitive effects of concussion. *Neurosurgery* 50 (5):1032–1040.

McCrory, P., K. Johnston, W. Meeuwisse, M. Aubry, R. Cantu, J. Dvorak, T. Graf-Baumann, J. Kelly, M. Lovell, P. Schamasch, and Sport international symposium on concussion in. 2005a. Summary and agreement statement of the 2nd international conference on concussion in sport, Prague 2004. *Clinical Journal of Sport Medicine* 15 (2):48–55.

McCrory, P., M. Makdissi, G. Davis, and A. Collie. 2005b. Value of neuropsychological testing after head injuries in football. *British Journal of Sports Medicine* 39 (Suppl 1):i58–63. doi:10.1136/bjsm.2005.020776.

McCrory, P., W. H. Meeuwisse, M. Aubry, B. Cantu, J. Dvorak, R. J. Echemendia, L. Engebretsen et al. 2013. Consensus statement on concussion in sport: The 4th international conference on concussion in sport held in Zurich, November 2012. *British Journal of Sports Medicine* 47 (5):250–258. doi:10.1136/bjsports-2013-092313.

McCrory, P., W. Meeuwisse, J. Dvorak, M. Aubry, J. Bailes, S. Broglio, R.C. Cantu et al. 2017. Consensus statement on concussion in sport: The 5th international conference on concussion in sport held in Berlin, October 2016. *British Journal of Sports Medicine* (Online First: 26 April 2017). doi: 10.1136/bjsports-2017-097699.

McCrory, P., W. Meeuwisse, K. Johnston, J. Dvorak, M. Aubry, M. Molloy, and R. Cantu. 2009. Consensus statement on concussion in sport: The 3rd international conference on concussion in sport held in Zurich, November 2008. *British Journal of Sports Medicine* 43 (Suppl 1):i76–i90. doi:10.1136/bjsm.2009.058248.

McCrory, P. R., T. Ariens, and S. F. Berkovic. 2000. The nature and duration of acute concussive symptoms in Australian football. *Clinical Journal of Sport Medicine: Official Journal of the Canadian Academy of Sport Medicine* 10 (4):235–238.

Meehan, W. P., R. C. Mannix, M. J. O'Brien, and M. W. Collins. 2013. The prevalence of undiagnosed concussions in athletes. *Clinical Journal of Sport Medicine: Official Journal of the Canadian Academy of Sport Medicine* 23 (5):339–342. doi:10.1097/JSM.0b013e318291d3b3.

Pedraza, O., and D. Mungas. 2008. Measurement in cross-cultural neuropsychology. *Neuropsychology Review* 18 (3):184–193. doi:10.1007/s11065-008-9067-9.

Richardson, J. T. E. 1990. *Clinical and Neuropsychological Aspects of Closed Head Injury.* London, UK: Taylor & Francis Group.

Russell, W. R. and P. Nathan. 1946. Amnesia. *Brain* 69:280–300.

Russell, W. R. and A. Smith. 1961. Posttraumatic amnesia in closed head injury. *Archives of Neurology* 5:16–29.

Schatz, P. and A. Maerlender. 2013. A two-factor theory for concussion assessment using ImPACT: Memory and speed. *Archives of Clinical Neuropsychology* 28 (8):791–797. doi:10.1093/arclin/act077.

Schatz, P. and S. Robertshaw. 2014. Comparing post-concussive neurocognitive test data to normative data presents risks for under-classifying "above average" athletes. *Archives Clinical Neuropsychology* 29 (7):625–632. doi:10.1093/arclin/acu041.

Sciarra, D. 1984. Head injury. In H. H. Merritt and L. P. Rowland, (Eds.) *Merritt's Textbook of Neurology,* pp. 277–279. Philadelphia, PA: Lea & Febiger.

Shuttleworth-Edwards, A. B., V. J. Whitefield-Alexander, S. E. Radloff, A. M. Taylor, and M. R. Lovell. 2009. Computerized neuropsychological profiles of South African versus US athletes: A basis for commentary on cross-cultural norming issues in the sports concussion arena. *The Physician and Sportsmedicine* 37 (4):45–52. doi:10.3810/psm.2009.12.1741.

Vagnozzi, R et al. 2010. Assessment of metabolic brain damage and recovery following mild traumatic brain injury: A multicentre, proton magnetic resonance spectroscopic study in concussed patients. *Brain* 133 (11):3232–3242.

Willer, B., J. Leddy, D. Pendergast, and K. Kozlowski. 2009. Use of low-level exercise to improve the physiologic condition of individuals with post concussion syndrome. *Journal of Head Trauma Rehabilitation* 24 (5):397.

Wipfli, B. M., C. D. Rethorst, and D. M. Landers. 2008. The anxiolytic effects of exercise: A meta-analysis of randomized trials and dose-response analysis. *Journal of Sport and Exercise Psychology* 30 (4):392–410.

Youngstedt, S. D. 2005. Effects of exercise on sleep. *Clinics in Sports Medicine* 24 (2):355–365. doi:10.1016/j.csm.2004.12.003.

## chapter fifteen

# How to manage persistent problems
### What if I don't recover as quickly as I expected from a concussion?

*Isabelle Gagnon*

### Contents

## Introduction

No matter what we accomplish in early and proactive management, as with any other neurological condition, there will be individuals who present a more complex picture to their recovery and they will go on to have persisting difficulties after their concussion. In some individuals, the concussion could have triggered the onset of problems, which could be long lasting. These difficulties can occur in many domains with the commonality that they disrupt functioning and interfere with individuals' abilities to fully participate in what they want or like to do.

Although the majority of individuals would have clinically recovered in the first 2–3 weeks post-injury, persisting symptoms and other problems are not uncommon in the concussion population with 10%–15% of adults (McCrory et al. 2013) and up to 30% of children and youth reporting them 1 month post-injury (Zemek et al. 2016).

Some of the persisting problems encountered after a concussion can be system specific and can respond to focused therapeutic approaches, for example, vestibular or cervical impairments (see Chapter 8). More often, however, problems are likely to relate to the diffuse nature of the injury itself and will require a more global approach to intervention. The notion of continuing to rest is at a continually decreasing rate while waiting for *things to get better* is accepted, and interventions are now generally advocated (Leddy et al. 2016) in an attempt to promote return to premorbid or optimal levels of activity. In that, the field of sport-related concussion is catching up to that of (mild traumatic brain injury) mTBI, where earlier and gradual returns to activity have been promoted consistently and repeatedly in guidelines and systematic reviews (Borg et al. 2004, Nygren-de Boussard et al. 2014, Marshall et al. 2012b, 2015).

One of the difficulties encountered when trying to find a *curative* approach to the rehabilitation of individuals after concussion is the lack of direct apparent link between the proposed pathophysiology and the observed persisting problems, especially as time passes (Waljas et al. 2015). The complexity and variability of the *recovery profiles*, as they are sometimes referred to (Collins et al. 2014, 2016, Henry et al. 2016), thus call for treatment strategies that expand beyond single professional groups and require interdisciplinary assessment and management.

A way to approach this complexity is to view functioning problems after concussion with the lens of a biopsychosocial model, such as the International Classification of Functioning (ICF) (World Health Organization 2001), and then to use that perspective to design interventions. The ICF was developed within the framework of the World Health Organization definition of health, conceptualized as a state of physical and psychosocial well-being. It is meant to accompany the International Classification of Disease-10, which is focused on the etiology of health conditions, but has little reference to the individual consequences of conditions for the individuals. The ICF considers, for example, severity of the condition or the availability of resources and support to more accurately describe an individual's functioning. It provides a unified and standardized language for describing and classifying health domains and health-related states and hence to provide a common framework for health outcome measurement (Stucki 2005). In this biopsychosocial model, disability and functioning are viewed as the outcomes of interactions between health conditions (diseases, disorders, injuries and their consequences on body functions and structures, activities, and participation) and contextual factors (environmental context of the individual and his or her personal factors) (Figure 15.1).

The use of the ICF in TBI has been proposed in both research and clinical care, and efforts to select salient categories that are most pertinent to this condition have led to a TBI ICF CORE set (Bernabeu et al. 2009). Indeed, from more than 1400 categories of the ICF, 139 were retained as being essential to describe the comprehensive nature of functioning after a TBI forms a comprehensive core set, whereas 23 categories were derived from the comprehensive core set and serve as a minimal international standard for

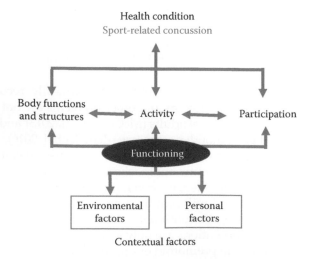

*Figure 15.1* ICF model (WHO, 2001) adapted to sport-related concussion.

reporting functioning through the continuum of care across sectors (see ICF Research Branch Website for details https://www.icf-research-branch.org/). Further work to validate the TBI CORE SET for milder types of TBI has been published (Sveen et al. 2013) confirming how persistent problems after mTBI and concussion can be multifaceted and complex. The line of evidence on prediction models and modifiers for persisting symptoms or slow recovery after concussion is further argumented for the use of biopsychosocial models. The quest for factors that can be used early to identify individuals who will go on to have persisting symptoms has had no choice but to move beyond factors that are related to the injury itself (Silverberg et al. 2015). These models usually not only include factors related to impairments of body functions and structures but also personal and environmental factors (Figure 15.2) (Barlow et al. 2010, McCrory, et al. 2013, Mac Donald et al. 2015, Corbin-Berrigan and Gagnon 2016, Zemek et al. 2016, McCrory et al. 2017). The recovery and intervention targets thus likely lie in the interaction between the identified difficulties or domains of impairments/activity limitations/participation restrictions and the person's environment or personal factors (what they bring to the condition).

We propose here to use the ICF to organize our approach to understand persistent problems and potential therapeutic options post-concussion. The ICF could account for the lack of direct relationship between identified lesions and overall functioning of individuals and would avoid the clinician thinking about simplistic ways to attack the problem one issue at a time. There may not be a single intervention that will help everyone and that, as with other neurotrauma, it is the individualization of treatment through the combination of evidence-based interventions that will likely yield the best results.

The next few pages will review interventions that have been proposed to individuals who have persisting symptoms after concussions. To do this, we will briefly review what

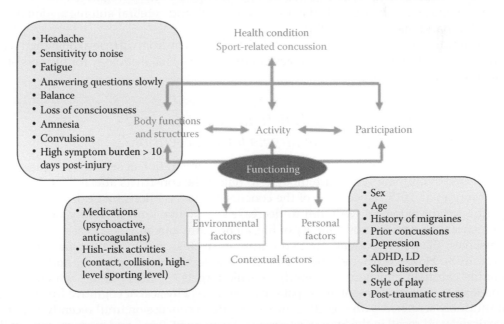

*Figure 15.2* Predictors for poor outcome from selected models and their relation to the ICF model. Models include variables classified as impairments of body functions and structures to personal and environmental factors. (From Zemek, R. et al., *JAMA*, 315, 1014–1025, 2016; Corbin-Berrigan, L.A. and Gagnon, J., *Clin. J. Sport Med.*, 27, 325–327, 2016; Mac Donald, C.L. et al., *Brain*, 138, 1314–1326, 2015; McCrory, P. et al., *Clin. J. Sport Med.*, 23, 89–117, 2013.)

we know about the pathophysiology of concussion that could contribute to longer lasting difficulties, how it could be targeted for intervention, and also discuss other factors that could be targeted.

## Body structures or the pathophysiology related to persistent symptoms

The exact mechanisms responsible for the persisting symptoms continue to elude clinicians and researchers in the field. The general pathophysiology has been described in terms of an acute *neurometabolic cascade* by Giza and Hovda (Giza and Difiori 2011, Giza and Hovda 2001, 2014). This chemical cascade is characterized by an initial injury to cellular membranes that lead to glutamate release and K+ leak into the extracellular space, thus causing the ionic pumps to work overtime and leading to ATP exhaustion. An influx of calcium follows the release of glutamate and makes the aerobic conversion of the initial glucose increase meant to match the pump activity demand inefficient for the cell. Glucose hypometabolism, decreased aerobic activity, and increased free radicals ensue and can last for days to weeks in mild TBI, but up to months after a severe TBI (Barkhoudarian et al. 2011). Tissue is thought to be vulnerable to a subsequent injury during this period. An eventual return to normal function is expected after a concussion; it is also suggested that cell apoptosis is possible in some cases. Giza and Hovda (2014) have suggested clinical correlates to these metabolic changes where the impaired neurotransmission and axonal injury would contribute to the observed persisting impaired cognition, slowed processing, and slowed reaction time (2014). Additional consequences include altered neural connectivity, vascular changes, and decreased cerebral blood flow, as well as decreased white matter volume, excitability, central autonomic control, and cerebral autoregulation (Choe et al. 2012, Barkhoudarian et al. 2016).

To summarize, whether from chemical disturbances or from diffuse axonal injury, the nature of the pathophysiological changes points to a very global etiology for the persistent post-concussion symptoms.

## Persisting problems in body functions, activities, and participation or what are the targets for intervention?

The cornerstone of concussion assessment is the administration of self-report scales grading selected symptoms, which are thought to reflect the constructs affected by the injury (Silverberg et al. 2015). Since most of the concussion interventions that exist or are in the pipeline for development, will aim to decrease symptoms, limit disability or participation restrictions, and improve quality of life, all domains can only be assessed by patients themselves, the use of patient-reported outcomes in this case is relevant and important (Black 2013). However, the addition of objective assessments for physical and cognitive domains can help clinicians to identify specific targets for intervention, which in turn could lead to an improvement of the patient experience. Physical or cognitive function was not routinely screened with objective measures after a concussion until recently. (e.g., balance or delayed recall in the Sport Concussion Assessment Test-3 and more recently in the Sport Concussion Assessment Test-5) (McCrory et al. 2013, Davis et al. 2017, Echemendia et al. 2017). Although the screening items such as the SCAT3 and more recently the SCAT5 represent a valid effort in identifying impairments, they remain of limited utility when planning interventions. Clinicians involved in concussion assessment and intervention need to recognize that, similar to any condition requiring rehabilitation interventions, thorough evaluations will be the key to intervention planning (Ring 2007).

## Self-reported problems

A plethora of papers have been published presenting common post-concussion symptoms reported by individuals beyond the initial recovery period (Marshall et al. 2012a, Leddy et al. 2015, Zemek et al. 2014, 2016). Usually grouped per their physical, cognitive, emotional, or sleep-related nature, symptoms are usually self-reported about their presence and severity when anchored to preinjury levels of the same symptoms, using a number of scales (Lovell 2010, McCrory et al. 2013, Gioia et al. 2009, McCrory et al. 2017). What persisting symptoms are usually reported is highly dependent on several factors, many of which are in the realm of personal factors. Studies relating the reporting of symptoms to imaging are contradictory, some finding clear correlations between image recovery and clinical recovery (Chen et al. 2008), whereas others find no such links (Waljas et al. 2015). In addition, symptom-reporting behaviors (presence and intensity) are found to vary according to age and gender, as well as to individuals' preexisting conditions (Iverson et al. 2015, Brown et al. 2015). Table 15.1 presents the most common symptoms included in current post-concussion scales.

Although symptoms are prominent in patient-reported outcomes after concussion, other areas of functioning that can only be ascertained through self-report can be affected beyond the initial recovery period. This is the case of emotional issues (Kontos et al. 2016, Ellis et al. 2015a) and quality of life, for example (Fineblit et al. 2016, Novak et al. 2016, Polster et al. 2016).

## Deficits observed and assessed

Beyond patient-reported symptoms, the post-concussion assessment includes objective measures of various domains affected by the injury. Those should usually complement what is reported by the patient but should not be limited to areas that are complained of by the patient as there could be deficits that are not reported by the patient (Leddy et al. 2015). Table 15.2 summarizes commonly documented persistent problems in various domains

*Table 15.1* Commonly reported post-concussion symptoms

| Physical symptoms | Cognitive symptoms | Emotional symptoms | Sleep-related symptoms |
|---|---|---|---|
| Headaches | Feeling slowed down | Irritability | Fatigue |
| Nausea | Feeling mentally foggy | Sadness | Trouble falling asleep |
| Vomiting | | Nervousness | |
| Balance problems | Difficulty concentrating | Feeling more emotional | Sleeping more than usual |
| Dizziness | | | |
| Sensitivity to light | Difficulty remembering | | Sleeping less than usual |
| Sensitivity to noise | | | |
| Numbness and tingling | | | Drowsiness |
| Visual problems | | | |
| Neck pain[a] | | | |

[a] Neck pain is sometimes added for a more comprehensive report of patient experience, although not related to the brain injury itself.

*Table 15.2* Commonly reported domains of persisting problems after
mTBI/concussion as per ICF model (order as per ICF codes)

| Body structures and functions | Activity and participation | Environmental factors | Personal factors |
|---|---|---|---|
| **Structures** | Reading | Products and | Previous mental health |
| Brain | Undertaking | technology used in | General physical health |
| Sympathetic and | multiple tasks | daily living | Age |
| parasympathetic | Conversations | Products and | Gender |
| system | Handling stress | technology for | Marital status |
| Eye, ear, and related | Walking | communication | Education and |
| structures | Driving | Sound | profession |
| Head and neck regions | Carrying out daily | Immediate family | Personality |
| **Functions** | routines | Friends | |
| Consciousness | Looking after one's | Community | |
| Temperament and | health | members | |
| personality | Assisting others | Health professionals | |
| Energy and drive | Informal social | People in positions | |
| Sleep | relationships | of authority | |
| Attention | Family relationships | Individual attitudes | |
| Memory | Complex | of family members | |
| Emotional | interpersonal | Individual attitudes | |
| Thought | relationships | of friends | |
| Higher level cognitive | Remunerative | Social security | |
| function | employment | services, systems, | |
| Seeing | Recreation and | and policies | |
| Vestibular | leisure | Health services, | |
| Pain (headache) | | systems, and | |
| | | policies | |

of functioning. The ICF provides us with the framework that is needed to articulate the holistic portrait of potential problems present after concussion.

## Nonpharmacological interventions for persistent problems after concussion

The current advocated early treatment for mTBI or concussion is supportive care with symptom management and avoidance of exertion that worsens symptoms, until the individual feels better or is thought to have recovered (McCrory et al. 2013, Silverberg and Iverson 2013, Zemek et al. 2014, Leddy et al. 2016, McCrory et al. 2017). Then a graded return to more vigorous physical activity and unrestricted sports participation is permitted, once academic and/or work activities are fully reintegrated. This management regime is guided in large part by symptom recovery but is often accompanied by exertional testing (see Chapters 5 through 7 for details on early management).

Individuals who do not recover in the expected timeline (within days up to 1 month post-injury) are often faced with clinicians who have little evidence-based strategies to offer (Zemek et al. 2014, Marshall et al. 2015). Previous chapters in this book have presented the role of various health-care professionals in addressing the multifactorial problems that are identified. Each group presented their perspective on tackling different but related issues. Here, we will not only summarize the existing evidence on interventions that are proposed specifically for problems persisting beyond the initial recovery period but also will highlight the gaps that are still found in the literature, despite intense work in this field over the past 10 years. Reviewing pharmacological interventions for individual symptoms is beyond the scope of this chapter as very little evidence exists in this area (Makdissi et al. 2013). Available consensus-based pharmacological algorithms are proposed for persisting post-traumatic headaches (Pinchefsky et al. 2015, Jensen 2016), sleep-related disorders, or depressive symptoms (Zemek et al. 2014, Marshall et al. 2015), but they have yet to be tested for effectiveness. Of note are the several randomized trials that are currently being conducted looking at the potential of specific molecules to improve headaches and other persistent symptoms (Burke et al. 2015).

Vestibular and cervical rehabilitation interventions have been presented in Chapter 8, whereas rest as a treatment option has been discussed in Chapter 6 and as psychosocial approaches in Chapter 9, thus will not be reviewed here. Instead, we will examine an approach that is more global in nature and will take advantage of the multiple benefits that are related to exercise as they apply to the nervous and cardio vascular systems and which can be viewed as a complement to any of the other treatment options that are already discussed.

## Aerobic exercise

Although it is promoted for daily practice in the general population (American College of Sports Medicine 2013, Pescatello et al. 2013) and its benefits are evident without doubt (Voss et al. 2013, Mann et al. 2014), aerobic exercise could also be an intervention with robust effects on multiple targets in concussion rehabilitation. Aerobic exercise has been used as a global intervention in many neurological conditions such as stroke (Pang et al. 2013, Austin et al. 2014), Parkinson's (Duchesne et al. 2016), brain tumors (Riggs et al. 2016), or severe TBI (Devine et al. 2016, Morris et al. 2016, Weinstein et al. 2017), for example, as well as for various assorted conditions with little commonalities such as migraines (Irby et al. 2015), depressive symptoms (Claesson et al. 2014, Cooney et al. 2014, Josefsson et al. 2014), or schizophrenia (Oertel-Knöchel et al. 2014). Exercise in older adults is associated with improved cognitive functioning (Smith et al. 2010), and there is some evidence that children with greater fitness levels show greater bilateral hippocampal volumes and better performance on a memory test than children with lower fitness levels (Etnier et al. 2006, Chaddock et al. 2010). Exercise is associated with higher ratings of self-esteem (Babic et al. 2014), and it has beneficial effects on sleep quality (Kredlow et al. 2015).

When specifically exploring the rationale to include aerobic activity to manage persistent symptoms and to improve overall functioning after concussion, the most direct preliminary evidence associates its performance with reduced symptom reporting in children, adolescents (Cordingley et al. 2016, Gagnon et al. 2009, 2016, Kurowski et al. 2016), and adults (Leddy et al. 2010a). The literatures regarding the intervention targets for aerobic exercise in the concussion population is organized around two broad lines of evidence: (1) using exercise in individuals who are present with apparent good recovery but who persist to have exercise intolerance, that is, symptoms that appear specifically when they engage in physical exertion; and (2) using exercise for its benefits on brain repair, on facilitating molecular markers of neuroplasticity, on cardiorespiratory function, and on metabolic function.

Exercise intolerance is proposed to be the result of physiological changes in the autonomic nervous system, responsible for cerebral blood flow autoregulation, as well as heart rate and blood pressure control during higher demand activities (Leddy et al. 2007,

2010b, Abaji et al. 2016). Exercise is thus presented as a retraining tool to prime the system into functioning or responding better to higher demands. It prepares it to return to more demanding physical activities. Some evidence suggests that subsymptom threshold aerobic exercises contribute to restore exercise tolerance to normal (Leddy et al. 2010b). Candidates to this treatment are identified through a treadmill exertion test (Baker et al. 2012), where symptom exacerbation is used as a marker during test. If no exacerbation is found, the individual is then thought to have symptoms of another origin and directed for alternative treatment, while being allowed to engage in noncontact physical activity (Leddy and Willer 2013, Ellis et al. 2015b).

Evidence suggests that in addition to restoring exercise tolerance, aerobic exercise can contribute to promoting recovery in a more global way (Wells et al. 2016). Animal models of concussive injury have revealed that aerobic exercise will increase levels of BDNF, a marker of neuroplasticity and will mediate cognitive function through neuroinflammatory and epigenetic responses (Lovatel et al. 2013), while improving spatial learning and memory through increased hippocampal neurogenesis and decreased stress (Li et al. 2013). These effects can be harnessed to promote recovery post-concussion in humans.

Almost 10 years ago, an intervention model, developed for children and adolescents but easily transferred to the general population, has put forward the use of aerobic exercise for all individuals, whether presenting exercise intolerance or not. The program is described extensively elsewhere (Gagnon et al. 2009, 2016, Iverson et al. 2012) but includes aerobic exercise, coordination, and sport-specific exercises, as well as mental imagery and education/reassurance. The latter components are added to specifically improve mood and self-efficacy in relation to the individuals' ability to return to more normal function. This program has shown promising results in not only improving the post-concussion symptoms but also in improving fatigue, mood, and overall quality of life (Gagnon et al. 2016, Gauvin-Lepage et al. 2016). More research is ongoing to examine which active ingredients are more essential to specific recovery profiles, and further work should also examine whether age or sex plays a role in the response.

## Could other types of exercises be useful?

Recent literature has explored other types of exercises including stretching or strengthening exercises in relation to brain health, and, not surprisingly, the benefits initially attributed to aerobic exercises are also suggested to take place in the presence of combinations of exercises, including strengthening and stretching (Gregory et al. 2013, Nouchi et al. 2014). These exercise modes have yet to be studied in the sport-concussion population.

## When should we start?

Concussion management research is now catching up to the TBI literature that has long advocated the return to light activity, including physical noncontact and low-risk activity as early as possible to post-injury (Carroll et al. 2004, Cancelliere et al. 2014, Nygren-de Boussard et al. 2014). Indeed, recent reports examining the early resumption of some form of activity after concussion show less detrimental effects than initially advocated (Grool et al. 2016). Animal models also propose to challenge this delay (Mychasiuk et al. 2016). Although no definitive conclusions can be brought forward, at this time, regarding this ideal delay, most would agree that participating in vigorous physical activity too early may be detrimental to neuroplasticity (Griesbach 2011), resting for long periods may also be detrimental (Thomas et al. 2015), but participating in high risk, contact activities before the *metabolic cascade* has resolved could lead to worse or even catastrophic outcomes. Lines of evidence regarding early activation and definitions of rest have been presented in Chapter 6 in detail and are now being advocated as part of most recent recommendations (McCrory et al. 2017).

Recent reports are suggesting that individuals who do not present with exercise-exacerbated symptoms should not be restricted in how much exercise they choose to participate, as long as it does not exacerbate their symptoms or pose a risk of reinjury (Collins et al. 2016, Leddy et al. 2016), whereas interventions of other nature should be initiated to promote recovery of impairments that are related to cognitive, emotional, or sleep-related dimensions. Interpretations of this *tolerance* level remain quite vague and, without direction, especially in immature adolescent risk-takers, individuals could choose to engage in risky activities.

In summary, management of persistent symptoms in concussion has evolved tremendously over the past 10 years. Experts in the field now recognize the need for a biopsychosocial approach to this issue, and it is only through the involvement of a multidisciplinary team of professionals that individuals sustaining concussions, just as in the case of other types of brain injury, will have optimal outcomes.

---

### Case study: Integrating exercise to intervention

#### SOFIA: 16-YEAR-OLD SOCCER PLAYER

Sofia is a 16-year-old female high-level soccer player who sustained a concussion while at a waterpark. When she was going down a ride in a tube (wearing a protective helmet), she fell out of her tube and hit the left side of her head against a cement wall. She was able to get back on the tube and complete her ride but was not feeling well. She went home at the end of the day. Her immediate symptoms included: unsteadiness, confusion (dazed), headache, pain, difficulty concentrating, and dizziness. She went on to be nauseous the next day but she still did not seek medical attention.

Her symptoms remained present but at low levels, until she reported an increase 2 weeks later when school started (increased cognitive demands). She had difficulty concentrating and completing her days at school. She consulted her pediatrician 3 weeks post-injury and was diagnosed with a concussion. Since she had not followed usual early management recommendations, she was placed on symptom-limited activity restrictions until she was seen for an initial assessment by her local Concussion Interdisciplinary Follow-up Program 2 days later.

##### INITIAL VISIT TO THE CONCUSSION FOLLOW-UP PROGRAM: 3 WEEKS POST-INJURY

Interview information

- Noted to be taking Ibuprofen (BID) since the injury.
- Post-concussion scale (from SCAT5) total score = 30.
  She complained of constant headache (4/6); pressure in the head (5/6); dizziness (1/6); sensitivity to light (3/6); sensitivity to noise (4/6); feeling slowed down (5/6); difficulty concentrating (5/6); and fatigue (5/6). Other items were at 0.
- She had no history of previous concussion, no history of migraines, or any mental health problems before the current concussion.

- The clinic coordinator (health-care professional)
  - Referred to neuropsychology to investigate the school difficulties.
  - Instructed her to stop Advil and initiated a protocol of vitamin B2 as per local headache management protocol.
  - Referred to physiotherapy to begin rehabilitation.
  - Reviewed early management instructions that had not been implemented: proper nutrition and hydration; sleep schedule, and activity management.
  - Letter to school with protocol regarding activity restrictions.

### INITIAL VISIT TO PHYSIOTHERAPY: SAME DAY (3 WEEKS POST-INJURY)

- Normal neurological screening exam; except for decreased coordination; average balance skills.
- No neck pain or dysfunction.
- No positive oculomotor or vestibular tests.
- Aerobic exercise initiated.
  - Tolerated stationary bike for 14 minutes, with heart rate maintained at 110–115 bpm; exertion level calibrated to heart rate target at 2.5/10 on a pediatric pictorial exertion scale.
  - Her headache remained at 4/6 before and during the activity; she reported some fatigue postexercise.
- Coordination exercises using a simple individual soccer drill were added to program.
- Same drill was used as a mental imagery exercise.
- She was sent home with home program including aerobic, coordination, and mental imagery exercises.
- Return in 1 week.

### INITIAL VISIT TO NEUROPSYCHOLOGY: 2 DAYS LATER

- Clinical interview performed.
- No formal testing deemed warranted at this time.
- Contact with school to personalize accommodations.
- Reviewed relaxation techniques and stress management strategies.

### FOLLOW-UP VISIT PHYSIOTHERAPY 4 WEEKS POST-INJURY

- PCS: total = 15. Headaches are much better (2/6), but she is becoming more anxious about making up school work and being away from soccer team; having more difficulty falling asleep (5/6—has begun taking 2-hour naps).
- Coordination skills have improved.
- Tolerated stationary bike for 20 minutes, HR 120–130; PCERT = 4/10. Her HA remained at 2/6 before and during but had disappeared 5 minutes after the end of exercise.
- Sent home with updated program.

### PHONE CONTACT BY CLINIC COORDINATOR 5 WEEKS POST-INJURY

- Symptom-free at rest.
- School return going well, taking exams with only *extended time* accommodations.

- Exercise program reported as being well tolerated and progressed to 30 minutes 70% max heart rate, corresponding to stage 2 of return to play protocol (RTP).

FOLLOW-UP VISIT PHYSIOTHERAPY 6 WEEKS POST-INJURY

- Symptom-free (PCS < 8) at rest and with school activities (including exams without accommodations).
- Completed stages 3–4 of RTP over past week.
- Exertion test administered in clinic, no symptoms elicited.
- Cleared for full return to play.

## References

Abaji, J. P., D. Curnier, R. D. Moore, and D. Ellemberg. 2016. Persisting effects of concussion on heart rate variability during physical exertion. *Journal of neurotrauma* 33 (9):811–817.

American College of Sports Medicine. 2013. *ACSM's Guidelines for Exercise Testing and Prescription.* Philadelphia, PA: Lippincott Williams & Wilkins.

Austin, M. W., M. Ploughman, L. Glynn, and D. Corbett. 2014. Aerobic exercise effects on neuroprotection and brain repair following stroke: A systematic review and perspective. *Neuroscience Research* 87:8–15. doi:10.1016/j.neures.2014.06.007.

Babic, M. J., P. J. Morgan, R. C. Plotnikoff, C. Lonsdale, R. L. White, and D. R. Lubans. 2014. Physical activity and physical self-concept in youth: Systematic review and meta-analysis. *Sports Medicine* 44 (11):1589–1601. doi:10.1007/s40279-014-0229-z.

Baker, J. G., M. S. Freitas, J. J. Leddy, K. F. Kozlowski, and B. S. Willer. 2012. Return to full functioning after graded exercise assessment and progressive exercise treatment of postconcussion syndrome. *Rehabilitation Research and Practice* 2012:705309. doi:10.1155/2012/705309.

Barkhoudarian, G., D. A. Hovda, and C. C. Giza. 2011. The molecular pathophysiology of concussive brain injury. *Clinics in Sports Medicine* 30 (1):33–48. doi:10.1016/j.csm.2010.09.001.

Barkhoudarian, G., D. A. Hovda, and C. C. Giza. 2016. The molecular pathophysiology of concussive brain injury-an update. *Physical Medicine and Rehabilitation Clinics of North America* 27 (2):373–393. doi:10.1016/j.pmr.2016.01.003.

Barlow, K. M., S. Crawford, A. Stevenson, S. S. Sandhu, F. Belanger, and D. Dewey. 2010. Epidemiology of postconcussion syndrome in pediatric mild traumatic brain injury. *Pediatrics* 126 (2):e374–e381. doi:10.1542/peds.2009-0925.

Bernabeu, M., S. Laxe, R. Lopez, G. Stucki, A. Ward, M. Barnes, N. Kostanjsek et al. 2009. Developing core sets for persons with traumatic brain injury based on the international classification of functioning, disability, and health. *Neurorehabilitation and Neural Repair* 23 (5):464–467. doi:10.1177/1545968308328725.

Black, N. 2013. Patient reported outcome measures could help transform healthcare. *BMJ: British Medical Journal* 346. doi:10.1136/bmj.f167.

Borg, J., L. Holm, P. M. Peloso, J. D. Cassidy, L. J. Carroll, H. von Holst, C. Paniak, and D. Yates. 2004. Nonsurgical intervention and cost for mild traumatic brain injury: Results of the WHO collaborating centre task force on mild traumatic brain injury. *Journal of Rehabilitation Medicine* suppl 43:76–83.

Brown, D. A., J. A. Elsass, A. J. Miller, L. E. Reed, and J. C. Reneker. 2015. Differences in symptom reporting between males and females at baseline and after a sports-related concussion: A systematic review and meta-analysis. *Sports Medicine* 45 (7):1027–1040. doi:10.1007/s40279-015-0335-6.

Burke, M. J., M. Fralick, N. Nejatbakhsh, M. C. Tartaglia, and C. H. Tator. 2015. In search of evidence-based treatment for concussion: Characteristics of current clinical trials. *Brain Injury* 29 (3):300–305. doi:10.3109/02699052.2014.974673.

Cancelliere, C., J. D. Cassidy, A. Li, J. Donovan, P. Cote, and C. A. Hincapie. 2014. Systematic search and review procedures: Results of the international collaboration on mild traumatic brain injury prognosis. *Archives of Physical Medicine and Rehabilitation* 95 (3 Suppl):S101–S131. doi:10.1016/j.apmr.2013.12.001.

Carroll, L. J., J. D. Cassidy, P. M. Peloso, J. Borg, H. von Holst, L. Holm, C. Paniak, and M. Pépin. 2004. Prognosis for mild traumatic brain injury: Results of the WHO collaborating center task force on mild traumatic brain injury. *Journal of Rehabilitation Medicine* suppl 43:84–105.

Chaddock, L., K. I. Erickson, R. S. Prakash, J. S. Kim, M. W. Voss, M. Vanpatter, M. B. Pontifex et al. 2010. A neuroimaging investigation of the association between aerobic fitness, hippocampal volume, and memory performance in preadolescent children. *Brain Research* 1358:172–183.

Chen, J. K., K. M. Johnston, M. Petrides, and A. Ptito. 2008. Neural substrates of symptoms of depression following concussion in male athletes with persisting postconcussion symptoms. *Archives of General Psychiatry* 65 :81–89.

Choe, M. C., T. Babikian, J. DiFiori, D. A. Hovda, and C. C. Giza. 2012. A pediatric perspective on concussion pathophysiology. *Current Opinion in Pediatrics* 24 (6):689–695. doi:10.1097/MOP.0b013e32835a1a44.

Claesson, I. M., S. Klein, G. Sydsjo, and A. Josefsson. 2014. Physical activity and psychological well-being in obese pregnant and postpartum women attending a weight-gain restriction programme. *Midwifery* 30 (1):11–16. doi:10.1016/j.midw.2012.11.006.

Collins, M. W., A. P. Kontos, D. O. Okonkwo, J. Almquist, J. Bailes, M. Barisa, J. Bazarian et al. 2016. Statements of agreement from the targeted evaluation and active management (TEAM) approaches to treating concussion meeting held in Pittsburgh, October 15–16, 2015. *Neurosurgery* 79 (6):912–929. doi:10.1227/NEU.0000000000001447.

Collins, M. W., A. P. Kontos, E. Reynolds, C. D. Murawski, and F. H. Fu. 2014. A comprehensive, targeted approach to the clinical care of athletes following sport-related concussion. *Knee Surgery, Sports Traumatology, Arthroscopy* 22 (2):235–246.

Cooney, G., K. Dwan, and G. Mead. 2014. Exercise for depression. *JAMA* 311 (23):2432–2433.

Corbin-Berrigan, L. A. and I. Gagnon. 2016. Postconcussion symptoms as a marker of delayed recovery in children and youth who recently sustained a concussion: A brief report. *Clinical Journal of Sport Medicine* 27 (3):325–327. doi:10.1097/JSM.0000000000000355.

Cordingley, D., R. Girardin, K. Reimer, L. Ritchie, J. Leiter, K. Russell, and M. J. Ellis. 2016. Graded aerobic treadmill testing in pediatric sports-related concussion: Safety, clinical use, and patient outcomes. *Journal of Neurosurgery: Pediatrics* 18 (6):693–702.

Davis, G. A., L. Purcell, K. J. Schneider, K. O. Yeates, G. A. Gioia, V. Anderson, R. G. Ellenbogen et al. 2017. The child sport concussion assessment tool 5th edition (Child SCAT5)." *British Journal of Sports Medicine* 51 (11). doi:10.1136/bjsports-2017-097492.

Devine, J. M., B. Wong, E. Gervino, A. Pascual-Leone, and M. P. Alexander. 2016. Independent, community-based aerobic exercise training for people with moderate-to-severe traumatic brain injury. *Archives of Physical Medicine and Rehabilitation* 97 (8):1392–1397.

Duchesne, C., F. Gheysen, A. Bore, G. Albouy, A. Nadeau, M. E. Robillard, F. Bobeuf et al. 2016. Influence of aerobic exercise training on the neural correlates of motor learning in Parkinson's disease individuals. *NeuroImage: Clinical* 12:559–569. doi:10.1016/j.nicl.2016.09.011.

Echemendia, R. J., W. Meeuwisse, P. McCrory, G. A. Davis, M. Putukian, J. Leddy, M. Makdissi et al. 2017. The sport concussion assessment tool 5th edition (SCAT5). *British Journal of Sports Medicine* 51 (11). doi:10.1136/bjsports-2017-097506.

Ellis, M. J., L. J. Ritchie, M. Koltek, S. Hosain, D. Cordingley, S. Chu, E. Selci, J. Leiter, and K. Russell. 2015a. Psychiatric outcomes after pediatric sports-related concussion. *Journal of Neurosurgery Pediatrics* 16 (6):709–718. doi:10.3171/2015.5.PEDS15220.

Ellis, M. J., J. J. Leddy, and B. Willer. 2015b. Physiological, vestibulo-ocular and cervicogenic post-concussion disorders: An evidence-based classification system with directions for treatment. *Brain Injury* 29 (2):238–248.

Etnier, J. L., P. M. Nowell, D. M. Landers, and B. A. Sibley. 2006. A meta-regression to examine the relationship between aerobic fitness and cognitive performance. *Brain Research Reviews* 52 (1):119–130.

Fineblit, S., E. Selci, H. Loewen, M. Ellis, and K. Russell. 2016. Health-related quality of life after pediatric mild traumatic brain injury/concussion: A systematic review. *Journal of Neurotrauma* 33 (17):1561–1568. doi:10.1089/neu.2015.4292.

Gagnon, I., C. Galli, D. Friedman, L. Grilli, and G. L. Iverson. 2009. Active rehabilitation for children who are slow to recover following sport-related concussion. *Brain Injury* 23 (12):956–964. doi:10.3109/02699050903373477.

Gagnon, I., L. Grilli, D. Friedman, and G. L. Iverson. 2016. A pilot study of active rehabilitation for adolescents who are slow to recover from sport-related concussion. *Scandinavian Journal of Medicine & Science in Sports* 26 (3):299–306. doi:10.1111/sms.12441.

Gauvin-Lepage, J., D. Friedman, L. Grilli, H. Kocilowicz, M. Sufrategui, C. DeMatteo, G. L. Iverson, and I. Gagnon. 2016. Active rehabilitation for youth who are slow to recover from concussion. *Brain Injury* 30 (5–6):551.

Gioia, G. A., J. C. Schneider, C. G. Vaughan, and P. K. Isquith. 2009. Which symptom assessments and approaches are uniquely appropriate for paediatric concussion? *British Journal of Sports Medicine* 43 (Suppl 1):i13–i22. doi:10.1136/bjsm.2009.058255.

Giza, C. C. and J. P. Difiori. 2011. Pathophysiology of sports-related concussion: An update on basic science and translational research. *Sports Health* 3 (1):46–51. doi:10.1177/1941738110391732.

Giza, C. C. and D. A. Hovda. 2001. The neurometabolic cascade of concussion. *Journal of Athletic Training* 36 (3):228–235.

Giza, C. C. and D. A. Hovda. 2014. The new neurometabolic cascade of concussion. *Neurosurgery* 75 (Suppl 4):S24–S33. doi:10.1227/NEU.0000000000000505.

Gregory, M. A, D. P. Gill, and R. J. Petrella. 2013. Brain health and exercise in older adults. *Current Sports Medicine Reports* 12 (4):256–271.

Griesbach, G. S. 2011. Exercise after traumatic brain injury: Is it a fouble-edged sword? *PM&R* 3 (Suppl 6):S64–S72. doi:10.1016/j.pmrj.2011.02.008.

Grool, A. M., M. Aglipay, F. Momoli, W. P. Meehan, S. B. Freedman, K. O. Yeates, J. Gravel et al. 2016. Association between early participation in physical activity following acute concussion and persistent postconcussive symptoms in children and adolescents. *JAMA* 316 (23):2504–2514. doi:10.1001/jama.2016.17396.

Henry, L. C, R. J. Elbin, M. W. Collins, G. Marchetti, and A. P. Kontos. 2016. Examining recovery trajectories after sport-related concussion with a multimodal clinical assessment approach. *Neurosurgery* 78 (2):232–241.

Irby, M. B., D. S. Bond, R. B. Lipton, B. Nicklas, T. T. Houle, and D. B Penzien. 2015. Aerobic exercise for reducing migraine burden: Mechanisms, markers, and models of change processes. *Headache: The Journal of Head and Face Pain* 56 (2):357–369.

Iverson, G. L., I. Gagnon, and G. S. Griesbach. 2012. Active rehabilitation for slow to recover children. In *Mild Traumatic Brain Injury in Children and Adolescents: From Basic Science to Clinical Management*, M. W. Kirkwood and K. O. Yeates, (Eds.). pp. 281–302. New York: Guilford Press.

Iverson, G. L., N. D. Silverberg, R. Mannix, B. A. Maxwell, J. E. Atkins, R. Zafonte, and P. D. Berkner. 2015. Factors associated with concussion-like symptom reporting in high school athletes. *JAMA Pediatrics* 169 (12):1132–1140. doi:10.1001/jamapediatrics.2015.2374.

Jensen, R. H. 2016. Pharmacological treatment of acute and chronic post-traumatic headache. In *Pharmacological Management of Headaches*, D. D. Mitsikostas and K. Paemeleire (Eds.). pp. 179–188. Cham, Switzerland: Springer.

Josefsson, T., M. Lindwall, and T. Archer. 2014. Physical exercise intervention in depressive disorders: Meta-analysis and systematic review. *Scandinavian Journal of Medicine & Science in Sports* 24 (2):259–272. doi:10.1111/sms.12050.

Kontos, A. P., J. M. Deitrick, and E. Reynolds. 2016. Mental health implications and consequences following sport-related concussion. *British Journal of Sports Medicine* 50 (3):139–140. doi:10.1136/bjsports-2015-095564.

Kredlow, M. A., M. C. Capozzoli, B. A. Hearon, A. W. Calkins, and M. W. Otto. 2015. The effects of physical activity on sleep: A meta-analytic review. *Journal of Behavioral Medicine* 38 (3):427–449. doi:10.1007/s10865-015-9617-6.

Kurowski, B. G, J. Hugentobler, C. Quatman-Yates, J. Taylor, P. J. Gubanich, M. Altaye, and S. L. Wade. 2016. Aerobic exercise for adolescents with prolonged symptoms after mild traumatic brain injury: An exploratory randomized clinical trial. *The Journal of Head Trauma Rehabilitation* 32:79–89.

Leddy, J. J., J. G. Baker, A. Merchant, J. Picano, D. Gaile, J. Matuszak, and B. Willer. 2015. Brain or strain? Symptoms alone do not distinguish physiologic concussion from cervical/vestibular injury. *Clinical Journal of Sports Medicine* 25 (3):237–242. doi:10.1097/JSM.0000000000000128.

Leddy, J. J., J. G. Baker, and B. Willer. 2016. Active rehabilitation of concussion and post-concussion syndrome. *Physics Medicine Rehabilitation Clinics of North America* 27 (2):437–454. doi:10.1016/j.pmr.2015.12.003.

Leddy, J. J., K. Kozlowski, J. P. Donnelly, D. R. Pendergast, L. H. Epstein, and B. Willer. 2010a. A preliminary study of subsymptom threshold exercise training for refractory post-concussion syndrome. *Clinical Journal of Sport Medicine* 20 (1):21–27.

Leddy, J. J., K. Kozlowski, J. P. Donnelly, D. R. Pendergast, L. H. Epstein, and B. Willer. 2010b. A preliminary study of subsymptom threshold exercise training for refractory post-concussion syndrome. *Clinical Journal of Sport Medicine* 20 (1):21–27. doi:10.1097/JSM.0b013e3181c6c22c.

Leddy, J. J., K. Kozlowski, M. Fung, D. R. Pendergast, and B. Willer. 2007. Regulatory and autoregulatory physiological dysfunction as a primary characteristic of post concussion syndrome: Implications for treatment. *NeuroRehabilitation* 22 (3):199–205.

Leddy, J. J., and B. Willer. 2013. Use of graded exercise testing in concussion and return-to-activity management. *Current Sports Medicine Reports* 12 (6):370–376.

Li, H., A. Liang, F. Guan, R. Fan, L. Chi, and B. Yang. 2013. Regular treadmill running improves spatial learning and memory performance in young mice through increased hippocampal neurogenesis and decreased stress. *Brain Research* 1531:1–8. doi:10.1016/j.brainres.2013.07.041.

Lovatel, G. A., V. R. Elsner, K. Bertoldi, C. Vanzella, S. Moyses Fdos, A. Vizuete, C. Spindler et al. 2013. Treadmill exercise induces age-related changes in aversive memory, neuroinflammatory and epigenetic processes in the rat hippocampus. *Neurobiology of Learning and Memory* 101:94–102. doi:10.1016/j.nlm.2013.01.007.

Lovell, M. R., Iverson, G. L., Collins, M. W., Podell, K., Johnston, K. M., Pardini, D., and Pardini, J. 2010. Measurement of symptoms following sports-related concussion: Reliability and normative data for the post-concussion scale. *Applied Neuropsychology* 13 (3):166–174. doi:10.1207/s15324826an1303_4.

Mac Donald, C. L., O. R. Adam, A. M. Johnson, E. C. Nelson, N. J. Werner, D. J. Rivet, and D. L. Brody. 2015. Acute post-traumatic stress symptoms and age predict outcome in military blast concussion. *Brain* 138 (Pt 5):1314–1326. doi:10.1093/brain/awv038.

Makdissi, M., R. C. Cantu, K. M. Johnston, P. McCrory, and W. H. Meeuwisse. 2013. The difficult concussion patient: What is the best approach to investigation and management of persistent (>10 days) postconcussive symptoms? *British Journal of Sports Medicine* 47 (5):308–313. doi:10.1136/bjsports-2013-092255.

Mann, S., C. Beedie, and A. Jimenez. 2014. Differential effects of aerobic exercise, resistance training and combined exercise modalities on cholesterol and the lipid profile: Review, synthesis and recommendations. *Sports Medicine* 44 (2):211–221.

Marshall, S., M. Bailey, S. McCullagh, D. Velikonja, and L. Berrigan. 2012a. Guide de pratique clinique pour les lésions cérébrales traumatiques légères et les symptômes persistants. *Canadian Family Physician* 58:e128–e140.

Marshall, S., M. Bayley, S. McCullagh, D. Velikonja, and L. Berrigan. 2012b. Clinical practice guidelines for mild traumatic brain injury and persistent symptoms. *Canadian Family Physician* 58 (3):257–267, e128–140.

Marshall, S., M. Bayley, S. McCullagh, D. Velikonja, L. Berrigan, D. Ouchterlony, K. Weegar, and T. B. I. Expert Consensus Group 2015. Updated clinical practice guidelines for concussion/mild traumatic brain injury and persistent symptoms. *Brain Injury* 29 (6):688–700. doi:10.3109/02699052.2015.1004755.

McCrory, P., W. Meeuwisse, M. Aubry, B. Cantu, J. Dvorak, R. J. Echemendia, L. Engebretsen et al. 2013. Consensus statement on concussion in sport—the 4th international conference on concussion in sport held in Zurich, November 2012. *Clinical Journal of Sport Medicine* 23 (2):89–117. doi:10.1097/JSM.0b013e31828b67cf.

McCrory, P., W. Meeuwisse, J. Dvorak, M. Aubry, J. Bailes, S. Broglio, R. C. Cantu et al. 2017. Consensus statement on concussion in sport-the 5th international conference on concussion in sport held in Berlin, October 2016. *British Journal of Sports Medicine* 51 (11). doi:10.1136/bjsports-2017-097699.

McCrory, P., W. H. Meeuwisse, M. Aubry, B. Cantu, J. Dvorak, R. J. Echemendia, L. Engebretsen et al. 2013. Consensus statement on concussion in sport: The 4th international conference on concussion in sport held in Zurich, November 2012. *British Journal of Sports Medicine* 47 (5):250–258. doi:10.1136/bjsports-2013-092313.

Morris, T., J. Gomes-Osman, D. Costa-Miserachs, and A. Pascual-Leone. 2016. The role of physical exercise in cognitive recovery after traumatic brain injury: A systematic review. *Restorative Neurology and Neuroscience* 34 (6):977–988.

Mychasiuk, R., H. Hehar, I. Ma, S. Candy, and M. J. Esser. 2016. Reducing the time interval between concussion and voluntary exercise restores motor impairment, short-term memory, and alterations to gene expression. *European Journal of Neuroscience* 44 (7):2407–2417.

Nouchi, R., Y. Taki, H. Takeuchi, A. Sekiguchi, H. Hashizume, T. Nozawa, H. Nouchi, and R. Kawashima. 2014. Four weeks of combination exercise training improved executive functions, episodic memory, and processing speed in healthy elderly people: Evidence from a randomized controlled trial. *Age* 36 (2):787–799.

Novak, Z., M. Aglipay, N. Barrowman, K. O. Yeates, M. H. Beauchamp, J. Gravel, S. B. Freedman et al. 2016. Association of persistent postconcussion symptoms with pediatric quality of life. *JAMA Pediatrics* 170 (12):e162900. doi:10.1001/jamapediatrics.2016.2900.

Nygren-de Boussard, C., L. W. Holm, C. Cancelliere, A. K. Godbolt, E. Boyle, B. M. Stalnacke, C. A. Hincapie, J. D. Cassidy, and J. Borg. 2014. Nonsurgical interventions after mild traumatic brain injury: A systematic review. Results of the international collaboration on mild traumatic brain injury prognosis. *Archives of Physical Medicine and Rehabilitation* 95 (Suppl 3):S257–S264. doi:10.1016/j.apmr.2013.10.009.

Oertel-Knöchel, V., P. Mehler, C. Thiel, K. Steinbrecher, B. Malchow, V. Tesky, K. Ademmer, D. Prvulovic, W. Banzer, and Y. Zopf. 2014. Effects of aerobic exercise on cognitive performance and individual psychopathology in depressive and schizophrenia patients. *European Archives of Psychiatry and Clinical Neuroscience* 264 (7):589–604.

Pang, M. Y., S. A. Charlesworth, R. W. Lau, and R. C. Chung. 2013. Using aerobic exercise to improve health outcomes and quality of life in stroke: Evidence-based exercise prescription recommendations. *Cerebrovascular Diseases* 35 (1):7–22. doi:10.1159/000346075.

Pescatello, L. S., R. Arena, D. Riebe, and P. D. Thompson. 2013. SNEAK PEEK: Preview of ACSM's guidelines for exercise testing and prescription, ninth edition. *ACSM's Health & Fitness Journal* 17 (2):16–20. doi:10.1249/FIT.0b013e318282a46d.

Pinchefsky, E., A. S. Dubrovsky, D. Friedman, and M. Shevell. 2015. Part II—Management of pediatric post-traumatic headaches. *Pediatric Neurology* 52 (3):270–280.

Polster, D. R., C. C. Giza, and T. Babikian. 2016. Health-related quality of life after concussion: How can we improve management of care? *JAMA Pediatrics* 170 (12):e162985. doi:10.1001/jamapediatrics.2016.2985.

Riggs, L., J. Piscione, S. Laughlin, T. Cunningham, B. W. Timmons, K. S. Courneya, U. Bartels et al. 2016. Exercise training for neural recovery in a restricted sample of pediatric brain tumor survivors: A controlled clinical trial with crossover of training versus no training. *Neuro Oncology* 19 (3):440–450. doi:10.1093/neuonc/now177.

Ring, H. 2007. Functional assessment in rehabilitation medicine: Clinical applications. *Eura Medicophysics* 43 (4):551–555.

Silverberg, N. D., A. J. Gardner, J. R. Brubacher, W. J. Panenka, J. J. Li, and G. L. Iverson. 2015. Systematic review of multivariable prognostic models for mild traumatic brain injury. *Journal of Neurotrauma* 32 (8):517–526. doi:10.1089/neu.2014.3600.

Silverberg, N. D. and G. L. Iverson. 2013. Is rest after concussion "the best medicine?": Recommendations for activity resumption following concussion in athletes, civilians, and military service members. *Journal of Head Trauma Rehabilitation* 28 (4):250–259. doi:10.1097/HTR.0b013e31825ad658.

Smith, P. J., J. A. Blumenthal, B. M. Hoffman, H. Cooper, T. A. Strauman, K. Welsh-Bohmer, J. N. Browndyke, and A. Sherwood. 2010. Aerobic exercise and neurocognitive performance: A meta-analytic review of randomized controlled trials. *Psychosomatic Medicine* 72 (3):239–252.

Stucki, G. 2005. International classification of functioning, disability, and health (ICF): A promising framework and classification for rehabilitation medicine. *American Journal of Physical Medicine & Rehabilitation* 84:733–740.

Sveen, U., S. Ostensjo, S. Laxe, and H. L. Soberg. 2013. Problems in functioning after a mild traumatic brain injury within the ICF framework: The patient perspective using focus groups. *Disability and Rehabilitation* 35 (9):749–757. doi:10.3109/09638288.2012.707741.

Thomas, D. G., J. N. Apps, R. G. Hoffmann, M. McCrea, and T. Hammeke. 2015. Benefits of strict rest after acute concussion: A randomized controlled trial. *Pediatrics* 135 (2):213–223. doi:10.1542/peds.2014-0966.

Voss, M. W., C. Vivar, A. F. Kramer, and H. van Praag. 2013. Bridging animal and human models of exercise-induced brain plasticity. *Trends in Cognitive Sciences* 17 (10):525–544.

Waljas, M., G. L. Iverson, R. T. Lange, U. Hakulinen, P. Dastidar, H. Huhtala, S. Liimatainen, K. Hartikainen, and J. Ohman. 2015. A prospective biopsychosocial study of the persistent post-concussion symptoms following mild traumatic brain injury. *Journal of Neurotrauma* 32 (8):534–547. doi:10.1089/neu.2014.3339.

Weinstein, A. A., L. M. K. Chin, J. Collins, D. Goel, R. E. Keyser, and L. Chan. 2017. Effect of aerobic exercise training on mood in people with traumatic brain injury: A pilot study. *The Journal of Head Trauma Rehabilitation* 32:E49–E56.

Wells, E. M., H. P. Goodkin, and G. S. Griesbach. 2016. Challenges in determining the role of rest and exercise in the management of mild traumatic brain injury. *Journal of Child Neurology* 31 (1):86–92. doi:10.1177/0883073815570152.

World Health Organization. 2001. *International Classification of Functioning, Disability and Health: ICF.* Geneva, Switzerland: World Health Organization.

Zemek, R., N. Barrowman, S. B. Freedman, J. Gravel, I. Gagnon, C. McGahern, M. Aglipay et al. 2016. Clinical risk score for persistent postconcussion symptoms among children with acute concussion in the ED. *JAMA* 315 (10):1014–1025. doi:10.1001/jama.2016.1203.

Zemek, R., S. Duval, C. DeMatteo, and I. Gagnon. 2014. *Guidelines for Diagnosing and Managing Pediatric Concussion.* Toronto, ON: Ontario Neurotrauma Foundation.

# chapter sixteen

# When the effects of concussions endure
## What are some of the longer term consequences?

**Robin Green and Charles Tator**

## Contents

## Introduction

Concussions were once considered innocuous, fully reversible events that in the context of contact sports were something to be simply *shaken off*, as in the proverbial *bell-ringer*. However, research in recent decades has shown that concussions are not always reversible and in some cases, are linked to enduring and deleterious consequences (Hiploylee et al. 2016).

Concussion symptoms that last beyond the expected period of recovery are known as post-concussion syndrome (PCS) or more recently as *persisting symptoms* (McCrory et al. 2017). Debate has revolved around the etiology of PCS, including the question of whether it reflects persisting organic effects of concussion—particularly in the case of a single concussion—or psychogenic and/or pre-injury factors, such as psychiatric dysfunction (Hoge et al. 2008, 2009, Lagarde et al. 2014, Lishman 1988). In this chapter, we will briefly address this debate, which is tied in part to the difficulties of objectively measuring persisting symptoms using conventional behavioral and imaging tools.

Concussions can also have much longer term effects, and there is increasing evidence of their negative influence on the aging process, which is the main focus of this chapter. We will discuss remote effects of concussion(s) sustained earlier in life, and their impact on brain and behavior decades after injury. We will also briefly discuss considerations for neurorehabilitation.

A comment on terminology: Much of the existing scientific literature uses the terms concussion and mild traumatic brain injury (mTBI) interchangeably. Both terms have multiple definitions associated; for example, Kristman et al. (2014) encountered more than 50 definitions of mTBI in a review spanning approximately a decade of research. We will use the term concussion in this chapter to refer to a traumatic brain injury induced by biomechanical forces, as is used to define a sport-related concussion in the recent consensus statement on concussion in sport (McCrory et al. 2017).

## Persisting symptoms following concussion

In most cases, concussions in adults resolve within 7–10 days when symptoms persist beyond this period, the concussed individual may be considered to be experiencing a failure of normal clinical recovery (McCrory et al. 2017). There has historically been a lack of consensus regarding the point at which recovery should be considered prolonged and anomalous, and this inconsistency is reflected in clinical practices: A recent poll of 2192 physician members of the American College of Sports Medicine (Rose et al. 2015) revealed cut-offs used for diagnosis of PCS ranging from less than 2 weeks to more than 3 months post-injury. The recent expert consensus statement on concussion in sport suggests a cutoff of 10–14 days. In addition, the statement uses the more descriptive and etiologically neutral term of *persisting symptoms* rather than PCS (McCrory et al. 2017).

As the literature reveals, understanding the nature of persisting symptoms – for example, whether they constitute a syndrome (i.e., with a consistent set of symptoms appearing and resolving synchronously)—has been challenging for a number of reasons. These include: the insensitivity of objective diagnostic approaches to the subtle cognitive and neurophysiological effects of the injury (e.g., neuropsychological performance-based testing; conventional neuroimaging); the nonspecific and heterogeneous array of persisting symptoms, many of which rely exclusively on self-report outcome measures (e.g., concentration problems, headache, light-sensitivity, and fatigue); and the range of premorbid individual differences that can moderate the manifestations of injury over time (Stein et al. 2016).

With regard to the limitations of neuropsychological assessment, even at the acute stages of injury, findings are often within the normal range. For example, an individual who scores in the 75th percentile pre-injury and drops 50 percentile points (i.e., > 1 z-score) is still scoring within the average range; thus, a true decline in capacity can be easily missed. Moreover, on self-report measures, current symptoms can be overestimated due to recall bias, for example, the misattribution of current symptoms to the concussion rather than to pre-injury factors. Sometimes known as the *good old days bias*, here the patient may inaccurately report pre-injury functioning as free of cognitive failures and mood problems, thereby overestimating (in relative terms) their post-injury problems (Silverberg et al. 2016). As well, since many persisting symptoms are nonspecific, there are high base-rates of such symptoms in those without concussion. For example, Wäljas et al. (2015) found that 31% of their healthy control sample met criteria for PCS using the International Classification of Diseases, Tenth Revision. Lastly, in some cases, a patient may show reduced engagement in testing, primary gain behaviors (i.e., subconsciously motivated distortion of symptoms in order to reduce an unpleasant psychological state), or volitional secondary gain behaviors (including malingering) that can confound measurement of the organic effects of injury or co-morbidities (Lange et al. 2010, Slick and Sherman 2012). Unfortunately, techniques to confirm or disconfirm such behaviors and motivations, known as *symptom validity* or *performance validity* testing, have notable limitations (Bigler 2014, Heilbronner et al. 2009).

With regard to neuroimaging, conventional approaches such as computed tomography (CT) and magnetic resonance imaging (MRI) do not reliably detect the neurophysiological changes of concussion (Dimou and Lagopoulos 2014). Diffusion tensor imaging (DTI) has emerged as a more promising imaging approach, one that is more sensitive to the microstructural changes of concussion, and use of which has found persistent positive findings in groups of patients who meet criteria for PCS (Smits et al. 2011). However, correlation between such imaging findings and persisting symptoms is observed inconsistently (Ross et al. 2012, Wäljas et al. 2015). This indicates either that behavioral outcome measures—known to be influenced by a host of biopsychosocial factors—cannot reliably measure persisting symptoms caused by concussion-related neural factors or alternatively that persisting symptoms are attributable to causes apart from the organic effects of concussion (Lishman 1988, Silverberg and Iverson 2011). The study of Ledwidge and Molfese (2016) speaks to the enduring neurological effects of concussion. Using electroencephalogram (EEG), they found positive event related potential findings (significantly larger N2 and P3b amplitudes than control, and longer P3b latencies) in athletes who were previously concussed on average four years earlier. These individuals showed normal cognitive performance on testing, but with evidence of compensatory neural recruitment. The findings suggest that greater resources and/or effort are needed for previously concussed individuals to maintain normal cognition. Such a finding has significant clinical import. They underscore the possibility that patients may be able to rise to the occasion of a neuropsychological assessment and perform *normally*, but still show erratic day-to-day functioning (since maintaining such increased effort would not be sustainable) as well as higher mental fatigue, and a need for more sleep. Compensatory neurological effects in the context of normal cognitive performance are observed even in more serious brain injuries (Turner et al. 2011). Such findings raise the question of whether the relationship between structural imaging changes and behavior might be masked by neurological compensation, thereby explaining the absence of correlation that is sometimes observed in studies of PCS (Wäljas et al. 2015).

In the absence of adequate sensitivity and specificity for imaging and neuropsychological measures, as well as varying definitions of concussion and of mTBI, debate continues as to whether there exists a true organic, mTBI-related etiology for PCS (Hoge et al. 2008, Lagarde et al. 2014). For example, Lagarde et al. (2014) argued that "persistent subjective symptoms frequently reported 3 months after MTBI are not specific enough to be identified as a unique PCS and should be considered part of the hyperarousal dimension of PTSD (post-traumatic stress disorder)." Others argue that preconcussion psychiatric disturbances account for the presence of PCS (Ettenhofer et al. 2013, Meares et al. 2008, Ponsford et al. 2012). Findings of acquired neuropsychiatric effects of mTBI do not support this explanation (Chen et al. 2008, Yurgil et al. 2014), nor do studies that have *not* observed a relationship between premorbid psychiatric status and PCS (Tator et al. 2016).

Indeed, quite extensive evidence for the enduring effects of concussion exists (Hiploylee et al. 2016). First, there are cumulative effects of concussions, with more severe symptoms and longer recovery times observed when successive concussions are sustained (Chrisman et al. 2013, Collins et al. 2002, Gronwall and Wrightson 1975, Guskiewicz et al. 2003, Terwilliger et al. 2016). Perhaps the strongest illustrations of the persisting behavioral effects of concussion come from studies that increase the cognitive and motor demands within experimental testing paradigms (Hurtubise et al. 2016). For example, Fait et al. (2013) found that one month post-injury, concussed athletes who were equivalent to controls on conventional neuropsychological testing and were fully recovered on the basis of return-to-play guidelines, showed abnormal performances on a more complex and challenging navigation task requiring integration of locomotor and cognitive functioning. Such findings suggest that behavioral (or neural) compensation may mask persisting symptoms unless a critical threshold of challenge is reached.

Despite evidence supporting the existence of organically based persisting symptoms in group studies, it remains a clinical challenge to reliably diagnose persisting organic effects of concussion at the single case level. As yet, clinical tools are not available to reliably discriminate persisting organic changes that are secondary to the concussion from symptoms that are attributable to: (1) premorbid (e.g., psychiatric) factors (Ponsford et al. 2012) or (2) organic effects that are psychologically amplified, either acutely or later (Lishman 1988, Silverberg and Iverson 2011). It is worth noting that the label *persisting symptoms* allows for any of these manifestations, and from a clinical point of view, there is an argument that hard distinctions between purely physiological versus purely psychological explanations of persisting symptoms are outmoded (Wood 2004).

## Remote effects of concussion

When it comes to measurement of the more remote effects of concussions on the aging process, ascertaining whether or how a prior concussion or multiple concussions is affecting current brain and behavior is even more challenging. Not only relevant are the medical/health-related and psychosocial histories that have transpired between the concussive event(s) and the present, but additional factors that influence the aging process, such as genetics and epi-genetics, as well as whether the acute effects of injury persist or have resolved (Bigler 2013, Ponsford et al. 2012).

Many older adults with a history of concussion feel anxiety when they or their family members become aware of declining cognitive function. A pressing clinical question is whether the individual is suffering from the ongoing effects of their initial injuries that may be worsening with age, or whether the cognitive symptoms are attributable to a neurodegenerative process. If the start-point of cognitive aging is lowered by the enduring cognitive effects of one or many concussions (e.g., persisting memory and attention problems), then in the context of a *normal* aging process, the point of functional disability (or dementia) stands to arrive earlier. In contrast to these additive effects, a synergistic relationship between concussions and aging predicts an even earlier point of functional disability, as described by Bigler in the context of more severe brain injuries (2013). An example of the latter would be the triggering or exacerbation by concussions of a neurodegenerative process.

## Neurodegeneration after a single concussion

A number of studies have shown an increased risk of dementia in patients with a history of moderate-severe TBI (Fleminger et al. 2003, Mortimer et al. 1991). However, in humans, even a single concussion can give rise to measurable early volumetric (Toth et al. 2013) and white matter changes (Gardner et al. 2012), and in animal models, a single concussion can show early deleterious effects that might interact with the aging process. For example, amyloid precursor protein (APP) is unregulated immediately after concussion (Giza and Hovda 2014); and one of its derivatives, beta-amyloid ($A\beta$; the main constituent of amyloid plaques that are the primary hallmark of Alzheimer's Disease) is further observed to accumulate in the weeks and months post-injury. Mediators and markers of APP cleavage into $A\beta$, including beta-secretase, presenilin-1, and caspase-3; along with cleaved tau (another common hallmark of neurodegenerative processes) are observed to accumulate up to 6 months after injury (Chen et al. 2004, Faden and Loane 2015). Such changes might play a causal role in the long-term neurodegenerative effects of injury, either by instigating neurodegeneration (Gerson et al. 2016, Shively et al. 2012) or by accelerating an established neurodegenerative cascade (Gardner and Yaffe 2014, Hobbs et al. 2016).

With regard to epidemiological studies of a single concussion and their remote effects, a small literature exists showing negative downstream effects. Most of the studies showing evidence of a link between a single concussion and dementia or neurodegenerative disease have had modest sample sizes (Graves et al. 1990, Schofield et al. 1997), and where sample sizes have been larger, confounds have been noted (Lee et al. 2013). For example, in one very large nationwide cohort study, the diagnosis of dementia after concussion was observed on average one year following injury, signaling a high likelihood of reverse causation, whereby concussion is caused by the as-yet undiagnosed dementia (Lee et al. 2013). In another large-scale study, Nordström et al. (2014) found only a small increased risk, which the authors surmised was attributable to confounds that had not yet been revealed. One large-scale study, which obviated many confounds of previous studies (e.g., including reverse causation, recall bias, inappropriate control group [e.g., comparison of concussion patients to nontrauma controls]), observed an increased risk of 22%–26% of dementia over the 5–7 years following concussion. However, this finding was restricted to patients who sustained their concussion at age 65 or older (Gardner et al. 2014). Recently, a large meta-analysis found an increased risk of Alzheimer's Disease, Parkinson's disease, Mild Cognitive Impairment, depression, mixed affective disorders, and bipolar disorder in individuals with a history of concussion that was not exclusive to older adults (Perry et al. 2016).

## Multiple concussions and neurodegeneration

The link between trauma to the head and neurodegeneration in the context of *multiple* blows is not new. In 1928 Martland, observed a relationship between blows to the head in boxing and a *punch drunk syndrome* (Martland 1928), a disorder later coined *dementia pugilistica* by Millspaugh (1937), based on the assumption that this relationship was restricted to boxing.

There is now extensive evidence for a link between multiple concussions (and subconcussions) and remote neurodegeneration (Hazrati et al. 2013, McKee et al. 2016, Omalu et al. 2006b). Chronic traumatic encephalopathy (CTE) was coined to describe an encephalopathy due to the effects of trauma that may include but is not exclusively due to boxing (Omalu et al. 2006a). CTE is a tauopathy with overlapping pathophysiology with other neurodegenerative diseases (Omalu et al. 2006a, McKee et al. 2013, Tartaglia et al. 2014). A recent paper presents the findings of the first consensus meeting of neuropathologists to produce neuropathological criteria for the diagnosis of CTE (McKee et al. 2016). The panel concluded there is indeed a unique pathognomonic lesion that distinguishes CTE from other tauopathies. The lesion comprises pathological perivascular accumulation of hyperphosphorylated tau at the depths of cortical sulci on neurons, astroglia and neuronal processes and that is generally distributed around small blood vessels, with an irregular spatial pattern of deposition (McKee et al. 2016).

In terms of the cause(s) of CTE, neuroinflammation is a candidate mechanism that is receiving increasing attention: neuroinflammation is observed in both the acute and chronic stages of injury (Faden et al. 2016), and has been shown to correlate with progressive behavioral decline in the chronic stages of illness (Mouzon et al. 2014). It has been suggested that acute injury leads to axonal injury, loss of microvascular integrity, and breach of the blood brain barrier, triggering an inflammatory cascade, with microglia and astrocyte activation – that leads eventually to CTE pathology (Lucke-Wold et al. 2014). Of interest, this mechanism is compatible with a recent explanation of persisting symptoms, where the authors have argued for a neuroinflammatory basis of explanation for persisting symptoms, recommending that PCS be classified as a *post-inflammatory brain syndrome* (Rathbone et al. 2015). A very recent human post-mortem study examined the relationship between microglial inflammation and hyperphosphorylated tau accumulation in CTE in 66 deceased American football players and found evidence that chronic activation of microglia mediated the effects of exposure to tau pathology and to CTE (Cherry et al. 2016). The finding provides human evidence of a link between early events (i.e., microglial activation that persists) and downstream neurodegeneration, evidence that encouragingly offers direction for treatment research.

An increased understanding of the connection between CTE and multiple concussions is actively being sought; answers to questions regarding the minimal dose or exposure (both for concussive and subconcussive events) necessary for disease, and resilience and risk factors are of high clinical and scientific import. Much of the human research to date on this topic has been limited by the case series methodology of studies, such as ascertainment bias, with many studies to date including predominantly patients who were neurologically symptomatic before they died. Not all individuals with a history of multiple concussions in the context of contact sport develop CTE (Hazrati et al. 2013). However, in their brain bank study, Bieniek et al. (2015) observed CTE only in former athletes who had participated in contact sports, with 21 of 66 of these individuals showing CTE pathology. Of the 198 individuals without a history of contact sports, including 33 with a history of a single TBI, CTE pathology was not observed.

It is of interest to note that neuropathological differences have been observed between single versus multiple events. For example, TDP-43 is notable in CTE (McKee et al. 2016). However, after a single moderate-severe TBI, pathological (phosphorylated) TDP-43 was not observed in a study by Johnson and colleagues (2011), although immunoreactivity to phosphorylation-independent TDP-43 both acutely and later post-injury was observed. Giza and Hovda (2014) raise the question whether occurrence of a second mTBI prior to full recovery, as occurs frequently in the context of contact sports, may instigate "…more lasting metabolic perturbations that may then trigger activation of intracellular proteases and the cascade that leads to apoptotic cell death." This offers an explanation for the pathophysiological differences of a single event versus multiple events in the case where the latter are sustained in close succession.

Finally, CTE is diagnosed post-mortem, but other post-trauma dementias are diagnosed clinically (though often confirmed post-mortem). Therefore it is possible that cases of mTBI-associated Alzheimer's Disease, Parkinson's Disease, and FTD would in fact on post-mortem analysis display CTE neuropathology or that CTE may contain co-occurring pathology. In a recent meta-analysis, Perry et al. (2016) found that multiple neurodegenerative and psychiatric disorders were associated with the same injury exposure. These findings raise mechanistic questions of shared vulnerability (e.g., predisposition to different dementias through common early mechanisms such as microglial activation or protein deposition), but also raise the question whether varying clinical presentations/phenotypes are actually the manifestation of a common underlying pathology (Perry et al. (2016)). More research, including longitudinal prospective studies with post-mortem examination of retired players of contact sports *without* neurological disorders, is needed in order to elucidate causal relationships between multiple concussions and CTE.

## Some neurorehabilitation considerations for the enduring effects of concussion(s)

Based on an understanding of underlying mechanisms of enduring effects of single and multiple concussions, promising treatment research is underway. For example, evidence of concussion effects on the autonomic nervous system (i.e., altered heart-rate variability and cerebrovascular coupling) (Gall et al. 2004a, 2004b, Goldstein et al. 1998, Leddy et al. 2007) has led to the subsymptom-threshold exercise regimen of Leddy et al. (2016). Here, exercise thresholds for eliciting concussion symptoms are individually determined, and an exercise regimen (below this threshold) is recommended. This approach has been demonstrated to improve tolerance of every-day activities including exercise.

In the context of aging, an important clinical question regarding the effects of single and multiple concussions is whether they are causing a neurodegenerative process. While the relationship between aging-related changes and concussions is ill-understood, predicting the outcome of concussion(s) in an *individual* is still more challenging. A wide range of factors with known neurological effects may negatively influence the physiological interactions between concussive events and the aging process, including systemic illnesses that compromise the brain (e.g., diabetes), substance use, sleep disturbance, mood disorders, and genetic and epigenetic factors (Chen et al. 2008, Ponsford et al. 2012). Conversely, even when a neurodegenerative process is present, there are factors that can temper its clinical manifestations. For example, higher cognitive reserve has been associated with normal clinical expression in individuals whose brains post-mortem revealed considerable neuropathology (Snowdon 2003).

Although we have only a very limited understanding of the additive and synergistic relationships between history of concussion, the aging process, and the countless subject and environmental factors that may contribute, it is essential nonetheless to be aware of *modifiable* factors that may help to protect current functioning and to stave off decline. Tomaszczyk et al. (2014) have argued that a person with an injured brain in the context of factors that can reduce cognitive, physical, and social stimulation (aka environmental enrichment)—such as aging-related vision and hearing loss and/or environmental changes (e.g., retirement)—may experience a more precipitous functional deterioration (Tomaszczyk et al. 2014). Such environmental and physical factors that increase isolation and withdrawal from family and communities (and thereby reduce ongoing cognitive and social stimulation)—should therefore be identified and managed appropriately (Tomaszczyk et al. 2014).

Certainly better management could be achieved if it were possible to prognosticate very long-term outcomes from the time of initial concussion(s). This would also allow for better research into early treatment options. An *in vivo* diagnostic tool for CTE (for which there is an increasing association with multiple concussions, though no definitive causal links as yet) would also increase treatment options. Positron emission tomography (PET) imaging with tau ligand is an imaging modality with the potential to make such determinations; this would allow for pharmacological agents that are in use with other tauopathies to be trialed in patients with CTE (Grüninger 2015, Karakaya et al. 2012).

Understanding the mechanistic relationship between concussion, PCS and these long-term outcomes is an important area of study. As noted earlier, there is increasing attention in the literature to neuroinflammation as one such mechanism in both animal (see Faden et al. (2016) for review) and human research (Cherry et al. 2016). Promising therapeutic studies to offset neuroinflammation in animals have now been reported, employing both exercise regimens and pharmacological interventions (e.g., the phosphodiesterase inhibitor ibudilast) in the *chronic* stages of injury, and ameliorative effects have been observed not only on chronic microglial activation, but also on later neurodegeneration and associated behavioral impairments (Piao et al. 2013, Rodgers et al. 2014).

Regarding behavioral interventions, there is evidence for atrophy and neurochemical (magnetic resonance spectroscopy) changes of the hippocampi not only in normal aging, but also due to the remote effects of aging plus multiple concussions (Aungst et al. 2014, Giza and Hovda 2014, Singh et al. 2014, Tremblay et al. 2013). Interventions that can affect hippocampal function and structure could therefore be harnessed. For example, Lövdén et al. (2012) found that 16 weeks of computerized allocentric navigation activities (tasks requiring virtual navigation from a bird's eye view) buffered against normal aging-related atrophy of the hippocampi over that period; others have demonstrated a positive relationship between hippocampal volume and allocentric spatial navigation in the context of neurological illness (Bohbot et al. 2004, Konishi and Bohbot 2013). Given the remote neuropsychiatric effects in those with a history of multiple concussions (Goswami et al. 2016, Hart et al. 2013), cognitive behavior therapy and mindfulness meditation are tried-and-true therapies for mood disorders as well as emotion regulation/anger problems (Fann et al. 2015, Hsieh et al. 2012, Johansson et al. 2012). Importantly, such therapies can be delivered remotely, even in people with severe cognitive impairments (Arundine et al. 2012, Bradbury et al. 2008, Fann et al. 2015), which would allow for greater access to therapy.

## Conclusion

In sum, there is extensive evidence that single and multiple mTBIs give rise to enduring and deleterious consequences to brain and behavior, from months to decades after injury. The extensive research into this area has begun to elucidate our understanding of the characteristics and mechanisms of these enduring effects. Encouragingly, some of these mechanisms may be modifiable, and promising treatment research that harnesses advances from this basic research is underway.

## Acknowledgments

The authors wish to thank Carmela Tartaglia, Brenda Colella, Bhanu Sharma, and Alana Changoor for their help with preparation of this book chapter.

## References

Arundine, A., C. L. Bradbury, K. Dupuis, D. R. Dawson, L. A. Ruttan, and R. E. Green. 2012. Cognitive behavior therapy after acquired brain injury: Maintenance of therapeutic benefits at 6 months posttreatment. *The Journal of Head Trauma Rehabilitation* 27 (2):104–112. doi:10.1097/HTR.0b013e3182125591.

Aungst, S. L., S. V. Kabadi, S. M. Thompson, B. A. Stoica, and A. I. Faden. 2014. Repeated mild traumatic brain injury causes chronic neuroinflammation, changes in hippocampal synaptic plasticity, and associated cognitive deficits. *Journal of Cerebral Blood Flow & Metabolism* 34 (7):1223–1232. doi:10.1038/jcbfm.2014.75.

Bieniek, K. F., O. A. Ross, K. A. Cormier, R. L. Walton, A. Soto-Ortolaza, A. E. Johnston, P. DeSaro et al. 2015. Chronic traumatic encephalopathy pathology in a neurodegenerative disorders brain bank. *Acta Neuropathologica* 130 (6):877–889.

Bigler, E. D. 2013. Traumatic brain injury, neuroimaging, and neurodegeneration. *Frontiers in Human Neuroscience* 7:395.

Bigler, E. D. 2014. Effort, symptom validity testing, performance validity testing and traumatic brain injury. *Brain Injury* 28 (13–14):1623–1638.

Bohbot, V. D., G. Iaria, and M. Petrides. 2004. Hippocampal function and spatial memory: Evidence from functional neuroimaging in healthy participants and performance of patients with medial temporal lobe resections. *Neuropsychology* 18 (3):418–425. doi:10.1037/0894-4105.18.3.418.

Bradbury, C. L., B. K. Christensen, M. A. Lau, L. A. Ruttan, A. L. Arundine, and R. E. Green. 2008. The efficacy of cognitive behavior therapy in the treatment of emotional distress after acquired brain injury. *Archives of Physical Medicine and Rehabilitation* 89 (12 Suppl):S61–S68. doi:10.1016/j.apmr.2008.08.210.

Chen, J. K., K. M. Johnston, M. Petrides, and A. Ptito. 2008. Neural substrates of symptoms of depression following concussion in male athletes with persisting postconcussion symptoms. *Archives of General Psychiatry* 65 (1):81–89.

Chen, X. H., R. Siman, A. Iwata, D. F. Meaney, J. Q. Trojanowski, and D. H. Smith. 2004. Long-term accumulation of amyloid-beta, beta-secretase, presenilin-1, and caspase-3 in damaged axons following brain trauma. *The American Journal of Pathology* 165 (2):357–371.

Cherry, J. D, Y. Tripodis, V. E. Alvarez, B. Huber, P. T. Kiernan, D. H. Daneshvar, J. Mez, P. H. Montenigro, T. M. Solomon, and M. L. Alosco. 2016. Microglial neuroinflammation contributes to tau accumulation in chronic traumatic encephalopathy. *Acta Neuropathologica Communications* 4 (1):112.

Chrisman, S. P, F. P. Rivara, M. A. Schiff, C. Zhou, and R. D. Comstock. 2013. Risk factors for concussive symptoms 1 week or longer in high school athletes. *Brain Injury* 27 (1):1–9.

Collins, M. W., M. R. Lovell, G. L. Iverson, R. C. Cantu, J. C. Maroon, and M. Field. 2002. Cumulative effects of concussion in high school athletes. *Neurosurgery* 51 (5):1175–1181.

Dimou, S. and J. Lagopoulos. 2014. Toward objective markers of concussion in sport: A review of white matter and neurometabolic changes in the brain after sports-related concussion. *Journal of Neurotrauma* 31 (5):413–424.

Ettenhofer, M. L., L. E. Reinhardt, and D. M. Barry. 2013. Predictors of neurobehavioral symptoms in a university population: A multivariate approach using a postconcussive symptom questionnaire. *Journal of the International Neuropsychological Society* 19 (9):977–985. doi:10.1017/S1355617713000763.

Faden, A. I. and D. J. Loane. 2015. Chronic neurodegeneration after traumatic brain injury: Alzheimer disease, chronic traumatic encephalopathy, or persistent neuroinflammation? *Neurotherapeutics* 12 (1):143–150. doi:10.1007/s13311-014-0319-5.

Faden, A. I., J. Wu, B. A. Stoica, and D. J. Loane. 2016. Progressive inflammation-mediated neurodegeneration after traumatic brain or spinal cord injury. *British Journal of Pharmacology* 173 (4):681–691.

Fait, P., B. Swaine, J. F. Cantin, J. Leblond, and B. J. McFadyen. 2013. Altered integrated locomotor and cognitive function in elite athletes 30 days postconcussion: A preliminary study. *The Journal of Head Trauma Rehabilitation* 28 (4):293–301.

Fann, J. R., C. H. Bombardier, S. Vannoy, J. Dyer, E. Ludman, S. Dikmen, K. Marshall, J. Barber, and N. Temkin. 2015. Telephone and in-person cognitive behavioral therapy for major depression after traumatic brain injury: A randomized controlled trial. *Journal of Neurotrauma* 32 (1):45–57. doi:10.1089/neu.2014.3423.

Fleminger, S., D. L. Oliver, S. Lovestone, S. Rabe-Hesketh, and A. Giora. 2003. Head injury as a risk factor for Alzheimer's disease: The evidence 10 years on; a partial replication. *Journal of Neurology, Neurosurgery & Psychiatry* 74 (7):857–862.

Gall, B., W. Parkhouse, and D. Goodman. 2004a. Heart rate variability of recently concussed athletes at rest and exercise. *Medicine and Science in Sports and Exercise* 36 (8):1269–1274.

Gall, B., W. S. Parkhouse, and D. Goodman. 2004b. Exercise following a sport induced concussion. *British Journal Sports Medicine* 38 (6):773–777. doi:10.1136/bjsm.2003.009530.

Gardner, A., F. Kay-Lambkin, P. Stanwell, J. Donnelly, W. H. Williams, A. Hiles, P. Schofield, C. Levi, and D. K. Jones. 2012. A systematic review of diffusion tensor imaging findings in sports-related concussion. *Journal of Neurotrauma* 29 (16):2521–2538. doi:10.1089/neu.2012.2628.

Gardner, R. C. and K. Yaffe. 2014. Traumatic brain injury may increase risk of young onset dementia. *Annals of Neurology* 75 (3):339.

Gardner, R. C., J. F. Burke, J. Nettiksimmons, A. Kaup, D. E. Barnes, and K. Yaffe. 2014. Dementia risk after traumatic brain injury vs nonbrain trauma: The role of age and severity. *JAMA Neurology* 71 (12):1490–1497. doi:10.1001/jamaneurol.2014.2668.

Gerson, J., D. L. Castillo-Carranza, U. Sengupta, R. Bodani, D. S. Prough, D. S. DeWitt, B. E. Hawkins, and R. Kayed. 2016. Tau oligomers derived from Traumatic Brain Injury cause cognitive impairment and accelerate onset of pathology in Htau mice. *Journal of Neurotrauma* 33 (22):2034–2043.

Giza, C. C. and D. A. Hovda. 2014. The new neurometabolic cascade of concussion. *Neurosurgery* 75 (4):S24.

Goldstein, B., D. Toweill, S. Lai, K. Sonnenthal, and B. Kimberly. 1998. Uncoupling of the autonomic and cardiovascular systems in acute brain injury. *American Journal of Physiology-Regulatory, Integrative and Comparative Physiology* 275 (4 Pt 2):R1287–R1292.

Goswami, R., P. Dufort, M. C. Tartaglia, R. E. Green, A. Crawley, C. H. Tator, R. Wennberg, D. J. Mikulis, M. Keightley, and K. D. Davis. 2016. Frontotemporal correlates of impulsivity and machine learning in retired professional athletes with a history of multiple concussions. *Brain Structure and Function* 221 (4):1911–1925.

Graves, A. B., E. White, T. D. Koepsell, B. V. Reifler, G. van Belle, E. B. Larson, and M. Raskind. 1990. The association between head trauma and Alzheimer's disease. *American Journal of Epidemiology* 131 (3):491–501.

Gronwall, D. and P. Wrightson. 1975. Cumulative effect of concussion. *The Lancet* 306 (7943):995–997.

Grüninger, F. 2015. Invited review: Drug development for tauopathies. *Neuropathology and Applied Neurobiology* 41 (1):81–96.

Guskiewicz, K. M, M. McCrea, S. W. Marshall, R. C. Cantu, C. Randolph, W. Barr, J. A. Onate, and J. P. Kelly. 2003. Cumulative effects associated with recurrent concussion in collegiate football players: The NCAA Concussion Study. *Jama* 290 (19):2549–2555.

Hart, J., Jr., M. A. Kraut, K. B. Womack, J. Strain, N. Didehbani, E. Bartz, H. Conover, S. Mansinghani, H. Lu, and C. M. Cullum. 2013. Neuroimaging of cognitive dysfunction and depression in aging retired National football league players: A cross-sectional study. *JAMA Neurology* 70 (3):326–335. doi:10.1001/2013.jamaneurol.340.

Hazrati, L. N., M. C. Tartaglia, P. Diamandis, K. Davis, R. E. A. Green, R. Wennberg, J. C. Wong, L. Ezerins, and C. H. Tator. 2013. Absence of chronic traumatic encephalopathy in retired football players with multiple concussions and neurological symptomatology. *Frontiers in Human Neuroscience* 7:222.

Heilbronner, R. L., J. J. Sweet, J. E. Morgan, G. J. Larrabee, S. R. Millis, and Conference Participants 1. 2009. American academy of clinical neuropsychology consensus conference statement on the neuropsychological assessment of effort, response bias, and malingering. *The Clinical Neuropsychologist* 23 (7):1093–1129.

Hiploylee, C., P. A. Dufort, H. S. Davis, R. A. Wennberg, M. C. Tartaglia, D. Mikulis, L. N. Hazrati, and C. H. Tator. 2016. Longitudinal study of postconcussion syndrome: Not everyone recovers. *Journal of Neurotrauma* 34 (8):1511–1523.

Hobbs, J. G., J. S. Young, and J. E. Bailes. 2016. Sports-related concussions: Diagnosis, complications, and current management strategies. *Neurosurgical Focus* 40 (4):E5. doi:10.3171/2016.1.FOCUS15617.

Hoge, C. W., H. M. Goldberg, and C. A. Castro. 2009. Care of war veterans with mild traumatic brain injury—flawed perspectives. *The New England Journal of Medicine* 360 (16):1588–1591. doi:10.1056/NEJMp0810606.

Hoge, C. W., D. McGurk, J. L. Thomas, A. L. Cox, C. C. Engel, and C. A. Castro. 2008. Mild traumatic brain injury in U.S. Soldiers returning from Iraq. *The New England Journal of Medicine* 358 (5):453–463. doi:10.1056/NEJMoa072972.

Hsieh, M. Y., J. Ponsford, D. Wong, M. Schonberger, A. McKay, and K. Haines. 2012. A cognitive behaviour therapy (CBT) programme for anxiety following moderate-severe traumatic brain injury (TBI): Two case studies. *Brain Injury* 26 (2):126–138. doi:10.3109/02699052.2011.635365.

Hurtubise, J., D. Gorbet, Y. Hamandi, A. Macpherson, and L. Sergio. 2016. The effect of concussion history on cognitive-motor integration in elite hockey players. *Concussion* 1 (3):CNC17.

Johansson, B., H. Bjuhr, and L. Ronnback. 2012. Mindfulness-based stress reduction (MBSR) improves long-term mental fatigue after stroke or traumatic brain injury. *Brain Injury* 26 (13–14):1621–1628. doi:10.3109/02699052.2012.700082.

Johnson, V. E, W. Stewart, J. Q. Trojanowski, and D. H. Smith. 2011. Acute and chronically increased immunoreactivity to phosphorylation-independent but not pathological TDP-43 after a single traumatic brain injury in humans. *Acta Neuropathologica* 122 (6):715–726.

Karakaya, T., F. Fußer, D. Prvulovic, and H. Hampel. 2012. Treatment options for tauopathies. *Current Treatment Options in Neurology* 14 (2):126–136.

Konishi, K. and V. D. Bohbot. 2013. Spatial navigational strategies correlate with gray matter in the hippocampus of healthy older adults tested in a virtual maze. *Frontiers in Aging Neuroscience* 5:1. doi:10.3389/fnagi.2013.00001.

Kristman, V. L., J. Borg, A. K. Godbolt, L. R. Salmi, C. Cancelliere, L. J. Carroll, L. W. Holm et al. 2014. Methodological issues and research recommendations for prognosis after mild traumatic brain injury: Results of the international collaboration on mild traumatic brain injury prognosis. *Archives of Physical Medicine and Rehabilitation* 95 (3 Suppl):S265–S277. doi:10.1016/j.apmr.2013.04.026.

Lagarde, E., L. R. Salmi, L. W. Holm, B. Contrand, F. Masson, R. Ribereau-Gayon, M. Laborey, and J. D. Cassidy. 2014. Association of symptoms following mild traumatic brain injury with post-traumatic stress disorder vs. postconcussion syndrome. *JAMA Psychiatry* 71 (9):1032–1040. doi:10.1001/jamapsychiatry.2014.666.

Lange, R. T., G. L. Iverson, and A. Rose. 2010. Post-concussion symptom reporting and the "good-old-days" bias following mild traumatic brain injury. *Archives Clinical Neuropsychology* 25 (5):442–450. doi:10.1093/arclin/acq031.

Leddy, J. J., K. Kozlowski, M. Fung, D. R. Pendergast, and B. Willer. 2007. Regulatory and autoregulatory physiological dysfunction as a primary characteristic of post concussion syndrome: Implications for treatment. *NeuroRehabilitation* 22 (3):199–205.

Leddy, J., A. Hinds, D. Sirica, and B. Willer. 2016. The role of controlled exercise in concussion management. *PM & R* 8 (3 Suppl):S91–S100. doi:10.1016/j.pmrj.2015.10.017.

Ledwidge, P. S. and D. L. Molfese. 2016. Long-term effects of concussion on electrophysiological indices of attention in varsity college athletes: An event-related potential and standardized low-resolution brain electromagnetic tomography approach. *Journal of Neurotrauma* 33 (23):2081–2090. doi:10.1089/neu.2015.4251.

Lee, Y. K., S. W. Hou, C. C. Lee, C. Y. Hsu, Y. S. Huang, and Y. C. Su. 2013. Increased risk of dementia in patients with mild traumatic brain injury: A nationwide cohort study. *PloS One* 8 (5):e62422.

Lishman, W. A. 1988. Physiogenesis and psychogenesis in the 'post-concussional syndrome'. *The British Journal of Psychiatry* 153:460–469.

Lövdén, M., S. Schaefer, H. Noack, N. C. Bodammer, S. Kühn, H. J. Heinze, E. Düzel, L. Bäckman, and U. Lindenberger. 2012. Spatial navigation training protects the hippocampus against age-related changes during early and late adulthood. *Neurobiology of Aging* 33 (3):620. e9–620, e22.

Lucke-Wold, B. P., R. C. Turner, A. F. Logsdon, J. E. Bailes, J. D. Huber, and C. L. Rosen. 2014. Linking traumatic brain injury to chronic traumatic encephalopathy: Identification of potential mechanisms leading to neurofibrillary tangle development. *Journal of Neurotrauma* 31 (13):1129–1138. doi:10.1089/neu.2013.3303.

Martland, H. S. 1928. Punch drunk. *Journal of the American Medical Association* 91 (15):1103–1107.

McCrory, P., W. Meeuwisse, J. Dvorak, M. Aubry, J. Bailes, S. Broglio, R. C. Cantu et al. 2017. Consensus statement on concussion in sport-the 5th international conference on concussion in sport held in Berlin, October 2016. *British Journal of Sports Medicine* doi:10.1136/bjsports-2017-097699.

McKee, A. C., N. J. Cairns, D. W. Dickson, R. D. Folkerth, C. D. Keene, I. Litvan, D. P. Perl, T. D. Stein, J. P. Vonsattel, and W. Stewart. 2016. The first NINDS/NIBIB consensus meeting to define neuropathological criteria for the diagnosis of chronic traumatic encephalopathy. *Acta Neuropathologica* 131 (1):75–86.

McKee, A. C., R. A. Stern, C. J. Nowinski, T. D. Stein, V. E. Alvarez, D. H. Daneshvar, H. S. Lee et al. 2013. The spectrum of disease in chronic traumatic encephalopathy. *Brain* 136 (Pt 1):43–64. doi:10.1093/brain/aws307.

Meares, S., E. A. Shores, A. J. Taylor, J. Batchelor, R. A. Bryant, I. J. Baguley, J. Chapman et al. 2008. Mild traumatic brain injury does not predict acute postconcussion syndrome. *Journal of Neurology, Neurosurgery & Psychiatry* 79 (3):300–306. doi:10.1136/jnnp.2007.126565.

Millspaugh, J. A. 1937. Dementia pugilistica. *Unites States Naval Medical Bulletin* 35 (297):e303.

Mortimer, J. A., C. M. Van Duijn, V. Chandra, L. Fratiglioni, A. B. Graves, A. Heyman, A. F. Jorm, E. Kokmen, K. Kondo, and W. A. Rocca. 1991. Head trauma as a risk factor for Alzheimer's disease: A collaborative re-analysis of case-control studies. *International Journal of Epidemiology* 20 (Supplement 2):S28–S35.

Mouzon, B. C., C. Bachmeier, A. Ferro, J. O. Ojo, G. Crynen, C. M. Acker, P. Davies, M. Mullan, W. Stewart, and F. Crawford. 2014. Chronic neuropathological and neurobehavioral changes in a repetitive mild traumatic brain injury model. *Annals of Neurology* 75 (2):241–254. doi:10.1002/ana.24064.

Nordström, P., K. Michaëlsson, Y. Gustafson, and A. Nordström. 2014. Traumatic brain injury and young onset dementia: A nationwide cohort study. *Annals of Neurology* 75 (3):374–381.

Omalu, B. I., S. T. DeKosky, R. L. Minster, M. I. Kamboh, R. L. Hamilton, and C. H. Wecht. 2006a. Chronic traumatic encephalopathy in a National Football League Player. *Neurosurgery* 58 (5):E1003. doi:10.1093/neurosurgery/58.5.E1003.

Omalu, B. I., S. T. DeKosky, R. L. Hamilton, R. L. Minster, M. I. Kamboh, A. M. Shakir, and C. H. Wecht. 2006b. Chronic traumatic encephalopathy in a national football league player: Part II. *Neurosurgery* 59 (5):1086–1093.

Perry, D. C., V. E. Sturm, M. J. Peterson, C. F. Pieper, T. Bullock, B. F. Boeve, B. L. Miller, K. M. Guskiewicz, M. S. Berger, and J. H. Kramer. 2016. Association of traumatic brain injury with subsequent neurological and psychiatric disease: A meta-analysis. *Journal of Neurosurgery* 124 (2):511–526.

Piao, C. S., B. A. Stoica, J. Wu, B. Sabirzhanov, Z. Zhao, R. Cabatbat, D. J. Loane, and A. I. Faden. 2013. Late exercise reduces neuroinflammation and cognitive dysfunction after traumatic brain injury. *Neurobiology of Disease* 54:252–263. doi:10.1016/j.nbd.2012.12.017.

Ponsford, J., P. Cameron, M. Fitzgerald, M. Grant, A. Mikocka-Walus, and M. Schonberger. 2012. Predictors of postconcussive symptoms 3 months after mild traumatic brain injury. *Neuropsychology* 26 (3):304–313. doi:10.1037/a0027888.

Rathbone, A. T. L., S. Tharmaradinam, S. Jiang, M. P. Rathbone, and D. A. Kumbhare. 2015. A review of the neuro-and systemic inflammatory responses in post concussion symptoms: Introduction of the "post-inflammatory brain syndrome" PIBS. *Brain, Behavior, and Immunity* 46:1–16.

Rodgers, K. M., Y. K. Deming, F. M. Bercum, S. Y. Chumachenko, J. L. Wieseler, K. W. Johnson, L. R. Watkins, and D. S. Barth. 2014. Reversal of established traumatic brain injury-induced, anxiety-like behavior in rats after delayed, post-injury neuroimmune suppression. *Journal of Neurotrauma* 31 (5):487–497. doi:10.1089/neu.2013.3090.

Rose, S. C., A. N. Fischer, and G. L. Heyer. 2015. How long is too long? The lack of consensus regarding the post-concussion syndrome diagnosis. *Brain Injury* 29 (7–8):798–803.

Ross, D. E., A. L. Ochs, J. M. Seabaugh, M. F. Demark, C. R. Shrader, J. H. Marwitz, and M. D. Havranek. 2012. Progressive brain atrophy in patients with chronic neuropsychiatric symptoms after mild traumatic brain injury: A preliminary study. *Brain Injury* 26 (12):1500–1509. doi:10.3109/02699052.2012.694570.

Schofield, P. W., M. Tang, K. Marder, K. Bell, G. Dooneief, M. Chun, M. Sano, Y. Stern, and R. Mayeux. 1997. Alzheimer's disease after remote head injury: An incidence study. *Journal of Neurology Neurosurgery & Psychiatry* 62 (2):119–124.

Shively, S., A. I. Scher, D. P. Perl, and R. Diaz-Arrastia. 2012. Dementia resulting from traumatic brain injury: What is the pathology? *Archives of Neurology* 69 (10):1245–1251. doi:10.1001/archneurol.2011.3747.

Silverberg, N. D. and G. L. Iverson. 2011. Etiology of the post-concussion syndrome: Physiogenesis and psychogenesis revisited. *NeuroRehabilitation* 29 (4):317–329.

Silverberg, N. D., G. L. Iverson, J. R. Brubacher, E. Holland, L. C. Hoshino, A. Aquino, and R. T. Lange. 2016. The nature and clinical significance of preinjury recall bias following mild traumatic brain injury. *The Journal of Head Trauma Rehabilitation* 31 (6):388–396.

Singh, R., T. B. Meier, R. Kuplicki, J. Savitz, I. Mukai, L. Cavanagh, T. Allen et al. 2014. Relationship of collegiate football experience and concussion with hippocampal volume and cognitive outcomes. *JAMA* 311 (18):1883–1888. doi:10.1001/jama.2014.3313.

Slick, D. and M. Sherman. 2012 Differential diagnosis of malingering (in ed. Dominic A Carone) In D. A. Carone (Eds.) *Mild Traumatic Brain Injury: Symptom Validity Assessment and Malingering.* New York: Springer Publishing Company.

Smits, M., G. C. Houston, D. W. Dippel, P. A. Wielopolski, M. W. Vernooij, P. J. Koudstaal, M. G. Hunink, and A. van der Lugt. 2011. Microstructural brain injury in post-concussion syndrome after minor head injury. *Neuroradiology* 53 (8):553–563. doi:10.1007/s00234-010-0774-6.

Snowdon, D. A. 2003. Healthy aging and dementia: Findings from the Nun Study. *Annals of Internal Medcine* 139 (5 Pt 2):450–454.

Stein, M. B., R. J. Ursano, L. Campbell-Sills, L. J. Colpe, C. S. Fullerton, S. G. Heeringa, M. K. Nock, N. A. Sampson, M. Schoenbaum, and X. Sun. 2016. Prognostic indicators of persistent post-concussive symptoms after deployment-related mild traumatic brain injury: A prospective longitudinal study in US Army soldiers. *Journal of Neurotrauma* 33 (23):2125–2132.

Tartaglia, M. C., L. N. Hazrati, K. D. Davis, R. E. A. Green, R. Wennberg, D. Mikulis, L. J. Ezerins, M. Keightley, and C. Tator. 2014. Chronic traumatic encephalopathy and other neurodegenerative proteinopathies. *Frontiers in Human Neuroscience* 8:30.

Tator, C. H., H. S. Davis, P. A. Dufort, M. C. Tartaglia, K. D. Davis, A. Ebraheem, and C. Hiploylee. 2016. Postconcussion syndrome: Demographics and predictors in 221 patients. *Journal of Neurosurgery* 125 (5):1206–1216.

Terwilliger, V. K., L. Pratson, C. G. Vaughan, and G. A. Gioia. 2016. Additional post-concussion impact exposure may affect recovery in adolescent athletes. *Journal of Neurotrauma* 33 (8):761–765.

Tomaszczyk, J. C., N. L. Green, D. Frasca, B. Colella, G. R. Turner, B. K. Christensen, and R. E. A. Green. 2014. Negative neuroplasticity in chronic traumatic brain injury and implications for neurorehabilitation. *Neuropsychology Review* 24 (4):409–427.

Toth, A., N. Kovacs, G. Perlaki, G. Orsi, M. Aradi, H. Komaromy, E. Ezer, P. Bukovics, O. Farkas, and J. Janszky. 2013. Multi-modal magnetic resonance imaging in the acute and sub-acute phase of mild traumatic brain injury: Can we see the difference? *Journal of Neurotrauma* 30 (1):2–10.

Tremblay, S., L. De Beaumont, L. C. Henry, Y. Boulanger, A. C. Evans, P. Bourgouin, J. Poirier, H. Theoret, and M. Lassonde. 2013. Sports concussions and aging: A neuroimaging investigation. *Cereb Cortex* 23 (5):1159–1166. doi:10.1093/cercor/bhs102.

Turner, G. R., A. R. McIntosh, and B. Levine. 2011. Prefrontal compensatory engagement in TBI is due to altered functional engagement of existing networks and not functional reorganization. *Frontiers in Systems Neuroscience* 5:9. doi:10.3389/fnsys.2011.00009.

Wäljas, M., G. L. Iverson, R. T. Lange, U. Hakulinen, P. Dastidar, H. Huhtala, S. Liimatainen, K. Hartikainen, and J. Öhman. 2015. A prospective biopsychosocial study of the persistent post-concussion symptoms following mild traumatic brain injury. *Journal of Neurotrauma* 32 (8):534–547.

Wood, R. L. 2004. Understanding the 'miserable minority': A diathesis-stress paradigm for post-concussional syndrome. *Brain Injury* 18 (11):1135–1153. doi:10.1080/02699050410001675906.

Yurgil, K. A., D. A. Barkauskas, J. Vasterling, C. M. Nievergelt, G. E. Larson, N. J. Schork, B. Litz, W. P. Nash, and D. G. Baker. 2014. Association between traumatic brain injury and risk of post-traumatic stress disorder in active-duty marines. *JAMA Psychiatry* 71 (2):149–157.

*section four*

---

*Additional considerations*

## chapter seventeen

# Team and high risk sports: The baseline model

## Is it useful to measure an athlete's abilities before the sport season?

**Gillian Hotz and Danielle Ransom**

### Contents

## Introduction

Preinjury baseline testing is considered to be an important part of the return-to-play decision for athletes recovering from sport-related concussion (Iverson and Schatz 2014). A comprehensive concussion management program starts before an injury has occurred with preventative measures, including concussion education and baseline testing. Some clinicians liken the assessment to *investing in insurance* for each individual athlete in the event of a suspected injury. Given the role of the sport medicine professional in safely returning an athlete to play, individual baseline testing results can be a useful tool to determine an athlete's level of post-injury functioning and to assist with clinical management and decision-making (Aubry et al. 2002; McCrory et al. 2005, 2009, 2013). Currently, baseline testing is mandatory in the NHL, MLS, MLB, NBA, NASCAR, US National Soccer Team, the NCAA, the Department of Defense, and many high-school programs. With respect to our institution, beginning in 2011, the University of Miami Concussion Program (UConcussion) partnered with the Miami Dade County School Board Athletics Program to develop a Countywide Concussion Management program, which includes six steps for Safe Play. Step #1 includes baseline testing (ImPACT) (Lovell 2007) for all high-school athletes who play contact sports, in addition to a sideline screening (King Devick) (Galetta et al. 2011a) for football players (Hotz et al. 2014, 2015a, 2015b).

Despite the apparent clinical advantage of having data unique to the patient, questions remain regarding the value added by obtaining individual baseline assessment and its utility above and beyond comparing post-injury scores to normative standards. The influence of practice effects on reliability and validity, potentially variable motivation on the part of the athlete, logistical challenges in coordinating group-based testing, and poor adherence to administration procedures can lead to diminished test validity, thus producing potentially invalid and subsequently misleading results (Levin et al. 1989; Macciocchi 1990; Collie et al. 2003; Broglio et al. 2007a; Moser et al. 2011; Vaughan et al. 2014). Findings from the research on the benefits and limitations of baseline testing underscore the importance of obtaining an *accurate and valid* measure of an athlete's preseason baseline performance using tools demonstrated to be sensitive and specific to the effects of concussion. When taken together, the role of baseline testing continues to be a controversial topic in the field of sport concussion.

This chapter will (1) review the current baseline model, emphasizing key domains (i.e., neuropsychological assessment, self-reported symptoms, and postural control) and measures to be assessed during the baseline evaluation, (2) highlight benefits and limitations inherent to the baseline testing model, and (3) summarize commonly used baseline assessment tools. For the purpose of this chapter, the baseline assessment model refers to the comprehensive evaluation of neuropsychological performance, self-reported symptoms and preinjury history, and postural stability. Primary emphasis is often placed on neuropsychological test results when considering pre-/post-injury testing; however, it is important to note that these data should be considered in the context of a multidisciplinary evaluation alongside the other domains discussed next. While retrospective report of preinjury baseline functioning may suffice, we advocate for true-baseline assessment of each key domain noted below, when resources allow, in accordance with best practice denoted in by the Concussion in Sport Group (McCrory et al. 2017).

## *The baseline model*

According to the International Conference on Concussion in Sport held in Zurich in 2012, concussion signs (those noticed by coaches, parents, and teammates) and symptoms (feelings or problems experienced by the athlete) fall into six main groups (McCrory et al. 2013):

1. *Symptoms*
   a. Somatic (e.g., headache, nausea, vomiting, dizziness, visual problems, sensitivity to light/noise, balance problems)
   b. Cognitive (e.g., feeling mentally *foggy,* feeling slowed down, difficulty concentrating and remembering)
   c. Emotional (e.g., lability, involuntary crying or uncontrollable episodes of crying and/or laughing)
2. *Physical signs* (e.g., loss of consciousness, amnesia, etc.)
3. *Balance impairment* (e.g., gait unsteadiness)
4. *Behavioral changes* (e.g., irritability, sadness, nervousness, feeling more emotional)
5. *Cognitive impairments* (e.g., slowed reaction times, etc.)
6. *Sleep/wake disturbance* (e.g., insomnia, drowsiness, sleeping less than usual, sleeping more than usual)

The premise of baseline testing is that standardized measures in key domains (e.g., symptoms, neuropsychological performance, balance, emotional functioning, etc.) are administered prior to a sports season before an athlete is exposed to any training or competition. Athletes, coaches, athletic trainers, and parents learn to recognize potential injuries and respond appropriately (i.e., remove from play, seek evaluation from a health-care professional), thereby minimizing potential post-injury consequences involved in prematurely returning an athlete to competition. If an injury is suspected, standardized baseline assessment of key domains allows for test results to be compared across pre- and post-injury time points to determine the relative change in an individual athlete. This individualized comparison has been theorized to provide a more reliable metric of change relative to group-based norms, as an athlete's own data is used by the clinician to guide post-injury management and return-to-play decisions.

Given the broad nature of symptoms present in concussion, a multidisciplinary post-injury evaluation is recommended when concussion is suspected (McCrory et al. 2017). Baseline testing can be useful for interpreting post-injury results obtained during such an evaluation and can assist with monitoring recovery progress. As noted earlier, it can also provide an opportunity for the physician/clinician to discuss the significance of the results with the patient in a context that is relevant to his/her own daily functioning. To capture important concussion signs and symptoms, measures of neuropsychological assessment, self-reported symptoms, and balance/postural stability are commonly assessed at baseline and post-injury time points. Each of these domains is discussed later, while specific measures are described at the end of the chapter.

## *Neuropsychological assessment*

Neuropsychological assessment has been a central component of concussion management since the University of Virginia studies in the 1980s (Barth et al. 1983; Levin et al. 1989; Macciocchi et al. 1996). Rather than employing a traditional full-length, neuropsychological assessment, Barth and colleagues implemented a model whereby college football players were administered an abbreviated paper/pencil screening battery prior to the season and were reassessed in the event of concussion. This longitudinal methodology established a foundation from which to study mild traumatic brain injury in the context of sports (sport as a laboratory assessment model—SLAM), and provided a new gold standard for understanding change in the athlete on an individual level by eliminating variance inherent to group normative comparisons (Levin et al. 1989; Webbe and Zimmer 2015).

The advent of computerized neuropsychological screening measures in the 1990s/early 2000s shifted the testing paradigm away from paper/pencil testing due to ease of test administration in group settings (Maroon et al. 2000). Traditional paper/pencil neuropsychological tests continue to be reliable, valid, and sensitive to the effects of concussion, but are not commonly used in baseline assessment due to the need for face-to-face administration, which requires resources and is highly labor-intensive when conducting group-based testing with athletes (Echemendia et al. 2013). A number of computerized neuropsychological test batteries have been developed for rapid pre-/post-injury assessment and can be quickly administered in a group setting (versus the 1:1 examiner to examinee test ratio required of traditional paper/pencil measures) and allow for portable, efficient data collection to facilitate the gathering and storage of large amounts of data (Echemendia et al. 2013). Preliminary research also suggests that computerized test administration may provide more precise measurement of reaction time in comparison to traditional neuropsychological test administration (Broglio et al. 2007b). These apparent advantages have spurred the growth of the baseline testing market at an exponential rate and now provide a broad range of athletes across all levels of sport access to individualized data in the event of an injury.

Over the past decade and a half, most position and consensus statements for the management of concussion in sport have incorporated neuropsychological assessment as a cornerstone of concussion management programs (Aubry et al. 2002; McCrory et al. 2005, 2009, 2013; AAN 2013). To date, there have been dozens of studies demonstrating that both traditional and computerized neuropsychological measures are sensitive to the acute effects of concussion (Barth et al. 1983; Macciocchi 1990; Maroon et al. 2000; Collins et al. 2003; Erlanger et al. 2003; Iverson et al. 2003; Lovell et al. 2003; Lovell et al. 2004; Broshek et al. 2005; Collie et al. 2006; Iverson et al. 2006; McClincy et al. 2006; Van Kampen et al. 2006; Broglio et al. 2007b; Fazio et al. 2007; Iverson 2007; AAN 2013; Echemendia et al. 2013; Webbe and Zimmer 2015).

## Self-reported symptoms

Concussion symptoms are relatively nonspecific and can be reported in conditions apart from concussion (e.g., whiplash, affective disorders such as depression, inner ear problems such as vertigo and dizziness). Individuals who sustain a blow to the head, however, often report that these symptoms are more frequent and severe in nature for a period of time (Mittenberg et al. 1992; Yeates et al. 1999; Taylor et al. 2010). Along with an evaluation of neuropsychological functioning, current guidelines highlight the importance of standardized symptom assessment in the management of sport-related concussion to ensure that athletes have returned to their preinjury baseline before returning to competition (Giza et al. 2013; McCrory et al. 2017). Self-reported symptom assessment of post-injury concussion symptoms, though well-intended have come under fire due to variable diagnostic efficiency and reliance on subjective symptom report. Very few scales have followed standard scale development processes (Standards for Educational & Psychological Testing 2014) and have published psychometric properties validating their utility with clinical samples (Alla et al. 2009; McLeod and Leach 2012). As a result, many measures have inherent problems discriminating normal baseline rates of concussion-like symptoms from those directly attributed to an acute concussion (Piland et al. 2010).

There are select symptom rating scales that have been developed in a systematic manner and have published psychometric properties, as highlighted in the recent American Academy of Neurology guidelines and report by the Institute of Medicine (Giza et al. 2013; Institute of Medicine 2013). These measures have demonstrated adequate diagnostic efficiency, with sensitivity levels ranging from 64% to 89% and specificity levels ranging from 91% to 100% (Piland et al. 2003; Lovell et al. 2003, 2004; McCrea et al. 2005; Kampen et al. 2006; Van Kampen et al. 2006; Lau et al. 2009; Peterson et al. 2003). When true symptom ratings are obtained during preinjury baseline testing, results can assist clinicians in making individually-driven return-to-play decisions regarding an athlete's own level of symptoms (Piland et al. 2010). True baseline ratings are particularly important in the event that an athlete experienced some level of symptoms (e.g., fatigue, headache) prior to the concussion, as standard guidelines require an athlete to be asymptomatic prior to returning to competition. If these symptoms are captured before an injury has occurred, the clinician is better able to distinguish an individual athlete's own relative change in functioning and return to personal baseline. Although true baseline ratings can partially account for nonspecific symptoms that persist following concussion, further research is needed regarding the base rates of concussion-like symptoms in an uninjured, healthy control sample to better refine our current symptom assessment tools.

## Balance/postural stability and visual system

Balance/postural stability testing is also an important part of a comprehensive concussion assessment. Dizziness and balance impairments are commonly reported following an impact to the head caused by disruption of the central integration of the vestibular, visual, and somatosensory information. Furthermore, the visual system is commonly compromised with alteration of consciousness or post-concussion. The visual pathways part of brain functioning may be affected and impaired eye movements can be present even when athletes appear to be asymptomatic. There are specific assessments to be administered at baseline and post-injury time points described later on in this chapter.

## Limitations to the baseline model

Despite the benefits of a reliable, valid, and accurate assessment of an individual's preinjury functioning, challenges have arisen that question the utility of the baseline testing model (Randolph et al. 2005; Randolph and Kirkwood 2009). First, baseline testing can be expensive and labor-intensive, a concern often mitigated through group-based test administration with trained examiners. However, an additional set of issues inherent to group testing may impact the validity of the test results, particularly since athletes are tested individually following concussion (Moser et al. 2011; Vaughan et al. 2014). In group-based settings, individuals may be at greater risk for difficulty comprehending and adhering to computerized test administration procedures, given the increased supervisory demand on the test administrator. Standardized test administration may be compromised by environmental distractors (e.g., peers, external noises, etc.) or a potential lack of motivation outside of the context of the one-on-one setting. In addition, athletes may demonstrate lower levels of motivation during group baseline testing, in contrast to a higher level of motivation following a suspected injury (Iverson and Schatz 2014). There have also been reported instances of high-profile athletes purposefully under-performing on baseline testing so that the post-injury results would compare more favorably to their arbitrarily lowered baseline. These anecdotes are particularly troubling when coupled with survey data showing that over half (56%) of NFL players assessed would not report a concussion due to not wanting to be withheld from competition (NFL Poll 2016). Invalid performance can be detected in some athletes; however, current validity indicators are unable to determine the factors influencing diminished test results (i.e., deliberately poor performance, poor comprehension of test instructions, distractions in the test environment, or a combination of factors) (Iverson and Schatz 2014). Researches have demonstrated, however, that only a small percentage of students deliberately feigning impairment were able to escape detection (Erdal 2012; Schatz and Glatts 2013).

Moser et al. (2011) explored performance-based outcomes in baseline testing with high-school athletes and found significant differences in cognitive test performance compared with athletes who were tested individually. Vaughan et al. (2014) further explored the baseline environment and found no differences in cognitive performance for children and adolescents tested individually or in a group setting when the level of examiner training and standardization of administration procedures and supervision were consistent across both test environments. When taken together, group-based test administration may yield artificially lower scores than individual testing when the proper test environment conditions are not met, and in subpopulations of athletes (Moser et al. 2011; Vaughan et al. 2014). Further studies are needed to expand validity indicators and explore the impact of situational factors on baseline test performance.

A third concern is in regard to test psychometrics, as computerized measures are brief and rely on a select sample of cognitive performance (Echemendia et al. 2013). Furthermore, some tests used in concussion management have low to medium test–retest reliability, leading to difficulty in accurately assessing baseline and post-injury change scores (Randolph et al. 2005; Broglio et al. 2007a; Mayers and Redick 2012; Resch et al. 2013). The pre-/post-injury model of assessment has not been empirically examined to demonstrate greater diagnostic accuracy in comparison to post-injury testing alone, which has shown high sensitivity and specificity in identifying students with a clinically significant change based on comparison to normative values (1.5 SD units below expected mean) (Echemendia et al. 2012). Another psychometric concern is the long-term test–retest reliability for younger athletes (i.e., high school and earlier) who are considered to be in a period of rapid cognitive maturation. In the past, annual baseline evaluations have been recommended for all athletes; however, studies from Schatz (2010) and Elbin et al. (2011) have demonstrated considerable stability of computerized test data over a two-year period for college athletes and over a one-year period for high-school athletes, respectively.

Even in the context of these limitations, an accurate measure of preinjury baseline functioning is believed to be helpful for quantifying post-injury changes in functioning and for monitoring the athlete over the course of recovery (Echemendia et al. 2012; Iverson and Schatz 2014). The pre-/post-injury model of assessment provides an opportunity for a greater level of individual accuracy in measurement by reducing extraneous variance. In addition, utilizing multiple methods to assess recovery can provide clinicians with a greater level of assurance of an athlete's readiness to return to competition. Preinjury baseline testing is particularly useful for athletes who perform in the above average or below average range of functioning (Iverson and Schatz 2014), or those with a history of developmental disorders, such as ADHD or LD (Elbin et al. 2013). More research is needed to determine the quantifiable value added of preinjury baseline testing, aside from its assumed qualitative role in clinical management and decision-making.

## Current recommendations for baseline test administration

The validity of the post-injury to pre-injury assessment method is based on the assumption that test results have been collected in a standardized, accurate manner (Vaughan et al. 2014). The limitations discussed in the previous section underscore the need for a high level of care and consideration when developing a baseline testing program. Invalid preinjury test results can lead to inaccurate interpretation of post-injury testing scores, which may compromise an athlete's safety through premature return to play (Vaughan et al. 2014).

If a baseline testing model is employed, the integrity of the results must be maximized through standardized baseline test administration procedures conducted by trained examiners with an appropriate supervisor-to-examinee ratio in highly controlled settings (Echemendia et al. 2013). Group-based testing can be a practical method of baseline test administration in the context of a properly controlled testing environment that is well monitored by trained examiners. Large group baseline testing should be avoided due to a lack of control of the testing environment. Current recommendations include no more than a 5:1 athlete: proctor ratio to discourage purposeful suboptimal performance (e.g., sandbagging) and to ensure that all the athletes understand test instructions. When possible, it is recommended that the same computer and testing environment be used for posttesting to make the testing conditions as similar as possible. Collegiate and high-school athletes should undergo repeat baseline testing every two years (ImPACT) and annually for a sideline screening (KD), while younger children should be reassessed each year to account for developmental changes.

At the University of Miami, the UConcussion Program implements baseline testing prior to the season by certified athletic trainers (ATCs) who have been trained. Following a suspected concussion, athletes are retested on the KD immediately on the sideline, while ImPACT is administered within 72 hours by their ATC. Athletes are closely monitored over the course of their injuries and undergo repeat testing until their assessments and symptoms return to preinjury baseline levels.

## Summary

Baseline testing has served an important role in the management of sport-related concussion since it originated as a cornerstone of Barth's SLAM model. Pre-/post-injury assessment is theorized to provide an opportunity for a higher level of measurement accuracy by reducing extraneous variance associated with normative comparisons. This individualized comparison afforded in the baseline testing model, however, is costly and labor-intensive, and research has yet to quantify the benefits of the value added to concussion management. Furthermore, the baseline testing model is limited by a number of factors that could impact the reliability and validity of test results, potentially placing athletes at risk for premature return to play due to misleading data. When taken together, we believe that valid baseline testing administered by trained examiners adds an important component to the clinical management of sport-related concussion, particularly when it is considered alongside multiple methods of assessing recovery.

## Review of commonly used baseline measures

### Concussion assessment tools

*SAC*: The Standardized assessment of concussion (SAC) allows trained sideline personnel to assess immediate changes in athletes suspected of having sustained a concussion (McCrea et al. 1998; Barr and McCrea 2001). The SAC is administered in approximately five minutes and is used to measure four cognitive domains at baseline, including orientation, immediate memory, concentration, and delayed memory. Additional neurologic and exertional screening questions are available following suspected concussion. The highest possible score is 30 with a mean of 26.6. The SAC has been shown to have good sensitivity and specificity for identifying possible concussion within 48 hours of a suspected injury (McCrea 2001; McCrea et al. 2003) when the proper normative groups are referenced (Barr 2003; Valovich et al. 2006).

*SCAT5*: The Sport Concussion Assessment Tool-5 (SCAT5) is a brief, structured medical assessment for adolescents and adults aged 13+ that can be administered at baseline, on the sideline or health care provider's office following a suspected concussion. Although empirical evidence does not support a specific timeframe for administration of the SCAT5, completion of the test requires a minimum of 10 minutes and should be performed in the resting state (McCrory et al. 2017). This latest version of the SCAT incorporates the SAC, the Glasgow Coma Scale (GCS), modified Maddocks questions (Maddocks et al. 1995), a neck evaluation and balance assessment, a symptom checklist, questions regarding mechanism of injury, and preinjury history

(McCrory et al. 2017). Specific components of the SCAT have been shown most useful in differentiating concussed from nonconcussed athletes in the phase immediately post-injury and declines days (approximately 3–5) after injury (Echemendia et al. 2017). The Child SCAT5 has recently been developed for children aged 5–12 years that incorporates age-appropriate questions (McCrory et al. 2017). Efforts were made to minimize changes to the SCAT3 (immediate predecessor of the SCAT5) to emphasize continuity and viability of normative and baseline data (McCrory et al. 2017).

*King Devick test*: The King Devick (KD) test is a two-minute rapid number naming assessment that is used to assess impairments in processing speed, visual tracking, and saccadic eye movements that may indicate suboptimal brain function (Galetta et al. 2011b). It was initially developed in 1976 to assess reading ability, and over thirty years later it has been investigated in a number of studies as a potential rapid sideline screening test in a variety of contact sports. Prior to the season, the examiner records the time the athlete takes to read the three cards. If a concussion is suspected, the athlete is retested and if the recorded time exceeds the baseline by two or more seconds, the athlete should be removed immediately from play.

The KD appears sensitive to the acute effects of sport-related concussion (Galetta et al. 2011a, 2011b; King et al. 2012, 2013; Galetta et al. 2013), though sensitivity and specificity diminishes in patients who are evaluated several hours or more after a suspected injury, in the absence of preinjury baseline data (Silverberg et al. 2014). The KD has a growing body of literature; however, many studies of the KD to date involve very small sample sizes (<10 concussed athletes), which is too small to determine the test's diagnostic efficiency and limits available norms derived based on age and gender (Giza et al. 2013; Institute of Medicine 2013). Despite these limitations, the KD is currently being accepted as the leading objective sideline assessment to assist in removing athletes from play.

*Clinical reaction time test*: Also known as the *ruler-drop test*, the Clinical Reaction Time Test ($RT_{clin}$) is a simple, low-cost measure of reaction time commonly used by athletic trainers (Eckner et al. 2010). The task requires an athlete to catch a measuring stick that has been dropped and the distance traveled is recorded. The $RT_{clin}$ shows promise in the context of a multimodal test battery with college athletes (Eckner et al. 2014); however, poor test–retest reliability and validity were demonstrated with high-school athletes (Macdonald et al. 2015). For baseline administration, it is recommended that athletes have at least one practice session before baseline values are recorded to minimize variance associated with practice-related improvements (Del Rossi et al. 2014).

*Computerized neuropsychological tests*

*ANAM*: The Automated Neuropsychological Assessment Metrics (ANAM) is a computerized neuropsychological measure that is used to assess attention, concentration, reaction time, memory, processing speed, and decision-making. The ANAM has been shown to be sensitive in distinguishing the severity of traumatic brain injury (Levinson and Reeves 1997); however, the ANAM sports medicine battery has demonstrated variable test–retest reliability in serial concussion testing (Cernich et al. 2007; Segalowitz et al. 2007), as well as practice effects in five of six subtests (Eonta et al. 2011). A recent study by Nelson et al. (2016) found moderate differences between concussed patients and controls within 24 hours of injury, as well as variable test–retest reliability and poor ability to discriminate between groups. More research is necessary to determine the ANAM's utility with concussed patients, particularly those injured in sport.

*Axon:* Axon is a computerized neuropsychological screening battery used to measure processing speed, attention, learning/memory, and working memory through a series of eight *card games* (Falleti et al. 2006). Axon has demonstrated greater sensitivity to cognitive impairment than paper/pencil measures of neuropsychological functioning (Digit Symbol Substitution Test and Trail Making Test Part B) (Makdissi et al. 2001). A separate study revealed moderate differences were found between concussed patients and controls, but variable test–retest reliability and poor ability to discriminate between groups at 24-hours post-injury (Nelson et al. 2016). Given the recent publication of Axon, more research is warranted to determine its effectiveness for baseline/post-injury concussion evaluations.

*ImPACT:* The most commonly utilized computerized neuropsychological screening instrument is the Immediate Post-Concussion Assessment and Cognitive Testing (ImPACT) (Lovell 2007). ImPACT is a 25-minute online assessment that includes the following: three test sections include demographic/background information, a symptom checklist, and six neuropsychological measures used to assess processing speed, working memory, and memory recognition. ImPACT has been shown to have good sensitivity, specificity, and construct validity, but variable test–retest reliability (Iverson et al. 2003; Broglio et al. 2007a; Miller et al. 2007; Elbin et al. 2011). Alongside a thorough clinical examination, ImPACT can assist clinicians and ATCs in making return to play decisions. For the purpose of this chapter, we will not review the expansive literature on ImPACT, as it has been covered elsewhere in this book.

*Self-reported symptoms*

*Concussion Symptom Inventory (CSI):* The CSI was the first empirically derived scale designed for the purpose of monitoring subjective symptoms following concussion. Randolph et al. (2009) analyzed data from three separate case-controlled studies conducted at baseline, immediately post-injury, postgame, and at 1, 3, and 5 days following injury, resulting in a 12-item symptom scale. Receiver-operating characteristic analyses were used to demonstrate that reducing the number of scale items did not negatively impact sensitivity or specificity. The CSI can be administered by trained health professionals as a part of the concussion assessment. Due to the limited item set in the inventory, test authors recommend a more complete symptom inventory and thorough neurological assessment for health professionals guiding the return to play.

*Post-Concussion Symptom Inventory (PCSI):* The PCSI is a developmentally appropriate concussion symptom rating scale for children and adolescents (Sady et al. 2014). There are four versions of the PCSI, with 5 items for children 5–7 years (PCSI-SR5), 17 items for children 8–12 years (PCSI-SR8), 21 items for adolescents 13–18 years (PCSI-SR13), and 20 items for parent report (PCSI-P). The PCSI is used to assess cognitive, physical, sleep, and emotional symptom domains. The PCSI has demonstrated moderate to high interrater reliability, internal consistency, and predictive and discriminant validity.

*Post-Concussion Symptom Scale (PCSS):* The PCSS is a 21-item self-reported scale given to high-school and collegiate athletes to monitor post-concussion symptoms (Lovell and Collins 1998). Athletes are asked to rate the severity of symptoms on a 7-point Guttman scale within a few hours of a suspected injury and then daily until recovery has been determined. The PCSS has demonstrated moderate test–retest reliability and ability to detect reliable change (Iverson et al. 2003) as well as an ability to discriminate between concussed and nonconcussed athletes (Echemendia et al. 2001; Field et al. 2003; Iverson et al. 2003; Lovell et al. 2006; Schatz and Putz 2006). A revised factor structure showed post-injury symptoms have been reported in adolescents who showed a four-factor solution (cognitive/fatigue/migraine, affective, somatic, and sleep) and higher scores in female than male athletes (Kontos et al. 2012).

*Balance / Postural stability*

*BESS*: The Balance Error Scoring System (BESS) is a quantified version of the Romberg balance test and can be used to assess postural instability occurring post-concussion. The BESS is a reliable and valid addition to a comprehensive concussion assessment (Riemann and Guskiewicz 2000; Guskiewicz et al. 2001). The BESS consists of three stances on two different surfaces, lasting 20 seconds per stance, with eyes closed and hands on the iliac crests. The three stances include a double leg stance (feet shoulder-width apart), single leg stance, and tandem stance. The two different surfaces include a firm (ground) and a medium-density foam surface. The BESS is scored based on the number of errors across trials (e.g., moving hands of the hips, opening the eyes, step/stumble/fall, etc.). This is an inexpensive, easy to administer measure and takes about 5–7 minutes. The BESS has very good test–retest reliability (Riemann and Guskiewicz 2000) and high specificity in the diagnosis of concussion (Giza et al. 2013). Despite the low to moderate levels of sensitivity when used in isolation, the BESS' sensitivity improved when used in conjunction with the SAC and a graded symptom checklist within 48-hours post-injury (McCrea et al. 2003; Giza et al. 2013).

# References

Alla, S. et al. 2009. Self-report scales/checklists for the measurement of concussion symptoms: A systematic review. *Br. J. Sports Med.* **43**(Suppl 1), i3–i12 (2009).

American Academy of Neurology. 2013. Position statement on sports concussion.

Aubry, M., Cantu, R., Dvorak, J., Graf-Baumann, T., Johnston, K., Kelly, J., Lovell, M., McCrory, P., Meeuwisse, W., and Schamasch P. 2002. Summary and agreement statement of the First International Conference on Concussion in Sport, Vienna 2001. Recommendations for the improvement of safety and health of athletes who may suffer concussive injuries. *Br. J. Sports Med.* **36**, 6–10.

Barr, W. B. and McCrea, M. 2001. Sensitivity and specificity of standardized neurocognitive testing immediately following sports concussion. *J. Int. Neuropsychol. Soc. JINS* **7**, 693–702.

Barr, W. B. 2003. Neuropsychological testing of high school athletes. Preliminary norms and test-retest indices. *Arch. Clin. Neuropsychol. Off. J. Natl. Acad. Neuropsychol.* **18**, 91–101.

Barth, J. T., Macciocchi, S.N., Giordani, B., Rimel, R., Jane J. A., and Boll, T. J. 1983. Neuropsychological sequelae of minor head injury. *Neurosurgery* **13**, 529–533.

Broglio, S. P., Ferrara, M.S., Macciocchi, S.N., Baumgartner, T.A., and Elliott R. 2007a. Test-retest reliability of computerized concussion assessment programs. *J. Athl. Train.* **42**(4), 509–514.

Broglio, S. P., Macciocchi, S. N., and Ferrara, M. S. 2007b. Sensitivity of the concussion assessment battery. *Neurosurgery* **60**, 1050–1057–1058.

Broshek, D. K., Kaushik, T., Freeman, J.R., Erlanger, D., Webbe, F., and Barth, J. T. 2005. Sex differences in outcome following sports-related concussion. *J. Neurosurg.* **102**, 856–863.

Cernich, A., Reeves D., Sun W., and Bleiberg, J. 2007. Automated neuropsychological assessment metrics sports medicine battery. *Arch. Clin. Neuropsychol.* **22**(1), S101–S114.

Collie, A., Maruff, P., Darby, D.G., and McSTEPHEN, M.I. 2003. The effects of practice on the cognitive test performance of neurologically normal individuals assessed at brief test-retest intervals. *J. Int. Neuropsychol. Soc.* **9**, 419–428.

Collie, A., Makdissi, M., Maruff, P., Bennell, K., and McCrory, P. 2006. Cognition in the days following concussion: Comparison of symptomatic versus asymptomatic athletes. *J. Neurol. Neurosurg. Psychiatry* **77**, 241–245.

Collins, M. W. Iverson, G.L., Lovell, M.R., McKeag, D.B., Norwig, J., and Maroon, J. 2003. On-field predictors of neuropsychological and symptom deficit following sports-related concussion. *Clin. J. Sport Med. Off. J. Can. Acad. Sport Med.* **13**, 222–229.

Del Rossi, G., Malaguti, A., and Del Rossi, S. 2014. Practice effects associated with repeated assessment of a clinical test of reaction time. *J. Athl. Train.* **49**, 356–359.

Echemendia, R. J., Putukian, M., Mackin, R. S., Julian L., and Shoss N. 2001. Neuropsychological test performance prior to and following sports-related mild traumatic brain injury. *Clin. J. Sport Med. Off. J. Can. Acad. Sport Med.* **11**, 23–31.

Echemendia, R. J., Bruce, J. M., Bailey, C. M., Sanders, J. F., Arnett, P., and Vargas, G. 2012. The utility of post-concussion neuropsychological data in identifying cognitive change following sports-related MTBI in the absence of baseline data. *Clin. Neuropsychol.* **26**, 1077–1091.

Echemendia, R. J., Iverson, G. L., McCrea, M., Macciocchi, S. N., Gioia, G. A., Putukian, M., and Comper, P. 2013. Advances in neuropsychological assessment of sport-related concussion. *Br. J. Sports Med.* **47**, 294–298.

Echemendia, R. J., Meeuwisse, W., McCrory, P., Davis, G. A., Putukian, M., Leddy, J., ... Herring, S. 2017. The sport concussion assessment tool 5th edition (SCAT5). *Br. J. Sports Med.* **51**, 848–850.

Eckner, J. T. Kutcher, J. S., and Richardson, J. K. 2010. Pilot evaluation of a novel clinical test of reaction time in national collegiate athletic association division I football players. *J. Athl. Train.* **45**, 327–332.

Eckner, J. T., Kutcher, J. S., Broglio, S. P., and Richardson, J. K. 2014. Effect of sport-related concussion on clinically measured simple reaction time. *Br. J. Sports Med.* **48**, 112–118.

Elbin, R. J., Schatz, P., and Covassin, T. 2011. One-year test-retest reliability of the online version of ImPACT in high school athletes. *Am. J. Sports Med.* **39**, 2319–2324.

Elbin, R. J., Kontos, A. P., Kegel, N., Johnson, E., Burkhart, S., and Schatz, P. 2013. Individual and combined effects of LD and ADHD on computerized neurocognitive concussion test performance: Evidence for separate norms. *Arch. Clin. Neuropsychol. Off. J. Natl. Acad. Neuropsychol.* **28**, 476–484.

Eonta, S.E., Carr, W., McArdle, J. J., Kain, J. M., Tate, C., Wesensten, N. J., Norris, J. N., Balkin, T. J. and Kamimori, G. H. 2011. Automated neuropsychological assessment metrics: Repeated assessment with two military samples. *Aviat. Space Env. Med.* **82**(1), 34–39.

Erdal, K. 2012. Neuropsychological testing for sports-related concussion: How athletes can sandbag their baseline testing without detection. *Arch. Clin. Neuropsychol.* **27**, 473–479.

Erlanger, D., Kaushik, T., Cantu, R., Barth, J. T., Broshek, D. K., Freeman, J. R., and Webbe, F. M. 2003. Symptom-based assessment of the severity of a concussion. *J. Neurosurg.* **98**, 477–484.

Falleti, M. G., Maruff, P., Collie, A., and Darby, D. G. 2006. Practice effects associated with the repeated assessment of cognitive function using the CogState battery at 10-minute, one week and one month test-retest intervals. *J. Clin. Exp. Neuropsychol.* **28**(7), 1095–1112.

Fazio, V. C., Lovell, M. R., Pardini, J. E., and Collins, M. W. 2007. The relation between post-concussion Symptoms and neurocognitive performance in concussed athletes. *NeuroRehabilitation* **22**, 207–216.

Field, M., Collins, M. W., Lovell, M. R., and Maroon, J. 2003. Does age play a role in recovery from sports-related concussion? A comparison of high school and collegiate athletes. *J. Pediatr.* **142**, 546–553.

Galetta, K. M. et al. 2011a. The King-Devick test and sports-related concussion: Study of a rapid visual screening tool in a collegiate cohort. *J. Neurol. Sci.* **309**, 34–39.

Galetta, K. M. et al. 2011b. The King-Devick test as a determinant of head trauma and concussion in boxers and MMA fighters. *Neurology* **76**, 1456–1462.

Galetta, M. S., Galetta, K. M., McCrossin, J., Wilson, J. A., Moster, S., Galetta, S. L., Balcer, L. J., Dorshimer, G. W. and Master, C. L. 2013. Saccades and memory: Baseline associations of the King-Devick and SCAT2 SAC tests in professional ice hockey players. *J. Neurol. Sci.* **328**, 28–31.

Giza, C. C. et al. 2013. Summary of evidence-based guideline update: Evaluation and management of concussion in sports Report of the Guideline Development Subcommittee of the American Academy of Neurology. *Neurology* **80**, 2250–2257.

Guskiewicz, K. M., Ross, S. E., and Marshall, S. W. 2001. Postural stability and neuropsychological deficits after concussion in collegiate athletes. *J. Athl. Train.* **36**, 263–273.

Hotz, G. et al. 2014. A countywide program to manage concussions in high school sports. *Sports J.* **19**, 1–9.

Hotz, G. et al. 2015a. The challenges of providing concussion education to high school football players. *Curr. Res. Concussion* **2**, 103–108.

Hotz, G., Crittenden, R., Baker, L., Hurley, E., Duerr, E., Golden, C., Page, C., and Nedd, K. 2015b. Countywide concussion injury surveillance system. *Curr. Res. Concussion* **2**, 11–16.

Institute of Medicine. Sports-Related Concussions in Youth: Improving the Science, Changing the Culture. Institute of Medicine (2013). Retrieved from http://www.iom.edu/Reports/2013/Sports-Related-Concussions-in-Youth-Improving-the-Science-Changing-the-Culture.aspx. (Accessed: November 4, 2014)

Iverson, G. L., Lovell, M. R., and Collins, M. W. 2003. Interpreting change on ImPACT following sport concussion. *Clin. Neuropsychol.* **17**, 460–467.

Iverson, G. L., Brooks, B. L., Collins, M. W., and Lovell, M. R. 2006. Tracking neuropsychological recovery following concussion in sport. *Brain Inj.* **20**, 245–252.

Iverson, G. 2007. Predicting slow recovery from sport-related concussion: The new simple-complex distinction. *Clin. J. Sport Med. Off. J. Can. Acad. Sport Med.* **17**, 31–37.

Iverson, G. L. and Schatz, P. 2014. Advanced topics in neuropsychological assessment following sport-related concussion. *Brain Inj.* 1–13. doi:10.3109/02699052.2014.965214.

King, D., Clark, T., and Gissane, C. 2012. Use of a rapid visual screening tool for the assessment of concussion in amateur rugby league: A pilot study. *J. Neurol. Sci.* **320**, 16–21.

King, D., Brughelli, M., Hume, P., and Gissane, C. 2013. Concussions in amateur rugby union identified with the use of a rapid visual screening tool. *J. Neurol. Sci.* **326**, 59–63.

Kontos, A. P., Elbin, R. J., Schatz, P., Covassin, T., Henry, L., Pardini, J., and Collins, M. W. 2012. A revised factor structure for the post-concussion symptom scale: Baseline and postconcussion factors. *Am. J. Sports Med.* **40**, 2375–2384.

Lau, B., Lovell, M. R., Collins, M. W., and Pardini, J. 2009. Neurocognitive and symptom predictors of recovery in high school athletes. *Clin. J. Sport Med. Off. J. Can. Acad. Sport Med.* **19**, 216–221.

Levin, H. S., Eisenberg, H. M., and Benton, A. L. 1989. *Mild Head Injury*. New York: Oxford University Press.

Levinson, D. M. and D. L. Reeves. 1997. Monitoring recovery from traumatic brain injury using Automated Neuropsychological Assessment Metrics (ANAM V1.0). *Arch. Clin. Neuropsychol.* **12**(2), 155–166.

Lovell, M. R. and Collins, M. 1998. Neuropsychological assessment of the college football player. *J. Head Trauma Rehabil.* **13**, 9–26.

Lovell, M. R. et al. 2003. Recovery from mild concussion in high school athletes. *J. Neurosurg.* **98**, 296–301.

Lovell, M. R., Collins, M. W., Iverson, G. L., Johnston, K. M., and Bradley, J. P. 2004. Grade 1 or 'ding' concussions in high school athletes. *Am. J. Sports Med.* **32**, 47–54.

Lovell, M. R., Iverson, G. L., Collins, M. W., Podell, K., Johnston, K. M., Pardini, D., Pardini, J., Norwig, J., and Maroon, J. C. 2006. Measurement of symptoms following sports-related concussion: Reliability and normative data for the post-concussion scale. *Appl. Neuropsychol.* **13**, 166–174.

Lovell, M. ImPACT 2007 (6.0)Clinical Interpretation Manual. Retrieved from http://impacttest.com/assets/pdf/2005ClinicalInterpretationManual.pdf.

Macciocchi, S. N., Barth, J. T., Alves, W., Rimel, R. W., and Jane, J. A. 1996. Neuropsychological functioning and recovery after mild head injury in collegiate athletes. *Neurosurgery* **39**, 510–514.

Macciocchi, S. N. 1990. 'Practice makes perfect:' retest effects in college athletes. *J. Clin. Psychol.* **46**, 628–631.

Macdonald, L., Wilson, J., Young, J., Duerson, D., Swisher, G., Collins, C. L., and Meehan III, W. P. 2015. Evaluation of a simple test of reaction time for baseline concussion testing in a population of high school athletes. *Clin. J. Sport Med.* **25**, 43–48.

Maddocks, D. L., Dicker, G. D., and Saling, M. M. 1995. The assessment of orientation following concussion in athletes. *Clin. J. Sport Med. Off. J. Can. Acad. Sport Med.* **5**, 32–35.

Makdissi, M., Collie, A., Maruff, P., Darby, D. G., Bush, A., McCrory, P., and Bennell, K. 2001. Computerized cognitive assessment of concussed Australian Rules footballers. *Br. J. Sports Med.* **35**, 354–360.

Maroon, J. C., Lovell, M. R., Norwig, J., Podell, K., Powell, J. W., and Hartl, R. 2000. Cerebral concussion in athletes: Evaluation and neuropsychological testing. *Neurosurgery* **47**, 659–669, discussed 669–672.

Mayers, L. B. and Redick, T. S. 2012. Clinical utility of ImPACT assessment for postconcussion return-to-play counseling: Psychometric issues. *J. Clin. Exp. Neuropsychol.* **34**, 235–242.

McClincy, M. P., Lovell, M. R., Pardini, J., Collins, M. W., and Spore, M. K. 2006. Recovery from sports concussion in high school and collegiate athletes. *Brain Inj.* **20**, 33–39.

McCrea, M., Kelly, J. P., Randolph, C., Kluge, J., Bartolic, E., Finn, G., and Baxter, B. 1998. Standardized assessment of concussion (SAC): On-site mental status evaluation of the athlete. *J. Head Trauma Rehabil.* **13**, 27–35.

McCrea, M. 2001. Standardized mental status testing on the sideline after sport-related concussion. *J. Athl. Train.* **36**, 274–279.

McCrea, M. Barr, W. B., Guskiewicz, K., Randolph, C., Marshall, S. W., Cantu, R., Onate, J. A., and Kelly, J. P. 2005. Standard regression-based methods for measuring recovery after sport-related concussion. *J. Int. Neuropsychol. Soc. JINS* **11**, 58–69.

McCrory, P. et al. 2005. Summary and agreement statement of the 2nd International Conference on Concussion in Sport, Prague 2004. *Br. J. Sports Med.* **39**, 196–204.

McCrory, P. et al. 2009. Consensus statement on concussion in sport - The 3rd international conference on concussion in sport held in Zurich, November 2008. *PMR* **1**, 406–420.

McCrory, P. et al. 2013. Consensus statement on concussion in sport: The 4th international conference on concussion in sport held in Zurich, November 2012. *Br. J. Sports Med.* **47**, 250–258.

McCrory, P. et al. 2017. Consensus statement on concussion in sport: The 5th international conference on concussion in sport held in Berlin, October 2016. *Br. J. Sports Med.* **51**, 838–847.

McLeod, T. C. V. and Leach, C. 2012. Psychometric properties of self-report concussion scales and checklists. *J. Athl. Train.* **47**, 221–223.

Miller, J. R., Adamson, G. J., Pink, M. M., and Sweet, J. C. 2007. Comparison of preseason, midseason, and postseason neurocognitive scores in uninjured collegiate football players. *Am. J. Sports Med.* **35**(8), 1284–1288.

Mittenberg, W., DiGiulio, D. V., Perrin, S., and Bass, A. E. 1992. Symptoms following mild head injury: Expectation as aetiology. *J. Neurol. Neurosurg. Psychiatry* **55**, 200–204.

Moser, R. S., Schatz, P., Neidzwski, K., and Ott, S.D. 2011. Group versus individual administration affects baseline neurocognitive test performance. *Am. J. Sports Med.* **39**, 2325–2330.

Nelson, L. D., LaRoche, A. A., Pfaller, A. Y., Lerner, E. B., Hammeke, T. A., Randolph, C., … McCrea, M. A. 2016. Prospective, head-to-head study of three computerized neurocognitive assessment tools (CNTs): Reliability and validity for the assessment of sport-related concussion. *J. Int. Neuropsychol. Soc. JINS* **22**, 24–37.

NFL concussion poll: 56 percent of players would hide symptoms to stay on field | NFL | Sporting News. Retrieved from http://www.sportingnews.com/nfl-news/4309119-nfl-concussions-players-hide-symptoms-sporting-news-midseason-poll. (Accessed: June 27, 2016)

Peterson, C. L., Ferrara, M. S., Mrazik, M., Piland, S., and Elliott, R., 2003. Evaluation of neuropsychological domain scores and postural stability following cerebral concussion in sports. *Clin. J. Sport Med. Off. J. Can. Acad. Sport Med.* **13**, 230–237.

Piland, S. G., Motl, R. W., Ferrara, M. S., and Peterson, C. L. 2003. Evidence for the factorial and construct validity of a self-report concussion symptoms scale. *J. Athl. Train.* **38**, 104–112.

Piland, S. G., Ferrara, M. S., Macciocchi, S. N., Broglio, S. P., and Gould, T. E. 2010. Investigation of baseline self-report concussion symptom scores. *J. Athl. Train.* **45**, 273–278.

Randolph, C., McCrea, M., and Barr, W. B. 2005. Is neuropsychological testing useful in the management of sport-related concussion? *J. Athl. Train.* **40**, 139–152.

Randolph, C. and Kirkwood, M. W. 2009. What are the real risks of sport-related concussion, and are they modifiable? *J. Int. Neuropsychol. Soc. JINS* **15**, 512–520.

Randolph, C., Millis, S., Barr, W. B., McCrea, M., Guskiewicz, K. M., Hammeke, T. A., and Kelly, J. P. 2009. Concussion symptom inventory: An empirically derived scale for monitoring resolution of symptoms following sport-related concussion. *Arch. Clin. Neuropsychol. Off. J. Natl. Acad. Neuropsychol.* **24**, 219–229.

Resch, J., Driscoll, A., McCaffrey, N., Brown, C., Ferrara, M. S., Macciocchi, S., Baumgartner, T., and Walpert, K. 2013. ImPact test-retest reliability: Reliably unreliable? *J. Athl. Train.* **48**, 506–511.

Riemann, B. L. and Guskiewicz, K. M. 2000. Effects of mild head injury on postural stability as measured through clinical balance testing. *J. Athl. Train.* **35**, 19–25.

Sady, M. D., Vaughan, C. G., and Gioia, G. A. 2014. Psychometric characteristics of the postconcussionsymptom inventory in children and adolescents. *Arch. Clin. Neuropsychol. Off. J. Natl. Acad. Neuropsychol.* **29**, 348–363.

Schatz, P. and Putz, B. O. 2006. Cross-validation of measures used for computer-based assessment of concussion. *Appl. Neuropsychol.* **13**, 151–159.

Schatz, P. 2010. Long-term test-retest reliability of baseline cognitive assessments using ImPACT. *Am. J. Sports Med.* **38**, 47–53.

Schatz, P. and Glatts, C. 2013. 'Sandbagging' baseline test performance on ImPACT, without detection, is more difficult than it appears. *Arch. Clin. Neuropsychol. Off. J. Natl. Acad. Neuropsychol.* **28**, 236–244.

Segalowitz, S., Mahaney, P., Santesso, D. L., MacGregor, L., Dywan, J., and Willer, B. 2007. Retest reliability in adolescents of a computerized neuropsychological battery used to assess recovery from concussion. *NeuroRehabilitation* **22**(3), 243–251.

Silverberg, N. D., Luoto, T. M., Öhman, J., and Iverson, G.L. 2014. Assessment of mild traumatic brain injury with the King-Devick test in an emergency department sample. *Brain Inj.* **28**, 1590–1593.

Standards for Educational & Psychological Testing (2014 ed). Retrieved from http://www.aera.net/Standards14. (Accessed: June 29, 2016).

Taylor, H. G., Dietrich, A., Nuss, K., Wright, M., Rusin, J., Bangert, B., Minich, N., and Yeates, K. O. 2010. Post-concussive symptoms in children with mild traumatic brain injury. *Neuropsychology* **24**, 148–159.

Valovich McLeod, T. C., Barr, W. B., McCrea, M., and Guskiewicz, K. M. 2006. Psychometric and measurement properties of concussion assessment tools in youth sports. *J. Athl. Train.* **41**, 399–408.

Van Kampen, D. A., Lovell, M. R., Pardini, J. E., Collins, M. W., and Fu, F. H. 2006. The 'value added' of neurocognitive testing after sports-related concussion. *Am. J. Sports Med.* **34**, 1630–1635.

Vaughan, C. G., Gerst, E. H., Sady, M. D., Newman, J. B., and Gioia, G. A. 2014. The relation between testing environment and baseline performance in child and adolescent concussion assessment. *Am. J. Sports Med.* **42**, 1716–1723.

Webbe, F. M. and Zimmer, A. 2015. History of neuropsychological study of sport-related concussion. *Brain Inj.* **29**, 129–138.

Yeates, K. O., Luria, J., Bartkowski, H., Rusin, J., Martin, L., and Bigler, E. D. 1999. Postconcussive symptoms in children with mild closed head injuries. *J. Head Trauma Rehabil.* **14**, 337–350.

*chapter eighteen*

# On-field diagnosis and management of concussion

## What should be done while I am still on the field?

*J. Scott Delaney and Ammar Al-Kashmiri*

## Contents

## Introduction

The on-field evaluation of an athlete who has sustained a head injury is very different than assessing a patient in an office setting. Each sport and field of play are unique, and sport medicine professionals must be prepared to adapt to the environment at hand. In a game or practice setting, there are many factors which can impede an ideal concussion evaluation. These may include crowd and ambient noise, inclement weather conditions, lack of physical space for an ideal evaluation, many interested observers in the evaluation process, and cameras in certain situations. All of these can make the evaluation of a possibly concussed athlete more difficult and can create more stress for the sport medicine team. The sideline or on-field evaluation is also often occurring during a game or competition when the injured athlete, teammates, coaches, and frequently parents are in the competition mindset. During this time, athletes and other interested parties can be less receptive to a thorough concussion evaluation and the potential news that an athlete is being removed from the competition. Preparation for what can and might occur in the evaluation of a head injured athlete is vital and whenever possible, preapproved standardized protocols should be activated or followed. This ensures that the medical team caring for the athlete is not forced to improvise at the moment of the evaluation when the stress level for all involved is likely to be high.

## Preseason and pre-event preparation and preparedness

Taking the time to prepare in advance for event or game coverage is essential. All parties that may be involved in the medical care of an injured athlete should be aware of the emergency medical procedures and their roles in the process (American College of Sports 2004, Delaney and Drummond 2002). Although an extensive review of all advanced medical operations, emergency action plans, equipment necessary for event coverage, and so on, is beyond the scope of this chapter, it is essential that preparation for a worst-case scenario involving an athlete who has sustained a head injury be anticipated (Casa et al. 2012). When evaluating an athlete who has sustained a head injury, prolonged unconsciousness, a spinal injury, or deterioration of the athlete's overall condition is always possible. In most circumstances, on-field and sideline care are not expected to function at an advanced trauma level. As such, evacuation and transfer of an injured athlete to more definitive care at an emergency department must be anticipated. Preparation with local emergency medical services (EMS) is essential (Andersen et al. 2002). Some events will require on-site EMS and ambulance(s) whereas others may rely on activation of the local EMS system for transfer to more definitive care in an emergency department. At a minimum, preparation with on-site medical staff and EMS should include an EMS action plan with the stadium or event address, directions to the stadium, stadium GPS coordinates, entry point to the stadium or event, the distance to the nearest hospital (or designated hospital, if applicable), security personnel to direct and/or accompany the EMS on arrival to the event, communication protocols, stadium maps with automatic external defibrillator (AED) locations, and the roles of first responders and other on-site medical staff (American College of Sports 2004, Andersen et al. 2002).

## Standardized concussion evaluation procedures and disposition decisions

Event coverage is provided by many different professionals with diverse medical backgrounds and skill sets (Delaney et al. 2011, 2012). Depending on protocols and availabilities, the evaluation of a potentially concussed athlete may be undertaken by sport medicine physicians, primary care physicians, emergency physicians, orthopedic surgeons, athletic trainers, physical therapists, or student learners. As such, it is imperative for each group or organization providing coverage for an athlete, team, or event to have a pre-approved standardized approach that will be utilized by all those who may be called on to evaluate a possible concussion. The concussion evaluation process should be discussed and approved in the preseason, or prior to competition, so that the staff, athletes, coaches, and parents are aware of the protocols and the time required to complete the process. All of the sport medicine staff involved in providing care should adhere to the same procedures. Disposition decisions for injured athletes should also be standardized and decided beforehand so that there is no confusion among the sport medicine team and the athletes when a diagnosis of a concussion is made. There may be league or association protocols for concussion management: both for evaluation and disposition decisions. Many jurisdictions also have laws that govern concussion management (Lowrey and Morain 2014, Mackenzie et al. 2015). It behooves the entire sport medicine team to be aware of the different laws and protocols and adhere to them, whenever possible, to avoid any future conflicts or liability (Broglio et al. 2014). Proper documentation of the evaluation, disposition, and follow-ups is mandatory and helps ensure continuity and adherence to the protocols.

## Initial assessment of the injured athlete

Rapidly identifying, evaluating, and managing athletes who have suffered a concussion or more severe brain injury is vital (Luke and Micheli 1999, Delaney et al. 2011, Broglio et al. 2014). Clinicians who identify and treat these athletes must address immediate safety concerns such as assessing the airway and breathing of an injured athlete, to eventually ruling out serious intracranial pathology. Although diagnosing a concussion is important, it is not the first priority when assessing an injured athlete. Other injuries take priority in management and hence require earlier recognition. To ensure this, the clinician must follow a systematic approach to the athlete's assessment that prioritizes injuries according to their urgency. The initial evaluation of any injured athlete must occur in an organized and systematic fashion to exclude life-threatening injuries and avoid overlooking other injuries. The latter may occur if the sport medicine professional *jumps* to the obvious injuries or initial concussion evaluation before completing a thorough overall assessment of the athlete. For example, a forearm deformed by a fracture, although very dramatic in appearance, should not be assessed and treated before a life-threatening condition such as an airway obstructed by a dislodged mouth guard.

The approach to the care of all patients injured in trauma has been standardized through the advanced trauma life support (ATLS) program set forth by the American College of Surgeons Committee on Trauma. This program has been widely adopted and accepted worldwide and has been consistently shown to have a positive impact on the outcome of the injured patient (Collicott and Hughes 1980, Walsh et al. 1989, Navarro et al. 2014). Although a detailed discussion of the entire ATLS program is beyond the scope of this chapter, certain elements should be highlighted. One of the keys to the success of the ATLS program is the systematic approach that it adopts in assessment, namely, the primary and secondary surveys. Although this program has been developed for hospital-based practitioners, the assessment approach can be easily applied to the injured athlete on the sport field. The primary survey is composed of the *ABCDE* assessment strategy that begins with an assessment of the airway (A) along with cervical spine (c-spine) protection, breathing (B), circulation (C), disability (D), exposure (E), and the secondary survey which employs a thorough assessment commencing from the head and ending at the toes. All medical and therapy staff attending to a sporting event should be familiar in assessing each of these components, even if the treatment of some conditions may be beyond the range of practice for many involved. It should also be reinforced that whenever an athlete is involved in a significant impact, it must always be assumed that there is a coexisting injury to the c-spine and immediate protection must be employed. An actual assessment of the c-spine can be done at a later stage during the secondary survey. As airway is being assessed, the c-spine is protected by inline immobilization. A rigid cervical collar should be applied if a c-spine injury cannot be ruled out.

## Concussion assessment

Once more serious injuries have been excluded, a thorough concussion evaluation may occur if necessary. The sport medicine team will need to decide WHO, HOW, WHEN, and WHERE an athlete should be evaluated.

### Who should be evaluated?

As discussed in previous chapters, there are numerous signs and symptoms that may be experienced by a concussed athlete (see Chapters 5, 15, 17). Making an accurate and prompt diagnosis is paramount for managing concussions properly and preventing further injury. Although the rare cases of concussion that result in a traumatically induced loss of consciousness may be overtly obvious to even a casual observer, in fact, there is no loss of consciousness and often no obvious external signs in the vast majority of sport-related concussions (Delaney et al. 2000, 2002, Gessel et al. 2007, Broglio and Puetz 2008, Halstead et al. 2010, McCrory et al. 2013a, 2013b, 2017, Echemendia et al. 2017c). In most cases, the process of evaluating and diagnosing a concussion begins with an athlete volunteering their symptoms to a member of the medical team. (Delaney et al. 2002, 2015).

#### Athletes who volunteer their symptoms

Athletes who volunteer that they do not feel well or are experiencing symptoms of a possible concussion should be evaluated. The concussion in sport group recommends that all athletes experiencing any signs or symptoms from a concussion be removed from play that day and be medically evaluated (McCrory et al. 2005, 2009, 2013a). Many of the signs or symptoms of a concussion can occur for other reasons, and those causes should be ruled out first. For example, blurred vision may occur from a traumatic eye injury such as a hyphema (blood in the anterior chamber of the eye), or feeling *light headed* may be due to low blood pressure and can be indicative of internal bleeding.

#### Athletes who do NOT volunteer their symptoms

In general, there are two main reasons that an athlete may not volunteer their symptoms to the medical staff. The first is unawareness that the symptoms he or she is experiencing are those of a concussion. An athlete who has sustained contact may not appreciate that, for example, the blurred or abnormal vision they are experiencing may be due to a brain injury (Delaney et al. 2000, 2002, McCrea et al. 2004, McCrory et al. 2005, Sullivan et al. 2009). Research in emergency department patients who had suffered a concussion revealed that it is not always the presence of individual symptoms that causes someone to seek medical evaluation; rather it is the severity of the symptoms (Delaney et al. 2005). For example, mild balance problems post-head injury may not cause an individual to seek medical evaluation, whereas severe dizziness may prompt the same patient to do so. These types of situations where an athlete does not recognize that they may be experiencing concussion symptoms may be considerably diminished by education programs (see Chapter 3 for prevention strategies) (McCrory et al. 2005, Goodman et al. 2006, Bagley et al. 2012, Bramley et al. 2012, Tator 2012). The use of preseason concussion *contracts* with athletes may also help to ensure they have read and understand the concussion information packages provided and comprehend the importance of being diagnosed and treated appropriately (Baugh et al. 2014). In an effort to ensure that players are constantly reminded, some leagues mandate that a poster or list of possible concussion signs and symptoms be in the dressing room area before each competition (Tator 2012, Prevention 2015). These posters are often in different languages so players from diverse backgrounds can understand the information (Delaney and McDonald [personal communication]).

The second reason that an athlete may not volunteer their symptoms to the medical team is if they do understand that they may have suffered a concussion, but do not wish to be removed from the field of play for the purpose of being evaluated (Caron et al. 2013, Delaney et al. 2015) (Kaut et al. 2003, McCrea et al. 2004). This may occur for many reasons, such as an athlete not believing that it is dangerous to continue playing with a concussion, wanting to continue playing, or fearing they may be restricted from future competition as part of the concussion treatment protocol (Delaney et al. 2015). Former professional ice hockey players who retired due to post-concussion symptoms revealed that they routinely hid their symptoms from teammates, coaches, and sport medicine team to continue playing (Caron et al. 2013). Many were only removed from competition by their coaches and medical professionals when they were no longer able to hide their concussion symptoms. Here again, preparticipation education may help avoid this from occurring by informing the athletes of the risks and potential consequences of continuing to play while still suffering symptoms from a concussion (McCrory et al. 2005, Goodman et al. 2006, Bagley et al. 2012, Bramley et al. 2012, Tator 2012).

### Spotters and sideline video review

It can be difficult for a medical staff to closely observe all athletes on the field of play. Very often there are many athletes involved in the competition; the field is large and athletes may be dozens of meters away from the medical staff. To help provide another set of eyes, several professional leagues now employ *spotters*, of which sole responsibility is to watch the competition for any visible signs (VS) of concussion or any concussion-like behavior or signs in participants (Seravalli 2015, Wagner-McGough 2015). These VS after contact may include loss of consciousness, motor incoordination, blank facial expression, difficulty or slowness to stand, or rubbing the head or helmet (Bruce et al. 2017, Echemendia et al. 2017a, 2017c). The spotters watch from the stands or watch the television feed for such behavior. If an athlete appears to be exhibiting signs and behaviors of a possible concussion, the spotter notifies the medical staff of the affected athlete. The medical staff can then observe and/or remove the athlete for further evaluation. Sideline access to video of the injury is becoming more common where available, and can allow the sport medicine team to visualize and review the mechanism of injury and the athlete's subsequent signs and behaviors (McCrory et al. 2017). Alternatively, valuable feedback on an athlete's behavior can be obtained from other players, coaches, equipment managers, and parents because most amateur leagues or teams will not have the resources to employ a designated spotter. Often these people know the affected competitor very well and can be attuned to subtle changes in personality and behavior. As such, any information provided by these individuals should be taken seriously and prompt an evaluation of the affected athlete.

Although most concussions will be evaluated and diagnosed after an athlete volunteers his or her symptoms to the medical staff, there are some VS and behaviors that can be observed by the medical staff, teammates, coaches, and parents that may help to identify a possible concussion. Although no list can account for all possible behaviors of a concussed

*Table 18.1* Visible signs and common behaviors of concussed athletes

Remains motionless on playing surface after contact

Slow to stand up after contact

Grabbing or rubbing head/helmet after contact

Change in the level of consciousness (seems sleepy or too quiet)

Dazed or stunned appearance

Confused

Unsure of score, game, opponent

Clumsy or uncoordinated

Answers questions more slowly than usual

Asks same questions repeatedly

Irritable, sad, or more emotional than usual

*Source:* McCrory, P. et al., *Br. J. Sports Med.* 47, 268–271, 2013b; Echemendia, R. J. et al., *Br. J. Sports Med.* 2017a; Aubry, M. et al., *Clin. J. Sport Med.*, 12, 6–11, 2002.

athlete, some VS or common behaviors which can be observed by others around them are listed in Table 18.1.

Athletes who show these behaviors should be removed from competition and be evaluated appropriately for a possible concussion.

## How should an athlete be evaluated?

After more serious injuries have been excluded, the athlete should be brought to the area selected for a concussion evaluation. It is important to notify the coach and/or parents that the player is being removed from competition for a concussion evaluation. There should be a pre-arranged understanding with the coach/coaches that the player is not to return or be expected to participate until the coach is informed by the sport medicine team. Ideally, the person who informs the coach that the player is being removed for a concussion evaluation should be the same person who will later update the coach on whether the athlete is able to return, or is being removed for the rest of the competition. This helps foster familiarity and routine so the coach knows and expects to be informed by that one person on a consistent basis. It also helps control the flow of information. Too many different people involved in updating the coach may lead to discordant messages and confusion.

Remembering that most athletes are competitive and will want to return to play as soon as possible, it is helpful to remove a vital piece of athletic gear from the athlete undergoing a concussion evaluation. This may be the helmet in American football, the stick in ice hockey, or the glove in baseball or softball. Removing and *hiding* a piece of required equipment will ensure that the athlete is unable to return to competition until given full medical clearance by the medical staff and the coach is informed. Once clearance has occurred, the player can have their gear returned to them. If they are not cleared for return to play, the gear should not be returned until the match is finished or the athlete has undressed and changed out of their athletic gear.

The four *pillars* of a sideline concussion evaluation are (1) general questioning, (2) the assessment of symptoms, (3) an evaluation of mental status and neurocognitive abilities, and (4) a focused physical examination (McCrory et al. 2009, Scorza et al. 2012, 2013a, Broglio et al. 2014). As mentioned earlier, the battery of tests to be used should be decided well in advance and be utilized by the entire sport medicine team consistently. There are sideline assessment tools that incorporate some or all of the four main elements of the concussion assessment. The standardized assessment of concussion (SAC) is a widely used tool that incorporates orientation, immediate memory, concentration, and delayed recall (McCrea 2001a, 2001b). Another widely used instrument is the sport concussion assessment tool (SCAT) in its different versions (SCAT-1 (McCrory et al. 2005), SCAT-2 (McCrory et al. 2009), SCAT-3 (McCrory et al. 2013a), and SCAT-5 (Echemendia et al. 2017b). The SCAT incorporates symptom assessment, targeted physical examination, and an evaluation of mental status and neurocognitive abilities.

Having baseline scores for the tests to be administered may be helpful in interpreting an athlete's performance (McCrory et al. 2013a, Bruce et al. 2016). Ideally, baseline testing should occur in the preseason or precompetition when the athlete is well rested and free from distracting injury or illness (Echemendia et al. 2009). Baseline data may help indicate that an athlete is performing well below their normal levels. It may also help interpretation of low performance by identifying areas of testing in which the athlete does not normally score well, even at baseline. If baseline data are to be compared with post-injury results, it is ideal if both tests were conducted under comparable conditions and in similar nondistracting environments (McCrory et al. 2017).

### General questioning

Before delving into specific concussion testing, the assessment of an athlete who is suspected of having suffered a concussion should first begin with open-ended questions such as "What happened?", "How are you feeling?", and "What do you remember?". Much information can be gathered from a few open-ended questions and can help identify how the player is feeling in general, the symptoms that are most obvious to him/her, if there was a loss of consciousness or amnesia, and what the mechanism of injury was. All of these are important in the evaluation process. While not always imperative to identify the mechanism of injury in the initial moments after an injury, the athlete, teammates, coaches, and eventually game film/video (if available) can help identify it. The mechanism of injury and the force involved are important in terms of future management. If the mechanism was rather innocuous, this may indicate a lowered threshold for concussion, that is, a concussion occurred with less force than would normally be expected. This lowering of the concussion threshold may occur if there is an active ongoing undiagnosed concussion at the time of the injury, or the threshold may be permanently lowered due to previous head injuries (Collins et al. 2002, Kutcher 2010, Simma et al. 2013). Both of these scenarios have implications in terms of disposition decisions.

### Assessment of symptoms

An evaluation of the athlete's post-injury symptoms is valuable. For athletes who are honest about their symptoms, their presence can be a sensitive tool for diagnosing an acute concussion (McCrea et al. 2005, Randolph et al. 2005, Broglio et al. 2007). The presence of concussive symptoms has been found to correlate well with abnormalities in brain function on advanced brain imaging (functional MRI) both acutely and during the recovery process (Chen et al. 2007, Ptito et al. 2007). Limitations of the symptoms assessment must be understood in that symptoms can be delayed in onset, can be denied by athletes who are experiencing them, may have been present at baseline, and/or may be due to other medical conditions (McCrory et al. 2017).

There are a number of symptom checklists that are available. These include the postconcussion symptom scale, head injury scale, concussion symptom inventory, McGill abbreviated concussion evaluation (ACE) post-concussion symptom score, concussion symptom inventory, and sport concussion assessment tool (SCAT) (Scorza et al. 2012, McCrory et al. 2013a, Giza et al. 2013, Makdissi et al. 2014, Echemendia et al. 2017b).

### Mental status and neurocognitive testing

The realities of an on-field concussion do not allow for prolonged assessment of mental status examination and neurocognitive abilities. As mentioned earlier, the SAC and different versions of the SCAT briefly assess these. While traditionally paper and pencil type testing has been used for on-field assessments, sideline computer tools are becoming more widely available. These often have the advantage of having immediate access to past testing and baseline measurement (Davis 2015). For a more detailed discussion of mental status and neurocognitive assessment tools available, the reader is referred back to Chapter 9.

### Physical examination

An organized and thorough initial approach to the injured athlete, as discussed earlier, will help ensure that serious and subtle injuries are identified. Although orientation and mental status exam will be conducted in the evaluation of mental status and neurocognitive abilities, a complete neurologic exam should be conducted including testing of the cranial nerves, sensation, motor strength, coordination with finger nose testing, and balance testing with the Romberg test. The Romberg test may be omitted if balance testing is evaluated in more detail using the Balance Error Scoring System (BESS). While not included in the different SCAT versions, an assessment of reaction time and ocular function and tracking may be included in the physical exam as well.

Although the assessment of balance in an office setting can be performed in a number of ways, often with specialized equipment, the assessment of balance on the sideline is usually done using the BESS, developed as an objective test to assess concussed athletes (Riemann and Guskiewicz 2000), (Guskiewicz et al. 2001). This test has been found to be a useful physical examination tool to help differentiate concussed from nonconcussed athletes, especially within the first few days following injury (McCrea et al. 2003). Although the traditional BESS testing is completed first on a firm then a foam surface, the modified version of the balance error scoring system (M-BESS) included in the SCAT-2, SCAT-3, and SCAT-5 only assesses balance on a firm surface (Glaviano et al. 2015, Snyder et al. 2014, Zimmer et al. 2014, Echemendia et al. 2017b). This is ideally performed on athletes who are barefoot, wearing no protective equipment, and dressed in shorts and a t-shirt. Sports with minimal equipment such as soccer lend themselves well to such an evaluation. In other sports, such as American football in which athletes wear a lot of equipment, this is more difficult. Nevertheless, the M-BESS scores appear to be reliable in athletes wearing athletic gear and cleats (Harmon et al. 2013) on a hard surface or a softer surface such as Fieldturf® (Azad et al. 2016). The decision of how the balance assessment will be performed is ultimately left up to the sport medicine staff performing the concussion evaluation. Ideally, this should be discussed with the entire team before the season or competition begins, and the procedure should be standardized for all those who may be called upon to perform a concussion evaluation.

The M-BESS requires balancing in three stances, that is, double leg, single leg, and tandem gait performed with eyes closed, hands placed on hips, and standing barefoot on a firm surface (Hunt et al. 2009). Balancing in each of the three stances is assessed with a maximum score of ten points each. Mistakes in each stance are subtracted from the maximum score of ten, making the total *mistake free* M-BESS score of 30 (Hunt et al. 2009). It should be noted that some clinicians prefer to score the number of mistakes on each stance instead. Although the normative scores for M-BESS have been published recently

(Snyder et al. 2014, Zimmer et al. 2014), clinical judgment prevails as the gold standard for diagnosing concussion (Guskiewicz et al. 2001, Furman et al. 2013). To date, definitive data are lacking on whether M-BESS scores reliably help rule in, or rule out, a concussion. Studies on the traditional version of the BESS test performed on both firm and foam surfaces indicate that performances can be influenced by gender (females better than males), training, bracing, injury, exercise, fatigue, and time since injury (Covassin et al. 2012, McCrea et al. 2013).

## When should an athlete be evaluated?

Only after more serious injuries have been excluded, a thorough initial concussion evaluation should take place. It is important to understand that the evaluation of an athlete who has possibly sustained a concussion is an ongoing process and is not limited to one encounter. All athletes who have been examined for a possible concussion should ideally be reevaluated within the next 5–10 minutes. This is especially true for those who have returned to competition. Some concussion signs and symptoms are not present or apparent immediately post-injury and may only become evident in the minutes, and sometimes hours after the first assessment (Aubry et al. 2002, McCrory et al. 2005, 2013a, 2017).

### Initial on-field concussion evaluation

The initial concussion evaluation should take place as soon as possible. Any athlete who is suspected of having suffered a concussion should not be permitted to continue playing or competing. Athletes who continue to play while symptomatic from a concussion are believed to be at risk for more severe injury, including second impact syndrome. Repeated concussions may also result in progressive and cumulative neurologic and neuropsychological impairment (McCrory and Berkovic 1998) (Tysvaer and Storli 1989) (Warren and Bailes 1998) (Kelly and Rosenberg 1997) (De Beaumont et al. 2009). Many jurisdictions have laws which mandate that athletes suspected of having suffered a concussion be removed from competition (Mackenzie et al. 2015) (Lowrey and Morain 2014) (Broglio et al. 2014).

Athletes who have just exited the field of play should be given a few minutes to recover physically. Initial questioning may take place, but the athlete should not begin the formal concussion evaluation if they are physically winded or exhausted. Physical exhaustion can affect the cognitive and physical performances (especially balance) of a concussion evaluation (Covassin et al. 2012, McCrea et al. 2013). It should also be noted that other symptoms can hamper a concussion evaluation (Scorza et al. 2012). These may include pain from a distracting injury and anxiety about the situation (Heyer et al. 2000, Moriarty et al. 2011, Robinson et al. 2013). Whenever possible, these symptoms should be assessed and treated before proceeding with the evaluation.

### Follow-up on-field concussion evaluations

Follow-up concussion evaluations should occur in all athletes after the initial assessment has been completed. The first should occur within the first 5–10 minutes after the initial evaluation. In all athletes, a follow-up evaluation is important to ensure that no new signs or symptoms that were not present on initial evaluation have appeared. Although some signs and symptoms can be delayed by minutes or even hours, others are not evident until exposure to certain stimuli (Aubry et al. 2002, McCrory et al. 2005, McCrory et al. 2013a, 2017). An athlete who is examined in a quiet environment may not realize that loud noises or bright lights are bothersome until they are placed in such an environment.

*Athletes removed from competition*   In athletes who have been removed from competition and diagnosed with a concussion, follow-up evaluations are done to ensure there is no worsening of the symptoms or progression of abnormalities detected at the time of the initial physical examination. All athletes who have been diagnosed with a concussion must be evaluated frequently to ensure signs and symptoms at least stabilize and do not continue to worsen (McCrory et al. 2005, 2009, 2013a, 2017). Those who are experiencing progressive and worsening signs or symptoms should be continuously monitored by the medical staff until their signs and symptoms stabilize or improve. If there is a continuing deterioration, the athlete may have to be transferred for more definitive testing and care.

*Athletes who return to competition*   Athletes who have been examined initially and cleared for return to competition should be reevaluated at the first possible opportunity. Even if the athlete is unable to leave the field of play for a formal evaluation, eye contact and hand signals (e.g., thumbs up for *feeling fine* or thumbs down for *feeling unwell*) can be used to get a general idea of how he/she is responding to competition. When a more thorough reevaluation may occur, it is often dependent on the sport itself. Soccer players may have to wait for half-time or the end of the match. Other athletes, such as ice hockey and American football players, can be examined at the first change of shift, or change of possession, respectively. They should be evaluated and questioned about any new onset of symptoms, their response to game or match play in general, and any contact in particular. They should be evaluated periodically throughout the competition, usually at breaks in the action such as half-time, in between periods or innings, and at the end of the competition or game.

It is not practical or likely that there will be compliance to perform a complete concussion evaluation at each encounter with the affected athlete. The follow-up evaluations do not need to take the form of a complete thorough concussion evaluation but can be a brief directed assessment of common signs and symptoms. There is evidence that repeating the same questions in a formal concussion evaluation may lead to a practice or learning effect (Broglio et al. 2007, 2014, Fazio et al. 2007).

No athlete who has been diagnosed with a concussion should initially be left unattended (McCrory et al. 2013a, Echemendia et al. 2017c). Ideally, a member of the medical staff should observe the athlete, but this is not always feasible. A teammate, parent, coach, or friend can help observe the player and often help him/her shower and get changed out of their athletic gear. Any observer should be briefed on the common symptoms and obvious signs of a concussion and asked to report back to the medical staff if there is any worsening or progression of the athlete's condition.

It is important for all medical staff, and even the athletes and coaches, to understand that even though an athlete has been cleared for return to competition after an initial concussion evaluation, the diagnosis can also be made at any point in the follow-up assessments. This does not mean that an improper initial evaluation was performed. Medical staff should not feel intimidated or embarrassed if the diagnosis of a concussion is made after an athlete returns to competition. This can be the natural presentation or evolution of a concussion. Some symptoms may have been delayed in onset, others only evident after exposure to certain stimuli for a period of time, and others still only evident after some contact. It is of utmost importance that the diagnosis be made as soon as it is recognized and that the athlete be removed from competition.

### Final on-field clearance concussion evaluation

A final thorough concussion evaluation should be administered to all athletes with a suspected concussion during competition, whether they were positively diagnosed or cleared for return to play. This may be carried out at the conclusion of the competition or when they have been cleared from the supervision of the medical team. It should be remembered that athletes who are experiencing progressive and worsening signs or symptoms should be continuously monitored by the medical staff until their signs and symptoms stabilize or improve. If there is a continuing deterioration, the athlete may have to be transferred for more definitive testing and care (see Section "Disposition").

## Where should an athlete be evaluated?

Examination of a potentially concussed athlete should preferably occur in a quiet space, removed from the distractions of the athletic environment (Guskiewicz et al. 2013, Echemendia et al. 2017b). This may be a locker room or another quiet space where the examiner and the athlete can speak and complete a through concussion evaluation. Too much noise can be distracting to everyone involved in the evaluation. Sounds from an ongoing competition may increase the stress level of a player who will constantly be reminded that they are absent from the field of play. A quiet evaluation room ensures that the athlete will not see the ongoing competition and will be more focused on the evaluation process and not on the score or the latest play. Some professional leagues now mandate that a concussion evaluation must take place in the *quiet room* or the *concussion room*, that is, in a quiet environment free from distraction and away from the bench or sidelines (Dixon 2011, NFL Head and Bradley 2013).

An evaluation room should have access to medical equipment to complete a thorough medical exam. It should be remembered that an athlete being evaluated for a concussion might have other unrelated injuries that mimic the signs and symptoms of a concussion. Characteristics of an ideal concussion evaluation room are listed in Table 18.2.

In reality, convenient access to a nearby room for an ideal evaluation area is not always possible. Pressure to complete a rapid assessment can come from the athletes themselves, coaches, other players, and sometimes parents. Some team sports such as American football and ice hockey allow for an easy in-game substitution during the medical evaluation so the team is not penalized by playing with fewer players during the evaluation process. This allows for more time to relocate to the dressing room or another less distracting environment. In contrast, soccer rules allow the game to continue with one team a player short until the evaluation process is completed. After the medical evaluation, the player is

*Table 18.2* Attributes of an ideal concussion evaluation room

Close proximity to field of play

Adjustable level of lighting

Closable door that will decrease outside noise and provide privacy during the examination

Table for an injured athlete to recline or sit on during the evaluation

Blood pressure cuff to assess blood pressure in light-headed athletes or in those who have suffered a loss of consciousness

Stethoscope to assess blood pressure and auscultate the heart, lungs and abdomen, if necessary

Ophthalmoscope to examine the eyes and assess pupillary reaction to light [a]

Otoscope to examine ears, throat and oral cavity [a]

Hard floor for balance examinations

Contains a medical kit for treatment of associated injuries

[a] A penlight can assess pupil reaction and help visualize the oral cavity and throat but does not allow a thorough examination of the eyes or the ears

allowed to return to play, or another player must be substituted. In these types of sports, a long trip to an ideal evaluation locale is less feasible, such that the evaluation is more likely to occur at the sidelines.

For an evaluation at the sidelines, the athlete should be examined as far away from the rest of the team as possible. This will provide a small measure of privacy and hopefully limit the number of interested observers from watching or interrupting the evaluation. It is useful to have any available helpers keep interested observers away from the ongoing evaluation. The examiner should face the field of play, whereas the athlete should be turned away from the competition. This is done to decrease the visual distraction of the player trying to follow the action on the field of play. Most events or teams will have access to a portable table or bench that the athlete can sit or lie on during the medical evaluation at the sidelines. A chair or another piece of sideline equipment can be used if no table or bench is available. It is best to have a player sitting during much of the concussion evaluation process so they are relaxed and better able to focus. Some teams or events have nearby medical tents that can be used. These tents provide some degree of privacy and protection from possible inclement weather. Access to a firm surface for balance assessment may be difficult on the sidelines. Often there is a firm surface around the field of play, whether this be a track, hallway, or nearby cement section of the facility.

## Disposition

The safety of an injured athlete is the overriding principle that should guide management and disposition decisions. While most concussed athletes can be managed by the on-site sport medicine team, others may need to be referred or transferred to an emergency department for more advanced investigations, neuroimaging, and definitive care. Having a predetermined plan for who should be referred to an emergency department will help avoid confusion at the time of injury. The sport medicine team should also have a standardized approach for discharge planning and follow-up for those athletes who have been concussed but do not require referral to an emergency department.

### When to refer to the emergency department

Once the clinician has completed the on-field assessment, a decision has to be made on whether the athlete needs to be transferred to an emergency department for further investigation, brain imaging, and definitive care. As much as possible, the decision should be made on an objective basis to only select those athletes who have the potential for having a serious traumatic brain injury (TBI). Clinical decision rules (CDRs) have been developed to aid clinicians decide which patients to send for brain imaging (Stiell et al. 2001a, 2001b). The rules were designed to help identify individuals who may have brain injuries that will require an emergent neurosurgical intervention. These injuries may include a subdural hemorrhage (SDH), epidural hemorrhage (EDH), and subarachnoid hemorrhage (SAH). Although these rules were devised to help identify individuals with serious brain injuries, they were also designed to identify unaffected players. Identifying those who do not have serious brain injuries helps limit unnecessary neuroimaging and unnecessary radiation exposure, primarily from cerebral CT scans. One widely accepted rule used to determine which patients who have sustained a head injury should undergo brain imaging is the Canadian CT head rule (Stiell et al. 2001c, 2001d) (Table 5.4). Although this rule has been developed for the emergency department setting, it can and should be utilized by the

*Table 18.3* Evaluating risk for serious cervical spine fracture

| |
|---|
| No posterior midline cervical spine tenderness is present |
| No evidence of intoxication is present |
| The patient has a normal level of alertness |
| No focal neurologic deficit is present |
| The patient does not have a painful distracting injury |

*Note:*   If these five criteria are met, there is no risk of serious cervical spine
fracture and imaging is not necessary.

sport medicine team for athletes who are 16 years of age and older. Implementing this rule provides an objective means for a safer disposition decision (Stiell et al. 2005).

Because there is a strong association between head injury and c-spine injuries (Mulligan et al. 2010), any athlete who has suffered a head injury should be assessed for a concomitant c-spine injury. If there is any suspicion of the latter, neck immobilization must be maintained and the athlete transported to the emergency department to obtain imaging studies of the c-spine. Similar to TBI, CDRs have been developed to guide clinicians in deciding who should undergo c-spine imaging. One of the widely accepted rules in clinical use is the NEXUS (National Emergency X-Radiography Utilization Study) criteria (Hoffman et al. 1998). The NEXUS rules have been shown to have a high sensitivity and specificity for the detection of serious fractures of the cervical spine in all age groups (Hoffman et al. 2000). Therefore, applying the NEXUS criteria on the sideline can help the sport clinician make an objective decision about the athlete's disposition (Table 18.3).

## Athletes who are not transferred to an emergency department

If the athlete is not transferred to an emergency department, he/she must be carefully observed for any worsening of signs or symptoms. To underscore the importance of frequent evaluations or continuous monitoring, it should be noted that for example, an EDH can appear to have a benign course initially. This condition usually results from a tear in the middle meningeal artery of the brain caused by a fracture to the temporal section of the skull. Classically, an athlete who has suffered an EDH post-head injury experiences a brief period of unconsciousness, followed by a period of lucidity. This period of lucidity can be falsely reassuring, as subsequent collapse and unconsciousness occurs 5–30 minutes later. An EDH is a neurosurgical emergency and the athlete would require a rapid surgical intervention to relieve the pressure on the brain by evacuating the compressing blood. With these worst-case scenarios in mind, the clinician should keep a high index of suspicion when dealing with a concussed athlete. For this reason, the concussed athlete must be monitored continuously or frequently reevaluated. Reevaluations should be done every 5 minutes for at least the first 15–30 minutes.

Once signs and symptoms have improved or stabilized with no evidence of worsening, the athlete can be sent home to rest. The first 24 hours after injury remain critical and observation at home should be continued. Therefore, the player should remain in the company of a responsible adult who can maintain the supervision and provide transport to medical attention if there are any signs of deterioration. Studies of head injured patients sent home from the emergency department in the care of others have shown that parents are the most likely to be compliant with discharge care and instructions (Cline and Whitley 1988). Discharge instructions must be clearly verbalized and, whenever possible, provided in a written format. The instructions should include the frequency of checks to be performed and which signs and symptoms to assess. There should also be clear instructions on whom to contact if there are doubts or concerns about any behaviors or symptoms. It should also be emphasized that excessive physical and/or cognitive activities can worsen symptoms and should be avoided as much as possible, until the athlete is reassessed at follow-up.

Follow-up care and evaluation by a qualified professional skilled in concussion assessment and management should occur the next day, or within a few days, to reassess the athlete and make further management decisions.

## *References*

American College of Sports, Medicine. 2004. Mass participation event management for the team physician: a consensus statement. *Med Sci Sports Exerc* 36 (11):2004–2008.

Andersen, J., R. W. Courson, D. M. Kleiner, and T. A. McLoda. 2002. National athletic trainers' association position statement: Emergency planning in athletics. *J Athl Train* 37 (1):99–104.

Aubry, M., R. Cantu, J. Dvorak, T. Graf-Baumann, K. M. Johnston, J. Kelly, M. Lovell et al. 2002. Summary and agreement statement of the 1st International Symposium on Concussion in Sport, Vienna 2001. *Clin J Sport Med* 12 (1):6–11.

Azad, A. M., S. Al Juma, J.A. Bhatti, and J. S. Delaney. 2016. Modified balance error scoring system (M-BESS) test scores in athletes wearing protective equipment and cleats. *BMJ Open Sport Exerc Med* 2 (1):e000117. doi:10.1136/bmjsem-2016-000117.

Bagley, A. F., D. H. Daneshvar, B. D. Schanker, D. Zurakowski, C. A. d'Hemecourt, C. J. Nowinski, R. C. Cantu, and K. Goulet. 2012. Effectiveness of the SLICE program for youth concussion education. *Clin J Sport Med* 22 (5):385–389. doi:10.1097/JSM.0b013e3182639bb4.

Baugh, C. M., E. Kroshus, A. P. Bourlas, and K. I. Perry. 2014. Requiring athletes to acknowledge receipt of concussion-related information and responsibility to report symptoms: a study of the prevalence, variation, and possible improvements. *J Law Med Ethics* 42 (3):297–313. doi:10.1111/jlme.12147.

Bramley, H., K. Patrick, E. Lehman, and M. Silvis. 2012. High school soccer players with concussion education are more likely to notify their coach of a suspected concussion. *Clin Pediatr (Phila)* 51 (4):332–336. doi:10.1177/0009922811425233.

Broglio, S. P., R. C. Cantu, G. A. Gioia, K. M. Guskiewicz, J. Kutcher, M. Palm, T. C. Valovich McLeod, and Association National Athletic Trainer's. 2014. National athletic trainers' association position statement: Management of sport concussion. *J Athl Train* 49 (2):245–265. doi:10.4085/1062-6050-49.1.07.

Broglio, S. P., S. N. Macciocchi, and M. S. Ferrara. 2007. Neurocognitive performance of concussed athletes when symptom free. *J Athl Train* 42 (4):504–508.

Broglio, S. P. and T. W. Puetz. 2008. The effect of sport concussion on neurocognitive function, self-report symptoms and postural control: A meta-analysis. *Sports Med* 38 (1):53–67.

Bruce, J., R. Echemendia, L. Tangeman, W. Meeuwisse, P. Comper, M. Hutchison, and M. Aubry. 2016. Two baselines are better than one: Improving the reliability of computerized testing in sports neuropsychology. *Appl Neuropsychol Adult* 23 (5): 336–342. doi:10.1080/23279095.2015.10 64002.

Bruce, J. M., R. J. Echemendia, W. Meeuwisse, M. G. Hutchison, M. Aubry, and P. Comper. 2017. Development of a risk prediction model among professional hockey players with visible signs of concussion. *Br J Sports Med*. doi:10.1136/bjsports-2016-097091.

Caron, J. G., G. A. Bloom, K. M. Johnston, and C. M. Sabiston. 2013. Effects of multiple concussions on retired national hockey league players. *J Sport Exerc Psychol* 35 (2):168–179.

Casa, D. J., K. M. Guskiewicz, S. A. Anderson, R. W. Courson, J. F. Heck, C. C. Jimenez, B. P. McDermott. et al. 2012. National athletic trainers' association position statement: Preventing sudden death in sports. *J Athl Train* 47 (1):96–118.

Chen, J. K., K. M. Johnston, A. Collie, P. McCrory, and A. Ptito. 2007. A validation of the post concussion symptom scale in the assessment of complex concussion using cognitive testing and functional MRI. *J Neurol Neurosurg Psychiatry* 78 (11):1231–1238. doi:10.1136/jnnp.2006.110395.

Cline, D. M. and T. W. Whitley. 1988. Observation of head trauma patients at home: A prospective study of compliance in the rural south. *Ann Emerg Med* 17 (2):127–131.

Collicott, P. E. and I. Hughes. 1980. Training in advanced trauma life support. *JAMA* 243 (11):1156–1159.

Collins, M. W., M. R. Lovell, G. L. Iverson, R. C. Cantu, J. C. Maroon, and M. Field. 2002. Cumulative effects of concussion in high school athletes. *Neurosurgery* 51 (5):1175–1179.

Covassin, T., R. J. Elbin, W. Harris, T. Parker, and A. Kontos. 2012. The role of age and sex in symptoms, neurocognitive performance, and postural stability in athletes after concussion. *Am J Sports Med* 40 (6):1303–1312. doi:10.1177/0363546512444554.

Davis, S. 2015. MLS to adopt new technology to curb concussions in soccer. Retrieved from http://worldsoccertalk.com/2015/01/15/mls-to-adopt-new-technology-to-curb-concussions-in-soccer/.

De Beaumont, L., H. Theoret, D. Mongeon, J. Messier, S. Leclerc, S. Tremblay, D. Ellemberg, and M. Lassonde. 2009. Brain function decline in healthy retired athletes who sustained their last sports concussion in early adulthood. *Brain* 132:695–708.

Delaney, J. S., F. Abuzeyad, J. A. Correa, and R. Foxford. 2005. Recognition and characteristics of concussions in the emergency department population. *J Emerg Med* 29 (2):189–197. doi:10.1016/j.jemermed.2005.01.020.

Delaney, J. S., A. Al-Kashmiri, P. J. Baylis, M. Aljufaili, and J. A. Correa. 2012. The effect of laryngoscope handle size on possible endotracheal intubation success in university football, ice hockey, and soccer players. *Clin J Sport Med* 22 (4):341–348. doi:10.1097/JSM.0b013e318257c9a8.

Delaney, J. S., A. Al-Kashmiri, P. J. Baylis, T. Troutman, M. Aljufaili, and J. A. Correa. 2011. The assessment of airway maneuvers and interventions in university Canadian football, ice hockey, and soccer players. *J Athl Train* 46 (2):117–125. doi:10.4085/1062-6050-46.2.117.

Delaney, J. S. and R. Drummond. 2002. Mass casualties and triage at a sporting event. *Br J Sports Med* 36 (2):85–88.

Delaney, J. S., V. J. Lacroix, S. Leclerc, and K. M. Johnston. 2000. Concussions during the 1997 Canadian football league season. *Clin J Sport Med* 10 (1):9–14.

Delaney, J. S., V. J. Lacroix, S. Leclerc, and K. M. Johnston. 2002. Concussions among university football and soccer players. *Clin J Sport Med* 12 (6):331–338.

Delaney, J. S., C. Lamfookon, G. A. Bloom, A. Al-Kashmiri, and J. A. Correa. 2015. Why university athletes choose not to reveal their concussion symptoms during a practice or game. *Clin J Sport Med* 25 (2):113–125. doi:10.1097/JSM.0000000000000112.

Delaney, J. S. and K. McDonald. Personal communication. Concussion Posters for Canadian Football League. April 27, 2016.

Dixon, R. 2011. Clarifying procedure in the NHL's concussion "quiet room". Last Modified May 26, 2011. Retrieved from http://www.thehockeynews.com/articles/40479-Inside-the-NHLs-concussion-quiet-room.html Accessed April 27, 2016.

Echemendia, R. J., J. M. Bruce, W. Meeuwisse, M. G. Hutchison, P. Comper, and M. Aubry. 2017a. Can visible signs predict concussion diagnosis in the National Hockey League? *Br J Sports Med.* doi:10.1136/bjsports-2016-097090.

Echemendia, R. J., S. Herring, and J. Bailes. 2009. Who should conduct and interpret the neuropsychological assessment in sports-related concussion? *Br J Sports Med* 43 Suppl 1:i32–i35. doi:10.1136/bjsm.2009.058164.

Echemendia, R. J., W. Meeuwisse, P. McCrory, G. A. Davis, M. Putukian, J. Leddy, M. Makdissi et al. 2017b. The sport concussion assessment tool 5th edition (SCAT5). *Br J Sports Med.* doi:10.1136/bjsports-2017-097506.

Echemendia, R. J., W. Meeuwisse, P. McCrory, G. A. Davis, M. Putukian, J. Leddy, M. Makdissi et al. 2017c. The concussion recognition tool 5th edition (CRT5). *Br J Sports Med.* doi:10.1136/bjsports-2017-097508.

Fazio, V. C., M. R. Lovell, J. E. Pardini, and M. W. Collins. 2007. The relation between post concussion symptoms and neurocognitive performance in concussed athletes. *NeuroRehabilitation* 22 (3):207–216.

Furman, G. R., C. C. Lin, J. L. Bellanca, G. F. Marchetti, M. W. Collins, and S. L. Whitney. 2013. Comparison of the balance accelerometer measure and balance error scoring system in adolescent concussions in sports. *Am J Sports Med* 41 (6):1404–1410. doi:10.1177/0363546513484446.

Gessel, L. M., S. K. Fields, C. L. Collins, R. W. Dick, and R. D. Comstock. 2007. Concussions among United States high school and collegiate athletes. *J Athl Train* 42 (4):495–503.

Giza, C. C., J. S. Kutcher, S. Ashwal, J. Barth, T. S. Getchius, G. A. Gioia, G. S. Gronseth et al. 2013. Summary of evidence-based guideline update: Evaluation and management of concussion in sports: Report of the guideline development subcommittee of the American academy of neurology. *Neurology* 80 (24):2250–2257. doi:10.1212/WNL.0b013e31828d57dd.

Glaviano, N. R., S. Benson, H. P. Goodkin, D. K. Broshek, and S. Saliba. 2015. Baseline SCAT2 assessment of healthy youth student-athletes: Preliminary evidence for the use of the child-SCAT3 in children younger than 13 years. *Clin J Sport Med*. 25 (4):373–379.

Goodman, D., N. L. Bradley, B. Paras, I. J. Williamson, and J. Bizzochi. 2006. Video gaming promotes concussion knowledge acquisition in youth hockey players. *J Adolesc* 29 (3):351–360. doi:10.1016/j.adolescence.2005.07.004.

Guskiewicz, K. M., J. Register-Mihalik, P. McCrory, M. McCrea, K. Johnston, M. Makdissi, J. Dvorak, G. Davis, and W. Meeuwisse. 2013. Evidence-based approach to revising the SCAT2: Introducing the SCAT3. *Br J Sports Med* 47 (5):289–293.

Guskiewicz, K. M., S. E. Ross, and S. W. Marshall. 2001. Postural stability and neuropsychological deficits after concussion in collegiate athletes. *J Athl Train* 36 (3):263–273.

Halstead, M. E., K. D. Walter, Medicine Council on Sports, and Fitness. 2010. American academy of pediatrics. Clinical report--sport-related concussion in children and adolescents. *Pediatrics* 126 (3):597–615. doi:10.1542/peds.2010-2005.

Harmon, K. G., J. A. Drezner, M. Gammons, K. M. Guskiewicz, M. Halstead, S. A. Herring, J. S. Kutcher, A. Pana, M. Putukian, and W. O. Roberts. 2013. American medical society for sports medicine position statement: Concussion in sport. *Br J Sports Med* 47 (1):15–26. doi:10.1136/bjsports-2012-091941.

Heyer, E. J., R. Sharma, C. J. Winfree, J. Mocco, D. J. McMahon, P. A. McCormick, D. O. Quest et al. 2000. Severe pain confounds neuropsychological test performance. *J Clin Exp Neuropsychol* 22 (5):633–639. doi:10.1076/1380-3395(200010)22:5;1-9;FT633.

Hoffman, J. R., W. R. Mower, A. B. Wolfson, K. H. Todd, and M. I. Zucker. 2000. Validity of a set of clinical criteria to rule out injury to the cervical spine in patients with blunt trauma. National emergency x-radiography utilization study group. *N Engl J Med* 343 (2):94–99. doi:10.1056/NEJM200007133430203.

Hoffman, J. R., A. B. Wolfson, K. Todd, and W. R. Mower. 1998. Selective cervical spine radiography in blunt trauma: Methodology of the national emergency x-radiography utilization study (NEXUS). *Ann Emerg Med* 32 (4):461–469.

Hunt, T. N., M. S. Ferrara, R. A. Bornstein, and T. A. Baumgartner. 2009. The reliability of the modified balance error scoring system. *Clin J Sport Med* 19 (6):471–475. doi:10.1097/JSM.0b013e3181c12c7b.

Kaut, K. P., R. DePompei, J. Kerr, and J. Congeni. 2003. Reports of head injury and symptom knowledge among college athletes: Implications for assessment and educational intervention. *Clin J Sport Med* 13 (4):213–221.

Kelly, J. P. and J. H. Rosenberg. 1997. Diagnosis and management of concussion in sports. *Neurology* 48 (3):575–580.

Kutcher, J. S. 2010. Management of the complicated sports concussion patient. *Sports Health* 2 (3):197–202. doi:10.1177/1941738109357305.

Lowrey, K. M. and S. R. Morain. 2014. State experiences implementing youth sports concussion laws: Challenges, successes, and lessons for evaluating impact. *J Law Med Ethics* 42 (3):290–296. doi:10.1111/jlme.12146.

Luke, A. and L. Micheli. 1999. Sports injuries: emergency assessment and field-side care. *Pediatr Rev* 20 (9):291–301.

Mackenzie, B., P. Vivier, S. Reinert, J. Machan, C. Kelley, and E. Jacobs. 2015. Impact of a state concussion law on pediatric emergency department visits. *Pediatr Emerg Care* 31 (1):25–30. doi:10.1097/PEC.0000000000000325.

Makdissi, M., G. Davis, and P. McCrory. 2014. Updated guidelines for the management of sports-related concussion in general practice. *Aust Fam Physician* 43 (3):94–99.

McCrea, M. 2001a. Standardized mental status assessment of sports concussion. *Clin J Sport Med* 11 (3):176–181.

McCrea, M. 2001b. Standardized mental status testing on the sideline after sport-related concussion. *J Athl Train* 36 (3):274–279.

McCrea, M., W. B. Barr, K. Guskiewicz, C. Randolph, S. W. Marshall, R. Cantu, J. A. Onate, and J. P. Kelly. 2005. Standard regression-based methods for measuring recovery after sport-related concussion. *J Int Neuropsychol Soc* 11 (1):58–69. doi:10.1017/S1355617705050083.

McCrea, M., K. M. Guskiewicz, S. W. Marshall, W. Barr, C. Randolph, R. C. Cantu, J. A. Onate, J. Yang, and J. P. Kelly. 2003. Acute effects and recovery time following concussion in collegiate football players: The NCAA concussion study. *JAMA* 290 (19):2556–2563. doi:10.1001/jama.290.19.2556.

McCrea, M., T. Hammeke, G. Olsen, P. Leo, and K. Guskiewicz. 2004. Unreported concussion in high school football players: Implications for prevention. *Clin J Sport Med* 14 (1):13–17.

McCrea, M., G. L. Iverson, R. J. Echemendia, M. Makdissi, and M. Raftery. 2013. Day of injury assessment of sport-related concussion. *Br J Sports Med* 47 (5):272–284. doi:10.1136/bjsports-2013-092145.

McCrory, P., K. Johnston, W. Meeuwisse, M. Aubry, R. Cantu, J. Dvorak, T. Graf-Baumann et al. 2005. Summary and agreement statement of the 2nd international conference on concussion in sport, Prague 2004. *Clin J Sport Med* 15 (2):48–55.

McCrory, P., W. Meeuwisse, M. Aubry, B. Cantu, J. Dvorak, R. J. Echemendia, L. Engebretsen et al. 2013a. Consensus statement on concussion in sport--the 4th international conference on concussion in sport held in Zurich, November 2012. *Clin J Sport Med* 23 (2):89–117. doi:10.1097/JSM.0b013e31828b67cf.

McCrory, P., W. Meeuwisse, J. Dvorak, M. Aubry, J. Bailes, S. Broglio, R. C. Cantu et al. 2017. Consensus statement on concussion in sport-the 5th international conference on concussion in sport held in Berlin, October 2016. *Br J Sports Med.* doi:10.1136/bjsports-2017-097699.

McCrory, P., W. H. Meeuwisse, R. J. Echemendia, G. L. Iverson, J. Dvorak, and J. S. Kutcher. 2013b. What is the lowest threshold to make a diagnosis of concussion? *Br J Sports Med* 47 (5):268–271. doi:10.1136/bjsports-2013-092247.

McCrory, P., W. Meeuwisse, K. Johnston, J. Dvorak, M. Aubry, M. Molloy, and R. Cantu. 2009. Consensus statement on concussion in sport 3rd international conference on concussion in sport held in Zurich, November 2008. *Clin J Sport Med* 19 (3):185–200. doi:10.1097/JSM.0b013e3181a501db.

McCrory, P. R. and S. F. Berkovic. 1998. Second impact syndrome. *Neurology* 50 (3):677–683.

Moriarty, O., B. E. McGuire, and D. P. Finn. 2011. The effect of pain on cognitive function: A review of clinical and preclinical research. *Prog Neurobiol* 93 (3):385–404. doi:10.1016/j.pneurobio.2011.01.002.

Mulligan, R. P., J. A. Friedman, and R. C. Mahabir. 2010. A nationwide review of the associations among cervical spine injuries, head injuries, and facial fractures. *J Trauma* 68 (3):587–592. doi:10.1097/TA.0b013e3181b16bc5.

Navarro, S., S. Montmany, P. Rebasa, C. Colilles, and A. Pallisera. 2014. Impact of ATLS training on preventable and potentially preventable deaths. *World J Surg* 38 (9):2273–2278. doi:10.1007/s00268-014-2587-y.

NFL Head, Neck and Spine Committee, and B Bradley. 2013. NFL's 2013 protocol for players with concussions. Last Modified August 22, 2014. Retrieved from http://www.nfl.com/news/story/0ap2000000253716/article/nfls-2013-protocol-for-players-with-concussions Accessed April 27, 2016.

Prevention, Centers for Disease Control and. 2015. Partnership spotlight: NFL. Last Modified February 16, 2015. Retrieved from http://www.cdc.gov/headsup/partners/nfl.html.

Ptito, A., J. K. Chen, and K. M. Johnston. 2007. Contributions of functional magnetic resonance imaging (fMRI) to sport concussion evaluation. *NeuroRehabilitation* 22 (3):217–227.

Randolph, C., M. McCrea, and W. B. Barr. 2005. Is neuropsychological testing useful in the management of sport-related concussion? *J Athl Train* 40 (3):139–152.

Riemann, B. L. and K. M. Guskiewicz. 2000. Effects of mild head injury on postural stability as measured through clinical balance testing. *J Athl Train* 35 (1):19–25.

Robinson, O. J., K. Vytal, B. R. Cornwell, and C. Grillon. 2013. The impact of anxiety upon cognition: Perspectives from human threat of shock studies. *Front Hum Neurosci* 7:203. doi:10.3389/fnhum.2013.00203.

Scorza, K. A., M. F. Raleigh, and F. G. O'Connor. 2012. Current concepts in concussion: Evaluation and management. *Am Fam Physician* 85 (2):123–132.

Seravalli, F. 2015. NHL to use concussion spotters at all games. Last Modified September 15, 2015. Retrieved from http://www.tsn.ca/nhl-to-use-concussion-spotters-at-all-games-this-season-1.360322 Accessed April 27, 2016.

Simma, B., J. Lutschg, and J. M. Callahan. 2013. Mild head injury in pediatrics: Algorithms for management in the ED and in young athletes. *Am J Emerg Med* 31 (7):1133–1138. doi:10.1016/j.ajem.2013.04.007.

Snyder, A. R., R. M. Bauer, and Impacts for Florida Network Health. 2014. A normative study of the sport concussion assessment tool (SCAT2) in children and adolescents. *Clin Neuropsychol* 28 (7):1091–1103. doi:10.1080/13854046.2014.952667.

Stiell, I. G., C. M. Clement, B. H. Rowe, M. J. Schull, R. Brison, D. Cass, M. A. Eisenhauer et al. 2005. Comparison of the Canadian CT head rule and the new orleans criteria in patients with minor head injury. *JAMA* 294 (12):1511–1518. doi:10.1001/jama.294.12.1511.

Stiell, I. G., H. Lesiuk, G. A. Wells, D. Coyle, R. D. McKnight, R. Brison, C. Clement et al. 2001a. Canadian CT head rule study for patients with minor head injury: Methodology for phase II (validation and economic analysis). *Ann Emerg Med* 38 (3):317–322. doi:10.1067/mem.2001.116795.

Stiell, I. G., H. Lesiuk, G. A. Wells, R. D. McKnight, R. Brison, C. Clement, M. A. Eisenhauer et al. 2001b. The Canadian CT head rule study for patients with minor head injury: Rationale, objectives, and methodology for phase I (derivation). *Ann Emerg Med* 38 (2):160–169. doi:10.1067/mem.2001.116796.

Stiell, I. G., G. A. Wells, K. Vandemheen, C. Clement, H. Lesiuk, A. Laupacis, R. D. McKnight et al. 2001c. The Canadian CT head rule for patients with minor head injury. *Lancet* 357 (9266):1391–1396.

Stiell, I. G., G. A. Wells, K. L. Vandemheen, C. M. Clement, H. Lesiuk, V. J. De Maio, A. Laupacis et al. 2001d. The Canadian C-spine rule for radiography in alert and stable trauma patients. *JAMA* 286 (15):1841–1848.

Sullivan, S. J., L. Bourne, S. Choie, B. Eastwood, S. Isbister, P. McCrory, and A. Gray. 2009. Understanding of sport concussion by the parents of young rugby players: A pilot study. *Clin J Sport Med* 19 (3):228–230. doi:10.1097/JSM.0b013e3181a41e43.

Tator, C. 2012. Sport Concussion education and Prevention. *J Clin Sport Psychol* 6:293–301.

Tysvaer, A. T. and O. V. Storli. 1989. Soccer injuries to the brain. A neurologic and electroencephalographic study of active football players. *Am J Sports Med* 17 (4):573–578.

Wagner-McGough, S. 2015. New NFL rule gives concussion spotters power to stop games. Last Modified August 9, 2015. Retrieved from http://www.cbssports.com/nfl/eye-on-football/25264465/new-nfl-rule-gives-concussion-spotters-power-to-stop-games_green Accessed April 27, 2016.

Walsh, D. P., G. R. Lammert, and J. Devoll. 1989. The effectiveness of the advanced trauma life support system in a mass casualty situation by non-trauma-experienced physicians: Grenada 1983. *J Emerg Med* 7 (2):175–180.

Warren, W. L. Jr. and J. E. Bailes. 1998. On the field evaluation of athletic neck injury. *Clin Sports Med* 17 (1):99–110.

Zimmer, A., J. Marcinak, S. Hibyan, and F. Webbe. 2014. Normative values of major SCAT2 and SCAT3 components for a college athlete population. *Appl Neuropsychol Adult*:1–9. doi:10.1080/23279095.2013.867265.

# chapter nineteen

# Emerging diagnosis technology
## What is coming up in terms of the use of biomarkers of concussion?

*Linda Papa*

## Contents

## Introduction

### Discovery of acute traumatic brain injury biomarkers

Discovery of biomarkers that are specific for traumatic brain injury (TBI) is a quest that has been ongoing for several decades. The pursuit of these elusive markers has been most intense over the last twenty years (Papa 2012, Papa et al. 2015a). Unlike other organ-based diseases in which rapid diagnosis employing biomarkers from blood tests are clinically essential to guide diagnosis and treatment, such as for myocardial ischemia or kidney and liver dysfunction, there are no rapid, definitive diagnostic tests for TBI. Currently, the selection of TBI biomarkers has been based on anatomic location such as axonal, neuronal (cell body, dendritic, synaptic), and astroglial areas of the brain, as well as on mechanisms of injury induced by trauma such as neuroinflammation and ischemia. Initial exploration of TBI biomarkers began using animal models which have been very helpful in providing histologic and pathophysiologic information on potential biomarkers. A number of promising biomarkers have since progressed to human trials. Initial human trials examined only severe TBI, and now, there is mounting research on milder injuries, including concussion (Papa 2016).

Although there are no validated biomarkers for concussion as yet, there is potential for biomarkers to provide diagnostic, prognostic, and monitoring information post-injury. Key features that would make a TBI biomarker clinically useful include (1) a high sensitivity (come from the brain) and specificity (low or undetectable in blood in noninjury states) for brain injury; (2) the ability to stratify patients by severity of injury (concentration of the biomarker should increase with worsening injury); (3) rapid appearance in accessible biological fluid such as serum, saliva, or urine; (4) a well-defined time course; (5) ability to monitor injury and response to treatment; (6) ability to predict functional outcome; and (7) easy measurement (Papa et al. 2008).

The release of substances and potential biomarkers after an injury is not a static process. Understanding the biokinetic and temporal profile of a biomarker is critical for understanding the release pattern and *optimum* time for measurement (Papa and Wang 2017). The temporal profile may be affected by factors such as: source of the sample (serum, CSF, and urine), lesion type (mass lesion versus diffuse injury), location of injury, presence of concomitant intracranial and extracranial injuries (fractures and solid organ injuries), and secondary insults (hypotension and hypoxia). For instance, contusions could demonstrate different kinetic parameters from subdural hematomas and, thus, may produce different quantities of a marker with different peaks and rates of decay. Secondary insults may also contribute to secondary elevations in a marker, altering its sensitivity and specificity at different time points. For markers measured in blood, the level of a biomarker may also reflect the extent of blood–brain barrier disruption. Furthermore, extracranial sources of the biomarker that may be present in serum may limit its specificity by creating false positives, thus compromising its clinical utility. For example, if a TBI biomarker is released into the serum from other traumatized tissues, then the level of the marker would not accurately reflect a brain injury. This would hamper its clinical value in the setting of polytrauma. Another possible situation in which false positive marker values could occur is in the presence of a preexisting disease state that may alter the metabolism or clearance of the marker, as with kidney or liver disease.

## Why brain injury biomarkers for mild TBI and concussion

Traditionally, TBI has been separated into three very broad categories: mild, moderate, and severe. The severity of TBI is initially based on the Glasgow Coma Scale (GCS) score which uses ocular, verbal, and motor responses to determine central nervous system impairment. A GCS score of less than 8 is considered severe; a GCS score of 9–12 is considered moderate; and a GCS score of 13–15 mild. The accuracy of the GCS score can be impeded by cerebral perfusion, intoxication from drugs or alcohol, sedative medications, and other distracting injuries. Therefore, this classification scheme fails to capture the spectrum of TBI and the different types of injuries associated with it. The presence of a severe TBI is usually evident on initial examination, but the severity of milder injury is more difficult to determine, particularly within the first few hours after injury when the neurological examination is of restricted value. Individuals who incur a mild TBI are acutely at risk for intracranial bleeding and diffuse axonal injury. Structural brain abnormalities from trauma can be detected using techniques such as computed tomography (CT) or standard magnetic resonance imaging (MRI).

CT is the standard imaging modality for assessing damage in TBI during the acute phase of injury. CT scan can detect macroscopic traumatic lesions such as skull fractures, intracranial hematomas, contusions, subarachnoid hemorrhages, and swelling. However, the more subtle injuries associated with mild TBI are often not demonstrated by this imaging modality. This discrepancy is evidenced by the lack of CT abnormalities in patients with cognitive, physical, and behavioral dysfunction following a mild TBI. Therefore, CT does not have sufficient sensitivity to detect damage incurred in mild TBI. This group of TBI patients represents the greatest challenge to accurate diagnosis and outcome prediction.

In light of the importance of timeliness, accuracy, and risk stratification in the diagnostic and treatment processes, serum biomarkers with reliable sensitivity and specificity would be welcomed tools. This is especially so in settings limited by acute care resources such as in rural settings and nonhospital environments such as the playing field, battlefield, and primary care practices.

A recent systematic review of biomarkers in sports concussion showed that there have been at least eleven different biomarkers assessed in athletes (Papa et al. 2015b). These include S100β, glial fibrillary acidic protein, neuron-specific enolase, tau, neurofilament, amyloid beta, and brain-derived neurotrophic factor. Some correlate with the number of hits to the head (soccer), acceleration/deceleration forces (jumps, collisions, and falls), post-concussive symptoms, trauma to the body versus the head, and dynamics of injury (Papa et al. 2015b). Some of these and other novel markers are discussed below.

## Biomarkers of astroglial injury

### S100β

S100β is expressed in astrocytes, and it helps to regulate intracellular levels of calcium. It is considered a marker of astrocyte injury or death. Of note, it can also be found in cells that are not neuronal such as adipocytes, chondrocytes, and melanoma cells, and therefore, it is not brain specific (Zimmer et al. 1995, Olsson et al. 2011). Despite this, S100β is one of the most extensively studied biomarkers for TBI (Papa et al. 2013, 2015b, Schulte et al. 2014). Elevated concentrations of S100β in serum have been associated with increased incidence of post-concussive symptoms, problems with cognition and traumatic abnormalities on MRI (Ingebrigtsen and Romner 1996, 1997, Waterloo et al. 1997, Ingebrigtsen et al. 1999, Heidari et al. 2015a). However, there are also a number of studies negating these findings (Bazarian et al. 2006, Lima et al. 2008, Metting et al. 2012, Dorminy et al. 2015). Because many of these results have been inconsistently reproduced, the clinical value of S100β in TBI, particularly mild TBI and concussion, is still controversial. A number of studies have found correlations between elevated serum levels of S100β and CT abnormalities in adults and children (Papa et al. 2013, Heidari et al. 2015b). Unfortunately, its utility in the setting of polytrauma remains controversial because it is also elevated in trauma patients with peripheral trauma who had no direct head trauma (Pelinka et al. 2004b, Papa et al. 2014, 2016b).

### Glial fibrillary acid protein

Glial fibrillary acidic protein (GFAP) is a protein found in astroglial skeleton of both white and gray brain matter. Trauma and disease-induced cellular damage in the brain are known to augment GFAP levels. Serum GFAP concentrations have been shown to increase with neurodegenerative disorders (Baydas et al. 2003, Mouser et al. 2006), stroke

(Herrmann et al. 2000, Foerch et al. 2006), and brain tumors (Tichy et al. 2016). GFAP has also been shown to correlate well with outcome following severe TBI (Missler et al. 1999, van Geel et al. 2002, Pelinka et al. 2004a, 2004b, Nylen et al. 2006, Vos et al. 2010, Mondello et al. 2011). Moreover, compared with S100β, GFAP appears to be much more brain specific in the setting of trauma (Pelinka et al. 2004a, Papa et al. 2012a, 2014, 2016b), and it is a particularly interesting brain-specific glial-derived biomarker for mild TBI and concussion, both in adults and children (Papa et al. 2012a, 2014, 2015d, 2016a, 2016b, Metting et al. 2012, Diaz-Arrastia et al. 2014, Welch et al. 2016).

Most recently, the temporal profile of GFAP was evaluated in a large cohort of 584 trauma patients seen at the emergency department. GFAP performed consistently over 7 days in identifying concussion and mild to moderate TBI, detecting traumatic intracranial lesions on head CT, and predicting neurosurgical intervention (Papa et al. 2016a). This study of the pathophysiological kinetics of GFAP renders a promising contender for clinical use for mild TBI and concussion diagnosis within a week of injury (Papa et al. 2016a). GFAP is released into serum following a mild TBI within an hour of injury and remains elevated for several days after (Papa et al. 2012a, 2014, 2016a).

Serum GFAP levels distinguish mild TBI patients from trauma patients without TBI and detect intracranial lesions on CT with a sensitivity of 94%–100% in children and 97%–100% in adults (Papa et al. 2012a, 2014, 2015d, 2016a, 2016b). Moreover, GFAP outperforms S100β in detecting CT lesions in the setting of multiple trauma when extracranial fractures are present (Papa et al. 2014, 2015d), and it also predicts the need for neurosurgical intervention in patients presenting with a GCS of 15 (Papa et al. 2012a, 2016a).

## Biomarkers of neuronal injury

### Neuron-specific enolase

Neuron specific enolase (NSE), an isozyme of the glycolytic enzyme enolase, is found in central and peripheral neuronal cell bodies. It increases in serum following cell injury (Skogseid et al. 1992) and has a biological half-life of about 48 hours. Notably, it is also present in erythrocytes and endocrine cells (Schmechel et al. 1978). NSE is passively released into the extracellular space only under pathological conditions during cell destruction. Several studies have been published examining serum NSE following mild TBI (Skogseid et al. 1992, Yamazaki et al. 1995, Ross et al. 1996, Ergun et al. 1998, Fridriksson et al. 2000). Many of these reports noted its limited utility as a marker of neuronal damage after trauma, but they used inadequate control groups. Early levels of NSE concentrations have been correlated with outcome in children, particularly those under 4 years of age (Varma et al. 2003, Bandyopadhyay et al. 2005, Berger et al. 2005, 2007). In the setting of diffuse axonal injury (DAI) in severe TBI, levels of NSE at 72 hours of injury have shown an association with unfavorable outcome (Chabok et al. 2012). One of the limitations of NSE is the occurrence of false positive results within hemolysis (Johnsson et al. 2000, Ramont et al. 2005).

### Ubiquitin C-terminal hydrolase

Another promising candidate biomarker for TBI currently under investigation is Ubiquitin C-terminal Hydrolase-L1 (UCH-L1). This protein is involved in the addition and removal of ubiquitin from proteins that are destined for metabolism (Tongaonkar et al. 2000, Gong and Leznik 2007). UCH-L1 was previously used as a histological marker for neurons because it is so copious (Jackson and Thompson 1981). Clinical studies performed in humans with severe TBI have established that the UCH-L1 protein is significantly elevated in human CSF and is detectable very early after injury (Siman et al. 2009, Papa et al. 2010, 2015c). Concentrations of UCH-L1 remain significantly elevated for at least 7 days post-injury (Papa et al. 2010, 2015c), and there is very good correlation between CSF and serum levels (Brophy et al. 2011). Serum UCH-L1 is also elevated in children with moderate and severe TBI (Berger et al. 2012). Most recently, UCH-L1 was detected in the serum of mild TBI patients within an hour of injury (Papa et al. 2012b, 2016a). Serum levels of UCH-L1 discriminated concussion patients from uninjured and nonhead injured trauma control patients that had orthopedic injuries or motor vehicle trauma without head injury (Papa et al. 2012b, 2016a). A handful of studies have shown serum UCH-L1 levels to be significantly higher in those with intracranial lesions on CT than those without lesions (Papa et al. 2012b, 2016a, Diaz-Arrastia et al. 2014, Welch et al. 2016) and to be much higher in those eventually requiring a neurosurgical intervention (Papa et al. 2012b, 2016a). The temporal profile of UCH-L1 was evaluated in a large cohort of emergency department trauma patients; UCH-L1 rose rapidly and peaked at 8 hours after injury and declined rapidly over 48 hours (Papa et al. 2016a). It appears to be a very early marker of mild TBI.

## Biomarkers of axonal injury

### Alpha-II spectrin breakdown products

Alpha-II spectrin is a 280 kDa protein that is an important structural component of the cortical membrane cytoskeleton and is plentiful in axons and presynaptic terminals (Riederer et al. 1986, Goodman et al. 1995). This compound serves as a substrate for calpain-2 and caspase-3 cysteine proteases (McGinn et al. 2009). These proteases (caspase-3 and calpain-2) cleave cytoskeletal αII-spectrin (Pike et al. 2004, Ringger et al. 2004) into spectrin breakdown products (SBDPs). These SBDPs have been reported in CSF from adults with severe TBI, and they have shown a significant relationship with severity of injury and clinical outcome (Papa et al. 2004, 2005, 2006, 2015c, Cardali and Maugeri 2006, Pineda et al. 2007, Brophy et al. 2009, Mondello et al. 2010). The time course of calpain-mediated SBDP150 and SBDP145 (markers of necrosis) differs from that of caspase-3 mediated SBDP120 (marker of apoptosis) and has been shown to correlate with severity of injury, CT scan findings, and outcome at 6 months post-injury (Brophy et al. 2009, Papa et al. 2015c). These findings were similar in children with moderate to severe TBI (Papa et al. 2005). More recently, serum levels of SBDP150 measured in mild TBI patients have shown a significant association with acute measures of injury severity, such as GCS score, intracranial injuries on CT, and neurosurgical intervention (Berger et al. 2012). In this study, serum SBDP150 levels were much higher in patients with concussion than other trauma patients who did not have a head injury (Papa et al. 2005).

### Tau protein

Tau is an intracellular, microtubule-associated protein that is amplified in axons and is involved with assembling axonal microtubule bundles and participating in anterograde axoplasmic transport (Teunissen et al. 2005). Tau lesions are apparently related to axonal disruption such as in trauma or hypoxia (Kosik and Finch 1987, Higuchi et al. 2002). After release, it is proteolytically cleaved at the N- and C-terminals. The C-Tau has been investigated as a potential biomarker of CNS injury. Initial elevated CSF C-Tau levels in severe TBI patients have been shown to predict elevations in intracranial pressure and to be associated with poor clinical outcome (Zemlan et al. 2002). In a study by Shaw et al., an elevated level of C-Tau was associated with a poor outcome at hospital discharge and with an increased chance of an intracranial injury on head CT (Shaw et al. 2002). However, these findings were not reproducible when C-Tau was measured in peripheral blood in mild TBI (Chatfield et al. 2002). Two additional studies showed that C-Tau was a poor predictor of CT lesions and a poor predictor of post-concussive syndrome (Bazarian et al. 2006, Ma et al. 2008).

Total tau (T-Tau) has also been found to be correlated with severity of injury in severe TBI (Sjogren et al. 2001, Franz et al. 2003, Ost et al. 2006, Marklund et al. 2009). Ost et al. (2006) found that T-Tau measured in CSF on days 2–3 discriminated between TBI and controls with normal pressure hydrocephalus and also between good and bad outcomes at one year per dichotomized GOS score. Unfortunately, T-Tau was not detected in serum at any time point during the study, only in the CSF. More recently, a study of professional hockey players showed that serum T-Tau outperformed S-100B and NSE in detecting concussion at 1 hour after injury, and that levels were significantly higher in post-concussion samples at all times compared with preseason levels (Shahim et al. 2014). T-Tau at 1 hour after concussion also correlated with the number of days it took for concussion symptoms to resolve. Accordingly, T-Tau remained significantly elevated at 144 hours in players with post-concussive symptoms (PCS) lasting more than 6 days versus players with PCS for less than 6 days (Shahim et al. 2014).

Phosphorylated-Tau (P-Tau) is also being examined following head trauma and may have some association with chronic encephalopathy, but further study is needed (Puvenna et al. 2016).

## Conclusion

Biomarkers measured through a simple blood test have the potential to (1) provide invaluable information about the management of acute mild TBI and concussion; (2) facilitate diagnosis and risk stratification of these patients; (3) offer timely information about the pathophysiology of injury to allow for monitoring and assessment of progression and recovery; (4) furnish major opportunities for drug target identification; and (5) guide the conduct of clinical research as surrogate outcome measures. As technology advances and integrates neuroproteomics, metabolomics, bioinformatics, genetics, and neuroimaging, characterization and validation of potential TBI biomarkers will occur more quickly. The development of a clinical tool to help health-care providers manage TBI patients more effectively and improve patient care is the ultimate goal.

## References

Bandyopadhyay, S., H. Hennes, M. H. Gorelick, R. G. Wells, and C. M. Walsh-Kelly. 2005. Serum neuron-specific enolase as a predictor of short-term outcome in children with closed traumatic brain injury. *Acad Emerg Med* 12 (8):732–738. doi:10.1197/j.aem.2005.02.017.

Baydas, G., V. S. Nedzvetskii, M. Tuzcu, A. Yasar, and S. V. Kirichenko. 2003. Increase of glial fibrillary acidic protein and S-100B in hippocampus and cortex of diabetic rats: Effects of vitamin E. *Eur J Pharmacol* 462 (1–3):67–71.

Bazarian, J. J., F. P. Zemlan, S. Mookerjee, and T. Stigbrand. 2006. Serum S-100B and cleaved-tau are poor predictors of long-term outcome after mild traumatic brain injury. *Brain Inj* 20 (7):759–765. doi:10.1080/02699050500488207.

Berger, R. P., P. D. Adelson, M. C. Pierce, T. Dulani, L. D. Cassidy, and P. M. Kochanek. 2005. Serum neuron-specific enolase, S100B, and myelin basic protein concentrations after inflicted and noninflicted traumatic brain injury in children. *J Neurosurg* 103 (1 Suppl):61–68. doi:10.3171/ped.2005.103.1.0061.

Berger, R. P., S. R. Beers, L. Papa, and M. Bell. 2012. Common data elements for pediatric traumatic brain injury: Recommendations from the biospecimens and biomarkers workgroup. *J Neurotrauma* 29 (4):672–677. doi:10.1089/neu.2011.1861.

Berger, R. P., S. R. Beers, R. Richichi, D. Wiesman, and P. D. Adelson. 2007. Serum biomarker concentrations and outcome after pediatric traumatic brain injury. *J Neurotrauma* 24 (12):1793–1801. doi:10.1089/neu.2007.0316.

Brophy, G. M., J. A. Pineda, L. Papa, S. B. Lewis, A. B. Valadka, H. J. Hannay, S. C. Heaton et al. 2009. alphaII-Spectrin breakdown product cerebrospinal fluid exposure metrics suggest differences in cellular injury mechanisms after severe traumatic brain injury. *Neurotrauma* 26 (4):471–479. doi:10.1089/neu.2008.0657.

Brophy, G., S. Mondello, L. Papa, S. Robicsek, A. Gabrielli, J. Tepas III, A. Buki, C. Robertson, F. C. Tortella, and K. K. Wang. 2011. Biokinetic analysis of ubiquitin C-terminal hydrolase-L1 (Uch-L1) in severe traumatic brain injury patient biofluids. *J Neurotrauma.* doi:10.1089/neu.2010.1564.

Cardali, S. and R. Maugeri. 2006. Detection of alphaII-spectrin and breakdown products in humans after severe traumatic brain injury. *J Neurosurg Sci* 50 (2):25–31.

Chabok, S. Y., A. D. Moghadam, Z. Saneei, F. G. Amlashi, E. K. Leili, and Z. M. Amiri. 2012. Neuron-specific enolase and S100BB as outcome predictors in severe diffuse axonal injury. *J Trauma Acute Care Surg* 72 (6):1654–1667. doi:10.1097/TA.0b013e318246887e.

Chatfield, D. A., F. P. Zemlan, D. J. Day, and D. K. Menon. 2002. Discordant temporal patterns of S100beta and cleaved tau protein elevation after head injury: A pilot study. *Br J Neurosurg* 16 (5):471–476.

Diaz-Arrastia, R., K. K. Wang, L. Papa, M. D. Sorani, J. K. Yue, A. M. Puccio, P. J. McMahon et al. 2014. Acute biomarkers of traumatic brain injury: Relationship between plasma levels of ubiquitin C-terminal hydrolase-L1 and glial fibrillary acidic protein. *J Neurotrauma* 31 (1):19–25. doi:10.1089/neu.2013.3040.

Dorminy, M., A. Hoogeveen, R. T. Tierney, M. Higgins, J. K. McDevitt, and J. Kretzschmar. 2015. Effect of soccer heading ball speed on S100B, sideline concussion assessments and head impact kinematics. *Brain Inj* 1–7. doi:10.3109/02699052.2015.1035324.

Ergun, R., U. Bostanci, G. Akdemir, E. Beskonakli, E. Kaptanoglu, F. Gursoy, and Y. Taskin. 1998. Prognostic value of serum neuron-specific enolase levels after head injury. *Neurol Res* 20 (5):418–420.

Foerch, C., I. Curdt, B. Yan, F. Dvorak, M. Hermans, J. Berkefeld, A. Raabe, T. Neumann-Haefelin, H. Steinmetz, and M. Sitzer. 2006. Serum glial fibrillary acidic protein as a biomarker for intracerebral haemorrhage in patients with acute stroke. *J Neurol Neurosurg Psychiatry* 77 (2):181–184. doi:10.1136/jnnp.2005.074823.

Franz, G., R. Beer, A. Kampfl, K. Engelhardt, E. Schmutzhard, H. Ulmer, and F. Deisenhammer. 2003. Amyloid beta 1-42 and tau in cerebrospinal fluid after severe traumatic brain injury. *Neurology* 60 (9):1457–1461.

Fridriksson, T., N. Kini, C. Walsh-Kelly, and H. Hennes. 2000. Serum neuron-specific enolase as a predictor of intracranial lesions in children with head trauma: A pilot study. *Acad Emerg Med* 7 (7):816–820.

Gong, B. and E. Leznik. 2007. The role of ubiquitin C-terminal hydrolase L1 in neurodegenerative disorders. *Drug News Perspect* 20 (6):365–370. doi:10.1358/dnp.2007.20.6.1138160.

Goodman, S. R., W. E. Zimmer, M. B. Clark, I. S. Zagon, J. E. Barker, and M. L. Bloom. 1995. Brain spectrin: Of mice and men. *Brain Res Bull* 36 (6):593–606.

Heidari, K., S. Asadollahi, M. Jamshidian, S. N. Abrishamchi, and M. Nouroozi. 2015a. Prediction of neuropsychological outcome after mild traumatic brain injury using clinical parameters, serum S100B protein and findings on computed tomography. *Brain Inj* 29 (1):33–40. doi:10.3109/02699052.2014.948068.

Heidari, K., A. Vafaee, A. M. Rastekenari, M. Taghizadeh, E. G. Shad, R. Eley, M. Sinnott, and S. Asadollahi. 2015b. S100B protein as a screening tool for computed tomography findings after mild traumatic brain injury: Systematic review and meta-analysis. *Brain Inj* 1–12. doi:10.3109/02699052.2015.1037349.

Herrmann, M., P. Vos, M. T. Wunderlich, C. H. de Bruijn, and K. J. Lamers. 2000. Release of glial tissue-specific proteins after acute stroke: A comparative analysis of serum concentrations of protein S-100B and glial fibrillary acidic protein. *Stroke* 31 (11):2670–2677.

Higuchi, M., V. M. Lee, and J. Q. Trojanowski. 2002. Tau and axonopathy in neurodegenerative disorders. *Neuromolecular Med* 2 (2):131–150.

Ingebrigtsen, T. and B. Romner. 1996. Serial S-100 protein serum measurements related to early magnetic resonance imaging after minor head injury. Case report. *J Neurosurg* 85 (5):945–948.

Ingebrigtsen, T. and B. Romner. 1997. Management of minor head injuries in hospitals in Norway. *Acta Neurol Scand* 95 (1):51–55.

Ingebrigtsen, T., K. Waterloo, E. A. Jacobsen, B. Langbakk, and B. Romner. 1999. Traumatic brain damage in minor head injury: Relation of serum S-100 protein measurements to magnetic resonance imaging and neurobehavioral outcome. *Neurosurgery* 45 (3):468–475.

Jackson, P. and R. J. Thompson. 1981. The demonstration of new human brain-specific proteins by high-resolution two-dimensional polyacrylamide gel electrophoresis. *J Neurol Sci* 49 (3):429–438.

Johnsson, P., S. Blomquist, C. Luhrs, G. Malmkvist, C. Alling, J. O. Solem, and E. Stahl. 2000. Neuron-specific enolase increases in plasma during and immediately after extracorporeal circulation. *Ann Thorac Surg* 69 (3):750–754.

Kosik, K. S. and E. A. Finch. 1987. MAP2 and tau segregate into dendritic and axonal domains after the elaboration of morphologically distinct neurites: An immunocytochemical study of cultured rat cerebrum. *J Neurosci* 7 (10):3142–3153.

Lima, D. P., C. Simao Filho, C. Abib Sde, and L. F. de Figueiredo. 2008. Quality of life and neuropsychological changes in mild head trauma. Late analysis and correlation with S100B protein and cranial CT scan performed at hospital admission. *Injury* 39 (5):604–611. doi:10.1016/j.injury.2007.11.008.

Ma, M., C. J. Lindsell, C. M. Rosenberry, G. J. Shaw, and F. P. Zemlan. 2008. Serum cleaved tau does not predict postconcussion syndrome after mild traumatic brain injury. *Am J Emerg Med* 26 (7):763–768. doi:10.1016/j.ajem.2007.10.029.

Marklund, N., K. Blennow, H. Zetterberg, E. Ronne-Engstrom, P. Enblad, and L. Hillered. 2009. Monitoring of brain interstitial total tau and beta amyloid proteins by microdialysis in patients with traumatic brain injury. *J Neurosurg* 110 (6):1227–1237. doi:10.3171/2008.9.JNS08584.

McGinn, M. J., B. J. Kelley, L. Akinyi, M. W. Oli, M. C. Liu, R. L. Hayes, K. K. Wang, and J. T. Povlishock. 2009. Biochemical, structural, and biomarker evidence for calpain-mediated cytoskeletal change after diffuse brain injury uncomplicated by contusion. *J Neuropathol Exp Neurol* 68 (3):241–249. doi:10.1097/NEN.0b013e3181996bfe.

Metting, Z., N. Wilczak, L. A. Rodiger, J. M. Schaaf, and J. van der Naalt. 2012. GFAP and S100B in the acute phase of mild traumatic brain injury. *Neurology* 78 (18):1428–1433. doi:10.1212/WNL.0b013e318253d5c7.

Missler, U., M. Wiesmann, G. Wittmann, O. Magerkurth, and H. Hagenstrom. 1999. Measurement of glial fibrillary acidic protein in human blood: Analytical method and preliminary clinical results. *Clin Chem* 45 (1):138–141.

Mondello, S., L. Papa, A. Buki, R. Bullock, E. Czeiter, F. Tortella, K. K. Wang, and R. L. Hayes. 2011. Neuronal and glial markers are differently associated with computed tomography findings and outcome in patients with severe traumatic brain injury: A case control study. *Crit Care* 15 (3):R156. doi:10.1186/cc10286.

Mondello, S., S. A. Robicsek, A. Gabrielli, G. M. Brophy, L. Papa, J. Tepas, C. Robertson et al. 2010. alphaII-spectrin breakdown products (SBDPs): Diagnosis and outcome in severe traumatic brain injury patients. *J Neurotrauma* 27 (7):1203–1213. doi:10.1089/neu.2010.1278.

Mouser, P. E., E. Head, K. H. Ha, and T. T. Rohn. 2006. Caspase-mediated cleavage of glial fibrillary acidic protein within degenerating astrocytes of the Alzheimer's disease brain. *Am J Pathol* 168 (3):936–946. doi:10.2353/ajpath.2006.050798.

Nylen, K., M. Ost, L. Z. Csajbok, I. Nilsson, K. Blennow, B. Nellgard, and L. Rosengren. 2006. Increased serum-GFAP in patients with severe traumatic brain injury is related to outcome. *J Neurol Sci* 240 (1–2):85–91. doi:10.1016/j.jns.2005.09.007.

Olsson, B., H. Zetterberg, H. Hampel, and K. Blennow. 2011. Biomarker-based dissection of neurodegenerative diseases. *Prog Neurobiol* 95 (4):520–534. doi:10.1016/j.pneurobio.2011.04.006.

Ost, M., K. Nylen, L. Csajbok, A. O. Ohrfelt, M. Tullberg, C. Wikkelso, P. Nellgard, L. Rosengren, K. Blennow, and B. Nellgard. 2006. Initial CSF total tau correlates with 1-year outcome in patients with traumatic brain injury. *Neurology* 67 (9):1600–1604. doi:10.1212/01.wnl.0000242732.06714.0f.

Papa, L. 2012. Exploring the role of biomarkers for the diagnosis and management of traumatic brain injury patients. In T. K. Man and R. J. Flores (Eds.) *Poteomics—Human Diseases and Protein Functions*. In Tech Open Access Publisher, Rijeka, Croatia.

Papa, L. 2016. Potential blood-based biomarkers for concussion. *Sports Med Arthrosc* 24 (3):108–115.

Papa, L., L. Akinyi, M. C. Liu, J. A. Pineda, J. J. Tepas III, M. W. Oli, W. Zheng et al. 2010. Ubiquitin C-terminal hydrolase is a novel biomarker in humans for severe traumatic brain injury. *Crit Care Med* 38 (1):138–144. doi:10.1097/CCM.0b013e3181b788ab.

Papa, L., G. M. Brophy, R. D. Welch, L. M. Lewis, C. F. Braga, C. N. Tan, N. J. Ameli et al. 2016a. Time course and diagnostic accuracy of glial and neuronal blood biomarkers GFAP and UCH-L1 in a large cohort of trauma patients with and without mild traumatic brain injury. *JAMA Neurol* 73 (5):551–560. doi:10.1001/jamaneurol.2016.0039.

Papa, L., D. D'Avella, M. Aguennouz, F. F. Angileri, O. de Divitiis, A. Germano, A. Toscano et al. 2004. Detection of alpha-II spectrin and breakdown products in humans after severe traumatic brain injury [abstract]. *Acad Emerg Med* 11 (5):515.

Papa, L., D. Edwards, and M. Ramia. 2015a. Exploring serum biomarkers for mild traumatic brain injury. *Brain Neurotrauma: Molecular, Neuropsychological, and Rehabilitation Aspects*. Boca Raton, FL: CRC Press/Taylor & Francis Group.

Papa, L., L. M. Lewis, J. L. Falk, Z. Zhang, S. Silvestri, P. Giordano, G. M. Brophy et al. 2012a. Elevated levels of serum glial fibrillary acidic protein breakdown products in mild and moderate traumatic brain injury are associated with intracranial lesions and neurosurgical intervention. *Ann Emerg Med* 59 (6):471–483. doi:10.1016/j.annemergmed.2011.08.021.

Papa, L., L. M. Lewis, S. Silvestri, J. L. Falk, P. Giordano, G. M. Brophy, J. A. Demery et al. 2012b. Serum levels of ubiquitin C-terminal hydrolase distinguish mild traumatic brain injury from trauma controls and are elevated in mild and moderate traumatic brain injury patients with intracranial lesions and neurosurgical intervention. *J Trauma Acute Care Surg* 72 (5):1335–1344. doi:10.1097/TA.0b013e3182491e3d.

Papa, L., S. B. Lewis, S. Heaton, J. A. Demery, J. J. Tepas III, K. K. W. Wang, C. S. Robertson, and R. L. Hayes. 2006. Predicting early outcome using alpha-II spectrin breakdown products in human CSF after severe traumatic brain injury [abstract]. *Acad Emerg Med* 13 (5):S39–S40.

Papa, L., M. K. Mittal, J. Ramirez, M. Ramia, S. Kirby, S. Silvestri, P. Giordano et al. 2016b. In children and youth with mild and moderate traumatic brain injury, glial fibrillary acidic protein out-performs S100beta in detecting traumatic intracranial lesions on computed tomography. *J Neurotrauma* 33 (1):58–64. doi:10.1089/neu.2015.3869.

Papa, L., J. Pineda, K. K. W. Wang, S. B. Lewis, J. A. Demery, S. Heaton, J. J. Tepas III, and R. L. Hayes. 2005. Levels of alpha-II spectrin breakdown products in human CSF and outcome after severe traumatic brain injury [abstract]. *Acad Emerg Med* 12 (5 (Suppl 1)):139–140.

Papa, L., M. M. Ramia, D. Edwards, B. D. Johnson, and S. M. Slobounov. 2015b. Systematic review of clinical studies examining biomarkers of brain injury in athletes after sports-related concussion. *J Neurotrauma* 32 (10):661–673. doi:10.1089/neu.2014.3655.

Papa, L., M. M. Ramia, J. M. Kelly, S. S. Burks, A. Pawlowicz, and R. P. Berger. 2013. Systematic review of clinical research on biomarkers for pediatric traumatic brain injury. *J Neurotrauma* 30 (5):324–338. doi:10.1089/neu.2012.2545.

Papa, L., C. S. Robertson, K. K. Wang, G. M. Brophy, H. J. Hannay, S. Heaton, I. Schmalfuss, A. Gabrielli, R. L. Hayes, and S. A. Robicsek. 2015c. Biomarkers improve clinical outcome predictors of mortality following non-penetrating severe traumatic brain injury. *Neurocrit Care* 22 (1):52–64. doi:10.1007/s12028-014-0028-2.

Papa, L., G. Robinson, M. Oli, J. Pineda, J. Demery, G. Brophy, S. A. Robicsek et al. 2008. Use of bio-markers for diagnosis and management of traumatic brain injury patients. *Expert Opinion on Medical Diagnostics* 2 (8):937–945.

Papa, L., S. Silvestri, G. M. Brophy, P. Giordano, J. L. Falk, C. F. Braga, C. N. Tan et al. 2014. GFAP out-performs S100beta in detecting traumatic intracranial lesions on computed tomography in trauma patients with mild traumatic brain injury and those with extracranial lesions. *J Neurotrauma* 31 (22):1815–1822. doi:10.1089/neu.2013.3245.

Papa, L. and K. K. W. Wang. 2017. Raising the bar for traumatic brain injury biomarker research: Methods make a difference. *J Neurotrauma* 34 (13):2187–2189

Papa, L., M. R. Zonfrillo, J. Ramirez, S. Silvestri, P. Giordano, C. F. Braga, C. N. Tan, N. J. Ameli, M. Lopez, and M. K. Mittal. 2015d. Performance of glial fibrillary acidic protein in detecting traumatic intracranial lesions on computed tomography in children and youth with mild head trauma. *Acad Emerg Med* 22 (11):1274–1282. doi:10.1111/acem.12795.

Pelinka, L. E., A. Kroepfl, M. Leixnering, W. Buchinger, A. Raabe, and H. Redl. 2004a. GFAP ver-sus S100B in serum after traumatic brain injury: Relationship to brain damage and outcome. *J Neurotrauma* 21 (11):1553–1561. doi:10.1089/neu.2004.21.1553.

Pelinka, L. E., A. Kroepfl, R. Schmidhammer, M. Krenn, W. Buchinger, H. Redl, and A. Raabe. 2004b. Glial fibrillary acidic protein in serum after traumatic brain injury and multiple trauma. *J Trauma* 57 (5):1006–1012.

Pike, B. R., J. Flint, J. R. Dave, X. C. Lu, K. K. Wang, F. C. Tortella, and R. L. Hayes. 2004. Accumulation of calpain and caspase-3 proteolytic fragments of brain-derived alphaII-spectrin in cerebral spinal fluid after middle cerebral artery occlusion in rats. *J Cereb Blood Flow Metab* 24 (1):98–106.

Pineda, J. A., S. B. Lewis, A. B. Valadka, L. Papa, H. J. Hannay, S. C. Heaton, J. A. Demery et al. 2007. Clinical significance of alphaII-spectrin breakdown products in cerebrospinal fluid after severe traumatic brain injury. *J Neurotrauma* 24 (2):354–366.

Puvenna, V., M. Engeler, M. Banjara, C. Brennan, P. Schreiber, A. Dadas, A. Bahrami et al. 2016. Is phosphorylated tau unique to chronic traumatic encephalopathy? Phosphorylated tau in epileptic brain and chronic traumatic encephalopathy. *Brain Res* 1630:225–240. doi:10.1016/j.brainres.2015.11.007.

Ramont, L., H. Thoannes, A. Volondat, F. Chastang, M. C. Millet, and F. X. Maquart. 2005. Effects of hemolysis and storage condition on neuron-specific enolase (NSE) in cerebrospinal fluid and serum: Implications in clinical practice. *Clin Chem Lab Med* 43 (11):1215–1217. doi:10.1515/CCLM.2005.210.

Riederer, B. M., I. S. Zagon, and S. R. Goodman. 1986. Brain spectrin(240/235) and brain spectrin(240/235E): Two distinct spectrin subtypes with different locations within mamma-lian neural cells. *J Cell Biol* 102 (6):2088–2097.

Ringger, N. C., B. E. O'Steen, J. G. Brabham, X. Silver, J. Pineda, K. K. Wang, R. L. Hayes, and L. Papa. 2004. A novel marker for traumatic brain injury: CSF alphaII-spectrin breakdown product levels. *J Neurotrauma* 21 (10):1443–1456.

Ross, S. A., R. T. Cunningham, C. F. Johnston, and B. J. Rowlands. 1996. Neuron-specific enolase as an aid to outcome prediction in head injury. *Br J Neurosurg* 10 (5):471–476.

Schmechel, D., P. J. Marangos, and M. Brightman. 1978. Neurone-specific enolase is a molecular marker for peripheral and central neuroendocrine cells. *Nature* 276 (5690):834–836.

Schulte, S., L. W. Podlog, J. J. Hamson-Utley, F. G. Strathmann, and H. K. Struder. 2014. A systematic review of the biomarker S100B: Implications for sport-related concussion management. *J Athl Train* 49 (6):830–850. doi:10.4085/1062-6050-49.3.33.

Shahim, P., Y. Tegner, D. H. Wilson, J. Randall, T. Skillback, D. Pazooki, B. Kallberg, K. Blennow, and H. Zetterberg. 2014. Blood biomarkers for brain injury in concussed professional ice hockey players. *JAMA Neurol* 71 (6):684–692. doi:10.1001/jamaneurol.2014.367.

Shaw, G. J., E. C. Jauch, and F. P. Zemlan. 2002. Serum cleaved tau protein levels and clinical outcome in adult patients with closed head injury. *Ann Emerg Med* 39 (3):254–257.

Siman, R., N. Toraskar, A. Dang, E. McNeil, M. McGarvey, J. Plaum, E. Maloney, and M. S. Grady. 2009. A panel of neuron-enriched proteins as markers for traumatic brain injury in humans. *J Neurotrauma* 26 (11):1867–1877. doi:10.1089/neu.2009.0882.

Sjogren, M., M. Blomberg, M. Jonsson, L. O. Wahlund, A. Edman, K. Lind, L. Rosengren, K. Blennow, and A. Wallin. 2001. Neurofilament protein in cerebrospinal fluid: A marker of white matter changes. *J Neurosci Res* 66 (3):510–516. doi:10.1002/jnr.1242.

Skogseid, I. M., H. K. Nordby, P. Urdal, E. Paus, and F. Lilleaas. 1992. Increased serum creatine kinase BB and neuron specific enolase following head injury indicates brain damage. *Acta Neurochir (Wien)* 115 (3–4):106–111.

Teunissen, C. E., C. Dijkstra, and C. Polman. 2005. Biological markers in CSF and blood for axonal degeneration in multiple sclerosis. *Lancet Neurol* 4 (1):32–41. doi:10.1016/S1474-4422(04)00964-0.

Tichy, J., S. Spechtmeyer, M. Mittelbronn, E. Hattingen, J. Rieger, C. Senft, and C. Foerch. 2016. Prospective evaluation of serum glial fibrillary acidic protein (GFAP) as a diagnostic marker for glioblastoma. *J Neurooncol* 126 (2):361–369. doi:10.1007/s11060-015-1978-8.

Tongaonkar, P., L. Chen, D. Lambertson, B. Ko, and K. Madura. 2000. Evidence for an interaction between ubiquitin-conjugating enzymes and the 26S proteasome. *Mol Cell Biol* 20 (13):4691–4698.

van Geel, W. J., H. P. de Reus, H. Nijzing, M. M. Verbeek, P. E. Vos, and K. J. Lamers. 2002. Measurement of glial fibrillary acidic protein in blood: An analytical method. *Clin Chim Acta* 326 (1–2):151–154.

Varma, S., K. L. Janesko, S. R. Wisniewski, H. Bayir, P. D. Adelson, N. J. Thomas, and P. M. Kochanek. 2003. F2-isoprostane and neuron-specific enolase in cerebrospinal fluid after severe traumatic brain injury in infants and children. *J Neurotrauma* 20 (8):781–786. doi:10.1089/089771503767870005.

Vos, P. E., B. Jacobs, T. M. Andriessen, K. J. Lamers, G. F. Borm, T. Beems, M. Edwards, C. F. Rosmalen, and J. L. Vissers. 2010. GFAP and S100B are biomarkers of traumatic brain injury: An observational cohort study. *Neurology* 75 (20):1786–1793. doi:10.1212/WNL.0b013e3181fd62d2.

Waterloo, K., T. Ingebrigtsen, and B. Romner. 1997. Neuropsychological function in patients with increased serum levels of protein S-100 after minor head injury. *Acta Neurochir (Wien)* 139 (1):26–31.

Welch, R. D., S. I. Ayaz, L. M. Lewis, J. Unden, J. Y. Chen, V. H. Mika, B. Saville et al. 2016. Ability of serum glial fibrillary acidic protein, ubiquitin c-terminal hydrolase-L1, and S100B to differentiate normal and abnormal head computed tomography findings in patients with suspected mild or moderate traumatic brain injury. *J Neurotrauma* 33 (2):203–214. doi:10.1089/neu.2015.4149.

Yamazaki, Y., K. Yada, S. Morii, T. Kitahara, and T. Ohwada. 1995. Diagnostic significance of serum neuron-specific enolase and myelin basic protein assay in patients with acute head injury. *Surg Neurol* 43 (3):267–270.

Zemlan, F. P., E. C. Jauch, J. J. Mulchahey, S. P. Gabbita, W. S. Rosenberg, S. G. Speciale, and M. Zuccarello. 2002. C-tau biomarker of neuronal damage in severe brain injured patients: Association with elevated intracranial pressure and clinical outcome. *Brain Res* 947 (1):131–139.

Zimmer, D. B., E. H. Cornwall, A. Landar, and W. Song. 1995. The S100 protein family: History, function, and expression. *Brain Res Bull* 37 (4):417–429.

*chapter twenty*

---

# Emerging diagnosis technology
## What is coming up in terms of the use of imaging technology in concussion care?

*Rajeet Singh Saluja\*, Scott A. Holmes\*,*
*Jen-Kai Chen, and Guido Guberman*

## Contents

---

\* Rajeet Singh Saluja and Scott A. Holmes are co-first authors.

## Introduction

Brain imaging is a field that has progressed dramatically since one of the first attempts to look past the human skull of a living person using X-rays back in 1896 (Daniel 1896). Though this attempt was not successful, it represented the forward thinking and progressive attitude that has allowed for the continued development of new techniques with greater resolution. Since this time, the advent of new approaches has enabled novel insights into the brain, a greater understanding of how diseases of the brain function, and how the brain performs in the diseased state.

Concussions present a unique challenge for neuroimaging researchers. Though severe forms of brain injury are often accompanied by large alterations to the structure of the brain due to hemorrhage, skull fracture, or swelling, concussions are routinely devoid of such overt structural alterations. Rather, a concussion has been considered to have an impact predominantly on brain function. Indeed, evidence of functional alterations is abundant, as is demonstrated in both resting and active states of the brain. However, with the use of neuroimaging, techniques that specifically evaluate brain structure such as diffusion-weighted imaging (DWI) have shown possible differences between concussed patients and controls. Moreover, research has shown that metabolic alterations are present in persons with an mTBI that can be detected using techniques such as positron emission tomography and magnetic resonance spectroscopy. The modern application of these techniques has been to determine if they are sensitive to differences between patients with a concussion and those in a healthy state. Therefore, they have not yet reached the level of diagnostics. However, in recent years their use in supplementing clinical diagnostics alongside the rise of techniques such as machine learning has demonstrated the capacity for neuroimaging to play a dominant role in the diagnostic stage of concussions.

In Chapters 5 and 7, acute guidelines are presented for the use of CT scans to help rule out more severe forms of neurological injury and inform a clinician's diagnosis. The current chapter is intended to provide an introduction to, as well as a brief overview of the promising neuroimaging-based tools that have the capacity to differentiate mTBI from healthy subjects. This chapter ends with a discussion on how neuroimaging techniques may be used to supplement traditional diagnostic methods, and perhaps adopt a more formal role as a diagnostic marker for concussion. A summary of each technique is presented at the end of this chapter.

## Structural neuroimaging

Evaluating the presence of a concussion based on structural neuroimaging has been a long-standing focus of researchers and clinicians. Reporting of symptoms by the patient will at times contrast with absent findings using existing techniques such as CT, causing researchers to pursue advanced forms of existing technologies, and to develop new methods that evaluate different parts of the human brain. The following provides an overview of emerging methods in structural neuroimaging that are being pursued for the diagnosis of concussions.

### Diffusion-weighted imaging

DWI is an umbrella term that refers to all magnetic resonance imaging (MRI) techniques that measure water diffusion. The basic principle of DWI is to measure the diffusion of water molecules inside the brain (Mori and Zhang 2006) and determine whether water molecules are diffusing in an evenly-spread (*isotropic* diffusion) or in a directionally-skewed way (*anisotropic* diffusion). With their capacity to assess white matter integrity, DWI modalities can be used in the context of diffuse axonal injury, which would be otherwise undetectable by conventionally used MRI and CT methods (Shenton et al. 2012, Sundman et al. 2015).

One method of DWI is called diffusion tensor imaging (DTI), which consists of mapping the diffusion measurements in several directions using particular mathematic techniques to evaluate the directional selectivity of water diffusion (Basser et al. 1994). In the most comprehensive review of this method to date, Hulkower et al. (2013) reviewed 100 DTI studies, 30 of which focused specifically on mTBI. Overall, the majority of studies reported decreased fractional anisotropy (FA) as a result of mTBI with authors concluding that DTI can effectively be used to detect TBI, irrespective of severity. However, this finding is not uniform. In a meta-analysis of 15 DTI studies, Aoki et al. (2012) reported decreased FA ratios and increased mean diffusivity (MD) suggestive of microstructural damage to the white matter preventing diffusion of water along axons. Alternatively, research has reported increased FA ratios and decreased MD in mTBI, interpreted as axonal swelling (Cubon et al. 2011, Honce et al. 2016, Kraus et al. 2007, Kumar et al. 2009, Lipton et al. 2008, Messe et al. 2011, Niogi et al. 2008, Rutgers et al. 2008a, 2008b). Meanwhile, other papers reported mixed or no difference between DTI findings of mTBI subjects as compared to controls (Bazarian et al. 2007, Borich et al. 2013, Henry et al. 2010, Ling et al. 2012, Wilde et al. 2008). As such, although the general trend in the literature points toward decreased FA values as a result of concussion, there continues to be contentious findings that need to be resolved.

*Tractography* refers to the reconstruction of white matter tracts from the eigenvalues and eigenvectors recorded from diffusion tensor imaging data (Figure 20.1); it is capable of reconstructing white matter tracts such as the cingulum, uncinate fasciculus, and anterior commissure (Catani et al. 2002). As such, DTI enables analyses on specific white matter tracts and correlating within-tract DTI parameters to specific functional

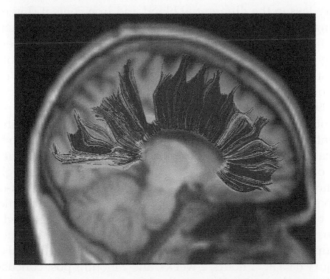

*Figure 20.1* White matter tracks eminating from the corpus callosum using difussion tensor imaging (DTI) superimposed on a standard T1 image. These tracks were generated using a region of interest extending from the genu to the splenium of the corpus callosum.

outcomes. For example, in a recent study by Goswami and colleagues (2016), subject-reported levels of impulsivity and aggression resulting from repeated concussions were associated with structural changes in the Uncinate Fasciculus (2016). Other research has shown that damage to white matter tracts including the arcuate fasciculus, inferior longitudinal fasciculus segments of the corpus callosum, and the fronto-occipital longitudinal fasciculi were associated with mood disorders after TBI (Spitz et al. 2016). Critically, the interpretation of such investigations is contingent upon accurate tract identification.

The presence of within-voxel directional hetereogeneity of white matter fibers presents a particular limitation to this technique (Le Bihan et al. 2006, Tuch 2004). That is, within any voxel, there exists a large number of neurons that point in nonuniform directions which, in DTI, are averaged out and lead to a loss of resolution. High definition fiber tracking (HDFT) attempts to reduce this limitation via the use of diffuse spectrum imaging, enhanced algorithms for imaging analysis, and increases the directional sensitivity of tractography-based analyses (Alexander and Barker 2005, Berman et al. 2013) to increase fiber resolution. While this technique has shown promise in the context of severe TBI (Presson et al. 2015), studies in the context of mTBI are still pending.

Together, data from DWI modalities have shown that in patients with mTBI, these imaging techniques have the capacity to identify differences between patients and controls, with data mainly reflecting damage to white matter structures of the brain. Although some studies find conflicting results (Ilvesmaki et al. 2014), the emerging consensus suggests that DTI is a promising tool for the assessment of mTBI (Hulkower et al. 2013). For most recent/comprehensive review (Hulkower et al. 2013.)

## Susceptibility weighted imaging

Different brain tissues have different magnetic susceptibilities (i.e., the degree to which the tissue is magnetized in a magnetic field) than its surrounding structures, which translate into differential phase shifts in MRI data (Haacke et al. 2004). A major source of tissue magnetic susceptibility lays in the differential blood and iron content (Liu et al. 2015), which makes this imaging technique particularly sensitive to cerebral micro-hemorrhages due to the paramagnetic nature of blood breakdown products such as hemosiderin. Susceptibility weighted imaging (SWI) takes advantage of this property as a source of contrast in MRI. Using this contrast method, SWI significantly increases the sensitivity of the sequence to detect micro-hemorrhages (Helmer et al. 2014).

Park et al. (2009) reported SWI findings on 21 mTBI patients without parenchymal hemorrhage on conventional MRI. Three quarters of these patients had positive hemorrhaging on SWI. Participants with evidence of micro-hemorrhages were found to have worse initial Glasgow Coma Scale (GCS) score and worse Glasgow Outcome Scale score than individuals without evidence of micro-hemorrhages one year post-injury. Interestingly, more than half of the patients who were positive for micro-hemorrhages reported post-concussive symptoms, whereas no symptoms were reported by patients negative for micro-hemorrhages, suggesting a link between the microscopic hemorrhagic lesions detected by SWI and persistent post-concussion symptoms. In a study by Helmer and colleagues (2014), baseline SWI data in a group of hockey players was acquired at the beginning and end of the season, as well as post-injury data at 72 hours, 2 weeks, and 2 months post-concussion. The authors introduced an automated quantification method for hypointensities associated with potential micro-hemorrhages and neural microstructural changes. They reported that, compared to the preseason baseline, concussed male athletes showed increased hypointensity burden

2 weeks post-injury. Female concussed athletes also showed a nonsignificant increase in hypointensity burden within the same time period. SWI have also been demonstrated in pediatric traumatic brain injury. Beauchamp et al. (2013) evaluated the relationship between SWI lesion number and volume with clinical and cognitive outcomes in a mostly mild TBI sample. SWI was acquired 2–8 weeks post-injury and cognitive testing was carried out 6 months post-injury. During the acute stage, SWI lesion size and volume correlated with clinical indices such as GCS and length of hospitalization. Greater number of SWI lesions also correlated with lower intellectual ability assessed 6 months post-injury, suggesting diffuse injury is more detrimental to cognitive function.

The utility of SWI in persons with a concussion is arguable. Indeed, it appears to have the potential to identify regions where brain micro-hemorrhage occurs, which has been correlated with the presence of post-concussion symptoms. However, bleeding is a product of significant forces to the brain, and as such, may have limited utility in terms of concussion diagnostics. Furthermore, a recent paper has suggested that some of these findings may be called into question as flawed methods in postprocessing manipulation of these images may have led to false positive results (Li et al. 2015). Thus, a standard method for micro-hemorrhage identification and quantification is yet to be developed and validated for its routine clinical use.

## Functional neuroimaging

The presence of a physical impact to the brain with a lack of structural lesions has inspired neuroimaging researchers to evaluate how the brain functions after a concussion. Work to date has demonstrated evidence to suggest that the brain may function in an abnormal state, displaying increased or decreased activity in regions that are active in healthy controls, as well as activity in regions that are otherwise not shown to be active in normal task performance, or resting state environments. The following is an overview of emerging neuroimaging methods that are focused on functional neuroimaging for the diagnosis of concussions or mTBI.

### Task-based functional magnetic resonance imaging

Functional MRI (fMRI) is a technique that evaluates the concentration of oxygenated versus deoxygenated hemoglobin based on how they interact with an induced magnetic field. In the confines of an MRI scanner, participants are exposed to multiple magnetic fields that vary in regard to specific protocols. The core feature of fMRI is that the oxygenated form of hemoglobin is *diamagnetic*, meaning that it interferes very little with the main magnetic field produced from the scanner. Alternatively, deoxyhemoglobin is *paramagnetic* and will produce a distortion with the magnetic field produced in the scanner. With this ability to differentiate oxygenated from deoxygenated hemoglobin, fMRI is able to evaluate the difference between the venous oxyhemoglobin and deoxyhemoglobin, a technique called blood oxygen level-dependent (BOLD) contrast. When a portion of the cortex becomes activated, following an initial drop in oxyhemoglobin levels from consumption, local cerebral blood flow to that area augments in response to the activation-related increased demand. This increased blood flow results in a relative rise in the concentration of oxyhemoglobin compared to deoxyhemoglobin. As these relative changes in concentration can be measured by the fMRI, areas that are activated will result in increased MRI signal using T2*-weighted imaging (Huettel et al. 2014).

There are several studies in the literature looking at the use of fMRI in concussion. FMRI was first used in the context of mTBI by McAllister et al. in two studies from 1999 and 2001. They used a working memory task that was an auditory version of a task known as n-back. Here, the subjects are tested for varying working memory loads ranging from 0-back to 3-back using a series of stimuli. In the 0-back paradigm, the subject simply had to answer whether the stimulus presented was the same as the one presented immediately before. In the 1-back, 2-back, and 3-back condition, the subject needed to determine if the stimulus was identical to the one presented before the last stimulus, two previous, or three previous, respectively. As a result, this test assesses varying working memory loads in a continuous manner (McAllister et al. 1999, 2001). In the two studies, McAllister and colleagues demonstrated that while the healthy control subjects demonstrated progressively increasing brain activation with increased working memory load, the mTBI subjects had an altered activation pattern with the increased load even though their performance was comparable to the normal controls in the task. The mTBI cohort had diminished brain activation compared to the control subjects in the low working memory load condition while with the moderate load (2-back > 1-back contrast), the mTBI subjects had more extensive brain activation, particularly in the right superior parietal and dorsolateral prefrontal cortex (DLPFC). With the highest load condition (3-back > 2-back contrast), the mTBI group did not show any further increase in brain activation, whereas the normal control subjects continued to show increased activation. The authors felt that these findings likely represented altered resource allocation in the mTBI subjects and that this led to altered brain activation patterns (McAllister et al. 1999, 2001). In these studies, however, the potential relationship between the altered activation patterns and symptomatology was not examined.

Soon after these initial studies, Chen and colleagues carried out three studies to further examine the use of fMRI in the context of concussion (Chen et al. 2004, 2007, 2008). An externally ordered working memory task that did not have varying working memory loads like the n-back was used. In this paradigm developed by Michael Petrides, the subjects were shown four items followed by a fifth item at a set interval. The subjects then had to answer whether this fifth item was a repeat of one of the first four or whether the fifth item was a novel one (Petrides 2013, 2005, Petrides et al. 2001). While this is also a working memory task, it is considered a discrete working memory task, whereas the n-back test is a continuous working memory task that requires constant surveillance of stimuli and, therefore, requiring a higher cognitive demand (Bryer et al. 2013). In their studies, Chen et al. (2004) demonstrated that, although concussed athletes performed just as well on the task as the normal controls, they had diminished task-specific percent BOLD signal increases usually seen in the typical areas of activation, particularly the DLPFC. Furthermore, it was noted that the concussed athletes had additional activation peaks in areas not typically activated with the task used (2004), suggesting possible recruitment of additional brain regions to compensate for those that were malfunctioning. This finding was later supported in another study (Pardini et al. 2010). In their follow-up paper in 2007, Chen and colleagues demonstrated that these percent BOLD signal alterations correlated well with levels of symptomatology as measured by the post-concussion symptom (PCS) scale—revised with increased PCS score correlating with diminished activation (Chen et al. 2007). Furthermore, with the aid of serial testing, Chen et al. were able to demonstrate that, as symptoms resolved, the activation patterns became similar to those seen with normal controls while subjects who remained symptomatic continued to have atypical activation patterns (Chen et al. 2008). Taken together, these studies demonstrate that fMRI, in addition to providing interesting insight into the pathophysiology behind concussions, has potential as a diagnostic tool in the assessment of concussion as well as in monitoring recovery.

There has been some debate whether the fMRI data in the literature is contradictory given that some working memory tasks produce hyperactivation (n-back) while others result in hypoactivation (Petrides task). The majority of studies in the literature investigating working memory has utilized the n-back task in various forms with relatively comparable results (Dettwiler et al. 2014, Lovell et al. 2007, McAllister et al. 2006, Smits et al. 2009, Stulemeijer et al. 2010, Pardini et al. 2010). In general, concussed subjects had increased activation with the low and moderate-load conditions, while at the highest load, they tended to not show as much increase as the normal controls. This is in stark contrast to the findings from studies using the Petrides externally ordered working memory task where hypoactivation was seen in the concussed individuals (Chen et al. 2004, 2007, 2008, Gosselin et al. 2011). The difference likely resides in the task construct. While both the n-back task and the Petrides task are meant to study working memory, the Petrides task can be seen as a discrete working memory task which has tended toward relative hypoactivation while the n-back task is considered a continuous working memory task which, particularly at higher loads, is considered to have a higher cognitive demand (Bryer et al. 2013). Furthermore, other studies have shown that, despite its common use as a working memory task, the n-back task itself has very weak correlations with other working memory tasks such as the working memory span task (Kane et al. 2007).

Other fMRI tasks that have been studied in concussion include auditory orienting tasks (Mayer et al. 2009), route learning (Slobounov et al. 2010), word listening (McAllister et al. 2006), counting Stroop (Smits et al. 2009), auditory oddball (Witt et al. 2010), and a combination of finger sequencing, serial calculation, and digit span (Jantzen et al. 2004). The differences in activation between concussion and healthy controls in these studies varied with some demonstrating concussion-related hypoactivation in regions of interest (Mayer et al. 2009, McAllister et al. 2006, Witt et al. 2010) and others showing hyperactivation (Slobounov et al. 2010, Smits et al. 2009, Jantzen et al. 2004). In the vast majority of studies in the literature, the performance measured on the tasks was no different between concussed subjects and healthy controls (McDonald et al. 2012). While some fMRI testing of mTBI subjects shows hyperactivation with some tasks and hypoactivation with others, it is likely that, similar to what is seen with the different working memory tasks the types of changes seen in mTBI are related to the nature and complexity of the tasks themselves. Regardless of how the activation is altered, either positively or negatively, there appears to be a preponderance of data demonstrating that there are clear functional changes that occur in the brains of patients after concussion.

Prior to 2014, only three papers in the literature addressed fMRI in children after concussion (Keightley et al. 2012). The three papers each used different tasks and had somewhat differing results. Yang et al. (2012) utilized an auditory orienting task in a group of 14 mTBI adolescents and 14 matched healthy controls to demonstrate significantly decreased task-related activation in various brain regions in mTBI adolescents compared to control subjects (2012). Another study by Krivitzky et al. (2011) examined a group of 13 mTBI subjects and matched controls using a tasks of executive control (TEC) paradigm which is a combination of the n-back task and the go/no-no task (testing inhibitory control) developed by their group. Here, the activation patterns did not differ between the two groups on the working memory portion of the TEC but increased activation with the mTBI group in the inhibitory control portion in the posterior cerebellum was documented (Krivitzky et al. 2011). In the third report by Talavage et al. (2014) the main thesis of the paper revolved around the finding that subjects with multiple subconcussive hits could develop similar activation patterns on fMRI to those with diagnosed concussions. fMRI findings of four patients with clinically diagnosed concussions using an n-back task demonstrated hyperactivation with the lower load memory tasks (2014). These findings are somewhat contradictory to those presented in the Krivitzky paper where no differences were found between mTBI patients and normal controls using the n-back portion of their task. Here again, none of these studies related fMRI findings to symptomatology.

In 2014, the group that carried out the previous adult studies using the Petrides externally-ordered working memory task applied the same paradigm to 15 concussed adolescents versus 15 age- and sex-matched controls (Keightley et al. 2014a). In this study, diminished task-related activation in various regions including the DLPFC in concussed subjects were noted, similar to the findings seen in concussed adults (Chen et al. 2004). However, unlike their adult counterparts, the children who were concussed had a task performance (as measured by accuracy of responses) that was significantly worse than that of healthy controls. Also of note, the concussed children did not have any additional activation peaks seen as compared to the normal controls (in the adult study, additional peaks were seen in the middle temporal gyrus). Keightley et al. (2014a) surmised that, taken together, these findings suggest that concussed children have a diminished capacity to recruit additional brain regions to help compensate for dysfunction in the areas normally activated for carrying out the working memory task.

In an another study, the same group examined the use of a novel navigational memory functional MRI task in the assessment of 15 adolescents post-concussion as compared to 15 healthy controls (Saluja et al. 2015). In this task paradigm, the subjects were required to learn the locations of various landmarks within a virtual three-dimensional environment prior to scanning. Once they were comfortable with the locations of the various landmarks (i.e., had created a cognitive map of the environment), they were then required to navigate from one location to another within the environment using the most efficient route possible while fMRI sequences were acquired. In this study, the concussed children had significantly diminished activation in various regions known to be activated in navigational memory recall including the posterior parahippocampal gyri (Figure 20.2) and

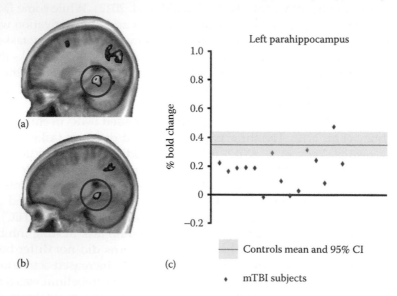

*Figure 20.2* fMRI t-maps displaying average activity in healthy controls (a) and in mTBI subjects (b) during a navigational memory task from Saluja (2015). Red circles illustrate activation peaks in the left parahippocampus for healthy controls (MNI x, y, z = −26, −44, −6) and for mTBI subjects (MNI x, y, z = −18, −40, −8). (c) demonstrates a scatter-plot showing % BOLD signal changes in the left Parahippocampus for each mTBI subject (red dots) compared to all healthy controls. Healthy control data is presented as the mean and 95% quantile (shaded area).

the retrosplenial regions. Furthermore, the concussed subjects had additional activations peaks seen in the left hippocampus and the right middle temporal gyrus as compared to the control group. An interesting aspect of this finding is that the left hippocampus is known to be important in the formation of the cognitive map based on previous studies (Spiers and Maguire 2007), suggesting that the concussed subjects were still trying to form the cognitive maps while attempting to complete the tasks.

In summary, in the last decade there has been an increased number of fMRI studies on concussion. They demonstrate that fMRI may provide unique insights into how the concussed brain operates. Observations have included both increased and decreased brain activity in regions normally activated in healthy controls, as well as brain activity in regions not typically observed in healthy persons. The meaning behind such abnormal brain activity is under debate and may be obscured by the diversity in imaging processing pipelines used as well as in the tasks performed in the scanner. For most recent/comprehensive review (McDonald et al. 2012).

## Resting state functional magnetic resonance imaging

Resting-state functional MRI (rs-fMRI) is a qualitative method of evaluating the brain's functional activity at rest. This technique focuses on low-frequency fluctuations of the BOLD signal while subjects are told to lie still in the scanner, not to think of anything, and to either leave their eyes open or closed (note: variability in protocols do exist). The use of such data has been applied toward understanding how regions of the brain are connected in terms of networks based on a similar pattern of BOLD signal fluctuations.

One of these methods is using *seed-based* connectivity. In this method, a region of interest is chosen from the brain (e.g., Broca's area) and regions that share the same temporal activation pattern to this region of interest are mapped. This information provides an indication as to the regions of the brain that share connectivity with the region of interest in its functional performance. For example, in a study by Banks and colleagues (2016), authors evaluated the functional connectivity of the thalamus and its relationship to post-concussion symptoms. Using 13 mTBI subjects and 11 healthy controls, increased functional connectivity between the thalamus and the default mode network, and decreased functional connectivity between the thalamus and the dorsal attention network, and frontoparietal control network were found in patients compared to controls. Alterations present in the thalamic functional connectivity after a concussion were reported to resolve alongside post-concussive symptoms (2016).

Another method of evaluating resting state fMRI data involves dividing the brain into distinct components that share similar activation patterns. Using statistical techniques such as independent component analysis, the brain can be divided into discrete components labeled as networks. These networks share a similar division to task-based areas of activation (Smith et al. 2009), the most commonly evaluated of which is the default mode network (DMN). In 2015, Zhu and colleagues (2015) evaluated the structural and functional connectivity of the default mode network. Using eight concussed student athletes and eleven control subjects, data was collected at 24 hours, 7 days, and 30 days after concussion. With no change in structural connectivity, there was evidence of reduced functional connectivity within the DMN from day 1 to day 7 in the concussed group that was partially recovered by day 30 (2015). In 2016, Orr and colleagues (2016) evaluated 16 young-adult ice hockey players with a history of concussion who had no subjective complaints versus teammates with any history of concussion. No difference was found between the two groups in neuropsychological performance despite evidence of structural abnormalities using DTI. Athletes also showed differences in the DMN through increased temporal correlation in the posterior aspect, decreased correlation in the anterior aspect, and increased correlation outside of the DMN. Thus, although no phenotypic difference was found between groups, a difference was found in terms of functional activity (2016).

Lastly, using more advanced methods, the brain can be evaluated based on the principles of *graph theory*. Graph theory is a technique that consists in understanding how regions in the brain relate to one another in the context of both small and large network-based systems. In a graph model, each node—or vertex—is represented by a region of the brain that can be defined either structurally or functionally. The connectivity between each node is defined as an edge value and will determine the global versus local connectivity profiles of each particular node. A common way of using graph theory is to evaluate small-worldness (Figure 20.3) as the balance between nodal-independence from other regions of the brain against nodal-integration with other regions of the brain. Other common metrics evaluated using graph theory include those reflecting segregation of a node, such as clustering coefficient and modularity, and those reflecting network integration such as betweenness centrality and global efficiency.

Messe and colleagues (2013) tested 17 individuals with post-concussion syndrome at 6 months post-injury, compared with 38 mTBI subjects with no post-concussion syndrome and 34 healthy controls. The authors found long-range functional network alterations in all mTBI patients; however, mTBI patients with post-concussion symptoms had greater alterations than patients who did not. It was found that alterations were mostly localized in the temporal and thalamic regions in the subacute stage (1–3 weeks post-injury) and frontal regions at the late phase (6 months post-injury) (2013). In another study, Zhou (2016) evaluated 30 patients with clinically defined mTBI and 45 age-matched healthy controls and showed that the mTBI patients had lower relative betweenness centrality but significantly higher clustering coefficient. Regions with lower betweenness centrality corresponded with regions of reduced FA. Also, global FA reduction correlated with betweenness centrality and clustering coefficient in mTBI patients. The author also found that significantly higher thalamocortical connectivity positively correlated with the clustering coefficient in mTBI participants.

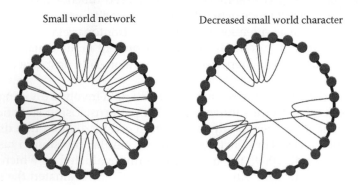

Small world network                    Decreased small world character

*Figure 20.3* The small world character is a method of describing the organization of networks such as those found in the brain. A commonly referenced example of a small world network is social networks and six-degrees of separation. In a small world, one individual (represented in the figure as a red dot) may not know an individual directly, but may know them through another individual. As the small worldness decreases, individuals become more isolated (image on the right). In terms of clinical neuroimaging, the small worldness of a network can be reduced through damage to white matter pathways that connect regions of the brain.

Hence, patients who had higher clustering coefficients tended to have lower PCS scores. As such, results demonstrated significant functional small-world properties in the patient who had an mTBI (2016). Decreased global efficiency was possibly due to diffuse axonal injury and local network up-regulation including increased thalamo-cortical connectivity.

The use of rs-fMRI in concussion has produced interesting results in terms of its ability to identify abnormal patterns of connectivity relative to a healthy state. The major limitation of this technique is in understanding the significance of such alterations and being able to replicate their occurrence. Moreover, some believe that alterations in functional connectivity are a derivative of structural damage, thus producing additive value in research already addressing the latter. The means through which limitations will be resolved is through collaborative decision-making when selecting imaging protocols, as well as through performing multi-modal analyses. For most recent/comprehensive review (McDonald et al. 2012).

## Functional near-infrared spectroscopy

Functional near-infrared spectroscopy (fNIRS) is a technology that makes use of near-infrared light from lasers or light emitting diodes (LED) and detectors placed on the surface of the subject's scalp to detect functional activation of the brain. The near-infrared light (700–1000 nm wavelength) is able to penetrate through the superficial layers including the scalp and skull to the surface of the brain. Built-in detectors are then able to differentiate between oxyhemoglobin and deoxyhemoglobin based on the unique absorptive properties of the individual molecules (Boas et al. 2003, Ferrari et al. 2004). As such, fNIRS is able to determine which areas of the brain are activated during task performance.

There are only a few studies that have used fNIRS in the context of mTBI. In one study, Helmich and colleagues (2015) had concussed subjects and age-matched controls tested with fNIRS using both verbal and nonverbal versions of the Petrides working memory task. In total, 17 concussed subjects (7 symptomatic, 10 minimally symptomatic) and 8 normal control subjects were included in the study. The results demonstrated that the symptomatic concussed subjects had decreased task-specific activation in the dorsolateral frontal cortex as compared to the minimally symptomatic and normal control groups (2015). Kontos et al. (2014) published a preliminary study with 9 mTBI subjects and 5 normal controls using tasks evaluating multiple cognitive processes including word memory, spatial design memory, digit-symbol substitution, and working memory (2014). They found decreased brain activation, particularly in frontal regions. The concussed subjects in this study did not perform as well on the tasks themselves as their control counterparts on all but the working memory task. Lastly, Urban and colleagues (2015) employed a resting-state and finger-tapping task synchronized to a 1-Hz metronome. In their study of 20 pediatric subjects (8 controls and 12 mTBI), Urban et al. (2015) showed that there was a difference in coherence between the two hemispheres in the mTBI subjects compared to controls (2015). As with the other studies, this was a preliminary investigation and no direct correlation with other testing modalities was carried out.

There are several advantages to this technique including it being noninvasive, portable, relatively inexpensive, and usable while subjects are performing dynamic tasks such as balance testing and exercising (Lareau et al. 2011, Sawan et al. 2013). The main disadvantage of this technology is its extremely limited reliability for assessing deeper structures in the brain, such as the thalamus (Boas et al. 2003, Ferrari et al. 2004). Furthermore, the spatial resolution of fNIRS (approximately 5 mm) is much lower than that of fMRI (Ferrari et al. 2004). Thus, fNIRS has shown the potential to show differences between concussed and healthy subjects; however, substantial research is required to improve its resolution and field of view.

## *Arterial spin labeling*

Arterial spin labeling (ASL) is capable of quantifying cerebral blood flow by using magnetically labeled water protons in arterial blood as an endogenous tracer (Petcharunpaisan et al. 2010, Wolf and Detre 2007). Quantification of perfusion is achieved by comparing two sets of images, a tag image (or flow image) and a control image (Petersen et al. 2006). To obtain the tag image, water protons in blood are first magnetically labeled outside of the imaging plane with a radiofrequency pulse that inverts the water proton. A delay, known as an inversion delay in pulsed ASL (postlabeling delay in continuous ASL), is then introduced to allow the labeled blood to flow into the tissue of interest (Petersen et al. 2006, Pollock et al. 2009). Because the tag image contains signals from both magnetically labeled blood and static tissues, while the control image contains only signal from static tissue, perfusion can be calculated by subtracting the control image from the tag image (Pollock et al. 2009), and the resulting signal provides a measure sensitive to local cerebral blood flow (Detre et al. 2009).

In one of the earliest studies using ASL in mTBI patients, Ge et al. (2009) showed that subjects had a significant decrease in CBF in the left and right thalamus compared to healthy controls. Furthermore reduced CBF was positively correlated with performance on several neuropsychological tests, including processing and response speed, memory, attention, word fluency, and executive functioning. In this study, the median time since the onset of the mTBI was 28.5 months, suggesting that hemodynamic impairment can persist years after the injury. Reduced CBF in the thalamus was also reported in a later study in a group of mTBI patients tested within 1 month post-injury, and at 9 months post-injury (Grossman et al. 2013). Interestingly, perfusion deficits in the thalamus coincided with DTI abnormalities as reduced FA and increased MD values. In addition to the thalamus, regional reduction in CBF has also been reported in frontal and occipital lobes during the subacute stage of the injury (Lin et al. 2016). Furthermore, the degree of hypoperfusion correlated with the severity of post-concussive symptoms. Perfusion deficits in the subacute and chronic stage have also been reported following pediatric concussion (Wang et al. 2015). Unlike previous studies with adults that showed deficits in the thalamus, adolescents tested 3–12 months post-injury showed reduced CBF in bilateral frontotemporal regions, while no change was reported in the subcortical regions.

Arterial spin labeling is a technique that has potential for future research in patients suffering a concussion. Experimental TBI animal models have shown that one of the most noteworthy markers of concussion is a perfusion deficit (Giza and Hovda 2014, Ginsberg et al. 1997, Pasco et al. 2007). ASL has provided evidence of altered levels of perfusion in both adult and pediatric samples and has several advantages including its noninvasive nature. However, a considerable limitation facing this technique is its complex postprocessing requirements.

## *Electroencephalography*

Electroencephalography (EEG) is a technique that is under continual reinvention. In its most basic form, EEG consists in applying electrodes to the scalp of individuals to measure small voltage changes that result from discharging neurons. EEG is believed to primarily measure dendritic postsynaptic potentials of pyramidal neurons in the cortex (Luck 2005), thus making it sensitive to discharging neurons during both resting and active states.

*Event-related potentials* (ERPs) are specific and reliable changes in voltage that occur in relation to particular events (e.g., presentation of a sensory stimulus), and, as such, are thought to reflect discrete brain processes (Luck 2005). Although the technique itself has been extensively reported on, more of late, ERPs have been shown to be a useful tool to study the link between TBI and cognitive impairments. For instance, usually in the context of oddball paradigms, both of the P3 components, the P3a and P3b—which are related to attentional processes (Polich 2007)—have shown alterations as a result of concussion, although the effect of TBI on P3a has been debated (Broglio et al. 2009, Gosselin et al. 2006) with some persistent changes seen despite symptom resolution (Gosselin et al. 2006). Changes in the P3 components as a result of TBI have also been observed in the context of executive control tasks (Di Russo and Spinelli 2010). Pontifex et al. (2009) evaluated the error-related negativity (ERN), observed after an error in a cognitive task is performed (Gehring et al. 2012) and found that mTBI subjects had lower ERN amplitudes than controls, despite no difference in task performance.

In an attempt to correlate fMRI findings with ERP, Gosselin and colleagues (2011) used the Petrides working memory task in both fMRI and ERP paradigms (2011). In their paper, they studied 14 mTBI subjects with persistent symptoms beyond 2 months post-injury (mean 5.7 ± 2.9 months). As in the previous studies by Chen et al. (2004, 2007) their data demonstrated that symptomatic subjects had hypoactivation in various regions including the mid-DLPFC. Furthermore, they measured ERPs using the same working memory task and noted decreased amplitudes in the N350 component in the frontal region. They concluded in their study that in patients with prolonged symptoms post-injury, there was evidence of continued cerebral dysfunction (Gosselin et al. 2011). Gosselin and colleagues (2012) followed up this study with an additional paper examining the use of ERP alone in 44 patients with mTBI. In this paper, they noted that similar ERP changes were seen in this group as well (2012). While ERP techniques may be very sensitive to abnormalities in the systems that give rise to them, they might not adequately capture the extensive heterogeneity that is associated with mTBI because of their task-specificity.

*Evoked potentials* (EP) are observed very quickly after a stimulus, and are thus thought to reflect the activity of neurons in the process of sensory perception (Luck 2005, Schmitt and Dichter 2015). In recent years, the frequency-following response (FFR) has been increasingly studied. In a recent study, Kraus et al. (2016) measured the FFR on children who had suffered concussions and found that, compared to controls, patients had disrupted auditory processing on a number of measures—timing, accuracy, and strength of encoding. In addition, they assessed whether they could use the FFR to correctly classify which individuals had suffered concussions. Their model was capable of correctly classifying the majority of individuals, achieving 90% sensitivity, 95% specificity, a positive predictive value of 94.7%, and a negative predictive value of 90.4%. Although the sample size in this study was fairly low (N = 20) and further research is needed to validate this technique, this study suggests that the FFR is a potential tool for identifying patients with an mTBI.

*Graph theory* is a mathematical technique that evaluates networks as a collection of nodes and edges represented by the electrodes and their connectivity, respectively. While studies using graph theory have been used to track recovery from severe TBI using EEG (Nakamura et al. 2009) as well as for finding epileptic foci as a result of severe TBI (Irimia et al. 2013), very few studies (Cao and Slobounov 2010, Tsirka et al. 2011) have applied this technique in persons with an mTBI. Tsirka et al. (2011) found that in a working memory task, mTBI patients displayed suboptimal network organization, as demonstrated by graph parameters. In another study, Cao and Slobounov (2010) studied 29 student-athletes who had sustained mTBI and found a significant decrease in long-distance connectivity, a significant increase in short-distance connectivity, as well as alterations in vertex degree and departure from small-world network configuration.

Research using EEG continues to show promising results in regards to its sensitivity to brain abnormalities present in persons with a concussion. EEG offers a considerable temporal resolution of 1ms (Luck 2005) and may be very portable, depending on its use.

However it is important to note that EEG suffers from issues relating to source location due to relatively poor spatial resolution. Despite the age of this technique, research is finding new ways to analyze and interpret EEG data that shows promise for diagnostics in concussion. As in other techniques, there is a need to determine optimal processing methods and analysis tools prior to EEG being adopted formally in the clinical setting. For most recent/comprehensive review (Rapp et al. 2015).

## Magnetoencephalography

Magnetocencephalography (MEG) is a technique sensitive to neuronal activity based on how neurons transmit information using electrical signals. As current passes through the cortex from discharging neurons, a magnetic field that projects radially can be detected, making this technique sensitive mainly to current flow that is tangential to the skull (Proudfoot et al. 2014). Therefore, MEG is a method capable of evaluating brain activity during both active and resting states.

*MEG studies using event-related fields (ERFs) or spectral analysis* have focused on evaluating abnormal activity during task-based performance. In a study by Robb Swan and colleagues (2015) authors evaluated 31 military and civilian participants with a history of mTBI and post-concussion symptoms as well as 33 matched healthy controls in the context of a cognitive battery and MEG. Authors reported decreased performance of concussion patients on tasks including information processing speed and a correlation between slow-wave activity on MEG and cognitive performance (2015). These findings suggest that neurocognitive deficits after a concussion are tied to altered neurological performance that can be detected by MEG. In a task-based study by da Costa and colleagues (2015), authors had a group of 16 adults with mTBI and 16 matched controls perform a neuropsychological battery and mental flexibility task (set-shifting) while in a MEG scanner. The study showed that despite similarities in performance (accuracy), patients with an mTBI had delayed reaction times and integrated regions of the brain into performance that were not observed in healthy controls (e.g., occipital lobe). The integration of atypical regions could point toward compensatory efforts (2015).

*Network based analyses* have produced interesting findings with regards to how brain organization may be perturbed following an mTBI. For example, Dimitriadis and colleagues (2015) evaluated 31 mTBI patients and 55 healthy controls using functional connectivity and graph theory under the premise that normal behavior may become disrupted in parallel with disruptions to the functional connectivity between brain regions. In contrast to controls that showed a brain profile focused on strong local connections, persons with an mTBI showed weak local connections and strong long-range connections. This research suggests that functional connectivity defined through MEG could be used as a potential biomarker in mTBI. In 2016, Alhourani and colleagues (2016) evaluated 9 mTBI subjects and 15 age matched controls using MEG in the context of a resting-state paradigm. In the mTBI group, decreased functional connectivity was observed in specific networks that included the default mode network. As well, graph-theory based measures suggested that reduced local efficiency was present in multiple brain regions in the mTBI subjects, demonstrating network abnormalities in the mTBI group (2016).

Together, data from MEG has shown interesting results in patients with an mTBI and its capacity to observe atypical brain activity relative to the healthy state. Because magnetic fields can pass essentially undisturbed through human tissues, MEG offers better spatial resolution than EEG (Lee and Huang 2014). Diagnostically, MEG has shown a lot of promise. Lewine et al. (2007) found that MEG detected abnormalities in 86% of patients with post-concussive cognitive impairments, a significantly higher sensitivity than the 40% from single-photon emission computed tomography (SPECT) and 18% from conventional MRI. Huang et al. (2009) studied 10 individuals with mTBI who had no CT or MRI abnormalities and found that MEG was able to detect abnormal delta waves in all patients. The main caveat of MEG is that it requires very specialized equipment that is not available widely. Hence, as research in MEG increases and more studies validate the results obtained thus far, efforts should be made to make MEG more accessible. For most recent/comprehensive review (Lee and Huang 2014).

## Neuroimaging and metabolomics

Metabolomics represents a promising field of neuroimaging research that is capable of evaluating the metabolic profile of a region of interest. Using these techniques can provide insight into the health of neurons, the presence of inflammatory molecules, quantities of neurotransmitters and other molecules relevant toward understanding optimal and suboptimal neuronal performance.

## Positron emission tomography

Positron emission tomography (PET) is an imaging modality that uses radio-labeled compounds that are injected intravenously. A positron is a form of anti-matter that has all the characteristics of an electron but with a positive charge instead of negative. Positrons only exist in our universe for fractions of seconds because immediately after they are created they collide with their electron counterparts resulting in the annihilation of the two particles and subsequent release of two gamma rays in opposite directions (i.e., 180° apart).

$^{18}F$-*fluorodeoxyglucose (FDG)* is a radiolabeled molecule that approximates the structure of glucose, replacing one of the hydroxyl groups with a radio-isotope of a fluorine atom. Because of the similitude between molecules, FDG will localize to tissues with higher glucose uptake due to higher metabolic demand (Bailey 2005, Meyer 1998). The first PET study on concussion was by Humayun et al. in 1989 where they compared, using FDG-based PET, 3 concussed subjects to 3 control subjects, within 3–12 months of injury. In their study, they found that concussed subjects had decreased FDG uptake in the medial temporal, posterior temporal, and posterior frontal regions (Humayun et al. 1989). The majority of studies looking at PET findings in the context of concussion demonstrated changes in the temporal and frontal lobes that correlated with worse outcome (Roberts et al. 1995, Umile et al. 2002), though one study demonstrated decreased cerebellar uptake in 12 mTBI soldiers who experienced blast injuries (Peskind et al. 2011). Studies have observed alterations in specific regions such as the midtemporal, anterior cingulate, precuneus, anterior temporal, frontal white, and corpus callosum brain regions (Gross et al. 1996, Ruff et al. 1994, Umile et al. 2002). A trend however appears to be present wherein hypometabolism is found in the frontal and temporal regions (Byrnes et al. 2014).

The use of PET in mTBI research has been a growing field. Other radiolabeled compounds such as *[(11)C]DPA-713* have been used to bind to translocator protein (TSPO), a marker of brain injury and repair, showing increased levels in retired athletes from the national football league (Coughlin et al. 2015). Furthermore, *[11C](R)PK11195(PK)* has been used to evaluate activated microglia, a cell-type involved in the immune response, showing binding in thalamus that was associated with more severe cognitive impairment in persons who had suffered severe brain injuries (Ramlackhansingh et al. 2011). Finally, *[18F]T807/AV1451* has been used to evaluate tau aggregates for individuals at risk of developing chronic traumatic encephalopathy showing increased values at the gray matter–white matter junction in the bilateral cingulate, occipital and orbitofrontal cortices, and several temporal areas (Dickstein et al. 2016).

Accordingly, PET research in patients with a concussion is continuing to evolve and follows the successful development of new tracers. Using molecules that mimic prominent biological molecules implicated in concussion can and have provided insight into functional as well as metabolic disturbances. Importantly, PET involves radiation, and thus may have limited potential in vulnerable populations such as pediatrics. Regardless, future research using PET should be considered in terms of concussion diagnostics.

## Magnetic resonance spectroscopy

Magnetic resonance spectroscopy (MRS) is a technique sensitive to how individual atoms in a molecule respond to their unique chemical environment. For example, Figure 20.4 highlights a molecule of the neurotransmitter GABA. In this figure, the hydrogen atoms will be exposed to unique chemical environments and therefore will be sensitive to different frequencies. A list of molecules that can be detected using MRS are outlined in Table 20.1 and include ones that can reflect the health of mitochondria, the amount of immune activity, and cellular energy. Thus, MRS is capable of providing insight into the health of the brain through metabolomics in a noninvasive manner.

The most commonly reported form of MRS focuses on the hydrogen atom. Proton-MRS ($^1$H-MRS) studies focused on the caudate, globus pallidus, putamen, and thalamus has

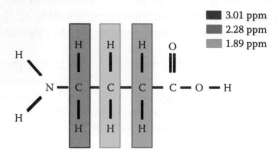

*Figure 20.4* Molecule of GABA showing the three different sets of hydrogen atoms (in the red, green, blue rectangles) that give rise to the three unique peaks in MRS (upper right). GABA has a unique frequency signature that can differentiate it from other compounds in the brain.

*Table 20.1* Metabolites that can be evaluated with MRS

| Metabolite | Frequency (ppm) | Marker |
|---|---|---|
| Creatine | 3.02 | Energy metabolism |
| Choline | 3.21 | Cellular membrane |
| GABA | 1.89; 2.28; 3.01 | Neurotransmitter |
| Glx | 2.12–2.35; 3.74–3.75 | Neurotransmitter |
| Lactate | 1.33 | Energy metabolism |
| Macromolecules | 0.93, 1.24, 1.43, 1.72, 2.05, 2.29, 3.00 | Lipids |
| Myo-inositol | 3.52 | Gliosis |
| NAA | 2.02 | Neuronal marker |

*Source:* Gardner, A. et al., *J. Neurotrauma*, 31, 1–18, 2014; Henry, L.C. et al., *J. Neurotrauma*, 27, 65–76, 2010.

found increased myo-inositol (MI), myo-inositol/creatinine ratio (MI/Cr), and glutamate/creatinine ratio (Glx/Cr) in patients after mTBI compared with healthy controls, which may point toward a glial and excitatory response to injury (Kierans et al. 2014). ¹H-MRS measures of neuronal health via N-acetylaspartate (NAA) have been correlated with damage to white matter tracts using DTI (Grossman et al. 2015). In a study by Johnson et al. (2012), the authors demonstrated that in the subacute stage of mTBI there is a decrease in the level of N-acetylaspartate/choline ratio (NAA/Cho) and NAA/Cr and that metabolic abnormalities persisted despite the return of clinical symptoms to baseline (2012). Importantly, after the resolution of symptoms, ¹H-MRS has shown in a group of mTBI subjects that there may be a temporal window wherein the brain is more vulnerable to injury. Vagnozzi and colleagues (2008) evaluated NAA levels at 2, 15, and 30 days post-injury. Initially, NAA values were lower post-injury, but returned to normal after 30 days; however, reported symptoms resolved between 3 and 15 days suggesting a disconnect between pathology and symptoms (2008). A similar finding was observed by Johnson et al. (2012) where the point of symptom resolution did not coincide with metabolite levels returning to normal levels.

Other forms of spectroscopy have also been applied including phosphorus-31 MRS. Whereas ¹H-MRS evaluates the neurochemical environment of proton containing compounds, phosphorous-based MRS focuses on compounds such as nucleoside triphosphate, and other energy-based compounds. In 2015, Sikoglu and colleagues (2015) evaluated 14 concussion patients and found significantly lower gamma-NTP levels in athletes after concussion despite normal performance on neuropsychological testing (2015).

Data obtained from research using MRS suggest that this technique may prove valuable in terms of identifying individuals who are continuing to recover despite having normal neuropsychological performance and no symptoms. Research has shown abnormalities predominately focused around NAA levels; however, energy-related and inflammatory compounds have also been identified by multiple studies. It is clear that MRS provides a unique way of understanding the brain post-concussion. For most recent/comprehensive review (Gardner et al. 2014).

## Neuroimaging in the diagnosis of concussion

The accurate diagnosis of a concussion is something that continues to elude researchers and clinicians. As outlined in Chapter 2 of this book, diagnostic criteria for a concussion largely focus around subjective symptoms, which are by nature inherently variable. As outlined in this chapter, results using neuroimaging to date have a similar pattern of variability. It remains unclear what, if any, measure is the best one to use for diagnostic purposes. The answer to this question may lie in an emerging field of neuroimaging based on machine learning.

### Machine learning

Machine learning is a method of developing functions to help delineate data trends and distinguish groups within a set of data without the explicit oversight from a user or, in the case of medicine, a clinician. As outlined in Figure 20.5, this technique involves discrete stages of data input, development of discriminate functions, and output. The types of discriminate models that can be used include support vector machines, logistic regression, and neuronal networks. Importantly, machine learning in the context of concussion research makes use of existing neuroimaging techniques and applies their data toward determining accurate discriminate functions.

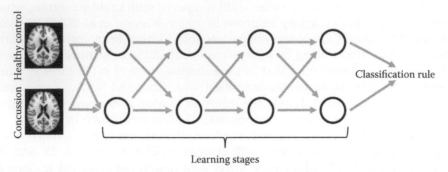

*Figure 20.5* A schematic representation of the stages of a neuronal network that can be used in machine learning. These networks can be used to develop a classification rule to divide groups based on criteria that are created at the input stage. Learning stages, also known as the hidden layer, is where the machine learns how to best apply variables to divide the proposed population.

Research using machine learning in the context of concussions has shown potential, with relatively high accuracy, sensitivity, and specificity values. In Table 20.2, exemplar studies that use machine learning in conjunction with imaging techniques outlined in this chapter are provided. As can be appreciated, a diverse range of subject numbers is present in each study; the higher the number of individuals in the training set, the more accurate data classifiers are.

The use of machine learning in the context of mTBI has not only received attention from academic institutions, but also from commercial entities building proprietary algorithms for diagnostic purposes. For example, one group has begun using such learning algorithms in combination with EEG to develop classifiers for persons with a concussion and achieving notable results with sensitivity of 80.5% and specificity of 73.9% (Prichep et al. 2012). These findings, in addition to the results presented in Table 20.2, are encouraging but they represent only preliminary findings from a field that has not yet reached consensus on how data should be acquired or preprocessed. Continued exploration using machine learning could provide invaluable contributions to the field of neuroimaging and concussion research.

*Table 20.2* Summary of results from the investigations making use of machine learning algorithms

| Study | Modality | Training set size | Accuracy | Sensitivity | Specificity |
|---|---|---|---|---|---|
| Yadav et al. (2016) | CT | 995 HC/84 mTBI | NR | 0.90 | 0.92 |
| Mitra et al. (2016) | DTI | 146 HC/179 mTBI | 0.68 | 0.8 | NR |
| Karamzadeh et al. (2016) | fNIRS | 31 HC/20 TBI | 0.85 | 0.85 | 0.84 |
| Vergara et al. (2017) | rs-fMRI | 50 HC/50 mTBI | 0.84 | 0.89 | 0.79 |
| Cao et al. (2008) | EEG | 31 HC/30 mTBI | 0.77 | 0.97 | 0.69 |
| Vakorin et al. (2016) | MEG | 21 HC/20 mTBI | 0.88 | 0.85 | 0.90 |
| Lui et al. (2014) | Multiple | 26 HC/24 mTBI | 0.80 | 0.75 | 0.85 |

*Note:* CT, Computer tomography; DTI, diffusion tensor imaging; fNIRS, functional near infrared spectroscopy; rs-fMRI, resting statefunctional magnetic resonance imaging; EEG, electroencephalography; MEG, magnetoencephalography; NR, not reported.

# Special considerations

## Sample variance

When evaluating persons with mTBI or concussion, research has demonstrated that not all populations respond to a concussion the same way. For example, it has been shown that individuals with higher education are able to moderate the impact of head trauma better than those of lower education (Mathias and Wheaton 2015, Sumowski et al. 2013). Gender is another issue requiring address as females have been shown to have an increased risk of developing post-concussion symptoms (Preiss-Farzanegan et al. 2009) and may display different brain activity patterns in relation to males during task-based functional neuroimaging (Hsu et al. 2015). One possible explanation of the discrepancy with regards to gender is that women tend to have less neck strength than men. In a recent study, it was noted that weaker neck strength correlated with increased risk of concussion and it was felt that this could explain higher rates of concussion amongst women compared to men in various sports (Collins et al. 2014).

Also, post-concussion symptoms are reported to be higher in individuals with a personal or family history of mood disorders or other psychiatric illnesses (Morgan et al. 2015). Accordingly, any research attempting to evaluate the presence or impact of a concussion should account for such variability in their analysis.

## Pediatrics

Children cannot simply be thought of as *little adults*, particularly when it comes to the brain, as extensive development (either through enlargement or refinement) occurs with respect to white (Giedd et al. 1999) and gray matter density (Giedd et al. 1999, Sowell et al. 2001). Some studies in animal models suggest that the lack of myelinated nerve fibers may put children at increased risk for brain damage, relative to adults (Ajao et al. 2012). Also, there is evidence to suggest that pediatric subjects have longer recovery times than adults (Choe et al. 2012). Specific network organization (Casey et al. 2005, Luna et al. 2010, Paus 2005) and cerebral blood flow patterns have been noted in pediatric subjects (Mandera et al. 2002). Furthermore, preprocessing strategies such as image registration can become distorted when attempting to use an adult template in a pediatric cohort (Wilke et al. 2003). As such, it cannot be assumed that research findings from adults can be extrapolated to the pediatric setting. Age-specific analyses are warranted.

## High magnetic fields

One of the major advances in neuroimaging is the continued development of higher magnetic field environments for MRI scanners. Currently, the strength of MRI scanners in clinical and research use is either 1.5 or 3 Tesla in strength. However, 7 Tesla scanners are becoming more frequently applied to evaluate clinical populations in a research setting. For persons with concussions or mTBIs, the greater resolution offered by higher-field environments translates into greater resolution for brain segmentation (Deng et al. 2016) that can impact measures such as cortical thickness (Lusebrink et al. 2013). This is very relevant as studies, such as that by Keightley et al. (2014b), have demonstrated cortical thinning in regions of the cortex after a concussion. Moreover, higher field environments offer greater resolution for fMRI based analyses (Vu et al. 2016) and metabolic quantification with magnetic resonance spectroscopy (Pradhan et al. 2015). Therefore, it is possible that a greater understanding of concussions can be obtained as the field strength of scanners continues to grow.

## *Discordance between neuroimaging and symptoms*

A significant limitation to concussion research is that the condition itself is subject to an evolving definition. Accordingly, any attempts to ascertain the value of neuroimaging toward the diagnosis of a concussion are limited by modern diagnostic criteria. This presents a significant problem toward optimizing the use of neuroimaging, especially in the context of research that has shown evidence of brain abnormalities after symptoms have resolved (Barr et al. 2012, Broglio et al. 2009, Gosselin et al. 2006, McCrea et al. 2010) as well as subconcussive events that are not significant enough to warrant a concussion diagnosis but are still capable of producing brain abnormalities (Bazarian et al. 2014, Breedlove et al. 2012, Koerte et al. 2012, McAllister et al. 2014, Taber et al. 2015, Talavage et al. 2014). To resolve these issues, future neuroimaging research should continue to evaluate patients after symptoms have resolved and emphasize factors such as mechanism of injury, especially in the absence of symptoms, to determine the clinical significance of abnormal brain data.

## *Future directions*

One of the foremost challenges of neuroimaging research is the methods required to acquire the imaging scans and process their contents to have quantifiable results. Indeed, each of the presented methods in this chapter currently requires explicit user expertise. If a method such as resting-state fMRI were to be used as a diagnostic test, there would have to be large-scale consensus on what imaging parameters should be used (e.g., echo time and repetition time), as well as how the data should be interpreted. For example, the default mode network is a very commonly used network but is vulnerable to methodological factors regarding how the brain is divided into discrete networks (Wang et al. 2015). As such, to see neuroimaging as a diagnostic tool, there must be *a large-scale convergence of imaging protocols and processing methods*.

Concussions have been the subject of an evolving definition. They were once believed to represent a primarily functional injury; however recent research has shown that some structural and metabolic alterations can be present. Their potential for alterations does not however imply that structural or functional abnormalities are always present, and there may be situations where there may be little to no evidence of structural injury despite the presence of atypical functional activity. Alternatively, it is possible that false-positives may be present, at which point we should be able to identify them. Under such situations, and not having the capacity for knowing a priori which method to use, *adopting a multi-modal approach* is likely the most effective for not only detecting anomalous data, but also providing a comprehensive report of what is known to be altered in persons who have had a concussion.

The ability to reliably identify an individual as belonging to one group versus another is critically dependent on a thorough knowledge of both groups. That is, to be able to accurately diagnose a patient with a concussion requires extensive knowledge not only of the variability inherent in a concussed population, but also the natural variability in healthy persons. The optimal use of neuroimaging as a diagnostic tool for concussion will depend on obtaining large datasets for evaluation to acquire a comprehensive understanding of the diversity of this population. Several groups have begun to form multi-center studies to expand their subject pools, including the TRACK-TBI group in the University of California who collected data from multiple US cities on 3000 TBI subjects (https://tracktbi.ucsf.edu) and the CENTER-TBI project aiming to collect data from 5400 TBI patients across Europe and Israel (Maas et al., 2015). Similar projects must be pursued to develop a comprehensive understanding of concussions at the structural, functional, and metabolic levels. To accomplish this task, inter-institutional and professional collaborations, as well as open-source data projects are essential.

| Modality | Target (Functional/ Structural/ Metabolic) | mTBI-related target (e.g., MRS and metabolic abnormalities) | Advantages | Disadvantages | Clinical considerations |
|---|---|---|---|---|---|
| Diffusion Weighted Imaging | Structural | Damaged white matter pathways | Sensitive to damage in white matter regions of the brain | Analysis of specific fiber pathways requires a high level of anatomical knowledge (lack of a standardized approach to define ROIs) | May be sensitive to diffuse axonal injury in persons with a concussion |
| Susceptibility Weighted Imaging | Structural | Minor brain hemorrhages | Able to detect small bleeds in the brain | Requires radiologist intervention | May detect bleeding too subtle for other imaging techniques such as CT scanning |
| fMRI—Task-based | Functional | Abnormal cortical activity | Able to show compensatory use of brain regions and monitor recovery of brain activity | Task must be sensitive to the damage that was sustained from the concussion | May show abnormal cortical and subcortical activity patterns |
| fMRI—Resting-state | Functional | Abnormal cortical activity | Noninvasive/ visualization-quantification of networks not involved in task-based performance | Nonstandard methods of preprocessing data | Requires participant to not actively be engaging in thought processes |

*(Continued)*

| Modality | Target (Functional/ Structural/ Metabolic) | mTBI-related target (e.g., MRS and metabolic abnormalities) | Advantages | Disadvantages | Clinical considerations |
|---|---|---|---|---|---|
| Electroencephalography | Functional | Abnormal cortical activity | Portable/Highly adaptable/Low cost/Very time-sensitive to information processing in the brain | Difficult to determine source of EEG signals | May show abnormal cortical activity patterns |
| Magnetoencephalography | Functional | Abnormal cortical activity | Better spatial resolution than EEG with similar temporal resolution | Requires highly specialized and expensive equipment | May show abnormaliteis in information processing and the use of atypical brain activity |
| Arterial Spin Labeling | Functional | Changes in cerebral blood flow | May provide greater resolution than fMRI/Sensitive to brain perfusion | Young technique— unclear what is optimal processing pipeline | May show abnormal cortical and subcortical activity patterns |
| Functional Near Infrared Spectroscopy | Functional | Abnormal cortical activity | Portable/Price (relative to MRI-based measures) | Resolution limited to peripheral areas of the cortex/Low spatial resolution | Ability to evaluate motor tasks such as balance |
| Positron Emission Tomography | Functional/ Metabolic | Functional adaptation of brain regions/ Build-up of tau proteins | Specificity to particular metabolites | Resolution of images | Requires use of radiation— may limit application in pediatric patients |
| Magnetic Resonance Spectroscopy | Metabolic | Energy metabolism/ Neuronal death/ Inflammation | Noninvasive | Nonstandard methods of processing | Trade-off between sensitivity of method and knowing region of interest for analysis |

# Conclusion

The accurate diagnosis of a concussion is something that continues to elude and attract clinicians and researchers alike. The disability and symptoms experienced by patients with a concussion were once dispelled, but with the use of neuroimaging tools, researchers have shown that their symptoms have an organic basis. Moreover, neuroimaging tools have identified individuals who have specific structural, functional, and/or metabolic alterations without corresponding symptoms or neuropsychological deficits. Despite these advances, the field of neuroimaging has considerable ground to cover before becoming a reliable contributor in the diagnosis of concussions. Machine learning and the use of data classifiers has demonstrated the feasibility of such methods as DTI, functional MRI, or EEG to eventually be used in such a capacity. However, it is important to keep an open mind that neuroimaging in the context of a diagnostic method may be best used in conjunction with existing neuropsychological testing, the use of symptom reporting, or physiological biomarkers (see Chapter 19). As the definition of a concussion continues to evolve, evidence from neuroimaging should not be overlooked and is likely to play a future role in the diagnosis and clinical care of concussed patients.

# References

Ajao, D. O., V. Pop, J. E. Kamper, A. Adami, E. Rudobeck, L. Huang, R. Vlkolinsky et al. 2012. Traumatic brain injury in young rats leads to progressive behavioral deficits coincident with altered tissue properties in adulthood. *J Neurotrauma* 29 (11):2060–2074. doi:10.1089/neu.2011.1883.

Alexander, D. C. and G. J. Barker. 2005. Optimal imaging parameters for fiber-orientation estimation in diffusion MRI. *Neuroimage* 27 (2):357–367. doi:10.1016/j.neuroimage.2005.04.008.

Alhourani, A., T. A. Wozny, D. Krishnaswamy, S. Pathak, S. A. Walls, A. S. Ghuman, D. N. Krieger, D. O. Okonkwo, R. M. Richardson, and A. Niranjan. 2016. Magnetoencephalography-based identification of functional connectivity network disruption following mild traumatic brain injury. *J Neurophysiol* 116 (4):1840–1847. doi:10.1152/jn.00513.2016.

Aoki, Y., R. Inokuchi, M. Gunshin, N. Yahagi, and H. Suwa. 2012. Diffusion tensor imaging studies of mild traumatic brain injury: A meta-analysis. *J Neurol Neurosurg Psychiatr* 83(9):83:870–876. doi: 10.1136/jnnp-2012-302742.

Bailey, D. L. 2005. *Positron Emission Tomography: Basic Sciences.* New York: Springer.

Banks, S. D., R. A. Coronado, L. R. Clemons, C. M. Abraham, S. Pruthi, B. N. Conrad, V. L. Morgan, O. D. Guillamondegui, and K. R. Archer. 2016. Thalamic functional connectivity in mild traumatic brain injury: Longitudinal associations with patient-reported outcomes and neuropsychological tests. *Arch Phys Med Rehabil* 97 (8):1254–1261. doi:10.1016/j.apmr.2016.03.013.

Barr, W. B., L. S. Prichep, R. Chabot, M. R. Powell, and M. McCrea. 2012. Measuring brain electrical activity to track recovery from sport-related concussion. *Brain Inj* 26 (1):58–66. doi:10.3109/02699052.2011.608216.

Basser, P. J., J. Mattiello, and D. LeBihan. 1994. MR diffusion tensor spectroscopy and imaging. *Biophys J* 66 (1):259–267. doi:10.1016/S0006-3495(94)80775-1.

Bazarian, J. J., J. Zhong, B. Blyth, T. Zhu, V. Kavcic, and D. Peterson. 2007. Diffusion tensor imaging detects clinically important axonal damage after mild traumatic brain injury: A pilot study. *Journal of Neurotrauma* 24 (9):1447–1459. doi:10.1089/neu.2007.0241.

Bazarian, J. J., T. Zhu, J. Zhong, D. Janigro, E. Rozen, A. Roberts, H. Javien, K. Merchant-Borna, B. Abar, and E. G. Blackman. 2014. Persistent, long-term cerebral white matter changes after sports-related repetitive head impacts. *PLoS One* 9 (4):e94734. doi:10.1371/journal.pone.0094734.

Beauchamp, M. H., R. Beare, M. Ditchfield, L. Coleman, F. E. Babl, M. Kean, L. Crossley, C. Catroppa, K. O. Yeates, and V. Anderson. 2013. Susceptibility weighted imaging and its relationship to outcome after pediatric traumatic brain injury. *Cortex* 49 (2):591–598. doi:10.1016/j.cortex.2012.08.015.

Berman, J. I., M. R. Lanza, L. Blaskey, J. C. Edgar, and T. P. Roberts. 2013. High angular resolution diffusion imaging probabilistic tractography of the auditory radiation. *AJNR Am J Neuroradiol* 34 (8):1573–1578. doi:10.3174/ajnr. A3471.

Boas, D. A., G. Strangman, J. P. Culver, R. D. Hoge, G. Jasdzewski, R. A. Poldrack, B. R. Rosen, and J. B. Mandeville. 2003. Can the cerebral metabolic rate of oxygen be estimated with near-infrared spectroscopy? *Phys Med Biol* 48 (15):2405–2418.

Borich, M., N. Makan, L. Boyd, and N. Virji-Babul. 2013. Combining whole-brain voxel-wise analysis with in vivo tractography of diffusion behavior after sports-related concussion in adolescents: A preliminary report. *J Neurotrauma* 30 (14):1243–1249. doi:10.1089/neu.2012.2818.

Breedlove, E. L., M. Robinson, T. M. Talavage, K. E. Morigaki, U. Yoruk, K. O'Keefe, J. King, L. J. Leverenz, J. W. Gilger, and E. A. Nauman. 2012. Biomechanical correlates of symptomatic and asymptomatic neurophysiological impairment in high school football. *J Biomech* 45 (7):1265–1272. doi:10.1016/j.jbiomech.2012.01.034.

Broglio, S. P., M. B. Pontifex, P. O'Connor, and C. H. Hillman. 2009. The persistent effects of concussion on neuroelectric indices of attention. *J Neurotrauma* 26 (9):1463–1470. doi:10.1089/neu.2008-0766.

Bryer, E. J., J. D. Medaglia, S. Rostami, and F. G. Hillary. 2013. Neural recruitment after mild traumatic brain injury is task dependent: A meta-analysis. *J Int Neuropsychol Soc* 19 (7):751–762. doi:10.1017/S1355617713000490.

Byrnes, K. R., C. M. Wilson, F. Brabazon, R. von Leden, J. S. Jurgens, T. R. Oakes, and R. G. Selwyn. 2014. FDG-PET imaging in mild traumatic brain injury: A critical review. *Front Neuroenergetics* 5:13. doi:10.3389/fnene.2013.00013.

Cao, C. and S. Slobounov. 2010. Alteration of cortical functional connectivity as a result of traumatic brain injury revealed by graph theory, ICA, and sLORETA analyses of EEG signals. *IEEE Trans Neural Syst Rehabil Eng* 18 (1):11–19. doi:10.1109/TNSRE.2009.2027704.

Cao, C., R. L. Tutwiler, and S. Slobounov. 2008. Automatic classification of athletes with residual functional deficits following concussion by means of EEG signal using support vector machines. *IEEE Trans Neural Syst Rehabil Eng* 16 (4):327–335.

Casey, B. J., N. Tottenham, C. Liston, and S. Durston. 2005. Imaging the developing brain: What have we learned about cognitive development? *Trends Cogn Sci* 9 (3):104–110. doi:10.1016/j.tics.2005.01.011.

Catani, M., R. J. Howard, S. Pajevic, and D. K. Jones. 2002. Virtual in vivo interactive dissection of white matter fasciculi in the human brain. *Neuroimage* 17 (1):77–94.

Chen, J. K., K. M. Johnston, A. Collie, P. McCrory, and A. Ptito. 2007. A validation of the post concussion symptom scale in the assessment of complex concussion using cognitive testing and functional MRI. *J Neurol Neurosurg Psychiatry* 78 (11):1231–1238. doi:10.1136/jnnp.2006.110395.

Chen, J. K., K. M. Johnston, S. Frey, M. Petrides, K. Worsley, and A. Ptito. 2004. Functional abnormalities in symptomatic concussed athletes: An fMRI study. *Neuroimage* 22 (1):68–82. doi:10.1016/j.neuroimage.2003.12.032.

Chen, J. K., K. M. Johnston, M. Petrides, and A. Ptito. 2008. Recovery from mild head injury in sports: Evidence from serial functional magnetic resonance imaging studies in male athletes. *Clin J Sport Med* 18 (3):241–247.

Choe, M. C., T. Babikian, J. Difiori, D. A. Hovda, and C. C. Giza. 2012. A pediatric perspective on concussion pathophysiology. *Curr Opin Pediatr* 24 (6):689–695. doi:10.1097/MOP.0b013e32835a1a44.

Collins, C. L., E. N. Fletcher, S. K. Fields, L. Kluchurosky, M. K. Rohrkemper, R. D. Comstock, and R. C. Cantu. 2014. Neck strength: A protective factor reducing risk for concussion in high school sports. *J Prim Prev* 35 (5):309–319. doi:10.1007/s10935-014-0355-2.

Coughlin, J. M., Y. Wang, C. A. Munro, S. Ma, C. Yue, S. Chen, R. Airan et al. 2015. Neuroinflammation and brain atrophy in former NFL players: An in vivo multimodal imaging pilot study. *Neurobiol Dis* 74:58–65. doi:10.1016/j.nbd.2014.10.019.

Cubon, V. A., M. Putukian, C. Boyer, and A. Dettwiler. 2011. A diffusion tensor imaging study on the white matter skeleton in individuals with sports-related concussion. *J Neurotrauma* 28 (2):189–201. doi:10.1089/neu.2010.1430.

da Costa, L., A. Robertson, A. Bethune, M. J. MacDonald, P. N. Shek, M. J. Taylor, and E. W. Pang. 2015. Delayed and disorganised brain activation detected with magnetoencephalography after mild traumatic brain injury. *J Neurol Neurosurg Psychiatry* 86 (9):1008–1015. doi:10.1136/jnnp-2014-308571.

Daniel, J. 1896. The x-rays. *Science* 3 (67):562–563. doi:10.1126/science.3.67.562.

Deng, M., R. Yu, L. Wang, F. Shi, P. T. Yap, D. Shen, and Initiative Alzheimer's Disease Neuroimaging. 2016. Learning-based 3T brain MRI segmentation with guidance from 7T MRI labeling. *Med Phys* 43 (12):6588–6597. doi:10.1118/1.4967487.

Detre, J. A., J. Wang, Z. Wang, and H. Rao. 2009. Arterial spin-labeled perfusion MRI in basic and clinical neuroscience. *Curr Opin Neurol* 22 (4):348–355. doi:10.1097/WCO.0b013e32832d9505.

Dettwiler, A., M. Murugavel, M. Putukian, V. Cubon, J. Furtado, and D. Osherson. 2014. Persistent differences in patterns of brain activation after sports-related concussion: A longitudinal functional magnetic resonance imaging study. *J Neurotrauma* 31 (2):180–188. doi:10.1089/neu.2013.2983.

Di Russo, F. and D. Spinelli. 2010. Sport is not always healthy: Executive brain dysfunction in professional boxers. *Psychophysiology* 47 (3):425–434. doi:10.1111/j.1469-8986.2009.00950.x.

Dickstein, D. L., M. Y. Pullman, C. Fernandez, J. A. Short, L. Kostakoglu, K. Knesaurek, L. Soleimani et al. 2016. Cerebral [18 F]T807/AV1451 retention pattern in clinically probable CTE resembles pathognomonic distribution of CTE tauopathy. *Transl Psychiatry* 6 (9):e900. doi:10.1038/tp.2016.175.

Dimitriadis, S. I., G. Zouridakis, R. Rezaie, A. Babajani-Feremi, and A. C. Papanicolaou. 2015. Functional connectivity changes detected with magnetoencephalography after mild traumatic brain injury. *Neuroimage Clin* 9:519–531. doi:10.1016/j.nicl.2015.09.011.

Ferrari, M., L. Mottola, and V. Quaresima. 2004. Principles, techniques, and limitations of near infrared spectroscopy. *Can J Appl Physiol* 29 (4):463–487.

Gardner, A., G. L. Iverson, and P. Stanwell. 2014. A systematic review of proton magnetic resonance spectroscopy findings in sport-related concussion. *J Neurotrauma* 31 (1):1–18. doi:10.1089/neu.2013.3079.

Ge, Y., M. B. Patel, Q. Chen, E. J. Grossman, K. Zhang, L. Miles, J. S. Babb, J. Reaume, and R. I. Grossman. 2009. Assessment of thalamic perfusion in patients with mild traumatic brain injury by true FISP arterial spin labelling MR imaging at 3T. *Brain Inj* 23 (7):666–674. doi:10.1080/02699050903014899.

Gehring, W. J., Y. Liu, J. M. Orr, and J. Carp. 2012. The error-related negativity (ERN/Ne). *Oxford Handbook of Event-Related Potential Components* 231–291.

Giedd, J. N., J. Blumenthal, N. O. Jeffries, F. X. Castellanos, H. Liu, A. Zijdenbos, T. Paus, A. C. Evans, and J. L. Rapoport. 1999. Brain development during childhood and adolescence: A longitudinal MRI study. *Nat Neurosci* 2 (10):861–863. doi:10.1038/13158.

Ginsberg, M. D., W. Zhao, O. F. Alonso, J. Y. Loor-Estades, W. D. Dietrich, and R. Busto. 1997. Uncoupling of local cerebral glucose metabolism and blood flow after acute fluid-percussion injury in rats. *Am J Physiol* 272:H2859–H2868.

Giza, C. C. and D. A. Hovda. 2014. The new neurometabolic cascade of concussion. *Neurosurgery* 75:S24–S33. doi:10.1227/NEU.0000000000000505.

Gosselin, N., C. Bottari, J. K. Chen, S. C. Huntgeburth, L. De Beaumont, M. Petrides, B. Cheung, and A. Ptito. 2012. Evaluating the cognitive consequences of mild traumatic brain injury and concussion by using electrophysiology. *Neurosurg Focus* 33 (6):E7: 1–7. doi:10.3171/2012.10.FOCUS12253.

Gosselin, N., C. Bottari, J. K. Chen, M. Petrides, S. Tinawi, E. de Guise, and A. Ptito. 2011. Electrophysiology and functional MRI in post-acute mild traumatic brain injury. *J Neurotrauma* 28 (3):329–241. doi:10.1089/neu.2010.1493.

Gosselin, N., M. Theriault, S. Leclerc, J. Montplaisir, and M. Lassonde. 2006. Neurophysiological anomalies in symptomatic and asymptomatic concussed athletes. *Neurosurgery* 58 (6):1151–1161. doi:10.1227/01.NEU.0000215953.44097.FA.

Goswami, R., P. Dufort, M. C. Tartaglia, R. E. Green, A. Crawley, C. H. Tator, R. Wennberg, D. J. Mikulis, M. Keightley, and K. D. Davis. 2016. Frontotemporal correlates of impulsivity and machine learning in retired professional athletes with a history of multiple concussions. *Brain Struct Funct* 221 (4):1911–1925. doi:10.1007/s00429-015-1012-0.

Gross, H., A. Kling, G. Henry, C. Herndon, and H. Lavretsky. 1996. Local cerebral glucose metabolism in patients with long-term behavioral and cognitive deficits following mild traumatic brain injury. *J Neuropsychiatry Clin Neurosci* 8 (3):324–334. doi:10.1176/jnp.8.3.324.

Grossman, E. J., J. H. Jensen, J. S. Babb, Q. Chen, A. Tabesh, E. Fieremans, D. Xia, M. Inglese, and R. I. Grossman. 2013. Cognitive impairment in mild traumatic brain injury: A longitudinal diffusional kurtosis and perfusion imaging study. *AJNR Am J Neuroradiol* 34 (5):951–957, S1–S3. doi:10.3174/ajnr. A3358.

Grossman, E. J., Kirov, II, O. Gonen, D. S. Novikov, M. S. Davitz, Y. W. Lui, R. I. Grossman, M. Inglese, and E. Fieremans. 2015. N-acetyl-aspartate levels correlate with intra-axonal compartment parameters from diffusion MRI. *Neuroimage* 118:334–343. doi:10.1016/j.neuroimage.2015.05.061.

Haacke, E. M., Y. Xu, Y. C. Cheng, and J. R. Reichenbach. 2004. Susceptibility weighted imaging (SWI). *Magn Reson Med* 52 (3):612–618. doi:10.1002/mrm.20198.

Helmer, K. G., O. Pasternak, E. Fredman, R. I. Preciado, I. K. Koerte, T. Sasaki, M. Mayinger et al. 2014. Hockey concussion education project, part 1. Susceptibility-weighted imaging study in male and female ice hockey players over a single season. *J Neurosurg* 120 (4):864–872. doi:10.3171/2013.12.JNS132093.

Helmich, I., R. S. Saluja, H. Lausberg, M. Kempe, P. Furley, A. Berger, J. K. Chen, and A. Ptito. 2015. Persistent postconcussive symptoms are accompanied by decreased functional brain oxygenation. *J Neuropsychiatry Clin Neurosci* 27 (4):287–298. doi:10.1176/appi.neuropsych.14100276.

Henry, L.C., S. Tremblay, Y. Boulanger, D. Ellemberg, and M. Lassonde. 2010. Neurometabolic change in the acute phase after sports concussion correlate with symptom severity. *J Neurotrauma* 27 (1):65–76.

Honce, J. M., E. Nyberg, I. Jones, and L. Nagae. 2016. Neuroimaging of concussion. *Phys Med Rehabil Clin N Am* 27 (2):411–428. doi:10.1016/j.pmr.2016.01.002.

Hsu, H. L., D. Y. Chen, Y. C. Tseng, Y. S. Kuo, Y. L. Huang, W. T. Chiu, F. X. Yan, W. S. Wang, and C. J. Chen. 2015. Sex differences in working memory after mild traumatic brain injury: A functional MR imaging study. *Radiology* 276 (3):828–835. doi:10.1148/radiol.2015142549.

Huang, M. X., R. J. Theilmann, A. Robb, A. Angeles, S. Nichols, A. Drake, J. D'Andrea et al. 2009. Integrated imaging approach with MEG and DTI to detect mild traumatic brain injury in military and civilian patients. *J Neurotrauma* 26 (8):1213–1226. doi:10.1089/neu.2008.0672.

Huettel, S. A., A. W. Song, and G. McCarthy. 2014. *Functional Magnetic Resonance Imaging* (3rd ed). Sunderland, MA: Sinauer Associates, Inc., Publishers.

Hulkower, M. B., D. B. Poliak, S. B. Rosenbaum, M. E. Zimmerman, and M. L. Lipton. 2013. A decade of DTI in traumatic brain injury: 10 years and 100 articles later. *AJNR Am J Neuroradiol* 34 (11):2064–2074. doi:10.3174/ajnr. A3395.

Humayun, M. S., S. K. Presty, N. D. Lafrance, H. H. Holcomb, H. Loats, D. M. Long, H. N. Wagner, and B. Gordon. 1989. Local cerebral glucose abnormalities in mild closed head injured patients with cognitive impairments. *Nucl Med Commun* 10 (5):335–344.

Ilvesmaki, T., T. M. Luoto, U. Hakulinen, A. Brander, P. Ryymin, H. Eskola, G. L. Iverson, and J. Ohman. 2014. Acute mild traumatic brain injury is not associated with white matter change on diffusion tensor imaging. *Brain* 137 (Pt 7):1876–1882. doi:10.1093/brain/awu095.

Irimia, A., S. Y. Goh, C. M. Torgerson, N. R. Stein, M. C. Chambers, P. M. Vespa, and J. D. Van Horn. 2013. Electroencephalographic inverse localization of brain activity in acute traumatic brain injury as a guide to surgery, monitoring and treatment. *Clin Neurol Neurosurg* 115 (10):2159–2165. doi:10.1016/j.clineuro.2013.08.003.

Jantzen, K. J., B. Anderson, F. L. Steinberg, and J. A. S. Kelso. 2004. A prospective functional MR imaging study of mild traumatic brain injury in college football players. *AJNR Am J Neuroradiol* 25 (5):738–745.

Johnson, B., K. Zhang, M. Gay, T. Neuberger, S. Horovitz, M. Hallett, W. Sebastianelli, and S. Slobounov. 2012. Metabolic alterations in corpus callosum may compromise brain functional connectivity in MTBI patients: An 1H-MRS study. *Neurosci Lett* 509 (1):5–8. doi:10.1016/j.neulet.2011.11.013.

Kane, M. J., A. R. Conway, T. K. Miura, and G. J. Colflesh. 2007. Working memory, attention control, and the N-back task: A question of construct validity. *J Exp Psychol Learn Mem Cogn* 33 (3):615–622. doi:10.1037/0278-7393.33.3.615.

Karamzadeh, N., F. Amyot, K. Kenney, A. Anderson, F. Chowdhry, H. Dashtestani, E. M. Wassermann et al. 2016. A machine learning approach to identify functional biomarkers in human prefrontal cortex for individuals with traumatic brain injury using functional near-infrared spectroscopy. *Brain Behav* 6 (11):e00541. doi:10.1002/brb3.541.

Keightley, M. L., J. K. Chen, and A. Ptito. 2012. Examining the neural impact of pediatric concussion: A scoping review of multimodal and integrative approaches using functional and structural MRI techniques. *Curr Opin Pediatr* 24 (6):709–716. doi:10.1097/MOP.0b013e3283599a55.

Keightley, M. L., R. S. Saluja, J. K. Chen, I. Gagnon, G. Leonard, M. Petrides, and A. Ptito. 2014a. A functional magnetic resonance imaging study of working memory in youth after sports-related concussion: Is it still working? *J Neurotrauma* 31 (5):437–451. doi:10.1089/neu.2013.3052.

Keightley, M., K. J. Sinopoli, J. K. Chen, A. Ptito, T. Taha, G. Wells, and P. Fait. 2014b. Cortical thinning following sports-related mTBI: The relationship between MRI findings and dual-task performance in youth. *Arch Phys Med Rehabil* 95:e68.

Kierans, A. S., Kirov, II, O. Gonen, G. Haemer, E. Nisenbaum, J. S. Babb, R. I. Grossman, and Y. W. Lui. 2014. Myoinositol and glutamate complex neurometabolite abnormality after mild traumatic brain injury. *Neurology* 82 (6):521–528. doi:10.1212/WNL.0000000000000105.

Koerte, I. K., B. Ertl-Wagner, M. Reiser, R. Zafonte, and M. E. Shenton. 2012. White matter integrity in the brains of professional soccer players without a symptomatic concussion. *JAMA* 308 (18):1859–1861. doi:10.1001/jama.2012.13735.

Kontos, A. P., T. J. Huppert, N. H. Beluk, R. J. Elbin, L. C. Henry, J. French, S. M. Dakan, and M. W. Collins. 2014. Brain activation during neurocognitive testing using functional near-infrared spectroscopy in patients following concussion compared to healthy controls. *Brain Imaging Behav* 8 (4):621–634. doi:10.1007/s11682-014-9289-9.

Kraus, M. F., T. Susmaras, B. P. Caughlin, C. J. Walker, J. A. Sweeney, and D. M. Little. 2007. White matter integrity and cognition in chronic traumatic brain injury: A diffusion tensor imaging study. *Brain* 130 (Pt 10):2508–2519. doi:10.1093/brain/awm216.

Kraus, N., E. C. Thompson, J. Krizman, K. Cook, T. White-Schwoch, and C. R. LaBella. 2016. Auditory biological marker of concussion in children. *Sci Rep* 6:39009. doi:10.1038/srep39009.

Krivitzky, L. S., T. M. Roebuck-Spencer, R. M. Roth, K. Blackstone, C. P. Johnson, and G. Gioia. 2011. Functional magnetic resonance imaging of working memory and response inhibition in children with mild traumatic brain injury. *J Int Neuropsychol Soc* 17 (6):1143–1152. doi:10.1017/S1355617711001226.

Kumar, R., R. K. Gupta, M. Husain, C. Chaudhry, A. Srivastava, S. Saksena, and R. K. Rathore. 2009. Comparative evaluation of corpus callosum DTI metrics in acute mild and moderate traumatic brain injury: Its correlation with neuropsychometric tests. *Brain Inj* 23 (7):675–685. doi:10.1080/02699050903014915.

Lareau, E., F. Lesage, P. Pouliot, D. Nguyen, J. Le Lan, and M. Sawan. 2011. Multichannel wearable system dedicated for simultaneous electroencephalographynear-infrared spectroscopy real-time data acquisitions. *J Biomed Opt* 16 (9):096014. doi:10.1117/1.3625575.

Le Bihan, D., C. Poupon, A. Amadon, and F. Lethimonnier. 2006. Artifacts and pitfalls in diffusion MRI. *J Magn Reson Imaging* 24 (3):478–488. doi:10.1002/jmri.20683.

Lee, R. R. and M. Huang. 2014. Magnetoencephalography in the diagnosis of concussion. *Prog Neurol Surg* 28:94–111. doi:10.1159/000358768.

Lewine, J. D., J. T. Davis, E. D. Bigler, R. Thoma, D. Hill, M. Funke, J. H. Sloan, S. Hall, and W. W. Orrison. 2007. Objective documentation of traumatic brain injury subsequent to mild head trauma: Multimodal brain imaging with MEG, SPECT, and MRI. *J Head Trauma Rehabil* 22 (3):141–155. doi:10.1097/01.HTR.0000271115.29954.27.

Li, N., W. T. Wang, D. L. Pham, and J. A. Butman. 2015. Artifactual microhemorrhage generated by susceptibility weighted image processing. *J Magn Reson Imaging* 41 (6):1695–1700. doi:10.1002/jmri.24728.

Lin, C. M., Y. C. Tseng, H. L. Hsu, C. J. Chen, D. Y. Chen, F. X. Yan, and W. T. Chiu. 2016. Arterial spin labeling perfusion study in the patients with subacute mild traumatic brain injury. *PLoS One* 11 (2):e0149109. doi:10.1371/journal.pone.0149109.

Ling, J. M., A. Pena, R. A. Yeo, F. L. Merideth, S. Klimaj, C. Gasparovic, and A. R. Mayer. 2012. Biomarkers of increased diffusion anisotropy in semi-acute mild traumatic brain injury: A longitudinal perspective. *Brain* 135 (Pt 4):1281–1292. doi:10.1093/brain/aws073.

Lipton, M. L., E. Gellella, C. Lo, T. Gold, B. A. Ardekani, K. Shifteh, J. A. Bello, and C. A. Branch. 2008. Multifocal white matter ultrastructural abnormalities in mild traumatic brain injury with cognitive disability: A voxel-wise analysis of diffusion tensor imaging. *Journal of Neurotrauma* 25 (11):1335–1342. doi:10.1089/neu.2008.0547.

Liu, G., P. Ghimire, H. Pang, G. Wu, and H. Shi. 2015. Improved sensitivity of 3.0 Tesla susceptibility-weighted imaging in detecting traumatic bleeds and its use in predicting outcomes in patients with mild traumatic brain injury. *Acta Radiol* 56 (10):1256–1263. doi:10.1177/0284185114552883.

Lovell, M. R., J. E. Pardini, J. Welling, M. W. Collins, J. Bakal, N. Lazar, R. Roush, W. F. Eddy, and J. T. Becker. 2007. Functional brain abnormalities are related to clinical recovery and time to return-to-play in athletes. *Neurosurgery* 61 (2):352–360. doi:10.1227/01.neu.0000279985.94168.7f.

Luck, S. J. 2005. *An Introduction to Event-Related Potentials and their Neural Origins* (Chapter 1). Cambridge, MA: MIT Press.

Lui, Y. W., Y. Xue, D. Kenul, Y. Ge, R. I. Grossman, and Y. Wang. 2014. Classification algorithms using multiple MRI features in mild traumatic brain injury. *Neurology* 83:1235–1240.

Luna, B., A. Padmanabhan, and K. O'Hearn. 2010. What has fMRI told us about the development of cognitive control through adolescence? *Brain Cogn* 72 (1):101–113. doi:10.1016/j.bandc.2009.08.005.

Lusebrink, F., A. Wollrab, and O. Speck. 2013. Cortical thickness determination of the human brain using high resolution 3T and 7T MRI data. *Neuroimage* 70:122–131. doi:10.1016/j.neuroimage.2012.12.016.

Maas, A.I., D. K. Menon, E. W. Steyerberg, G. Citerio, F. Lecky, G. T. Manley, S. Hill, V. Legrand, A. Sorgner (on behalf of CENTER-TBI Participants and Investigators). 2015. Collaborative European neurotrauma effectiveness research in traumatic brain injury (Center-TBI): A prospective longitudinal observational study. *Neurosurgery* 76 (1):67–80.

Mandera, M., D. Larysz, and M. Wojtacha. 2002. Changes in cerebral hemodynamics assessed by transcranial Doppler ultrasonography in children after head injury. *Childs Nerv Syst* 18 (3–4):124–128. doi:10.1007/s00381-002-0572-5.

Mathias, J. L. and P. Wheaton. 2015. Contribution of brain or biological reserve and cognitive or neural reserve to outcome after TBI: A meta-analysis (prior to 2015). *Neurosci Biobehav Rev* 55:573–593. doi:10.1016/j.neubiorev.2015.06.001.

Mayer, A. R., M. V. Mannell, J. Ling, R. Elgie, C. Gasparovic, J. P. Phillips, D. Doezema, and R. A. Yeo. 2009. Auditory orienting and inhibition of return in mild traumatic brain injury: A FMRI study. *Hum Brain Mapp* 30 (12):4152–4166. doi:10.1002/hbm.20836.

McAllister, T. W., L. A. Flashman, B. C. McDonald, and A. J. Saykin. 2006. Mechanisms of working memory dysfunction after mild and moderate TBI: Evidence from functional MRI and neurogenetics. *J Neurotrauma* 23 (10):1450–1467. doi:10.1089/neu.2006.23.1450.

McAllister, T. W., J. C. Ford, L. A. Flashman, A. Maerlender, R. M. Greenwald, J. G. Beckwith, R. P. Bolander et al. 2014. Effect of head impacts on diffusivity measures in a cohort of collegiate contact sport athletes. *Neurology* 82 (1):63–69. doi:10.1212/01.wnl.0000438220.16190.42.

McAllister, T. W., A. J. Saykin, L. A. Flashman, M. B. Sparling, S. C. Johnson, S. J. Guerin, A. C. Mamourian, J. B. Weaver, and N. Yanofsky. 1999. Brain activation during working memory 1 month after mild traumatic brain injury. *Neurology* 53 (6):1300–1308.

McAllister, T. W., M. B. Sparling, L. A. Flashman, S. J. Guerin, A. C. Mamourian, and A. J. Saykin. 2001. Differential working memory load effects after mild traumatic brain injury. *Neuroimage* 14 (5):1004–1012. doi:10.1006/nimg.2001.0899.

McCrea, M., L. Prichep, M. R. Powell, R. Chabot, and W. B. Barr. 2010. Acute effects and recovery after sport-related concussion: A neurocognitive and quantitative brain electrical activity study. *J Head Trauma Rehabil* 25 (4):283–292. doi:10.1097/HTR.0b013e3181e67923.

McDonald, B. C., A. J. Saykin, and T. W. McAllister. 2012. Functional MRI of mild traumatic brain injury (mTBI): Progress and perspectives from the first decade of studies. *Brain Imaging Behav* 6 (2):193–207. doi:10.1007/s11682-012-9173-4.

Messe, A., S. Caplain, G. Paradot, D. Garrigue, J. F. Mineo, G. Soto Ares, D. Ducreux et al. 2011. Diffusion tensor imaging and white matter lesions at the subacute stage in mild traumatic brain injury with persistent neurobehavioral impairment. *Hum Brain Mapp* 32 (6):999–1011. doi:10.1002/hbm.21092.

Messe, A., S. Caplain, M. Pelegrini-Issac, S. Blancho, R. Levy, N. Aghakhani, M. Montreuil, H. Benali, and S. Lehericy. 2013. Specific and evolving resting-state network alterations in post-concussion syndrome following mild traumatic brain injury. *PLoS One* 8 (6):e65470. doi:10.1371/journal.pone.0065470.

Meyer, E. 1998. Personal communication: Basics of positron emission tomography.

Mitra, J., K. K. Shen, S. Ghose, P. Bourgeat, J. Fripp, O. Salvado, K. Pannek, D. J. Taylor, J. L. Mathias, and S. Rose. 2016. Statistical machine learning to identify traumatic brain injury (TBI) from structural disconnections of white matter networks. *Neuroimage* 129:247–259. doi:10.1016/j.neuroimage.2016.01.056.

Morgan, C. D., S. L. Zuckerman, Y. M. Lee, L. King, S. Beaird, A. K. Sills, and G. S. Solomon. 2015. Predictors of postconcussion syndrome after sports-related concussion in young athletes: A matched case-control study. *J Neurosurg Pediatr* 15 (6):589–598. doi:10.3171/2014.10.PEDS14356.

Mori, S. and J. Zhang. 2006. Principles of diffusion tensor imaging and its applications to basic neuroscience research. *Neuron* 51 (5):527–539. doi:10.1016/j.neuron.2006.08.012.

Nakamura, T., F. G. Hillary, and B. B. Biswal. 2009. Resting network plasticity following brain injury. *PLoS One* 4 (12):e8220. doi:10.1371/journal.pone.0008220.

Niogi, S. N., P. Mukherjee, J. Ghajar, C. Johnson, R. A. Kolster, R. Sarkar, H. Lee et al. 2008. Extent of microstructural white matter injury in postconcussive syndrome correlates with impaired cognitive reaction time: A 3T diffusion tensor imaging study of mild traumatic brain injury. *AJNR Am J Neuroradiol* 29 (5):967–973. doi:10.3174/ajnr. A0970.

Orr, C. A., M. D. Albaugh, R. Watts, H. Garavan, T. Andrews, J. P. Nickerson, J. Gonyea et al. 2016. Neuroimaging biomarkers of a history of concussion observed in asymptomatic young athletes. *J Neurotrauma* 33 (9):803–810. doi:10.1089/neu.2014.3721.

Pardini, J. E., D. A. Pardini, J. T. Becker, K. L. Dunfee, W. F. Eddy, M. R. Lovell, and J. S. Welling. 2010. Postconcussive symptoms are associated with compensatory cortical recruitment during a working memory task. *Neurosurgery* 67 (4):1020–1028. doi:10.1227/NEU.0b013e3181ee33e2.

Park, J., S. Park, S. Kang, T. Nam, B. Min, and S. Hwang. 2009. Detection of traumatic cerebral microbleeds by susceptiblity-weighted image of MRI. *J Korean Neurosurg Soc* 46:365–369.

Pasco, A., L. Lemaire, F. Franconi, Y. Lefur, F. Noury, J. P. Saint-Andre, J. P. Benoit, P. J. Cozzone, and J. J. Le Jeune. 2007. Perfusional deficit and the dynamics of cerebral edemas in experimental traumatic brain injury using perfusion and diffusion-weighted magnetic resonance imaging. *J Neurotrauma* 24 (8):1321–1330. doi:10.1089/neu.2006.0136.

Paus, T. 2005. Mapping brain maturation and cognitive development during adolescence. *Trends Cogn Sci* 9 (2):60–68. doi:10.1016/j.tics.2004.12.008.

Peskind, E. R., E. C. Petrie, D. J. Cross, K. Pagulayan, K. McCraw, D. Hoff, K. Hart et al. 2011. Cerebrocerebellar hypometabolism associated with repetitive blast exposure mild traumatic brain injury in 12 Iraq war Veterans with persistent post-concussive symptoms. *Neuroimage* 54 Suppl 1:S76–S82. doi:10.1016/j.neuroimage.2010.04.008.

Petcharunpaisan, S., J. Ramalho, and M. Castillo. 2010. Arterial spin labeling in neuroimaging. *World J Radiol* 2 (10):384–398. doi:10.4329/wjr.v2.i10.384.

Petersen, E. T., T. Lim, and X. Golay. 2006. Model-free arterial spin labeling quantification approach for perfusion MRI. *Magn Reson Med* 55 (2):219–232. doi:10.1002/mrm.20784.

Petrides, M. 2005. Lateral prefrontal cortex: Architectonic and functional organization. *Philos Trans R Soc Lond B Biol Sci* 360 (1456):781–795. doi:10.1098/rstb.2005.1631.

Petrides, M. 2013. The mid-dorsolateral prefronto-parietal network and the epoptic process. In Stuss, D. T. and R. T. Knight (Eds.). *Principles of Frontal Lobe Function*, pp. 79–89. New York: Oxford University Press.

Petrides, M., S. Frey, and J. K. Chen. 2001. Increased activation of the mid-dorsolateral frontal cortex during the monitoring of abstract visual and verbal stimuli. *Neuroimage* 13 (6):721. doi:10.1016/s1053-8119(01)92064-6.

Polich, J. 2007. Updating P300: An integrative theory of P3a and P3b. *Clin Neurophysiol* 118 (10):2128–2148. doi:10.1016/j.clinph.2007.04.019.

Pollock, J. M., H. Tan, R. A. Kraft, C. T. Whitlow, J. H. Burdette, and J. A. Maldjian. 2009. Arterial spin-labeled MR perfusion imaging: Clinical applications. *Magn Reson Imaging Clin N Am* 17 (2):315–338. doi:10.1016/j.mric.2009.01.008.

Pontifex, M. B., P. M. O'Connor, S. P. Broglio, and C. H. Hillman. 2009. The association between mild traumatic brain injury history and cognitive control. *Neuropsychologia* 47 (14):3210–3216. doi:10.1016/j.neuropsychologia.2009.07.021.

Pradhan, S., S. Bonekamp, J. S. Gillen, L. M. Rowland, S. A. Wijtenburg, R. A. Edden, and P. B. Barker. 2015. Comparison of single voxel brain MRS AT 3T and 7T using 32-channel head coils. *Magn Reson Imaging* 33 (8):1013–1018. doi:10.1016/j.mri.2015.06.003.

Preiss-Farzanegan, S. J., B. Chapman, T. M. Wong, J. Wu, and J. J. Bazarian. 2009. The relationship between gender and postconcussion symptoms after sport-related mild traumatic brain injury. *PM R* 1 (3):245–253. doi:10.1016/j.pmrj.2009.01.011.

Presson, N., D. Krishnaswamy, L. Wagener, W. Bird, K. Jarbo, S. Pathak, A. M. Puccio et al. 2015. Quantifying white matter structural integrity with high-definition fiber tracking in traumatic brain injury. *Mil Med* 180 (3 Suppl):109–121. doi:10.7205/MILMED-D-14-00413.

Prichep, L. S., A. Jacquin, J. Filipenko, S. G. Dastidar, S. Zabele, A. Vodencarevic, and N. S. Rothman. 2012. Classification of traumatic brain injury severity using informed data reduction in a series of binary classifier algorithms. *IEEE Trans Neural Syst Rehabil Eng* 20 (6):806–822. doi:10.1109/TNSRE.2012.2206609.

Proudfoot, M., M. W. Woolrich, A. C. Nobre, and M. R. Turner. 2014. Magnetoencephalography. *Pract Neurol* 14 (5):336–343. doi:10.1136/practneurol-2013-000768.

Ramlackhansingh, A. F., D. J. Brooks, R. J. Greenwood, S. K. Bose, F. E. Turkheimer, K. M. Kinnunen, S. Gentleman et al. 2011. Inflammation after trauma: Microglial activation and traumatic brain injury. *Ann Neurol* 70 (3):374–383. doi:10.1002/ana.22455.

Rapp, P. E., D. O. Keyser, A. Albano, R. Hernandez, D. B. Gibson, R. A. Zambon, W. D. Hairston, J. D. Hughes, A. Krystal, and A. S. Nichols. 2015. Traumatic brain injury detection using electrophysiological methods. *Front Hum Neurosci* 9:11. doi:10.3389/fnhum.2015.00011.

Robb Swan, A., S. Nichols, A. Drake, A. Angeles, M. Diwakar, T. Song, R. R. Lee, and M. X. Huang. 2015. Magnetoencephalography slow-wave detection in patients with mild traumatic brain injury and ongoing symptoms correlated with long-term neuropsychological outcome. *J Neurotrauma* 32 (19):1510–1521. doi:10.1089/neu.2014.3654.

Roberts, M. A., F. F. Manshadi, D. L. Bushnell, and M. E. Hines. 1995. Neurobehavioural dysfunction following mild traumatic brain injury in childhood: A case report with positive findings on positron emission tomography (PET). *Brain Inj* 9 (5):427–436.

Ruff, R. M., J. A. Crouch, A. I. Troster, L. F. Marshall, M. S. Buchsbaum, S. Lottenberg, and L. M. Somers. 1994. Selected cases of poor outcome following a minor brain trauma: Comparing neuropsychological and positron emission tomography assessment. *Brain Inj* 8 (4):297–308.

Rutgers, D. R., P. Fillard, G. Paradot, M. Tadie, P. Lasjaunias, and D. Ducreux. 2008a. Diffusion tensor imaging characteristics of the corpus callosum in mild, moderate, and severe traumatic brain injury. *AJNR Am J Neuroradiol* 29 (9):1730–1735. doi:10.3174/ajnr. A1213.

Rutgers, D. R., F. Toulgoat, J. Cazejust, P. Fillard, P. Lasjaunias, and D. Ducreux. 2008b. White matter abnormalities in mild traumatic brain injury: A diffusion tensor imaging study. *AJNR Am J Neuroradiol* 29 (3):514–519. doi:10.3174/ajnr. A0856.

Saluja, R. S., J. K. Chen, I. J. Gagnon, M. Keightley, and A. Ptito. 2015. Navigational memory functional magnetic resonance imaging: A test for concussion in children. *J Neurotrauma* 32 (10):712–722. doi:10.1089/neu.2014.3470.

Sawan, M., M. T. Salam, J. Le Lan, A. Kassab, S. Gelinas, P. Vannasing, F. Lesage, M. Lassonde, and D. K. Nguyen. 2013. Wireless recording systems: From noninvasive EEG-NIRS to invasive EEG devices. *IEEE Trans Biomed Circuits Syst* 7 (2):186–195. doi:10.1109/TBCAS.2013.2255595.

Schmitt, S. and M. A. Dichter. 2015. Electrophysiologic recordings in traumatic brain injury. *Handb Clin Neurol* 127:319–339. doi:10.1016/B978-0-444-52892-6.00021-0.

Shenton, M. E., H. M. Hamoda, J. S. Schneiderman, S. Bouix, O. Pasternak, Y. Rathi, M. A. Vu et al. 2012. A review of magnetic resonance imaging and diffusion tensor imaging findings in mild traumatic brain injury. *Brain Imaging Behav* 6 (2):137–192. doi:10.1007/s11682-012-9156-5.

Sikoglu, E. M., A. A. Liso Navarro, S. M. Czerniak, J. McCafferty, J. Eisenstock, J. H. Stevenson, J. A. King, and C. M. Moore. 2015. Effects of recent concussion on brain bioenergetics: A phosphorus-31 magnetic resonance spectroscopy study. *Cogn Behav Neurol* 28 (4):181–187. doi:10.1097/WNN.0000000000000076.

Slobounov, S. M., K. Zhang, D. Pennell, W. Ray, B. Johnson, and W. Sebastianelli. 2010. Functional abnormalities in normally appearing athletes following mild traumatic brain injury: A functional MRI study. *Exp Brain Res* 202 (2):341–354. doi:10.1007/s00221-009-2141-6.

Smith, S. M., P. T. Fox, K. L. Miller, D. C. Glahn, P. M. Fox, C. E. Mackay, N. Filippini et al. 2009. Correspondence of the brain's functional architecture during activation and rest. *Proc Natl Acad Sci U S A* 106 (31):13040–13045. doi:10.1073/pnas.0905267106.

Smits, M., D. W. Dippel, G. C. Houston, P. A. Wielopolski, P. J. Koudstaal, M. G. Hunink, and A. van der Lugt. 2009. Postconcussion syndrome after minor head injury: Brain activation of working memory and attention. *Hum Brain Mapp* 30 (9):2789–2803. doi:10.1002/hbm.20709.

Sowell, E. R., P. M. Thompson, K. D. Tessner, and A. W. Toga. 2001. Mapping continued brain growth and gray matter density reduction in dorsal frontal cortex: Inverse relationships during post-adolescent brain maturation. *J Neurosci* 21 (22):8819–8829.

Spiers, H. J. and E. A. Maguire. 2007. The neuroscience of remote spatial memory: A tale of two cities. *Neuroscience* 149 (1):7–27. doi:10.1016/j.neuroscience.2007.06.056.

Spitz, G., Y. Alway, K. R. Gould, and J. L. Ponsford. 2016. Disrupted white matter microstructure and mood disorders after traumatic brain injury. *J Neurotrauma* 34 (4):807–815. doi:10.1089/neu.2016.4527.

Stulemeijer, M., P. E. Vos, S. van der Werf, G. van Dijk, M. Rijpkema, and G. Fernandez. 2010. How mild traumatic brain injury may affect declarative memory performance in the post-acute stage. *J Neurotrauma* 27 (9):1585–1595. doi:10.1089/neu.2010.1298.

Sumowski, J. F., N. Chiaravalloti, D. Krch, J. Paxton, and J. Deluca. 2013. Education attenuates the negative impact of traumatic brain injury on cognitive status. *Arch Phys Med Rehabil* 94 (12):2562–2564. doi:10.1016/j.apmr.2013.07.023.

Sundman, M., P. M. Doraiswamy, and R. A. Morey. 2015. Neuroimaging assessment of early and late neurobiological sequelae of traumatic brain injury: Implications for CTE. *Front Neurosci* 9:334. doi:10.3389/fnins.2015.00334.

Taber, K. H., R. A. Hurley, C. C. Haswell, J. A. Rowland, S. D. Hurt, C. D. Lamar, and R. A. Morey. 2015. White matter compromise in veterans exposed to primary blast forces. *J Head Trauma Rehabil* 30 (1):E15–E25. doi:10.1097/HTR.0000000000000030.

Talavage, T. M., E. A. Nauman, E. L. Breedlove, U. Yoruk, A. E. Dye, K. E. Morigaki, H. Feuer, and L. J. Leverenz. 2014. Functionally-detected cognitive impairment in high school football players without clinically-diagnosed concussion. *J Neurotrauma* 31 (4):327–338. doi:10.1089/neu.2010.1512.

Tsirka, V., P. G. Simos, A. Vakis, K. Kanatsouli, M. Vourkas, S. Erimaki, E. Pachou, C. J. Stam, and S. Micheloyannis. 2011. Mild traumatic brain injury: Graph-model characterization of brain networks for episodic memory. *Int J Psychophysiol* 79 (2):89–96. doi:10.1016/j.ijpsycho.2010.09.006.

Tuch, D. S. 2004. Q-ball imaging. *Magn Reson Med* 52 (6):1358–1372. doi:10.1002/mrm.20279.

Umile, E. M., M. E. Sandel, A. Alavi, C. M. Terry, and R. C. Plotkin. 2002. Dynamic imaging in mild traumatic brain injury: Support for the theory of medial temporal vulnerability. *Arch Phys Med Rehabil* 83 (11):1506–1513.

Urban, K. J., K. M. Barlow, J. J. Jimenez, B. G. Goodyear, and J. F. Dunn. 2015. Functional near-infrared spectroscopy reveals reduced interhemispheric cortical communication after pediatric concussion. *J Neurotrauma* 32 (11):833–840. doi:10.1089/neu.2014.3577.

Vagnozzi, R., S. Signoretti, B. Tavazzi, R. Floris, A. Ludovici, S. Marziali, G. Tarascio et al. 2008. Temporal window of metabolic brain vulnerability to concussion: A pilot 1H-magnetic resonance spectroscopic study in concussed athletes-part III. *Neurosurgery* 62 (6):1286–1296. doi:10.1227/01.NEU.0000316421.58568.AD.

Vakorin, V. A., S. M. Doesburg, L. da Costa, R. Jetly, E. W. Pang, and M. J. Taylor. 2016. Detecting mild traumatic brain injury using resting state magnetoencephalographic connectivity. *PLoS Comput Biol* 12 (12):e1004914. doi:10.1371/journal.pcbi.1004914.

Vergara, V. M., A. R. Mayer, E. Damaraju, K. A. Kiehl, and V. Calhoun. 2017. Detection of mild traumatic brain injury by machine learning classification using resting state functional network connectivity and fractional anisotropy. *J Neurotrauma* 34 (5):1045–1053. doi:10.1089/neu.2016.4526.

Vu, A. T., K. Jamison, M. F. Glasser, S. M. Smith, T. Coalson, S. Moeller, E. J. Auerbach, K. Ugurbil, and E. Yacoub. 2016. Tradeoffs in pushing the spatial resolution of fMRI for the 7T human connectome project. *Neuroimage* 154:23–32. doi:10.1016/j.neuroimage.2016.11.049.

Wang, Y., J. D. West, J. N. Bailey, D. R. Westfall, H. Xiao, T. W. Arnold, P. A. Kersey, A. J. Saykin, and B. C. McDonald. 2015. Decreased cerebral blood flow in chronic pediatric mild TBI: An MRI perfusion study. *Dev Neuropsychol* 40 (1):40–44. doi:10.1080/87565641.2014.979927.

Wilde, E. A., S. R. McCauley, J. V. Hunter, E. D. Bigler, Z. Chu, Z. J. Wang, G. R. Hanten et al. 2008. Diffusion tensor imaging of acute mild traumatic brain injury in adolescents. *Neurology* 70:948–955.

Wilke, M., V. J. Schmithorst, and S. K. Holland. 2003. Normative pediatric brain data for spatial normalization and segmentation differs from standard adult data. *Magn Reson Med* 50 (4):749–757. doi:10.1002/mrm.10606.

Witt, S. T., D. W. Lovejoy, G. D. Pearlson, and M. C. Stevens. 2010. Decreased prefrontal cortex activity in mild traumatic brain injury during performance of an auditory oddball task. *Brain Imaging Behav* 4 (3–4):232–247. doi:10.1007/s11682-010-9102-3.

Wolf, R. L. and J. A. Detre. 2007. Clinical neuroimaging using arterial spin-labeled perfusion MRI. *Neurotherapeutics* 4 (3):346–359.

Yadav, K., E. Sarioglu, H. A. Choi, W. B. Cartwright, P. S. Hinds, and J. M. Chamberlain. 2016. Automated outcome classification of computed tomography imaging reports for pediatric traumatic brain injury. *Acad Emerg Med* 23 (2):171–178. doi:10.1111/acem.12859.

Yang, Z., R. A. Yeo, A. Pena, J. M. Ling, S. Klimaj, R. Campbell, D. Doezema, and A. R. Mayer. 2012. An FMRI study of auditory orienting and inhibition of return in pediatric mild traumatic brain injury. *Journal of Neurotrauma* 29 (12):2124–2136. doi:10.1089/neu.2012.2395.

Zhou, Y. 2016. Small world properties changes in mild traumatic brain injury. *J Magn Reson Imaging* 46 (2):518–527. doi:10.1002/jmri.25548.

Zhu, D. C., T. Covassin, S. Nogle, S. Doyle, D. Russell, R. L. Pearson, J. Monroe, C. M. Liszewski, J. K. DeMarco, and D. I. Kaufman. 2015. A potential biomarker in sports-related concussion: Brain functional connectivity alteration of the default-mode network measured with longitudinal resting-state fMRI over thirty days. *J Neurotrauma* 32 (5):327–341. doi:10.1089/neu.2014.3413.

*chapter twenty one*

# Emerging treatments
## What is coming up in terms of the use of technology for treatment of concussion?

*Lisa Koski*

## Contents

## Introduction

A bewildering array of interventions can be discovered by individuals who have suffered a head injury. Those affected by traumatic brain injury (TBI) are often frustrated by the limited support from the medical establishment for interventions that have not undergone rigorous scientific study to demonstrate their effectiveness at promoting recovery. On the plus side, increasing resources are being applied to studies aimed at investigating more novel treatment approaches, particularly those that modulate the central nervous system, with the goal of bringing them into the mainstream.

In this chapter, we present information on a wide variety of emerging therapies designed to directly stimulating the brain to improve health outcomes and quality of life for people with a TBI. We provide a brief explanation of the nature of each therapy and review the current state of evidence on its effectiveness in treating TBI. Some brain stimulation modalities have been tested in only very few individuals with TBI, whereas others have shown preliminary evidence of effectiveness in randomized sham-controlled trials. Very few studies involve milder forms of TBI, including concussion. As the quality of evidence for or against various interventions grows, health-care teams will be in a position to offer a wider range of treatment options to those who suffer the aftermath of TBI.

Research studying the effects of repetitive transcranial magnetic stimulation (rTMS) and transcranial direct current stimulation (tDCS) in people with TBI is presented in Tables 21.1 and 21.2. The literature was reviewed in detail in papers published in 2015 by Li et al. (2015) and Dhaliwal et al. (2015). Here, we provide an overview as well as a detailed description of the interim publications on the topic. We then present and discuss two newer electrical stimulation techniques: transcranial *alternating* current stimulation and transcranial random noise stimulation. We also touch on two distinctly different methods of brain stimulation: One method uses specific wavelengths of light to stimulate cellular mechanisms for recovery in the injured brain. The other uses electrical stimulation of the tongue to influence brain activity indirectly. The majority of research to date using these methods has studied their effects in healthy volunteers, with a smaller number of studies in clinical neurologic or psychiatric conditions. Although they have not yet been tested in people with TBI, it is worth developing an awareness of these methods and their current status within the toolbox of brain modulation techniques.

## Transcranial magnetic stimulation

### The procedure

Transcranial magnetic stimulation (TMS) is a noninvasive technique for modifying brain activity and function. It works by running a brief but intense current through a coil, which in turn generates a magnetic field with a rapid rise time. This time-varying magnetic field is capable of eliciting electric current in nearby conductors, of which brain tissue is one. Thus, the pulse delivered through the coil when positioned against the person's scalp causes firing of neurons located in close proximity to the coil. Repeated trains of stimulation delivered in specific patterns can have the longer term effect of either increasing or decreasing activity not only in a specific brain region but also in its connected neural networks located more distantly from the point of stimulation.

Patterns of stimulation using rTMS to *increase* activity in a brain region include short trains of stimulation at 10–20 Hz with tens of seconds between trains (conventional high-frequency rTMS), or more complex patterns of pulses involving triplets of very

*Table 21.1* TMS studies in TBI

| Reference | Study type | TBI severity | Time since TBI | N | Age (yrs) | Outcome measure | Stimulation target | Stimulation protocol | Stimulation intensity | # Sessions | Result |
|---|---|---|---|---|---|---|---|---|---|---|---|
| (Bonni et al. 2013) | Case | Severe | 2 yrs | 1 | 20 | Spatial attention test, fMRI, and MEP cortical activity | L posterior parietal | cTBS | 80% MT | 20 | > spatial attention; > Fr-Par connectivity; < Lpar-M1 excitability |
| (Cosentino et al. 2010) | Case | n.s. | 10 mos | 1 | 63 | Musical hallucination intensity, duration; FDG-PET | R posttemporal cortex | rTMS 1 Hz | 90% MT | 10 | No hallucination ×4 mos; Normalize R posttemporal lobe hyperactivity post-rTMS |
| (Fitzgerald et al. 2011) | Case | Mild | 14 yrs | 1 | 41 | MADRS depression rating; disability | DLPFC | rTMS R: 1 Hz L: 10 Hz | 110% MT | 20 | MADRS < by 50%; < disability |
| (Kreuzer et al. 2013) | Case | Severe | 5 yrs | 1 | 53 | Tinnitus questionnaire and rating scales | L auditory cortex | 1 Hz | 110% MT | 10 × 5 over 3 yrs | < tinnitus severity |
| (Nielson et al. 2015) | Blinded rTMS only | Severe | 5 yrs | 1 | 48 | HAM-D, standard tests of depression, anxiety, cognition | R DLPFC | 1 Hz | 110% MT | 30 | HAM-D < 23%, < anhedonia, > function |
| (Pachalska et al. 2011) | Case | Severe | ~3 yrs | 1 | 26 | Executive function tests; Frontal Behavior Inventory | Fronto-temporal | rTMS R: 1 Hz L: 5 Hz | n.s. | 20* | > cognition; improved frontal behaviors; normalize ERPs |

*(Continued)*

*Table 21.1 (Continued)* TMS studies in TBI

| Reference | Study type | TBI severity | Time since TBI | N | Age (yrs) | Outcome measure | Stimulation target | Stimulation protocol | Stimulation intensity | # Sessions | Result |
|---|---|---|---|---|---|---|---|---|---|---|---|
| (Martino et al. 2015) | Case | 2-mos coma after TBI | 44 mos | 1 | ~29 | Standardized tests of motor, balance, and gate function | R lateral cerebellum | iTBS[a] | 80% aMT | 30 | Improved motor and balance scores |
| (George et al. 2014) | RCT | *Mild* in suicidal inpatient ± PTSD | n.s. | 13 real, 11 sham | 42.5 ± 15.7 | Beck Scale and visual analog scales of suicidal ideation | L prefrontal | rTMS 10 Hz | 120% MT | 3/d × 3d (54,000 pulses) | < suicidal ideation real = sham; 1-day response to real |
| (Koski et al. 2015) | Open label | Mild, GCS 13–15 | >6 mos | 15 | 20–60 | Post-concussion Symptoms Scale, task-related BOLD signal | L DLPFC | rTMS 10 Hz | 110% MT | 20 | 12 complete; 9 respond; < PCS score; > DLPFC and < rostral ACC activity |
| (Pistoia et al. 2013) | Case series | VS | 5–8 mos | 3 | 70, 19, 38 | MEP facilation; Behavioral responsiveness | L motor cortex | 15 pulses × 10 trains (ISI 10 sec) × 3 conditions | 110% MT | 3 (1/condition) | > MEPs during observation to imitate; > Sustained eye opening and tracking; motor response to command |
| (Leung et al. 2016a) | Case series | Mild TBI w/ constant Headache | 1.5–7 yrs | 6 | 38–60 | Headache Intensity, Frequency, Duration | L motor cortex and L DLPFC alternating/session | rTMS 10 Hz | 80% MT | 4 | Intensity: 53% <; Exacerbation frequency: 79% <; < medication use |
| (Leung et al. 2016b) | RCT | Mild w/ Headache | 33–580 mos | 12 real 12 sham | 25–69 | Headache intensity, duration; Ham-D, CPT | L motor cortex | rTMS 10 Hz | 80% MT | 3 | Real>Sham for < intensity and exacerbation, and improved CPT |

*(Continued)*

*Table 21.1 (Continued)* TMS studies in TBI

| Reference | Study type | TBI severity | Time since TBI | N | Age (yrs) | Outcome measure | Stimulation target | Stimulation protocol | Stimulation intensity | # Sessions | Result |
|---|---|---|---|---|---|---|---|---|---|---|---|
| (Cincotta et al. 2015) | Random sham-controlled cross-over | VS | 31 and 85 mos | 2 | 47 and 65 | Coma Recovery Scale-Revised; Clinical Global Impression scale | Motor cortex | rTMS 20 Hz | 90% rMT or 60% MSO | 5 real 5 sham | No effect on clinical or EEG measures |
| (Tremblay et al. 2015) | Case series | Grade 2–3 concussion | 2 and 6 wks | 5 | 22–44 | Cortical excitability (MEP) | L motor cortex | cTBS | 80% aMT | 1 at 2 wks, 1 at 6 wks | MEP response (synaptic plasticity) absent at 2 wks, present at 6 wks |

*Notes:* >, increase; <, decrease; RCT, randomized sham-controlled parallel groups trial; L, left hemisphere; R, right hemisphere; Ctbs, continuous theta-burst stimulation; rTMS, repetitive transcranial magnetic stimulation; d, day(s); wk, week; mo, month; MSO, intensity as a percent of maximum stimulator output; n.s., not specified; VS, vegetative state after severe TBI; DLPFC, dorsolateral prefrontal cortex; GCS, Glasgow Coma Scale; BOLD, blood oxygenation level-dependent signal measured with functional magnetic resonance imaging; MADRS, Montgomery-Asberg Depression Rating Scale; Ham-D, Hamilton Rating Scale for Depression; CPT, Continuous Performance Test of attention; fMRI, functional magnetic resonance imaging; EEG = electroencephalography used to measure patterns of electrical activity coming from the brain; FDG-PET, regional cerebral glucose metabolism measured with positron emission tomography; MEP, motor evoked potentials; rMT, resting motor threshold; aMT, active motor threshold.

[a] iTBS combined with *neuromotor therapy*

*Table 21.2* rDCS studies in TBI

| Ref | Study type | TBI severity | Time since TBI | N | Age (years) | Outcome measure | Stimulation target | Stimulus intensity | Durations (min) | # Simulation sessions | Result |
|---|---|---|---|---|---|---|---|---|---|---|---|
| (Middleton et al. 2014) | Open label | Unspecified (motor deficits) | 9 and 206 mos | 1 TBI, 1 TBI + stroke | 38, 39 | Feasibility; Box and Block Test, Purdue Pegboard, Stroke Impact Scale-16 | An: ipsilesional M1; Cath: contralesional M1 | 1.5 mA[a], | 15 | 24 (3/wk) | Transient improvement Sustained > in arm use |
| (Angelakis et al. 2014) | Sham and dose-controlled fixed order | Severe (MC/VS) | Chronic | 5 | 19–44 | JFK Coma Recovery Scale-Revised | An: L SM1 or L DLPFC Cath: RSO | Sham, 1 mA, 2 mA | 20 | 5 per intensity | Slight improvement in 3 |
| (Thibaut et al. 2014) | Sham-controlled rand crossover | Severe (MCS/VS/UWS) | Stable 28 d–26 yr | 19 MCS, 6 VS/UWS | 15–55 | JFK Coma Recovery Scale-Revised | An: L DLPFC, Cath: RSO | 2 mA | 20 | 1 Real, 1 sham | MCS: Transient improvement |
| (Naro et al. 2015) | Sham-controlled rand crossover | Severe (MC/VS) | 4–72 mos | 5 MCS, 5 VS | 33–78 | MEP measures of cortical excitability and motor connectivity | An: Orbitofrontal; Cathode: Cz | 1 mA | 10 | 1 Real, 1 Sham | > excitability and connectivity in MCS but not in VS |
| (Kang et al. 2012) | Sham-controlled rand crossover | CHI w/ Attention deficit | 56–532 mos | 9 | 20–79 | Attention test: Reaction times and error rates | An: L DLPFC, Cath: RSO | 2 mA | 20 | 1 real, 1 sham | Transiently shorter RTs after real > sham tDCS |
| (Lesniak et al. 2014) | Sham-controlled parallel groups | Severe | 4–92 mos | 11 real, 10 sham | 18–45 | Attention and memory test, European Brain Injury Questionnaire | An: L DLPFC, Cath: RSO | 1 mA[b] | 10 | 15 | No significant group differences in response |

*(Continued)*

*Table 21.2 (Continued)* rDCS studies in TBI

| Ref | Study type | TBI severity | Time since TBI | N | Age (years) | Outcome measure | Stimulation target | Stimulus intensity | Durations (min) | # Simulation sessions | Result |
|---|---|---|---|---|---|---|---|---|---|---|---|
| (Ulam et al. 2015) | Sham-controlled, rand parallel-groups | Altered or LOC at injury | Real: 57 ± 38 d, Sham: 41 ± 21d | 13 real, 13 sham | Real: 31 ± 10; Sham 36 ± 15 | Resting EEG oscillations; cognitive test battery | An: L DLPFC, Cath: RSO | 1 mA | 20 | 10 | > cognition in both groups; Real: < delta activity correlated w/ > cognitive performance |
| (Sacco et al. 2016) | Sham-controlled rand parallel groups | GCS < 9 at injury | 3–17 yrs | 16 real, 16 sham | 18–66 | Divided attention test errors and RT, Task-based BOLD signal | An: Ipsilesional DLPFC, Cath: contralesional DLPFC; n = 6 bifrontal anodal tDCS | 2 mA[c] | 20 | 10 (2/d × 5d) | Improved RT and error rates in real > sham <BOLD during task performance (real) |
| (O'Neil-Pirozzi et al. 2016) | Sham- and montage controlled rand crossover | GCS = 3–7 at injury | 1.2–14 yrs | 4 TBI, 4 no-TBI control | TBI: 35–53 | EEG: P300 in oddball task; power; immediate word-list recall | 1) An: L DLPFC, Cath: RSO; 2) Cath: L DLPFC, An: RSO | 2 mA | 20 min | 1 anodal; 1 cathodal; 1 sham | > word recall and P300 in anodal > other conditions; |
| (Wilke et al. 2016) | Sham-controlled rand crossover | Mild recurrent | 7–54 mos | 17 TBI, 22 no-TBI controls | 24 ± 3 | GABA with MRS or MEP silent periods | An: L motor. cath: RSO | 1 mA | 20 | 2 Real vs. Sham by 2 MRS vs. MEP | No effects of tDCS in TBI or healthy controls |

*Notes:* >, increase; <, decrease; DLPFC, dorsolateral prefrontal cortex; L, left hemisphere; R, right hemisphere; d, day(s); wk, week; mo, month; RSO, R supraorbital location; rand, randomized assignment of treatment condition (crossover trials) or to treatment group (parallel groups trials); GCS, Glasgow Coma Scale; LOC, loss of consciousness; MEP, motor evoked potential; MRS, magnetic resonance spectroscopy; BOLD, blood oxygen level-dependent signal measured with functional magnetic resonance imaging.

[a] Paired with functional rehabilitation

[b] Paired with computerized cognitive rehabilitation

[c] Paired with computerized attention training

high-frequency (50 Hz) pulses presented in 5-Hz trains of triplets, with several seconds between trains (intermittent theta burst stimulation, or iTBS). Patterns of stimulation using rTMS to *decrease* or suppress activity in hyperactive brain regions include continuous 1-Hz stimulation for 10–30 minutes (conventional low-frequency stimulation) or triplets of very high-frequency (50 Hz) pulses delivered at 5 Hz for less than a minute (continuous theta-burst stimulation, or cTBS). Repeated sessions of stimulation can have effects on brain activity and associated behaviors that outlast the time of stimulation by several months. This is the principle underlying the proven benefits of rTMS over the frontal cortex for treatment of depression.

Placebo or *sham* stimulation procedures are used as a control condition in clinical trials to test the effects of rTMS on brain functioning. In sham rTMS, the stimulating coil is visually identical to that used in real rTMS, creates a comparable tactile sensation as it rests against the participant's head, and generates the same clicking sound as the real stimulation coil. There are subtle differences in the tactile sensations evoked on the scalp by the pulse from the two coils. As a result, experienced participants may be able to guess which intervention is being delivered (real vs. sham); however, participants who have not experienced rTMS before tend not to be able to guess correctly whether they are receiving real or sham stimulation.

## Effects of repetitive transcranial magnetic stimulation on people with traumatic brain injury

Fourteen published studies to date have reported on the effects of rTMS in the context of TBI (see Table 21.1 for references and study details). Of these, seven were case studies, four were open-label case series (n = 3 to 15), and three were sham-controlled trials. Six of these studies involved patients classified as having *mild* TBI (Fitzgerald et al. 2011, George et al. 2014, Koski et al. 2015, Leung et al. 2016a, 2016b, Tremblay et al. 2015), whereas the others involved moderate to severe TBI, or even persistent altered states of consciousness following a TBI.

The first applications in people with TBI occurred in the context of receiving rTMS treatment for depression. In single case studies of individuals with a remote history of TBI, depressive symptoms improved after low-frequency stimulation of the right dorsolateral prefrontal cortex (DLPFC), alone (Nielson et al. 2015) or in combination with high-frequency stimulation of the left DLPFC (Fitzgerald et al. 2011, Nielson et al. 2015). In two other case reports, low-frequency rTMS over the temporal cortex reduced tinnitus (Kreuzer et al. 2013) and musical hallucinations (Cosentino et al. 2010) associated with TBI.

Other studies using cognitive test performance as outcomes soon followed; however, these were typically in people with more severe head injuries. Decreasing activity in the left posterior parietal cortex using cTBS was effective in reducing spatial neglect in one case (Bonnì et al. 2013), while combining low-frequency and high-frequency rTMS over the left and right fronto-temporal regions, respectively, reduced symptoms of frontal lobe syndrome in patients treated years after a severe head injury (Pachalska et al. 2011). More recently, a paper by Martino et al. (2015) reported improvements in motor task and locomotor function after 30 sessions of intermittent theta burst stimulation to the right lateral cerebellum in an individual who had spent two months in a trauma-induced coma 3 years previously.

Three patients with severe TBI resulting in a vegetative state showed increased cortical excitability and increased behavioral responsiveness (visual tracking, response to commands) after a series of rTMS trains (Pistoia et al. 2013). One sham-controlled trial

(Cincotta et al. 2015) enrolled 11 patients in a vegetative state, in two of whom TBI was the cause. Each participant received both real 20-Hz and sham stimulation in a randomized order. No effect on clinical or physiological measures was seen in these patients.

Two open-label trials and one randomized sham-controlled trial are of more direct relevance to the treatment of concussion. These studies investigated the effects of rTMS on clinical outcomes in patients with a mild TBI rather than the more severe case studied previously. Nine out of 12 patients with mild TBI treated with 10-Hz rTMS over the left DLPFC showed a reduction in post-concussion symptoms (Koski et al. 2015). Moreover, this intervention was associated with a change in TBI-related patterns of brain activity in the DLPFC and rostral anterior cingulate regions as measured with functional magnetic resonance imaging (fMRI). A reduction in headache severity was the most consistently observed effect in that study.

This finding was recently replicated by another group of researchers, this time using rTMS over the motor cortex. First, a series of 6 veterans with persistent headaches associated with a mild TBI were studied (Leung et al. 2016a). More compellingly, these same authors (Leung et al. 2016b) also published the results of a randomized, sham-controlled trial in 24 veterans with chronic headache resulting from a remote, mild TBI. Half received three sessions of real 10-Hz rTMS delivered within one week whereas the other half received sham stimulation. The intensity of headache, the frequency, and the severity of exacerbation headaches were reduced to a greater extent in the group treated with active stimulation than in the group treated with sham stimulation. The active group also showed greater improvements on a computerized test of attention. This study provides strong support for the use of rTMS to treat concussion-related headaches.

One additional randomized sham-controlled treatment trial was conducted in 24 patients with a history of mild TBI (George et al. 2014). This study in veterans and active duty personnel with a history of mild TBI, who were admitted to an inpatient unit for severe depression, showed that an intense schedule (9 sessions in three days) of 10-Hz stimulation over the left prefrontal cortex had no impact on suicidal ideation when compared with sham stimulation. This study was not designed to compare the effects of rTMS on TBI-related physiological or clinical outcome; however, it demonstrates the safety of a more intensive stimulation schedule in the context of a mild TBI.

Very little is known about the effects of brain stimulation in the acute stages after a head injury, due to concerns about safety and the potential increased risk of seizures. A recent study safely used cTBS over the left motor cortex with the aim of evaluating the potential for induction of synaptic plasticity in the weeks following a mild TBI (Tremblay et al. 2015). The five participants had grade 2–3 concussion with no structural brain lesions. The motor potentials evoked by single pulses of TMS were measured before and after a single session of 600 pulses delivered in 200 bursts of three 50-Hz pulses, with a 200-ms interval. Plasticity, as measured by a change in the motor evoked potentials, was not present at two weeks post-injury and only emerged at 6-week follow-up. These results suggested that the brain might not be optimally sensitive to stimulation in the first few weeks after an injury, potentially limiting its use in the acute stages of recovery from a TBI.

## Future research on rTMS for concussion

Several randomized sham-controlled clinical trials of rTMS for mild TBI in military service personnel are registered as ongoing, targeting such primary outcomes as patient-reported concussion symptoms, cognitive impairment, and depression. There are, at this time, no published or registered trials evaluating the clinical benefits of rTMS for treating symptoms that follow one or more sport-related concussions.

# Transcranial direct current stimulation *studies in traumatic brain injury*

## *The procedure*

In transcranial direct current stimulation (tDCS), a 1–2 mA current flows through the head from a positively charged electrode (anode) to a negatively charged electrode (cathode) for 10–20 minutes. The procedure is painless. The skull absorbs much of the low-intensity current, but enough of it reaches the brain to increase excitability of the cortex underlying the anode while reducing excitability under the cathode, for 1–2 hours after the end of stimulation. Relatively large electrodes are used (25–35 cm²), and the stimulated area is less focal than in rTMS. In a majority of applications in which the goal is to promote activity in one brain region without suppressing activity in another, the cathode is positioned supraorbitally (on the forehead), and a larger electrode is used to disperse and diffuse the effect of the current.

Repeated sessions of tDCS over multiple days lead to increases in cortical excitability that may persist for many weeks. In the sham stimulation procedure, the current is turned on to evoke the initial mild tingling sensations of real stimulation but then extinguished soon thereafter, a process that cannot be detected by the participant.

## *Effects of* transcranial direct current stimulation *on people with traumatic brain injury*

Studies evaluating the effects of tDCS in TBI are detailed in Table 21.2. Nine papers reported on the effects of tDCS in moderate to severe TBI. These include one open trial in one patient with TBI and one with mixed TBI plus stroke (Middleton et al. 2014), five sham-controlled randomized cross-over trials (Angelakis et al. 2014, Kang et al. 2012, Naro et al. 2015, O'Neil-Pirozzi et al. 2016, Thibaut et al. 2014) and three parallel-group, randomized sham-controlled trials (Lesniak et al. 2014, Sacco et al. 2016, Ulam et al. 2015).

Three sham-controlled crossover studies enrolled patients who were in a minimally conscious (MCS) or vegetative state following severe TBI. Results suggest that a single session of anodal tDCS to the frontal lobe in MCS patients can produce brief increases in cortical excitability (Naro et al. 2015) and in behavioral responsiveness as measured by the coma recovery scale—revised (Thibaut et al. 2014) with some patients showing small but persistent clinical improvements after 5 daily sessions (Angelakis et al. 2014). There is no evidence that patients in a persistent vegetative state after TBI respond to tDCS.

In the open-label trial (Middleton et al. 2014), patients in a functional rehabilitation program who had motor impairments after TBI were given tDCS with the anode over the ipsilesional motor cortex and the cathode over the contralesional motor cortex. This intervention was paired with 24 sessions of rehabilitation targeting the upper extremity. They showed some temporary improvements in speed and accuracy on standardized tests of motor function and a more sustained increase in use of the arm. The study was designed to assess feasibility and safety of this combined intervention, and improvements could not be attributed to tDCS specifically.

Cognitive test performance was the primary clinical outcome in other studies. In a sham-controlled crossover study of nine participants with attention deficits in the subacute to chronic stages of closed head injury, a single session of tDCS, but not sham stimulation, led to transiently faster reaction times on a computerized attention test (Kang et al. 2012). In a study of four patients, studied >1 year after a severe TBI and four age-matched non-TBI controls, a single session of anodal tDCS over the left DLPFC, when compared with cathodal or sham stimulation, was associated with greater improvements on a word-learning task (O'Neil-Pirozzi et al. 2016). The TBI patients in this study also responded to anodal tDCS with an increase in the amplitude of the P300 evoked potential response.

When repeated sessions of tDCS were delivered in a sham-controlled parallel groups design, results in participants with severe TBI have been mixed. Changed scores on neuropsychological test batteries did not differ between groups receiving tDCS or sham (Lesniak et al. 2014, Ulam et al. 2015), although electroencephalogram (EEG) measures of brainwaves in one study showed decreased delta activity that correlated with the improvement on cognitive test scores in the real tDCS group only (Ulam et al. 2015). More promising results were found in a recent study in which 32 patients were studied in the chronic stages after a severe TBI, and the outcome targeted was divided attention impairment (Sacco et al. 2016). Participants were assigned to 10 sessions (twice daily) of either real or sham anodal tDCS over the ipsilesional DLPFC, with a cathodal electrode placed over the contralesional DLPFC. The tDCS sessions were combined with a computerized attention training intervention. The group treated with real tDCS showed more improvement in reaction time and error rates than the group receiving sham stimulation. Task-related fMRI scans obtained before and after the tDCS intervention showed a reduction in brain activations during task performance, which the authors interpreted as reflecting more efficient mental processing in response to treatment.

To date, there is only one published study of the effects of tDCS in mild TBI and this involved only physiological outcomes studied before and after single sessions of real or sham stimulation in a crossover design (Wilke et al. 2016). Seventeen patients studied 7–54 months after a mild TBI, and 22 healthy controls were assessed using magnetic resonance spectroscopy and motor evoked potential measures of the inhibitory neurotransmitter GABA. No effects of tDCS were found in either the patient or the control group.

## *The future of research on* transcranial direct current stimulation *for concussion*

We must look to the future for any evidence of the effectiveness of tDCS in treating clinical outcomes in concussion. Fortunately, several trials of tDCS in mild TBI are registered as currently in progress or recently completed. These trials use a sham-controlled parallel group design to evaluate effects on tests of working memory and other cognitive abilities. These studies should provide more definitive answers to the question of whether tDCS is an appropriate treatment modality for concussion-related cognitive impairments.

## *Transcranial alternating current stimulation (tACS)*

### *The procedure*

This relatively novel intervention delivers specific frequencies of alternating current to the head with the goal of modifying the brain's intrinsic electrical activity. Spontaneous electrical activity in the brain is composed of currents of varying strength that oscillate at different frequencies, often referred to as *brainwaves*. The relative size and strength of the oscillations within a specific range of frequencies can be linked to the behavioral state of an individual. Delta (<3 Hz) and theta (3–8 Hz) waves are predominant during sleep, alpha waves (8–12 Hz) during relaxed or meditative awake states, beta waves (12–30 Hz) during attentive, problem-focused states, and gamma waves (25–100 Hz) during rapid simultaneous processing of multiple sensory inputs. *Transcranial alternating current stimulation* delivered at a specific frequency over a specific area of the brain is capable of modifying brainwaves, particularly those within the same frequency band.

A recent review by Hamid and colleagues (2015) provides a description of the current state of knowledge regarding the brain modulating effects of tACS. In brief, physiological studies indicate that tACS induces or *entrains* activity within specific frequencies, increasing the coherence of neuronal firing while it is delivered and ultimately leading to an increase in synaptic strength within the brain networks where it is applied. These observations suggest that tACS could be used to enhance the functions or behaviors associated with specific oscillation frequencies within specific neural networks. For example, a study using fMRI gamma-frequency tACS over the motor cortex led to correlated changes in primary motor and frontomedial activity, which were in proportion to its beneficial effects on motor task performance (Moisa et al. 2016).

Human studies have been conducted in healthy volunteers with the goal of better understanding the effects of tACS on brain activity and behavior. Delivering tACS over the motor cortex can increase cortical excitability and improve motor task performance; however, these results have not been observed consistently across studies (Rjosk et al. 2016). Moreover, the effects observed at the physiological and behavioral levels are highly dependent on stimulation frequency, and changes in these parameters are not always associated with the same stimulation frequencies (Antal et al. 2008, Feurra et al. 2011a, Pollok et al. 2015). Stimulation frequency also determines whether tACS delivered while the person is engaged in a motor task has beneficial or noxious effects on behavioral performance measures (Joundi et al. 2012, Pogosyan et al. 2009, Wach et al. 2013). Although tACS is proposed to work by entraining activity at its specific frequency, one study found that combinations of frequencies may elicit the strongest effects on cortical excitability (Schutter and Hortensius 2011). Still others showed that increases in cortical excitability for up to one-hour poststimulation could be induced using high stimulation frequencies—even those beyond the physiological range (Chaieb et al. 2011, Moliadze et al. 2010).

## *Transcranial alternating current stimulation studies in the healthy human brain*

Other variables influencing the effects of tACS at both the physiological and behavioral levels include the phase as well as the frequency of stimulation (Nakazono et al. 2016) and the size and placement of the reference electrode (Mehta et al. 2015). Effects are even influenced by a person's behavior state (e.g., eyes open or closed (Neuling et al. 2013) and motor imagery (Feurra et al. 2013)). This is presumably because these activities influence the frequencies of oscillations that predominate in the brain and hence the effectiveness of the stimulation frequency. In 2013, Chaieb and colleagues (2014) reviewed the existing data on safety of tACS in healthy human subjects for frequencies as high as 5,000 Hz, with no adverse effects as yet noted.

A complicated set of results has emerged from recent research on the effects of tACS on other functional networks in a healthy brain. tACS has different effects, depending on the brain region underlying the electrodes. tACS over DLPFC enhanced working memory (Hoy et al. 2015, Jaušovec et al. 2014, Meiron and Lavidor 2014, Polanía et al. 2012) and problem solving (Lustenberger et al. 2015, Santarnecchi et al. 2013); over parietal cortex, it modified visual attention (Brignani et al. 2013, van Schouwenburg et al. 2016), and over the temporo-parietal cortex, it increased language learning (Antonenko et al. 2016). This suggests a potential use to treat deficits in executive functioning in individuals with concussion.

Yet caution is warranted because the story is not so straightforward. Another study showed an increase in risky decision-making after stimulation of the DLPFC in healthy subjects (Sela et al. 2012). Similarly, others have demonstrated induction of phosphenes and increased excitability of the visual cortex from occipital stimulation (Turi et al. 2013) and increased sensitivity to tactile sensation from somatosensory cortex stimulation (Feurra et al. 2011b). To be useful in treating symptoms of concussion, it may be necessary to identify a set of stimulation parameters that can reliably *decrease* sensitivity in individuals who report hypersensitivity to sensory input. Interestingly, the behavioral effects of tACS may also differ as a function of the age of the healthy brain. A recent study (Rufener et al. 2016) showed that 40-Hz (gamma) stimulation of the auditory cortex bilaterally disrupted performance on a phoneme perception task in younger adults but improved performance in adults aged 60–75 years. These observations also suggest a need to carefully distinguish between an intervention that simply increases the intensity of the input versus one that increases the ability to detect signal in noise.

## Studies of tACS in neurologic conditions

Nevertheless, this evidence from studies in healthy volunteers suggests the exciting possibility that tACS could be harnessed to strengthen damaged neural networks, or to enhance activity in compensatory networks, thus restoring function in individuals with a brain injury. Indeed, in patients with optic nerve damage, 10 sessions of alternating current stimulation delivered around the orbits of the eyes alter the visual pathway: enhancing alpha frequency brain oscillations at the occipital pole (visual cortex), increasing the size of the visual fields, and improving visual acuity (Fedorov et al. 2011).

To date, reports on the effects of tACS in clinical populations have been limited. In terms of positive outcomes, tACS over the motor cortex is effective at cancelling out the spontaneous oscillations associated with tremor in people with Parkinson's disease, when delivered at the beta frequency (Krause et al. 2013). Whether these effects could be prolonged beyond the time of stimulation with repeated stimulation sessions is unknown. Compared with usual rehabilitation, 15 days of adjunctive tACS delivered over the mastoids bilaterally within 15–60 days after stroke led to greater improvements in function as measured with the NIH stroke scale (Wu et al. 2016). The amount of recovery correlated with improvements in measures of cerebral blood flow. Finally, a reduction in negative symptoms and an increase in illness insight were reported in three schizophrenic patients treated with repeated sessions of theta-frequency tACS over the DLPFC (Kallel et al. 2016).

While these results appear promising, it is too early to conclude that tACS will benefit individuals with a neurologic condition. Vanneste and colleagues (2013) randomly assigned 50 chronic tinnitus sufferers to receive one session of brain stimulation over the DLPFC bilaterally using either tDCS or tACS targeting brainwaves in the alpha frequency. No effect of tACS was observed and only the tDCS group showed a reduction in tinnitus loudness and annoyance. A recent study in stroke patients (Naros and Gharabaghi 2016) compared the effects of beta-frequency tACS continuously before, versus intermittently during, a robotically controlled hand opening task with neurofeedback. Performance improved with the intermittent tACS during task performance (*online*) but not after the continuous tACS (offline), and there were no longer term effects of either intervention.

Recently, a session of gamma-frequency tACS was shown to modulate gamma oscillations in healthy participants and some individuals with mild cognitive impairment (MCI), but not in those diagnosed with Alzheimer's disease (Naro et al. 2016). An improvement in neuropsychological test performance was seen only among the healthy controls and some of the patients with MCI.

Finally, an increase in seizures was reported in an epileptic patient after undergoing 4 days of 1 mA 3-Hz stimulation over the frontoparietal cortex (San-Juan et al. 2016), highlighting the need for close monitoring of the safety of tACS, particularly in vulnerable clinical populations.

## *The future of tACS for treatment of* traumatic brain injury

We are in the very early stages of work aimed at determining the therapeutic potential of tACS in clinical populations. There are no published or registered trials investigating its effects in concussion or TBI. The results of studies to date in both healthy and clinical populations emphasize the key importance of an individual's intrinsic patterns of brain activity on the effectiveness of tACS, which may complicate the design of large-scale clinical trials.

## *Transcranial random noise stimulation*

Transcranial random noise stimulation (tRNS) is a form of tACS in which low-intensity alternating current is delivered to the brain at randomly varying frequencies and intensities. Studies using tRNS in healthy subjects were reviewed recently by Antal and Hermann (2016) and have demonstrated positive, neutral, or even negative effects on cognitive task performance. There are no published studies in animal models, and studies in clinical populations are sparse. As with other brain stimulation modalities, tRNS over auditory cortex appears to be beneficial in reducing tinnitus (Joos et al. 2015, Kreuzer et al.2017) and may be most effective when paired with bilateral tDCS over the DLPFC (To et al. 2016). In a randomized sham-controlled crossover study of 16 people with multiple sclerosis, tRNS but not sham improved pain ratings and decreased pain-related evoked potentials (Palm et al. 2016). Whether tRNS might also reduce pain associated with concussion-related headache remains to be studied. As with other forms of electrical brain stimulation, we are still far from understanding the mechanisms underlying the beneficial effects of tRNS or the optimal means for delivering such an intervention to people with TBI.

## *Low-level laser/LED therapy*

### *The procedure*

In low-level laser light or LED light therapy (LLLD or LED therapy), red or near infrared wavelengths of light are applied to the scalp or forehead. The stimulation imparts no heat, sound, or vibration. The light is applied with sufficient power to penetrate through the skull to the cortex. Although the size of the light clusters is quite small, the skin and skull serve to disperse laser light to a broader chunk of brain tissue than that underlying its source. The therapy activates light-sensitive receptors in mitochondria to produce a cascade of cellular-level events that reduce inflammation, reduce cell death, and enhance healing. LLLD with its low cost and ease of application is receiving growing interest as an emerging intervention for a variety of neurologic disorders including TBI.

### *Studies of LLLD/LED therapy for neurologic conditions*

This method of brain stimulation has been reviewed in recent publications by Hamblin and Naeser and colleagues (Hamblin 2016, Naeser et al. 2016). The use of transcranial light therapy for clinical trials in humans began in the field of stroke, where improved outcomes relative to sham therapy were observed in patients administered light therapy early after onset of an ischemic stroke (Lampl et al. 2007). Although a subsequent large-scale trial did not support the early promise of the initial studies (Zivin et al. 2014), it has been suggested that this is caused by individual differences in the complex dose–responses to the use of certain stimulation parameters (Hamblin 2016). For example, studies in animal models of brain injury have demonstrated a biphasic response to variations in parameters such as energy density (Huang et al. 2011) and the number of treatments given (Xuan et al. 2013).

## Studies of LLLD/LED therapy for TBI

Research on transcranial light therapy for TBI is still in its infancy. Only a decade has now passed since the first demonstrations that LLLD used in a rodent model of TBI was safe, reduced brain lesion volume, and had long-term benefits on behavior outcomes (McCarthy et al. 2010, Oron et al. 2007, Xuan et al. 2014). Pulsed rather than continuous light (Ando et al. 2011, Oron et al. 2012) and 810 or 660 nm wavelengths (Wu et al. 2012) were found to be the most effective parameters for enhancing brain recovery and reducing the behavioral impact of experimentally induced TBI. The information gained from such studies will allow for better determination of the optimal parameters for stimulation with light therapy in clinical trials for concussion.

The only published data on light therapy in human subjects with TBI come from open-label case studies. In the first report, nightly home use of LED therapy by two patients with chronic mild TBI was associated with symptom reduction and improvements in cognitive and occupational functioning (Naeser et al. 2011). Continued use of the treatment was required to maintain these gains.

In another report, three patients with persistent cognitive and sleep impairments after a *mild/moderate* TBI were treated with 18 sessions of transcranial (n = 2) or intranasal (n = 1) LED with a subsequent increase of 1 hour of sleep per night and improved performance on cognitive tests (Bogdanova et al. 2015).

Finally, in a case study of a patient in vegetative state after a severe head injury, LLLD over the forehead led to increased regional cerebral blood flow over the frontal lobes and was associated with a sign of increased behavioral responsiveness (Nawashiro et al. 2012).

## The future of LED therapy for mild TBI

The use of LED rather than low-level laser light for clinical applications is preferred for its lower cost and risk profile. However, the characteristics of the two light sources differ in ways that could influence therapeutic response (e.g., range of wavelengths), and further animal studies of the effects of LED therapy in animal models of TBI are needed. Preliminary support for the use of LED therapy led to the launch of a randomized sham-controlled clinical trial in military service personnel with a history of mild TBI or blast exposure, the results of which are expected late in 2018.

## Cranial nerve noninvasive neuromodulation

### The procedure

Several studies have shown that the tongue can be used as an effective interface for sending electrical signals to the central nervous system (Bach-y-Rita et al. 1998, Bach-y-Rita and Kercel 2003, Chebat et al. 2007, Sampaio et al. 2001, Tyler et al. 2003, Wildenberg et al. 2010, 2011).

Although the actual mechanism remains elusive, it is postulated that electrical stimulation to the tongue induces neuroplasticity by stimulating trigeminal (CN-V) and facial (CN-VII) nerves. This stimulation excites a natural flow of neural impulses to the brainstem (pons and medulla), and cerebellum via the lingual branch of the cranial nerve (CN-Vc), and chorda tympani branch of CN-VII, to effect changes in the function of these targeted brain structures (Wildenberg et al. 2010, 2011). Intensive activation of these structures is believed to initiate a sequential cascade of changes in neighboring and/or connected nuclei by direct collateral connections, brainstem interneuron circuitry, and/or passive transmission of biochemical compounds in the intercellular space. Cranial nerve noninvasive neuromodulation (CN-NINM) is a neurorehabilitation method based on this concept. It was conceptualized by the Tactile Communication and Neurorehabilitation Lab (TCNL) at the University of Wisconsin-Madison. The idea is to combine neurostimulation with a specific set of physical, cognitive, and/or mental exercises to promote neuroplasticity and to enhance functional recovery.

The device used to deliver electrical stimulation to the tongue is called portable neuromodulation stimulator (PoNS). This device is held lightly in place by the lips and teeth around the neck of the tab that goes into the mouth and rests on the anterior and superior parts of the tongue. The paddle-shaped tab of the system has a hexagonally patterned array of 144 gold-plated circular electrodes that delivers triplets of 0.4–60 μs wide pulses at 5 ms intervals (that is, 200 Hz) every 20 ms (50 Hz).

## Review of studies to date

Being a novel technology that is still under development, no data have been published on CN-NINM and mTBI. Unpublished data obtained from TCNL indicate a significant improvement in gait and balance problems in a group of moderate TBI patients after 5-day period of CN-NINM intervention (Figure 21.1).

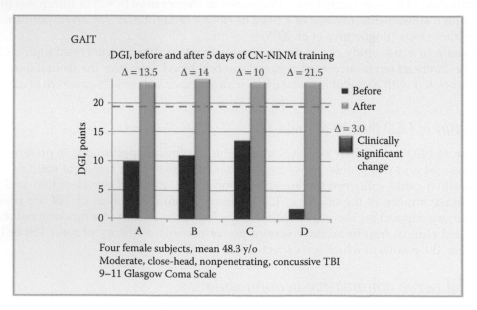

*Figure 21.1* Summary of results from dynamic gait index (DGI) for 4 subjects with nonpenetrating TBI. Changes greater than 3 points are considered clinically significant improvement in performance.

Studies with other diseases have also shown the rehabilitation potential of CN-NINM. Individuals with primary vestibular disorders who trained using electrical stimulation through the tongue coupled with head-position information demonstrated balance improvements that were sustained for weeks beyond the final stimulation session (Danilov et al. 2007, Kaczmarek 2011, Tyler et al. 2006). In another study, twenty chronic MS subjects with an identified gait disturbance were assigned to either an active or control group (Tyler et al. 2014). Both groups completed a 14-week intervention program using a standardized combination of exercise and the PoNS device that provided electrical stimulation to the tongue. At the end of the study, there were significant differences between the groups, with the active group showing statistically greater improvement relative to the control group on gait function. These authors concluded that MS patients demonstrated improved gait with CN-NINM training and suggested that tongue-based neurostimulation may amplify the benefits of exercise for improving gait in people with chronic MS. Recently, Leonard and colleague (2017) reported significant effect of CN-NINM interventions across the wide range of cognitive domains examined, both in the active and in the sham groups, albeit with a trend to greater improvements in the active group. Consistent with behavioral improvement, fMRI activation study using a working memory task also showed greater activation in prefrontal regions of interest in the active group after 14 weeks of CN-NINM intervention. In contrast, little change in brain activation was observed in the sham group postintervention.

## Summary and future directions

A wide variety of methods are available for stimulating the brain with the aim of improving function after injury. Of the brain stimulation modalities presented here, rTMS is the only one for which we currently have high-level evidence of effectiveness. Specifically, rTMS over the motor cortex was shown in a sham-controlled randomly assigned parallel groups study to be effective in treating headaches that persist for three months or more after mild TBI. Thus, it seems reasonable to support its use in treating sports concussion. Nevertheless, its safety and effectiveness in the more acute or subacute stages of recovery remain to be established.

Although a greater number of randomized sham-controlled trials have been conducted using tDCS, these studies were conducted in patients with moderate to severe TBI, and their relevance for the treatment of post-concussion symptoms is unknown. For both tDCS and rTMS, clinical recommendations for therapy await evidence demonstrating their efficacy in concussion from large trials that incorporate sensitive clinical and cognitive outcomes. In the meantime, participation in clinical trials using these modalities seems safe to recommend, at least in the postacute stage of recovery.

For safety, cost, and convenience of use in a home environment, transcranial light therapy using LED head caps seems the most attractive modality; however, evidence of its potential effectiveness is very limited at this time.

As yet we are far from being able to determine whether one stimulation modality is more clinically effective than another. Evidence on which individual patient factors might influence the relative efficacy of one treatment over another is the ultimate goal as we move toward an era of personalized care for TBI.

## References

Ando, T., W. Xuan, T. Xu, T. Dai, S. K Sharma, G. B. Kharkwal, Y. Y. Huang, Q. Wu, M. J. Whalen, and S. Sato. 2011. Comparison of therapeutic effects between pulsed and continuous wave 810-nm wavelength laser irradiation for traumatic brain injury in mice. *PLoS One* 6 (10):e26212.

Angelakis, E., E. Liouta, N. Andreadis, S. Korfias, P. Ktonas, G. Stranjalis, and D. E. Sakas. 2014. Transcranial direct current stimulation effects in disorders of consciousness. *Archives of Physical Medicine and Rehabilitation* 95 (2):283–289.

Antal, A., K. Boros, C. Poreisz, L. Chaieb, D. Terney, and W. Paulus. 2008. Comparatively weak after-effects of transcranial alternating current stimulation (tACS) on cortical excitability in humans. *Brain Stimulation* 1 (2):97–105.

Antal, A. and C. S. Herrmann. 2016. Transcranial alternating current and random noise stimulation: Possible mechanisms. *Neural Plasticity* 2016:3616807. doi: 10.1155/2016/3616807.

Antonenko, D., M. Faxel, U. Grittner, M. Lavidor, and A. Flöel. 2016. Effects of transcranial alternating current stimulation on cognitive functions in healthy young and older adults. *Neural Plasticity* 2016:4274127. doi: 10.1155/2016/4274127.

Bach-y-Rita, P., Kaczmarek K. A., and Meier K. 1998. The tongue as a man-machine interface: A wireless communication system. In *Proceedings of International Symposium on Information Theory and Its Application (ISITA 1998)*, October 14–16, Mexico City, IEEE, pp. 79–81.

Bach-y-Rita, P. and W. Kercel. 2003. Sensory substitution and the human-machine interface. *Trends Cognitive Sciences* 7 (12):541–546.

Bogdanova, Y., P. I. Martin, M. D. Ho, M. K. Yee, V. T. Ho, and J. A. Knight. 2015. Improved sleep and cognition post transcranial or intranasal, red/near-infrared LED treatments in chronic TBI: Pilot case series. *The Journal of Head Trauma Rehabilitation* 30:E61–E116.

Bonnì, S., C. Mastropasqua, M. Bozzali, C. Caltagirone, and G. Koch. 2013. Theta burst stimulation improves visuo-spatial attention in a patient with traumatic brain injury. *Neurological Sciences* 34 (11):2053–2056.

Brignani, D., M. Ruzzoli, P. Mauri, and C. Miniussi. 2013. Is transcranial alternating current stimulation effective in modulating brain oscillations? *PloS One* 8 (2):e56589.

Chaieb, L., A. Antal, A. Pisoni, C. Saiote, A. Opitz, G. G. Ambrus, N. Focke, and W. Paulus. 2014. Safety of 5 kHz tACS. *Brain Stimulation* 7 (1):92–96. doi:10.1016/j.brs.2013.08.004.

Chaieb, L., A. Antal, and W. Paulus. 2011. Transcranial alternating current stimulation in the low kHz range increases motor cortex excitability. *Restorative Neurology and Neuroscience* 29 (3):167–175.

Chebat, D. R., C. Rainville, R. Kupers, and M. Ptito. 2007. Tactile-'visual' acuity of the tongue in early blind individuals. *Neuroreport* 18 (18):1901–1904. doi:10.1097/WNR.0b013e3282f2a63.

Cincotta, M., F. Giovannelli, R. Chiaramonti, G. Bianco, M. Godone, D. Battista, C. Cardinali, A. Borgheresi, A. Sighinolfi, and A. M. D'Avanzo. 2015. No effects of 20 Hz-rTMS of the primary motor cortex in vegetative state: A randomised, sham-controlled study. *Cortex* 71:368–376.

Cosentino, G., G. Giglia, A. Palermo, M. L. Panetta, R. Lo Baido, F. Brighina, and B. Fierro. 2010. A case of post-traumatic complex auditory hallucinosis treated with rTMS. *Neurocase* 16 (3):267–272.

Danilov, Y. P., M. E. Tyler, K. L. Skinner, R. A. Hogle, and P. Bach-y-Rita. 2007. Efficacy of electrotactile vestibular substitution in patients with peripheral and central vestibular loss. *Journal of Vestibular Research* 17 (2–3):119–130.

Dhaliwal, S. K, B. P. Meek, and M. M. Modirrousta. 2015. Non-invasive brain stimulation for the treatment of symptoms following traumatic brain injury. *Frontiers in Psychiatry* 6:119.

Fedorov, A., S. Jobke, V. Bersnev, A. Chibisova, Y. Chibisova, C. Gall, and B. A. Sabel. 2011. Restoration of vision after optic nerve lesions with noninvasive transorbital alternating current stimulation: A clinical observational study. *Brain Stimulation* 4 (4):189–201.

Feurra, M., G. Bianco, E. Santarnecchi, M. Del Testa, A. Rossi, and S. Rossi. 2011a. Frequency-dependent tuning of the human motor system induced by transcranial oscillatory potentials. *Journal of Neuroscience* 31 (34):12165–12170.

Feurra, M., P. Pasqualetti, G. Bianco, E. Santarnecchi, A. Rossi, and S. Rossi. 2013. State-dependent effects of transcranial oscillatory currents on the motor system: What you think matters. *Journal of Neuroscience* 33 (44):17483–17489.

Feurra, M., W. Paulus, V. Walsh, and R. Kanai. 2011b. Frequency specific modulation of human somatosensory cortex. *Frontiers in Psychology* 2:13.

Fitzgerald, P. B., K. E. Hoy, J. J. Maller, S. Herring, R. Segrave, S. McQueen, A. Peachey, Y. Hollander, J. F. Anderson, and Z. J. Daskalakis. 2011. Transcranial magnetic stimulation for depression after a traumatic brain injury: A case study. *The Journal of ECT* 27 (1):38–40.

George, M. S., R. Raman, D. M. Benedek, C. G. Pelic, G. G. Grammer, K. T. Stokes, M. Schmidt et al. 2014. A two-site pilot randomized 3 day trial of high dose left prefrontal repetitive transcranial magnetic stimulation (rTMS) for suicidal inpatients. *Brain Stimulation* 7 (3):421–431. doi:10.1016/j.brs.2014.03.006.

Hamblin, M. R. 2016. Shining light on the head: Photobiomodulation for brain disorders. *BBA Clinical* 6:113–124. doi:10.1016/j.bbacli.2016.09.002.

Hamid, A. I., C. Gall, O. Speck, A. Antal, and B. A. Sabel. 2015. Effects of alternating current stimulation on the healthy and diseased brain. *Frontiers in Neuroscience* 9:391. doi: 10.3389/fnins.2015.00391.

Hoy, K. E, N. Bailey, S. Arnold, K. Windsor, J. John, Z. J. Daskalakis, and P. B. Fitzgerald. 2015. The effect of γ-tACS on working memory performance in healthy controls. *Brain and Cognition* 101:51–56.

Huang, Y. Y., S. K. Sharma, J. Carroll, and M. R. Hamblin. 2011. Biphasic dose response in low level light therapy–An update. *Dose-Response* 9 (4):602–618.

Jaušovec, N., K. Jaušovec, and A. Pahor. 2014. The influence of theta transcranial alternating current stimulation (tACS) on working memory storage and processing functions. *Acta Psychologica* 146:1–6.

Joos, K., D. De Ridder, and S. Vanneste. 2015. The differential effect of low-versus high-frequency random noise stimulation in the treatment of tinnitus. *Experimental Brain Research* 233 (5):1433–1440.

Joundi, R. A, N. Jenkinson, J. S. Brittain, T. Z. Aziz, and P. Brown. 2012. Driving oscillatory activity in the human cortex enhances motor performance. *Current Biology* 22 (5):403–407.

Kaczmarek, K. A. 2011. The tongue display unit (TDU) for electrotactile spatiotemporal pattern presentation. *Scientia Iranica* 18 (6):1476–1485. doi:10.1016/j.scient.2011.08.020.

Kallel, L., M. Mondino, and J. Brunelin. 2016. Effects of theta-rhythm transcranial alternating current stimulation (4.5 Hz-tACS) in patients with clozapine-resistant negative symptoms of schizophrenia: A case series. *Journal of Neural Transmission* 123 (10):1213–1217.

Kang, E. K., D. Y. Kim, and N. J. Paik. 2012. Transcranial direct current stimulation of the left prefrontal cortex improves attention in patients with traumatic brain injury: A pilot study. *Journal of Rehabilitation Medicine* 44 (4):346–350.

Koski, L., T. Kolivakis, C. Yu, J. K. Chen, S. Delaney, and A. Ptito. 2015. Noninvasive brain stimulation for persistent postconcussion symptoms in mild traumatic brain injury. *Journal of Neurotrauma* 32 (1):38–44.

Krause, V., C. Wach, M. Sudmeyer, S. Ferrea, A. Schnitzler, and B. Pollok. 2013. Cortico-muscular coupling and motor performance are modulated by 20 Hz transcranial alternating current stimulation (tACS) in Parkinson's disease. *Frontiers in Human Neuroscience* 7:928. doi:10.3389/fnhum.2013.00928.

Kreuzer, P. M., M. Landgrebe, E. Frank, and B. Langguth. 2013. Repetitive transcranial magnetic stimulation for the treatment of chronic tinnitus after traumatic brain injury: A case study. *The Journal of head trauma rehabilitation* 28 (5):386–389.

Kreuzer, P. M., Vielsmeier, V., Poeppl, T. B., Langguth, B. 2017. A case report on red ear syndrome with tinnitus successfully treated with transcranial random noise stimulation. *Pain Physician* 20:E199–E205.

Lampl, Y., J. A. Zivin, M. Fisher, R. Lew, L. Welin, B. Dahlof, P. Borenstein et al. 2007. Infrared laser therapy for ischemic stroke: a new treatment strategy: Results of the neurothera effectiveness and safety trial-1 (NEST-1). *Stroke* 38 (6):1843–1849. doi:10.1161/STROKEAHA.106.478230.

Lesniak, M., K. Polanowska, J. Seniów, and A. Czlonkowska. 2014. Effects of repeated anodal tDCS coupled with cognitive training for patients with severe traumatic brain injury: A pilot randomized controlled trial. *The Journal of Head Trauma Rehabilitation* 29 (3):E20–E29.

Leung, A., A. Fallah, S. Shukla, L. Lin, A. Tsia, D. Song, G. Polston, and R. Lee. 2016a. rTMS in alleviating mild TBI related headaches-A case series. *Pain Physician* 19 (2):E347–E354.

Leung, A., S. Shukla, A. Fallah, D. Song, L. Lin, S. Golshan, A. Tsai, A. Jak, G. Polston, and R. Lee. 2016b. Repetitive transcranial magnetic stimulation in managing mild traumatic brain injury-related headaches. *Neuromodulation: Technology at the Neural Interface* 19 (2):133–141.

Li, S., A. L. Zaninotto, I. S. Neville, W. S. Paiva, D. Nunn, and F. Fregni. 2015. Clinical utility of brain stimulation modalities following traumatic brain injury: Current evidence. *Neuropsychiatric Disease and Treatment* 11:1573–1586.

Lustenberger, C., M. R. Boyle, A. A. Foulser, J. M. Mellin, and F. Fröhlich. 2015. Functional role of frontal alpha oscillations in creativity. *Cortex* 67:74–82.

Martino, C. A., S. Bonnì, M. Iosa, V. Ponzo, A. Fusco, C. Caltagirone, and G. Koch. 2015. Clinical effects of non-invasive cerebellar magnetic stimulation treatment combined with neuromotor rehabilitation in traumatic brain injury. A single case study. *Functional Neurology* 31 (2):117–120.

McCarthy, T. J., L. De. Taboada, P. K. Hildebrandt, E. L. Ziemer, S. P. Richieri, and J. Streeter. 2010. Long-term safety of single and multiple infrared transcranial laser treatments in Sprague–Dawley rats. *Photomedicine and Laser Surgery* 28 (5):663–667.

Mehta, A. R., A. Pogosyan, P. Brown, and J. S. Brittain. 2015. Montage matters: The influence of transcranial alternating current stimulation on human physiological tremor. *Brain Stimulation* 8 (2):260–268.

Meiron, O. and M. Lavidor. 2014. Prefrontal oscillatory stimulation modulates access to cognitive control references in retrospective metacognitive commentary. *Clinical Neurophysiology* 125 (1):77–82.

Middleton, A., S. L. Fritz, D. M. Liuzzo, R. Newman-Norlund, and T. M. Herter. 2014. Using clinical and robotic assessment tools to examine the feasibility of pairing tDCS with upper extremity physical therapy in patients with stroke and TBI: A consideration-of-concept pilot study. *NeuroRehabilitation* 35 (4):741–754.

Moisa, M., R. Polania, M. Grueschow, and C. C. Ruff. 2016. Brain network mechanisms underlying motor enhancement by transcranial entrainment of gamma oscillations. *Journal of Neuroscience* 36 (47):12053–12065.

Moliadze, V., A. Antal, and W. Paulus. 2010. Boosting brain excitability by transcranial high frequency stimulation in the ripple range. *The Journal of Physiology* 588 (24):4891–4904.

Naeser, M. A., P. I. Martin, M. D. Ho, M. H. Krengel, Y. Bogdanova, J. A. Knight, M. K. Yee et al. 2016. Transcranial, red/near-infrared light-emitting diode therapy to improve cognition in chronic traumatic brain injury. *Photomedicine and Laser Surgery* 34 (12):610–626. doi:10.1089/pho.2015.4037.

Naeser, M. A., A. Saltmarche, M. H. Krengel, M. R. Hamblin, and J. A. Knight. 2011. Improved cognitive function after transcranial, light-emitting diode treatments in chronic, traumatic brain injury: Two case reports. *Photomedicine and Laser Surgery* 29 (5):351–358.

Nakazono, H., K. Ogata, T. Kuroda, and S. Tobimatsu. 2016. Phase and frequency-dependent effects of transcranial alternating current stimulation on motor cortical excitability. *PloS One* 11 (9):e0162521.

Naro, A., R. S. Calabrò, M. Russo, A. Leo, P. Pollicino, A. Quartarone, and P. Bramanti. 2015. Can transcranial direct current stimulation be useful in differentiating unresponsive wakefulness syndrome from minimally conscious state patients? *Restorative Neurology and Neuroscience* 33 (2):159–176.

Naro, A., F. Corallo, S. De Salvo, A. Marra, G. Di Lorenzo, N. Muscara, M. Russo, S. Marino, R. De Luca, and P. Bramanti. 2016. Promising role of neuromodulation in predicting the progression of mild cognitive impairment to dementia. *Journal of Alzheimer's Disease* 53 (4):1375–1388.

Naros, G. and A. Gharabaghi. 2016. Physiological and behavioral effects of β-tACS on brain self-regulation in chronic stroke. *Brain Stimulation* 10 (2):251–259.

Nawashiro, H., K. Wada, K. Nakai, and S. Sato. 2012. Focal increase in cerebral blood flow after treatment with near-infrared light to the forehead in a patient in a persistent vegetative state. *Photomedicine and Laser Surgery* 30 (4):231–233.

Neuling, T., S. Rach, and C. S. Herrmann. 2013. Orchestrating neuronal networks: Sustained after-effects of transcranial alternating current stimulation depend upon brain states. *Frontiers in Human Neuroscience* 7:161. doi:10.3389/fnhum.2013.00161.

Nielson, D. M., C. A. McKnight, R. N. Patel, A. J. Kalnin, and W. J. Mysiw. 2015. Preliminary guidelines for safe and effective use of repetitive transcranial magnetic stimulation in moderate to severe traumatic brain injury. *Archives of Physical Medicine and Rehabilitation* 96 (4):S138–S144.

O'Neil-Pirozzi, T. M., D. Doruk, J. M. Thomson, and F. Fregni. 2016. Immediate memory and electro-physiologic effects of prefrontal cortex transcranial direct current stimulation on neurotypical individuals and individuals with chronic traumatic brain injury: A pilot study. *International Journal of Neuroscience* 127:1–9.

Oron, A., U. Oron, J. Streeter, L. De Taboada, A. Alexandrovich, V. Trembovler, and E. Shohami. 2012. Near infrared transcranial laser therapy applied at various modes to mice following traumatic brain injury significantly reduces long-term neurological deficits. *Journal of Neurotrauma* 29 (2):401–407.

Oron, A., U. Oron, J. Streeter, L. De Taboada, A. Alexandrovich, V. Trembovler, and E. Shohami. 2007. Low-level laser therapy applied transcranially to mice following traumatic brain injury significantly reduces long-term neurological deficits. *Journal of Neurotrauma* 24 (4):651–656.

Pachalska, M., M. Lukowicz, J. D. Kropotov, I. Herman-Sucharska, and J. Talar. 2011. Evaluation of differentiated neurotherapy programs for a patient after severe TBI and long term coma using event-related potentials. *Medical Science Monitor* 17 (10):CS120–CS128.

Palm, U., M. A. Chalah, F. Padberg, T. Al-Ani, M. Abdellaoui, M. Sorel, D. Dimitri, A. Créange, J. P. Lefaucheur, and S. S. Ayache. 2016. Effects of transcranial random noise stimulation (tRNS) on affect, pain and attention in multiple sclerosis. *Restorative Neurology and Neuroscience* 34 (2):189–199.

Pistoia, F., S. Sacco, A. Carolei, and M. Sara. 2013. Corticomotor facilitation in vegetative state: Results of a pilot study. *Archives of Physical Medicine Rehabilitation* 94 (8):1599–606. doi:10.1016/j.apmr.2013.01.019.

Pogosyan, A., L. D. Gaynor, A. Eusebio, and P. Brown. 2009. Boosting cortical activity at beta-band frequencies slows movement in humans. *Current Biology* 19 (19):1637–1641.

Polanía, R., M. A Nitsche, C. Korman, G. Batsikadze, and W. Paulus. 2012. The importance of timing in segregated theta phase-coupling for cognitive performance. *Current Biology* 22 (14):1314–1318.

Pollok, B., A. C. Boysen, and V. Krause. 2015. The effect of transcranial alternating current stimulation (tACS) at alpha and beta frequency on motor learning. *Behavioural Brain Research* 293:234–240.

Rjosk, V., E. Kaminski, M. Hoff, C. Gundlach, A. Villringer, B. Sehm, and P. Ragert. 2016. Transcranial alternating current stimulation at beta frequency: Lack of immediate effects on excitation and interhemispheric inhibition of the human motor cortex. *Frontiers in Human Neuroscience* 10:560. doi: 10.3389/fnhum.2016.00560.

Rufener, K. S., M. S. Oechslin, T. Zaehle, and M. Meyer. 2016. Transcranial alternating current stimulation (tACS) differentially modulates speech perception in young and older adults. *Brain Stimulation* 9 (4):560–565.

Sacco, K., V. Galetto, D. Dimitri, E. Geda, F. Perotti, M. Zettin, and G. C. Geminiani. 2016. Concomitant use of transcranial direct current stimulation and computer-assisted training for the rehabili-tation of attention in traumatic brain injured patients: Behavioral and neuroimaging Results. *Frontiers in Behavioral Neuroscience* 10:57. doi: 10.3389/fnbeh.2016.00057.

Sampaio, E., S. Maris, and P. Bach-y-Rita. 2001. Brain plasticity: 'visual' acuity of blind persons via the tongue. *Brain Research* 908 (2):204–207.

San-Juan, D., C. I. Sarmiento, A. Hernandez-Ruiz, E. Elizondo-Zepeda, G. Santos-Vázquez, G. Reyes-Acevedo, H. Zúñiga-Gazcón, and C. M. Zamora-Jarquín. 2016. Transcranial alternating current stimulation: A potential risk for genetic generalized epilepsy patients (Study Case). *Frontiers in Neurology* 7:213. doi: 10.3389/fneur.2016.00213.

Santarnecchi, E., N. R. Polizzotto, M. Godone, F. Giovannelli, M. Feurra, L. Matzen, A. Rossi, and S. Rossi. 2013. Frequency-dependent enhancement of fluid intelligence induced by transcra-nial oscillatory potentials. *Current Biology* 23 (15):1449–1453.

Schutter, D. J. L. G. and R. Hortensius. 2011. Brain oscillations and frequency-dependent modulation of cortical excitability. *Brain Stimulation* 4 (2):97–103.

Sela, T., A. Kilim, and M. Lavidor. 2012. Transcranial alternating current stimulation increases risk-taking behavior in the balloon analog risk task. *Frontiers in Neuroscience* 6 (22). doi:10.3389/fnins.2012.00022.

Thibaut, A., M. A. Bruno, D. Ledoux, A. Demertzi, and S. Laureys. 2014. tDCS in patients with disorders of consciousness: Sham-controlled randomized double-blind study. *Neurology* 82 (13):1112–1118. doi:10.1212/WNL.0000000000000260.

To, W. T., J. Ost, J. Hart, D. De Ridder, and S. Vanneste. 2016. The added value of auditory cortex tran-scranial random noise stimulation (tRNS) after bifrontal transcranial direct current stimula-tion (tDCS) for tinnitus. *Journal of Neural Transmission* 124:1–10.

Tremblay, S., M. Vernet, S. Bashir, A. Pascual-Leone, and H. Théoret. 2015. Theta burst stimulation to characterize changes in brain plasticity following mild traumatic brain injury: A proof-of-principle study. *Restorative Neurology and Neuroscience* 33 (5):611–620.

Turi, Z., G. G. Ambrus, K. Janacsek, K. Emmert, L. Hahn, W. Paulus, and A. Antal. 2013. Both the cutaneous sensation and phosphene perception are modulated in a frequency-specific manner during transcranial alternating current stimulation. *Restorative Neurology and Neuroscience* 31 (3):275–285.

Tyler, M., Y. Danilov, and P. Bach-Y-Rita. 2003. Closing an open-loop control system: Vestibular substitution through the tongue. *Journal of Integrative Neuroscience* 2 (2):159–164.

Tyler, M. E., Y. P. Danilov, and P. Bach-Y-Rita. 2006. Systems and methods for altering vestibular biology. Google Patents.

Tyler, M. E., K. A. Kaczmarek, K. L. Rust, A. M. Subbotin, K. L. Skinner, and Y. P. Danilov. 2014. Non-invasive neuromodulation to improve gait in chronic multiple sclerosis: A randomized double blind controlled pilot trial. *Journal of Neuroengineering Rehabilitation* 11:79. doi:10.1186/1743-0003-11-79.

Ulam, F., C. Shelton, L. Richards, L. Davis, B. Hunter, F. Fregni, and K. Higgins. 2015. Cumulative effects of transcranial direct current stimulation on EEG oscillations and attention/working memory during subacute neurorehabilitation of traumatic brain injury. *Clinical Neurophysiology* 126 (3):486–496.

van Schouwenburg, M. R., T. Zanto, and A. Gazzaley. 2016. Spatial attention and the effects of frontoparietal alpha band stimulation. *Frontiers in Human Neuroscience* 10:658.

Vanneste, S., V. Walsh, P. Van De Heyning, and D. De Ridder. 2013. Comparing immediate transient tinnitus suppression using tACS and tDCS: A placebo-controlled study. *Experimental Brain Research* 226 (1):25–31.

Wach, C., V. Krause, V. Moliadze, W. Paulus, A. Schnitzler, and B. Pollok. 2013. Effects of 10Hz and 20Hz transcranial alternating current stimulation (tACS) on motor functions and motor cortical excitability. *Behavioural Brain Research* 241:1–6.

Wildenberg, J. C., M. E. Tyler, Y. P. Danilov, K. A. Kaczmarek, and M. E. Meyerand. 2010. Sustained cortical and subcortical neuromodulation induced by electrical tongue stimulation. *Brain Imaging and Behavior* 4 (3–4):199–211. doi:10.1007/s11682-010-9099-7.

Wildenberg, J. C., M. E. Tyler, Y. P. Danilov, K. A. Kaczmarek, and M. E. Meyerand. 2011. High-resolution fMRI detects neuromodulation of individual brainstem nuclei by electrical tongue stimulation in balance-impaired individuals. *Neuroimage* 56 (4):2129–2137. doi:10.1016/j. neuroimage.2011.03.074.

Wilke, S., J. List, R. Mekle, R. Lindenberg, M. Bukowski, S. Ott, F. Schubert, B. Ittermann, and A. Flöel. 2016. No effect of anodal transcranial direct current stimulation on gamma-aminobutyric acid levels in patients with recurrent mild traumatic brain injury. *Journal of Neurotrauma* 4 (2):281–290.

Wu, J., H. Wang, Y. Wu, F. Li, Y. Bai, P. Zhang, and C. C. Chan. 2016. Efficacy of transcranial alternating current stimulation over bilateral mastoids (tACSbm) on enhancing recovery of subacute post-stroke patients. *Topics in Stroke Rehabilitation* 23 (6):420–429.

Wu, Q., W. Xuan, T. Ando, T. Xu, L. Huang, Y. Y. Huang, T. Dai, S. Dhital, S. K Sharma, and M. J Whalen. 2012. Low-level laser therapy for closed-head traumatic brain injury in mice: Effect of different wavelengths. *Lasers in Surgery and Medicine* 44 (3):218–226.

Xuan, W., F. Vatansever, L. Huang, and M. R. Hamblin. 2014. Transcranial low-level laser therapy enhances learning, memory, and neuroprogenitor cells after traumatic brain injury in mice. *Journal of Biomedical Optics* 19 (10):108003–108003.

Xuan, W., F. Vatansever, L. Huang, Q. Wu, Y. Xuan, T. Dai, T. Ando, T. Xu, Y. Y. Huang, and M. R. Hamblin. 2013. Transcranial low-level laser therapy improves neurological performance in traumatic brain injury in mice: Effect of treatment repetition regimen. *PLoS One* 8 (1):e53454.

Zivin, J. A., R. Sehra, A. Shoshoo, G. W. Albers, N. M. Bornstein, B. Dahlof, S. E. Kasner et al. 2014. NeuroThera(R) Efficacy and Safety Trial-3 (NEST-3): A double-blind, randomized, sham-controlled, parallel group, multicenter, pivotal study to assess the safety and efficacy of transcranial laser therapy with the NeuroThera(R) Laser System for the treatment of acute ischemic stroke within 24 h of stroke onset. *International Journal of Stroke* 9 (7):950–955. doi:10.1111/j.1747-4949.2012.00896.x.

*section five*

---

# *Putting it all together*
*Complete concussion care*

*chapter twenty two*

---

# Putting it all together: The need for personalized care after concussion

*Isabelle Gagnon and Alain Ptito*

## Contents

"Alone we can do so little; together we can do so much."

This quote, by Helen Keller, truly captures what an effective post-concussion management program is about. Our journey through this book, exploring various options and perspectives for management of sport-related concussions, now brings us to highlight key elements of a concussion follow-up program which, in our opinion, could lead to optimized care provided to injured individuals. We propose to view recovery, and therefore care, after concussion as a multitiered process, separated in three broad phases: acute, subacute, and chronic.

## Acute phase

The acute phase post-injury corresponds broadly to the initial *metabolic cascade*, where within the first 48–72 hours many physiological processes are taking place. As enumerated in Chapters 6 and 7, management during this phase is organized around education/reassurance as well as general activity management, aimed at finding appropriate levels of activities, which will not be symptom provoking or will not increase current symptoms, and avoidance of risky activities, which could lead to injury. A key element of the acute phase is also the documentation of preinjury functioning and preinjury history related to risk factors, or modifiers, for protracted recovery. A discussion of those risk factors was specifically included in Chapter 7 as well as referred to in multiple chapters throughout the book. Figure 22.1 schematically represents key elements of the acute phase management.

## Subacute phase

The subacute phase corresponds approximately to the period spanning from 72 hours to 2–3 weeks post-injury. If recovery goes well, this will be the period in which the individual will reintegrate into play, school, and work protocols. If recovery is slow, this will be the time when additional assessments of comorbidities will be performed, and a more individualized approach to accommodations for work and learning will be implemented. Ongoing education, stress management, and reassurance continue to remain a key. Figure 22.2 illustrates the key points important for that period.

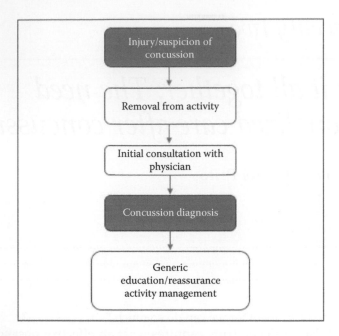

*Figure 22.1* Key elements proposed for concussion management in the acute phase.

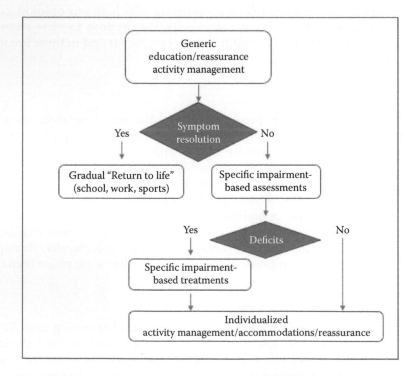

*Figure 22.2* Key elements proposed for concussion management in the subacute phase.

## Chronic phase

This chronic phase corresponds to the period of time beyond 2–3 weeks post-injury. Once symptoms and problems persist through that period, a more aggressive approach to intervention is warranted. This ranges from specific physical and/or cognitive interventions, to exercise-based programs acting on broader physiological processes. Chapters included in parts 2 and 3 of the book will provide the reader with ideas of what can be implemented at that stage. This is the period in which an interdisciplinary approach to care is essential and in which management by a sole professional may not optimize outcomes. Figure 22.3 summarizes recommendations for this period, whereas Figure 22.4 summarizes the trajectory in one single pathway.

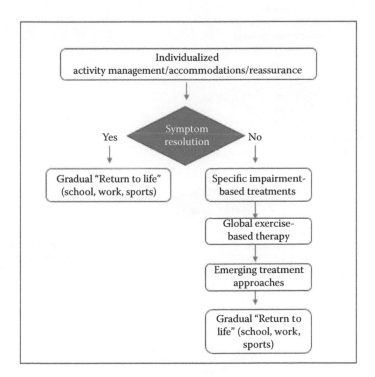

*Figure 22.3* Key elements proposed for concussion management in the chronic phase.

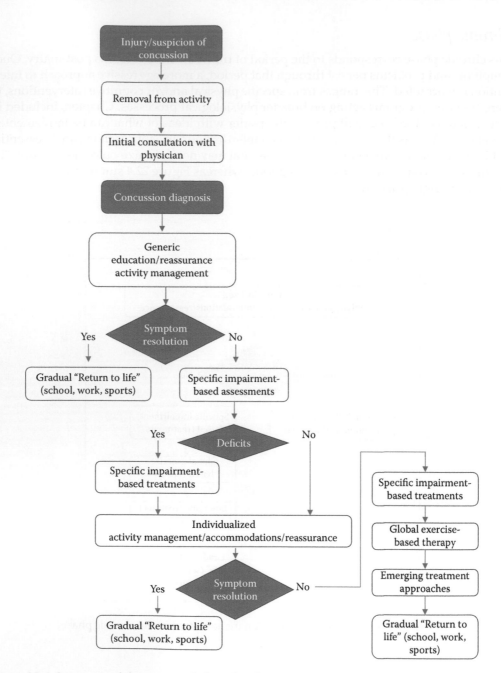

*Figure 22.4* Summary of the proposed algorithm for complete concussion management.

*chapter twenty three*

# Complex case studies

*Maude Laguë-Beauvais, Alain Ptito, and Isabelle Gagnon*

## Contents

Not all sport-related brain injuries lead to rapid recovering and short-lasting disruptions of function. In some cases, participating in sports can lead to more severe injuries. Although recovery times may be longer in those cases, we can learn from the multidisciplinary approach and the processes of care that lead to successful outcomes.

This chapter presents two simple cases and two additional more complex case studies. The first two cases report the recovery of pediatric patients who are present to their concussion follow-up program with various degrees of symptoms. The third case portrays the assessment and management of a female recreational synchronized skater, whose concussion, although in appearance uncomplicated, leads to a particularly long recovery, likely due to the delayed proactive management. The final case deals with a horseback-riding injury that leads to a moderate traumatic brain injury (TBI) with positive findings on neuroimaging and the accompanying hospital admission and rehabilitation. For this case, we present not only the problem list, in an effort to illustrate the depth of difficulties encountered in more severe injuries but also the problems that could arise in more complex concussions even without neuroimaging findings.

## Case #1: Andrew, rugby player

Andrew is a 16-year-old male who was injured while playing rugby. He was punched in the face, fell to the ground, and had lost consciousness for 30–60 seconds. He got up and continued to play despite feeling dizzy and confused. He finished the game. His confusion persisted for another few minutes, and then he felt a severe headache that continued throughout the week. He also complained of occasional ringing in his left ear and some visual disturbances when at school.

### Concussion clinic initial assessment (2 weeks post-injury)

Andrew was referred to a specialized concussion clinic about 2 weeks after his injury, and in the last week prior to the visit, his headache had improved to 3–4/10. On the day of visit, it was 6/10. His endurance was slowly improving, but he continued to be easily fatigued, and presented difficulty reading and concentrating. Despite minimal improvements, he remained symptomatic. There were no significant findings in his past medical history.

His neurological evaluation was unremarkable except for some slowness in coordination (good precision) and some increased swaying in single-leg stance with eyes closed.

After evaluation, the patient's headache persisted at 6/10 but he began to complain of dizziness. The patient was about 2 weeks post-injury and education of precautions, recommendations, and activity restrictions was given. It was suggested that he begins light walking for 15 minutes daily as long as his symptoms did not increase.

### Phone follow-up (3 weeks post-injury)

The patient was called the following week and he reported the doctor no dizziness but persistent headache at 3–4/10. The patient was walking without any difficulty. He was told to continue taking walks for about 15 minutes daily as long as the symptoms did not increase.

### Concussion clinic visit (4 weeks post-injury)

The patient was presented to clinic with persisting symptoms. His headaches were less intense with an average 3/10 but often less. He feels less fatigued and he is compliant with daily walk. Single-leg stance lasted now for 10 seconds with eyes closed without swaying.

*Exercise-based rehabilitation initiated*: Treadmill 3.8 km/hr 10 minutes. Working at about 60%–70% max heart rate; added push-ups 10; and light jumping drills.

*Postexercise*: Reported no increase in symptoms.

He has to continue with 15–20 minutes of light aerobic workout for the rest of the week as long as there is no increase in the symptoms.

## Concussion clinic visit (6 weeks post-injury)

About 2 weeks later, the patient was called and he reported that he was improving. He has no symptoms for some days and when he did, he had a mild headache at 1–2/10. The patient felt much more energetic and progressed to 20–30 minutes of workout including jogging, treadmill, and/or bicycle.

## Final visit (8 weeks post-injury)

Andrew reported that he had had no symptoms over the past week.

He was now tolerating almost 1 hour of aerobic and resistance training with no symptoms elicited. He continued to train to improve his fitness. He was happy with recovery and was looking forward to returning to sports. He was cleared for return to play and he was discharged from the program.

# Case #2: Patrick, outdoor hockey player

Patrick is a 13-year-old boy who was injured while playing hockey outdoors with no helmet. He hit another player head to head who was wearing a helmet.

He felt dizzy, so he stopped playing and returned home. He did not stop activities and was diagnosed 2 months post-injury with complaints of persistent headaches since the incident. He also complained of sensitivity to light and loud sounds. He presented to the emergency department with severe headaches. A CT scan was done (−ve), and he was given a dose of intravenous abortive headache medication with some relief.

## Initial concussion clinic visit (8 weeks post-injury)

He reported that he is slowly improving but often feels tired and misses playing hockey with his friends. His neurological exam was normal with good balance and coordination.

Exercise-based treatment was initiated with 15–20 minutes of light aerobic activity for 1 week. He did light jumps, push-ups, and treadmill for 10 mins, 60%–70% max in clinic, no symptoms increased, his headache remained at 2/10, but he felt good to move.

## Follow-up concussion clinic visit (9 weeks post-injury)

Patrick returned to clinic reporting improvements. His headaches were only present occasionally at a level of 2/10 and for a brief amount of time (minutes). There is no increase in symptoms with activity, and he felt more energetic. He was compliant with rehabilitation program.

The patient progressed to 20–30 minutes of workout with some sport-specific drills for soccer. He could do foot-handling drills with ball on his own. In clinic, he had no symptoms and did treadmill for 20 minutes, ball activities, and light-jumping drills.

*Phone follow-up (10 weeks post-injury)*

He has resumed his exams at school and reports some fatigue, but overall he is doing well and had been improving, with days in which there are no headaches, occasional brief H/A (1/10) for a minute or two, and then okay. He has progressed in the time of workout, doing 30–60 minutes of exercise. He is occasionally doing soccer drills with a partner. He worked out for 30 minutes with jumping activities, treadmill, and ball activities with no increase in symptoms. He was cleared for return to play protocol.

*Follow-up visit (11 weeks post-injury)*

The patient had a final visit to the clinic, and he reports that he is doing fine. He has returned to full practices after trying a few with no contact and is doing very well. There are no symptoms elicited with activity. He feels back to baseline energy levels and feels ready to return to play. The patient has been discharged from the program.

## Case #3: Mrs. M.—Recreational synchronized skater

Mrs. M. is a right-handed 47-year-old woman. She is married and is living with her two teenage sons. She has obtained a bachelor's degree and is working as a marketing manager. During her schooling, no difficulties were reported. On the contrary, she had an accelerated school career, finishing high school a year early. Mrs. M. describes a very active lifestyle, both mentally and physically, before her accident, training 4–5 times per week.

Mrs. M. fell from her own height while doing synchronized skating. One of her skate got caught in another partner's skate. She was not wearing a helmet at the time of the accident. She did not lose consciousness and has no amnesia of the event. Following her fall, she drove home in her car. She felt dazed but did not report suffering from any other symptoms in the first 24 hours post-injury.

The following day, Mrs. M. complained of headaches, dizziness, vertigo, and nausea. She consulted a doctor in a walk-in clinic, which resulted in a referral for physiotherapy at her local clinic. A cervical injury (nonspecified) was then diagnozed according to her. Furthermore, she had trouble reintegrating work in the following weeks due to difficulties concentrating and performing multiple tasks simultaneously, though she did not stop work officially until a month later following a consultation with her family doctor who recommended that she had to stay at home while minimizing all sensory stimulation. This then led to a decrease in her symptoms. Mrs. M. initiated weekly visits in chiropractic, which helped her symptoms to decrease according to her. However, going back to physical activities caused an increase in her symptoms.

Mrs. M. reported having had other concussions in the past (number unspecified), specifically during her teenage years while playing sports without any type of significant sequelae. She has a history of migraine and gastric reflux, but no psychiatric history.

*Initial intake concussion clinic (2 months post-injury)*

Due to the long course of her recovery, Mrs. M. was referred and assessed at the out-patient mTBI/concussion clinic of a tertiary care trauma center. A first phone screening done by a neuropsychologist two months following the accident revealed that the patient still reported headaches, dizziness, nausea, loss of balance problems, sensitivity to noise, fatigue, blurred vision, forgetfulness, difficulty finding words, lowered concentration, longer time to think, irritability, sadness, emotionality, and pain in her left ear.

## Rehabilitation medicine assessment (3 months post-injury)

An appointment was made with the program physiatrist, specialized in TBI, three months following her injury.

On the day of assessment, Mrs. M. was oriented but her effect showed mild anxiety. Cranial nerves, strength, sensation, and tendon reflexes were all within normal limits. Cerebellar function was also normal. A left C2–C3 tenderness was detected at the cervical spine level. Her score on the rivermead post-concussion symptoms questionnaire was 42/64 (severe levels). A recommendation to resume physical activities regularly and progressively was suggested. She was informed not to panic if there were headaches after exertion. A prescription of Elavil was increased from 10 to 20 mg, and diclofenac/misoprostol (50 mg BID) was also prescribed. A follow-up in 3–4 weeks was scheduled to reassess and plan progressive return to work.

## Follow-up rehabilitation medicine (4 months post-injury)

One month later at her follow-up, she still reported important migraines for which diclofenac/misoprostol (50 mg BID) was taken as needed. She was still on Elavil, which caused drowsiness, fatigue, and a decrease in attention and concentration. Even with a gradual improvement of her post-concussive symptoms, and a gradual and positive reinitiation of her physical activities, Mrs. M. complained of significant fatigue and drowsiness, and her Rivermead score remained at moderate levels of 28/64. However, she had reintegrated her pilates practice and was now walking twice per week. At that time, the intervention plan was to wean her off the Elavil and was to plan a progressive return to work starting two weeks later after the appointment at three half days for a week, half days the next week, five half days the next, and so on. Given the presence of significant symptoms and decreased function, a neuropsychology consultation was then done.

## Neuropsychological assessment (5 months post-injury)

A neuropsychological assessment was performed to document Mrs. M.'s residual difficulties and to orient her to further rehabilitation services to optimize the professional reintegration that she had initiated 11 days before the neuropsychological assessment (5 months following her initial concussion). Although her work environment was amenable to her gradually reintegrating her work, Mrs. M. still suffered from severe fatigue, drowsiness, and attention difficulties. At the time of the neuropsychological assessment, the patient described nausea and headaches. Daily functioning is marked by periods of inattention and trouble doing multiple tasks at once, which is different from that of her premorbid abilities. Psychologically, she reports irritability and frustration but no anxiety or depressive symptoms.

The neuropsychologist proceeded to formally evaluate her functioning using the California verbal learning test, 2nd edition (CVLT-II); D2—Test of attention; Digit span (Wechsler adult intelligence scale IV); mental control (Wechsler memory scale III); Rey Figure; Rivermead questionnaire; Stroop (D-KEFS); Tower of London, Drexel version, 2nd edition; trail making test A and B; verbal fluency—D-KEFS (animals and switching); and Wechsler abbreviated scale of intelligence II (WASI-II) block design and similarities (detailed results are found in Section "Details of Neuropsychological initial assessment").

Mrs. M.'s assessment revealed a cognitive profile of someone with an intellectual potential within the high average range, although somewhat heterogeneous. Nevertheless, very few weaknesses were revealed, other than some mild executive and memory vulnerabilities, tributary to her anxiety and post-concussive symptoms such as her fatigue. As such, her fatigue causes fluctuations in alertness making it harder to mobilize during tasks, to plan, to organize, and to autoregulate herself, thus corroborating her complaints related to having difficulties at work.

Her prognosis was considered positive, as her working environment allows her to adjust her work load accordingly and as she has strong support from her family. Mrs. M. was encouraged to continue her progressive return to work as her symptoms alleviate with no specific neuropsychological follow-up. If her reintegration at work and physical activities remained limited, a follow-up in psychotherapy should have been considered to learn about the potential physical exhibition of anxiety and how to compensate more effectively.

### Follow-up in rehabilitation medicine (5 months post-injury)

Two weeks after the neuropsychological assessment (five months postaccident), a follow-up in physiatry was done. She continued to be present with mild post-traumatic symptoms (Rivermead: 22/64) but was able to reintegrate work at 17.5 hours per week (two full days and one half day). She expresses that she is often exhausted but that she manages her schedule appropriately. She complains that she is unable to do multitasking and that she drops in attention and concentration, which was described as *absences* by her. She stopped taking Arthrotec and Elavil. She was recommended to continue working at that rhythm for another six weeks.

### Conclusion

Six weeks later, Mrs. M. was still improving albeit slowly. She remained with mild residual headaches and fatigue. Her score at the Rivermead remained in the mild range at 19/64, and she admitted being less anxious and having more attention capacity. The patient was encouraged to gradually increase her work schedule to a full load as tolerated, which she went on to implement in the following weeks. Residual headaches are now considered of the same type as the pretraumatic history of migraines.

Using reassurance and a progressive but sustained approach to return to activities, a small team of health-care professionals is sufficient to help an individual presenting with a mild uncomplicated TBI or concussion. Reassurance is used to ensure that patients, especially those who are present with anxious personalities, do not panic with the occurrence of symptoms during the gradual return to activities.

## Details of neuropsychological initial assessment

*Clinical Observations*: Mrs. M. is a smiling woman whose contact is easy and familiar. Visual contact is appropriately modulated. Her symptom is anxious, although mobilizable, and she seems hypervigilent, speaking really fast, and showing signs of performance anxiety. She collaborated very well during the interview. Judgment and insight capacities are preserved. Her appearance is well groomed.

As for the neuropsychological assessment, Mrs. M. makes all the necessary efforts to accomplish what is asked of her. No signs of motor hyperactivity or impulsivity are noted. Consequently, the results of the assessment are interpreted as valid.

*Intellectual Functioning Estimate*: Results obtained from two subtests of the WASI-II attest to an intellectual functioning estimated in the high average range. Her profile is somewhat heterogeneous as her performance in a visuoperceptual task (block design) is superior to average (92nd percentile), though her verbal abilities (similarities) are in the average range (60th percentile). Thus, Mrs. M. processes visuoperceptual and visuoconstructive information very efficiently.

*Attention and Working Memory*: Mrs. M. shows an efficient attentional control. Visual selective attention abilities (D2) are effective as to the number of targets detected across distractors. Her passive verbal span is in the high average (digit span forward = 8, WAIS-IV) as was her verbal (mental control) and visual (trail making test A) processing speeds. Mrs. M. had no working memory problems (digit span backwards = 6, WAIS-IV), and her performance was also in the high average range. Overall, attention abilities are preserved.

*Executive Functions*: Although mostly efficient, executive function performances are modulated downward by fatigue, resulting in fluctuations of her alertness. Thus, it becomes more difficult for Mrs. M. to mobilize when entering tasks. Nevertheless, she normally succeeds, which attests to good premorbid abilities.

Mental activation to access lexico-semantic information is excellent (verbal fluency, D-KEFS). No mental rigidity is observed in tasks requiring switching between two sets of information (trail making test B, Stroop D-KEFS—switching condition, verbal fluency D-KEFS—switching condition). Inhibition mechanisms are also intact (Stroop). Moreover, Mrs. M. demonstrates good reasoning abilities—both at the verbal level (Similarities) and at the visuoconstructive level (block design). Organization of complex visual information is also not a problem (Rey Figure copy) and she showed a global and integrated approach to the task. However, she has trouble in generating good learning strategies while learning a list of words (CVLT-II), where she renders the words randomly without strategies, such as semantic grouping. This weakness is also noticed in terms of her autoregulation when structured planning is required (Tower of London). Despite being adequate, her performance is below her potential that leads to her visual reasoning abilities.

*Learning and Memory*: No franc memory problems are observed, although some weaknesses have been found tributary to her anxiety and alertness fluctuations. Thus, her learning curve (CVLT-II) progresses normally across recalls (6-9-9-11-15/16). However, her immediate and delayed recalls are somewhat weak, and a mild retroactive interference is noted. The same has been observed in a visual memory task (Rey Figure), in which there are weaknesses in information retrieval during the immediate and delayed recalls. However, the performance was influenced by the rather quick exhibition of the figure due to her fast copy and her performance anxiety. The latter also influences her recognition performance that Mrs. M. prefers to answer "no" when uncertain, so as not to make any mistakes.

*Language*: Despite not being formally investigated, language abilities seem normal. Discourse is coherent, and oral comprehension is preserved.

## Case #4: Mrs. H. horseback riding

Mrs. H. is a right-handed 56-year-old woman. She lives with her husband, and she has no children. She has completed a bachelor's degree and is working as a research coordinator in the medical domain. As for her past medical history, there is nothing notable other than a shoulder tendinitis. She drinks one alcoholic beverage per day and does not smoke. She was independent in all instrumental activities of daily living, preinjury, and her home has 15 interior steps and 3 exterior steps. She is an avid horseback rider (rides 7 days per week).

Mrs. H. was horseback riding when she fell from her horse, but she was wearing a helmet during the accident. She was found two hours later, confused and disoriented walking along with her horse. She probably lost consciousness and her post-traumatic amnesia lasted more than 24 hours but less than 48 hours. Her Glasgow coma scale score varied between 13/15 and 15/15 when she was sent to a local hospital. After her CT scan, she was transferred to a tertiary trauma center where she was admitted. The CT scan that was done the same day revealed a left holohemispheric subdural hematoma, small bifrontal subdural hemorrhages, and inferior bifrontal subarachnoid foci. She did not suffer from any other traumatic injuries.

During her hospital stay, once deemed safe by neurosurgery, she was followed by an multidisciplinary team, such as a physiotherapist, an occupational therapist, a speech language pathologist, a social worker, a physiatrist, and a neuropsychologist as well as a complete nursing team.

## Patient's complaints (multiple disciplines)

At the moment of the assessment, the patient reported being agitated and feeling antsy. She noticed that she had some difficulty in finding her words. She admitted that she was feeling bored while being admitted to the hospital and having trouble doing nothing. She first complained of severe left-sided headaches which subsided. She denied vertigo, dizziness, and diplopia. She denied noticing any problems with memory.

## Clinical observations (multiple disciplines)

Mrs. H. was alert and aware during the initial team multidisciplinary assessment. Her social interactions were adequate: she was polite and maintained good visual contact. She did not resist answering questions, and she collaborated well with testing. She even tended to be overly jovial at times. However, her symptom was generally anxious, and she became somewhat defensive when confronted with her difficulties. Her anxiety was sometimes overwhelming, which seemed to cause a drop in her performance at times. Thus, her testing results had to be interpreted with caution. Moreover, some impulsivity was noted during the completion of tasks. Her judgment and insight were affected.

Her overall difficulties are summarized as follows (detailed report is given in Section "Detailed reports and recommendations"):

- Some confusion/impulsivity
- Moderate psychomotor slowness
- Mildly decreased balance in complex activities
- Requires supervision for ADLs (confusion, poor planning, poor judgment, and insight)
- Fluctuations while maintaining and manipulating verbal information
- Weakness in visual analysis/visual planning
- Impaired working memory
- Weakness in lexico-semantic access
- Mental rigidity/somewhat concrete thinking pattern.

## Final discharge plan

The patient refused in-patient rehabilitation categorically and threatened to leave against medical advice if she was sent to in-patient rehabilitation. An out-patient service was, thus, organized as the patient was still considered competent. She was able to resume all her pre-injury roles after discharge from rehabilitation services.

# Detailed reports and recommendations

## Social work recommendation and intervention plan

Patient will either require in- or out-patient rehabilitation. She has strong support from husband and extended family and friends. Mrs. H. expresses eagerness in returning home and may be minimizing the severity of her TBI condition. Ongoing support counselling with patient and family will be of benefit to encourage accepting the treatment team's rehabilitation recommendations.

## Rehabilitation medicine assessment

The patient was slow, somewhat confused, and was present with moderate psychomotor slowness. The examination of the cranial nerves (nerves I to XII), reflexes, and senses is normal. The patient shows no drift in her limbs. The Dix–Hallpike test was deferred because there were no dizziness complaints. Out-patient rehabilitation was recommended at first but was then changed to an in-patient rehabilitation recommendation following the TBI team's advice.

## Neurosurgery trauma assessment

Acute but stable subdural hematoma was confirmed with no complications and increased alertness and orientation. She tolerated oral feeding and remained hemodynamically stable throughout her hospitalization. The patient was advised to go to in-patient rehabilitation several times, but she was discharged to home with out-patient rehabilitation.

## Physiotherapy assessment

Patient was moving all limbs. She was cooperative and oriented to person and place. She was able to roll in bed, sit up from lying, stand up from sitting, and was able to go from the bed to her chair independently. Static and dynamic balances were good while sitting and standing. Her score at the Berg balance scale was 54/56. She tolerated walking well for a distance of 100 m with supervision. She was able to go up and down 20 steps using the railing by alternating her legs. Her range of motion and her strength were normal. In-patient rehabilitation was recommended due to her mental status and to further optimize her balance and functional independence.

## Occupational therapy assessment

*Functional assessment*: The patient showed that she was independent with modified structures for feeding and mobility transfers. She needed supervision for grooming, bathing, dressing her upper and lower body, and transferring in and out of the tub. As for instrumental activities of daily living, she required assistance for

household chores, meal preparation, groceries, driving, transportation, and medication. Finances could be done with some supervision.

*Physical components*: Her strength as measured by a dynamo was 20 kg on the right side
and 23 kg on the left side. She showed good finger to nose coordination.

*Cognitive-perceptual components*: Attention and scanning (Bells test) were slightly
impaired. The motor-free visual perception test (MVPT-III) showed a normal performance and verbal problem solving. The patient had trouble in recalling her age, and
her insight was poor.

Considering the severity of the TBI and her premorbid status, the patient was thought
to have benefited from functional intensive rehabilitation to maximize her independence in instrumental and domestic activities of daily living and to help her return to
baseline.

## Speech-language pathology assessment

*Administered Tests*:
- Boston naming test (BNT)—short form
- Selected subtests of the Boston diagnostic aphasia examination (BDAE)
- Arizona battery for communication disorders of dementia (ABCD)
- Detroit test of learning aptitude (DTLA)
- Scales of cognitive ability for TBI (SCATBI)
- Canadian adult achievement test (CAAT)
- Protocole Montréal d'évaluation de la communication (MEC)

There were no swallowing or hearing problems reported or observed. Her voice quality
was good, and there were no significant motor speech deficits noted.

*Auditory comprehension*: She missed a simple reasoning question and also did not understand inferential information from a short story (BDAE). Her score on the immediate
recall in a story-telling subtest (ABCD) was poor, and she could not mention any
of the elements of the story during a delayed recall. She correctly explained verbal
absurdities, except for one of six items (DTLA).

*Oral expression*: Performance for confrontation naming on the BNT was adequate. She
obtained 11/13 on orientation questions from the mental status subtest of the ABCD,
missing the current year and her age. Semantic category naming (semantic verbal
fluency) was below average for her age and level of education, whereas letter-cate-
gory naming (lexical verbal fluency) was poor. Procedural discourse for the recall
task steps subtest of the SCATBI was accurate. However, narrative discourse for the
description of a sequential picture story with six images, although accurate, failed
to include all salient details, and the patient omitted one image completely. In spontaneous conversation, the patient adequately understood concrete information, but
instructions for testing were needed to be repeated sometimes. The discourse checklist of the MEC revealed that the patient was generally able to express her needs and
discuss simple hospital-related topics adequately. However, the content tended to
reflect poor recall and occasional word-finding problems. A mildly decreased verbal
initiative was also noted as compared with norms.

*Reading comprehension*: The patient correctly answered all questions about a functional
reading text of the reading comprehension subtest of the CAAT (grade 7 to 10 level),
but she had significant difficulty for descriptive texts of a higher level, where she had
difficulty in understanding and recalling the information read.

*Clinical conclusions*: Mrs. H. is present with moderate to severe cognitive-communication deficits in auditory recall, whereas moderate problems were noted in reading comprehension and organization of narrative discourse. In addition, mild problems were found for verbal reasoning and production of conversational discourse. She senses changes in cognitive functioning without being able to identify what problems are there and does not fully appreciate the impact on return to work. Thus, a referral to a specialized in-patient rehabilitation center is recommended with intervention in speech-language pathology to improve cognitive-communication skills for optimal home and community reintegration.

## Results of the brief neuropsychological assessment

*Administered Tests*:

- Clock drawing
- Digit span (Wechsler adult intelligence scale IV)
- Frontal assessment battery (FAB)
- Gavelston orientation and amnesia test (GOAT)
- Mental control (Wechsler memory scale III)
- Similarities (Wechsler adult intelligence scale IV)
- Trail-making test A and B
- Repeatable battery for assessment of neuropsychological status (RBANS-A)

*Language*: Oral comprehension is preserved. Spontaneous discourse is coherent. No word-finding difficulties are noted, but the denomination task (RBANS) is poor and reveals trouble with lexical access as the patient produces two semantic paraphasias (e.g., bugle for trumpet).

*Attention and working memory*: Auditory selective attention is in the average range due to fluctuations in her performance because the length of the span is excellent (digit span forward = 9, RBANS-A). Moreover, Mrs. H. recites and manipulates overlearned information (e.g., reciting days of the week forward and backward, mental control—WMS-III) easily, and processing speed is adequate. Working memory, without bonus points for speed, is in the high average range (digit span backward = 8, WAIS-IV), but some fluctuations are also noted. Psychomotor speed is in the low average range as measured by the coding subtest (RBANS-A), in which the patient must write the right number associated with the right symbol. As for visual selective attention, her performance was normal for time of completion on the trail-making test A, and she did not make any mistakes. Although sustained attention was not formally assessed, Mrs. H. tolerated mental effort well, and the assessment was done in one session. Overall, attentional abilities are characterized by a mild weakness in psychomotor speed and fluctuation in maintaining and manipulating verbal information.

*Visuoperceptual and visuoconstructive abilities*: The ability to recognize images during a denomination task is normal and does not attest to any visual agnosia. However, a line orientation task (RBANS) reveals a performance in the low average range for visual analysis. Furthermore, the copy of a geometric figure (RBANS) is in the borderline range. The clock drawing test where the patient needs to draw a clock with all the numbers and the hands indicates 11:10. She produced many errors in organizing her numbers, and perseverations are observed. She was also doing these tasks impulsively, which was detrimental to her score.

*Learning and memory*: Concerning verbal memory, Mrs. H.'s learning curve of a 10-word list presented four times (RBANS-A) was somewhat weak (5–6/0 to 6–7/10). Moreover, the total amount of words recalled was in the low average range. She cannot recall any of these words during the delayed recall and the recognition task is also poor, although she does not produce any false positive. Mrs. H. also has trouble recalling a short story (RBANS) both at the immediate recall and the delayed recall. However, she obtained an almost perfect score at the GOAT, which suggests that she is oriented in person, time, and place. As for visual memory, her delayed recall is very poor that the patient is not reproducing any details, other than the figure's contour. Thus, a consolidation and retrieval of information deficits are observed, somewhat modulated by the patient's performance anxiety, especially during the delayed recalls.

*Executive functions*: Frontal efficiency, as assessed by the FAB, is poor. Verbal fluency under a semantic constraint (RBANS-A) was poor, given her age, whereas verbal fluency under a lexical constraint (FAB) was in the borderline range. Performances to the inhibition and inhibitory control tasks (FAB) were normal. She easily replicated the Luria motor sequence (FAB) while mirroring the assessor, but she could not maintain it alone. However, she did not show any prehension behavior (FAB). Concerning mental flexibility, her performance on a task in which she must link in order and by switching two overlearned sets (trail making test B) was poor, and she made two sequencing mistakes. Finally, her score on the similarities subtest (WAIS-IV), which measures verbal abstraction abilities, was in the low average range. Consequently, a weakness in lexico-semantic access is noted, and trouble in maintaining motor programming, mental rigidity, and a somewhat concrete thinking pattern are noted.

# Index

Note: Page numbers followed by f and t refer to figures and tables respectively.

Printed and bound by CPI Group (UK) Ltd, Croydon, CR0 4YY

01/11/2024

01782603-0009